Clinical Endocrinology

Clinical Endocrinology

Editor: Donovan Douglas

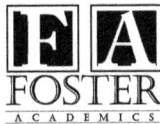

FA FOSTER ACADEMICS

www.fosteracademics.com

www.fosteracademics.com

FA FOSTER
ACADEMICS

Cataloging-in-Publication Data

Clinical endocrinology / edited by Donovan Douglas.
    p. cm.
Includes bibliographical references and index.
ISBN 978-1-63242-644-4
1. Endocrinology. 2. Endocrine glands--Diseases. I. Douglas, Donovan.
RC648 .C55 2019
6164--dc23

© Foster Academics, 2019

Foster Academics,
118-35 Queens Blvd., Suite 400,
Forest Hills, NY 11375, USA

ISBN 978-1-63242-644-4 (Hardback)

Contents

Preface XI

Chapter 1   **Idiopathic Basal Ganglia Calcification Presented with Impulse Control Disorder** 1
Cem Sahin, Mustafa Levent, Gulhan Akbaba, Bilge Kara, Emine Nese Yeniceri and
Betul Battaloglu Inanc

Chapter 2   **Paraganglioma Presenting as Postpartum Fever of Unknown Origin** 5
Shraddha Narechania, Amrita Bath, Laleh Ghassemi, Chetan Lokhande,
Abdo Haddad, Ali Mir Yousuf, Jessica Marquard and K. V. Gopalakrishna

Chapter 3   **A Case of Glucocorticoid Remediable Aldosteronism and Thoracoabdominal
Aneurysms** 9
Anahita Shahrrava, Sunnan Moinuddin, Prajwal Boddu and Rohan Shah

Chapter 4   **Cerebral Malaria: An Unusual cause of Central Diabetes Insipidus** 13
Resmi Premji, Nira Roopnarinesingh, Joshua Cohen and Sabyasachi Sen

Chapter 5   **46, XY Disorder of Sex Development caused by 17α-Hydroxylase/17, 20-Lyase
Deficiency due to Homozygous Mutation of *CYP17A1* Gene: Consequences of
Late Diagnosis** 17
Giampaolo Papi, Rosa Maria Paragliola, Paola Concolino, Carlo Di Donato,
Alfredo Pontecorvi and Salvatore Maria Corsello

Chapter 6   **Pegvisomant-Induced Cholestatic Hepatitis in an Acromegalic Patient with
UGT1A1*28 Mutation** 23
Maria Susana Mallea-Gil, Ignacio Bernabeu, Adriana Spiraquis, Alejandra Avangina,
Lourdes Loidi and Carolina Ballarino

Chapter 7   **Treatment of Ipilimumab Induced Graves' Disease in a Patient with
Metastatic Melanoma** 28
Umal Azmat, David Liebner, Amy Joehlin-Price, Amit Agrawal and Fadi Nabhan

Chapter 8   **Posaconazole-Induced Adrenal Insufficiency in a Case of Chronic
Myelomonocytic Leukemia** 32
Ann Miller, Lauren K. Brooks, Silpa Poola-Kella and Rana Malek

Chapter 9   **Adrenal Insufficiency under Standard Dosage of Glucocorticoid Replacement after
Unilateral Adrenalectomy for Cushing's Syndrome** 36
Kentaro Fujii, Kazutoshi Miyashita, Isao Kurihara, Ken Hiratsuka, Seiji Sato,
Kenichi Yokota, Sakiko Kobayashi, Hirotaka Shibata and Hiroshi Itoh

Chapter 10 **Acute Primary Adrenal Insufficiency after Hip Replacement in a Patient with
Acute Intermittent Porphyria** 40
Adele Latina, Massimo Terzolo, Anna Pia, Giuseppe Reimondo, Elena Castellano,
Micaela Pellegrino and Giorgio Borretta

Chapter 11   **A Large PROP1 Gene Deletion in a Turkish Pedigree** 44
Suheyla Gorar, Doga Turkkahraman and Kanay Yararbas

Chapter 12   **A Rapid Biochemical and Radiological Response to the Concomitant
Therapy with Temozolomide and Radiotherapy in an Aggressive ACTH
Pituitary Adenoma** 49
Ana Misir Krpan, Tina Dusek, Zoran Rakusic, Mirsala Solak, Ivana Kraljevic,
Vesna Bisof, David Ozretic and Darko Kastelan

Chapter 13   **Hypercalcemia of Malignancy in Thymic Carcinoma: Evolving Mechanisms of
Hypercalcemia and Targeted Therapies** 54
Cheng Cheng, Jose Kuzhively and Sanford Baim

Chapter 14   **A Novel T55A Variant of $G_s\alpha$ Associated with Impaired cAMP Production, Bone
Fragility and Osteolysis** 59
Kelly Wentworth, Alyssa Hsing, Ashley Urrutia, Yan Zhu, Andrew E. Horvai,
Murat Bastepe and Edward C. Hsiao

Chapter 15   **Isolated Liver Metastasis in Hürthle Cell Thyroid Cancer Treated with
Microwave Ablation** 65
Konstantinos Segkos, Carl Schmidt and Fadi Nabhan

Chapter 16   **Does the Intensity of IGG4 Immunostaining have a Correlation with the
Clinical Presentation of Riedel's Thyroiditis?** 69
C. A. Simões, M. R. Tavares, N. M. M. Andrade, T. M. Uehara, R. A. Dedivitis and
C. R. Cernea

Chapter 17   **Vasopressin Bolus Protocol Compared to Desmopressin (DDAVP) for Managing
Acute, Postoperative Central Diabetes Insipidus and Hypovolemic Shock** 73
Anukrati Shukla, Syeda Alqadri, Ashley Ausmus, Robert Bell,
Premkumar Nattanmai and Christopher R. Newey

Chapter 18   **Gigantomastia and Macroprolactinemia Responding to Cabergoline Treatment** 77
Fatma Dilek Dellal, Didem Ozdemir, Cevdet Aydin, Gulfem Kaya,
Reyhan Ersoy and Bekir Cakir

Chapter 19   **Hypocalciuric Hypercalcemia due to Impaired Renal Tubular Calcium
Excretion in a Type 2 Diabetic Patient** 82
Sihao Yang, Yan Ren, Xi Li, Haoming Tian, Zhenmei An and Tao Chen

Chapter 20   **An Ectopic ACTH Secreting Metastatic Parotid Tumour** 85
Thomas Dacruz, Atul Kalhan, Majid Rashid and Kofi Obuobie

Chapter 21   **Nonfunctioning Pituitary Adenoma That Changed to a Functional
Gonadotropinoma** 89
Gerson Geovany Andino-Ríos, Lesly Portocarrero-Ortiz, Carlos Rojas-Guerrero,
Alejandro Terrones-Lozano, Alma Ortiz-Plata and Alfredo Adolfo Reza-Albarrán

Chapter 22   **A Normotensive Patient with Primary Aldosteronism** 93
Xiao Lin, Xiaoyu Miao, Pengli Zhu and Fan Lin

Chapter 23   **Adrenocorticotropic Hormone Secreting Pheochromocytoma Underlying
Glucocorticoid Induced Pheochromocytoma Crisis** 97
Gil A. Geva, David J. Gross, Haggi Mazeh, Karine Atlan, Iddo Z. Ben-Dov and
Matan Fischer

Chapter 24 **Pituitary Adenoma and Hyperprolactinemia Accompanied by Idiopathic Granulomatous Mastitis** **101**
Sebahattin Destek, Vahit Onur Gul, Serkan Ahioglu and
Kursat Rahmi Serin

Chapter 25 **Severe Hyperthyroidism Complicated by Agranulocytosis Treated with Therapeutic Plasma Exchange** **104**
Vishnu Garla, Karthik Kovvuru, Shradha Ahuja, Venkatataman Palabindala,
Bharat Malhotra and Sohail Abdul Salim

Chapter 26 **Anaplastic Spindle Cell Squamous Carcinoma Arising from Tall Cell Variant Papillary Carcinoma of the Thyroid Gland** **110**
Darren K. Patten, Alia Ahmed, Owain Greaves, Roberto Dina, Rashpal Flora and
Neil Tolley

Chapter 27 **Recurrent Episodes of Thyrotoxicosis in a Man following Pregnancies of his Spouse with Hashimoto's Thyroiditis** **115**
Regina Belokovskaya and Alice C. Levine

Chapter 28 **Primary Mucosa-Associated Lymphoid Tissue Lymphoma of Thyroid with the Serial Ultrasound Findings** **119**
Eon Ju Jeon, Ho Sang Shon and Eui Dal Jung

Chapter 29 **Adrenal Ganglioneuroblastoma in Adults: A Case Report and Review of the Literature** **124**
Stefano Benedini, Giorgia Grassi, Carmen Aresta, Antonietta Tufano,
Luca Fabio Carmignani, Barbara Rubino, Livio Luzi and Sabrina Corbetta

Chapter 30 **Spontaneous Regression of Metastatic Papillary Thyroid Cancer in a Lymph Node** **131**
Jien Shim, Jianyu Rao and Run Yu

Chapter 31 **Hashimoto's Thyroiditis and Graves' Disease in One Patient: The Extremes of Thyroid Dysfunction Associated with Interferon Treatment** **135**
R. H. Bishay and R. C. Y. Chen

Chapter 32 **Recurrent Thyrotoxicosis due to both Graves' Disease and Hashimoto's Thyroiditis in the same Three Patients** **139**
Ashley Schaffer, Vidya Puthenpura and Ian Marshall

Chapter 33 **Diabetes Mellitus with Poor Glycemic Control as a Consequence of Inappropriate Injection Technique** **143**
Ramesh Sharma Poudel, Shakti Shrestha, Sushma Bhandari, Rano Mal Piryani and
Shital Adhikari

Chapter 34 **Remarkable Presentation: Anaplastic Thyroid Carcinoma Arising from Chronic Hyperthyroidism** **147**
Habib G. Zalzal, Jeffson Chung and Jessica A. Perini

Chapter 35 **DKA with Severe Hypertriglyceridemia and Cerebral Edema in an Adolescent Boy** **151**
Tansit Saengkaew, Taninee Sahakitrungruang, Suttipong Wacharasindhu and
Vichit Supornsilchai

Chapter 36   **Internal Spreading of Papillary Thyroid Carcinoma: A Case Report and Systemic Review** 155
Hui Jin, Huanhuan Yan, Huamei Tang, Miao Zheng, Chaojie Wu and Jun Liu

Chapter 37   **Bilateral Carotid-Cavernous Fistulas: An Uncommon Cause of Pituitary Enlargement and Hypopituitarism** 160
Anthony Liberatore and Ronald M. Lechan

Chapter 38   **A Case of Pneumothorax after Treatment with Lenvatinib for Anaplastic Thyroid Cancer with Lung Metastasis** 166
Haruhiko Yamazaki, Hiroyuki Iwasaki, Toshinari Yamashita, Tatsuya Yoshida, Nobuyasu Suganuma, Takashi Yamanaka, Katsuhiko Masudo, Hirotaka Nakayama, Kaori Kohagura, Yasushi Rino and Munetaka Masuda

Chapter 39   **A Case of Cushing's Syndrome due to Ectopic Adrenocorticotropic Hormone Secretion from Esthesioneuroblastoma with Long Term Follow-Up after Resection** 170
Leslee N. Matheny, Sudipa Sarkar, Hanyuan Shi, Jiun-Ruey Hu, Hannah Harmsen, Ty W. Abel, Shubhada M. Jagasia and Shichun Bao

Chapter 40   **A False Positive I-131 Metastatic Survey caused by Radioactive Iodine Uptake by a Benign Thymic Cyst** 175
Avneet K. Singh, Adina A. Bodolan and Matthew P. Gilbert

Chapter 41   **Lithium as an Alternative Option in Graves Thyrotoxicosis** 179
Ishita Prakash, Eric Sixtus Nylen and Sabyasachi Sen

Chapter 42   **Humoral Hypercalcemia of Malignancy with a Parathyroid Hormone-Related Peptide-Secreting Intrahepatic Cholangiocarcinoma Accompanied by a Gastric Cancer** 183
Katsushi Takeda, Ryosuke Kimura, Nobuhiro Nishigaki, Shinya Sato, Asami Okamoto, Kumiko Watanabe and Sachie Yasui

Chapter 43   **Identification of a Novel Mutation in a Family with Pseudohypoparathyroidism Type 1a** 189
Adelaide Moutinho, Rosa Carvalho, Rita Ferreira Reis and Sandra Tavares

Chapter 44   **Psychological Aspects of Androgen Insensitivity Syndrome: Two Cases Illustrating Therapeutical Challenges** 193
Filippa Pritsini, Georgios A. Kanakis, Ioannis Kyrgios, Eleni P. Kotanidou, Eleni Litou, Konstantina Mouzaki, Aggeliki Kleisarchaki, Dimitrios G. Goulis and Assimina Galli-Tsinopoulou

Chapter 45   **Mifepristone Improves Octreotide Efficacy in Resistant Ectopic Cushing's Syndrome** 198
Andreas G.Moraitis and Richard J. Auchus

Chapter 46   **Simultaneous Papillary Carcinoma in Thyroglossal Duct Cyst and Thyroid** 202
Gustavo Cancela e Penna, Henrique Gomes Mendes, Adele O. Kraft, Cynthia Koeppel Berenstein, Bernardo Fonseca, Wagner José Martorina, Andreise Laurian N. R. de Souza, Gustavo Meyer de Moraes, Kamilla Maria Araújo Brandão Rajão and Bárbara Érika Caldeira Araújo Sousa

Chapter 47   **False Positive Findings on I-131 WBS and SPECT/CT in Patients with History of Thyroid Cancer** 207
Zeina C. Hannoush, Juan D. Palacios, Russ A. Kuker and Sabina Casula

Chapter 48   **A Rare Complication following Thyroid Percutaneous Ethanol Injection: Plummer Adenoma** 212
Roberto Cesareo, Anda Mihaela Naciu, Valerio Pasqualini, Giuseppe Pelle, Silvia Manfrini, Gaia Tabacco, Angelo Lauria Pantano, Alessandro Casini, Roberto Cianni and Andrea Palermo

Chapter 49   **Normalization of Bilateral Adrenal Gland Enlargement after Treatment for Cryptococcosis** 216
Yuka Muraoka, Shintaro Iwama and Hiroshi Arima

Chapter 50   **A Novel RET D898Y Germline Mutation in a Patient with Pheochromocytoma** 220
Jin Wook Yi, Hye In Kang, Su-jin Kim, Chan Yong Seong, Young Jun Chai, June Young Choi, Moon-Woo Seong, Kyu Eun Lee and Sung Sup Park

Chapter 51   **An Atypical HNF4A Mutation which does not Conform to the Classic Presentation of HNF4A-MODY** 226
Andrew J. Spiro, Katherine N. Vu and Alicia Lynn Warnock

Chapter 52   **Asymptomatic Congenital Hyperinsulinism due to a Glucokinase-Activating Mutation, Treated as Adrenal Insufficiency for Twelve Years** 230
Kae Morishita, Chika Kyo, Takako Yonemoto, Rieko Kosugi, Tatsuo Ogawa and Tatsuhide Inoue

Chapter 53   **A Case Report of Dramatically Increased Thyroglobulin after Lymph Node Biopsy in Thyroid Carcinoma after Total Thyroidectomy and Radioiodine** 236
Mandana Moosavi and Stuart Kreisman

Chapter 54   **Atypical Parathyroid Adenoma Complicated with Protracted Hungry Bone Syndrome after Surgery** 240
Óscar Alfredo Juárez-León, Miguel Ángel Gómez-Sámano, Daniel Cuevas-Ramos, Paloma Almeda-Valdés, Manuel Alejandro López-Flores A La Torre, Alfredo Adolfo Reza-Albarrán and Francisco Javier Gómez-Pérez

Chapter 55   **Calcitonin-Secreting Neuroendocrine Carcinoma of Larynx with Metastasis to Thyroid** 248
Lauren LaBryer, Ravindranauth Sawh, Colby McLaurin and R. Hal Scofield

Chapter 56   **Early Onset Primary Hyperparathyroidism Associated with a Novel Germline Mutation in CDKN1B** 254
Marianne S. Elston, Goswin Y. Meyer-Rochow, Michael Dray, Michael Swarbrick and John V. Conaglen

Chapter 57   **A Rare Presentation of Transfusional Hemochromatosis: Hypogonadotropic Hypogonadism** 258
Rifki Ucler, Erdal Kara, Murat Atmaca, Sehmus Olmez, Murat Alay, Yaren Dirik and Aydin Bora

Permissions

List of Contributors

Index

Preface

The endocrine system is an organ system comprising of the endocrine glands, the hormones that they secrete and the feedback loops that control the release of these hormones. Some endocrine glands are pancreas, pituitary gland, adrenal gland, etc. These hormones are important for the regulation of the functions of various target organs and for the maintenance of homeostasis. Endocrinology is a branch of medicine and biology that deals with the study of the endocrine system, its diseases and endocrine hormones. Endocrine disorders may be subdivided into endocrine gland hypersecretion, endocrine gland hyposecretion and tumors. Some examples are hyperthyroidism and hypothyroidism, diabetes, goitre, hypogonadism, etc. This book is a valuable compilation of topics, ranging from the basic to the most complex advancements in the field of clinical endocrinology. It presents the complex subject of endocrinology in the most comprehensible and easy to understand language. With state-of-the-art inputs by acclaimed experts of this field, this book targets students and professionals.

This book has been the outcome of endless efforts put in by authors and researchers on various issues and topics within the field. The book is a comprehensive collection of significant researches that are addressed in a variety of chapters. It will surely enhance the knowledge of the field among readers across the globe.

It gives us an immense pleasure to thank our researchers and authors for their efforts to submit their piece of writing before the deadlines. Finally in the end, I would like to thank my family and colleagues who have been a great source of inspiration and support.

Editor

Idiopathic Basal Ganglia Calcification Presented with Impulse Control Disorder

Cem Sahin,[1] Mustafa Levent,[1] Gulhan Akbaba,[2] Bilge Kara,[3]
Emine Nese Yeniceri,[4] and Betul Battaloglu Inanc[4]

[1]Department of Internal Medicine, School of Medicine, Mugla Sıtkı Kocman University, Orhaniye Mahallesi, İsmet Catak Caddesi, 48000 Mugla, Turkey
[2]Department of Endocrinology, School of Medicine, Mugla Sıtkı Kocman University, Orhaniye Mahallesi, İsmet Catak Caddesi, 48000 Mugla, Turkey
[3]Department of Psychiatry, School of Medicine, Mugla Sıtkı Kocman University, Orhaniye Mahallesi, İsmet Catak Caddesi, 48000 Mugla, Turkey
[4]Department of Family Medicine, Faculty of Medicine, Mugla Sıtkı Kocman University, Orhaniye Mahallesi, İsmet Catak Caddesi, 48000 Mugla, Turkey

Correspondence should be addressed to Cem Sahin; cemsahin@mu.edu.tr

Academic Editor: Offie P. Soldin

Primary familial brain calcification (PFBC), also referred to as Idiopathic Basal Ganglia Calcification (IBGC) or "Fahr's disease," is a clinical condition characterized by symmetric and bilateral calcification of globus pallidus and also basal ganglions, cerebellar nuclei, and other deep cortical structures. It could be accompanied by parathyroid disorder and other metabolic disturbances. The clinical features are dysfunction of the calcified anatomic localization. IBGC most commonly presents with mental damage, convulsion, parkinson-like clinical picture, and neuropsychiatric behavior disorders; however, presentation with impulse control disorder is not a frequent presentation. In the current report, a 43-year-old male patient who has been admitted to psychiatry policlinic with the complaints of aggressive behavior episodes and who has been diagnosed with impulse control disorder and IBGC was evaluated in the light of the literature.

1. Introduction

The calcification of deep cortical structures and basal ganglions has been first defined histologically in 1855 by Bamberger. The disease is named by the name of German pathologist Karl Theodor Fahr who has first demonstrated the anatomical lesions. Fahr has first defined the disease in 1930 in an adult who had been under follow-up due to the symptoms of dementia and in which calcification had been detected in cerebral blood vessels in autopsy examination and has reported the disease as "idiopathic calcification in cerebral vessels" [1]. The radiological findings of the disease have been first defined by Modrego et al. in 2005 [2]. While the severity of calcification could be observed in direct roentgenograms, computerized tomography (CT) is a more sensitive modality than direct radiography in early diagnosis and demonstration of small calcifications.

Calcium deposits are histologically present in capillary vessels, media layer of small arteries, and vein and perivascular area. The disease is generally transmitted in an autosomal dominant pattern. Clinically Parkinsonism-like movement disorders, psychiatric symptoms, and radiologically nonatherosclerotic bilateral idiopathic calcification in basal ganglions are the necessary criteria for the diagnosis.

IBGC frequently begins between the fourth and the sixth decades. Generally calcium deposits appear in the first three decades of life and neurological impairment begins two decades later than calcium deposits. However, IBGC could rarely be observed in pediatric population also [3].

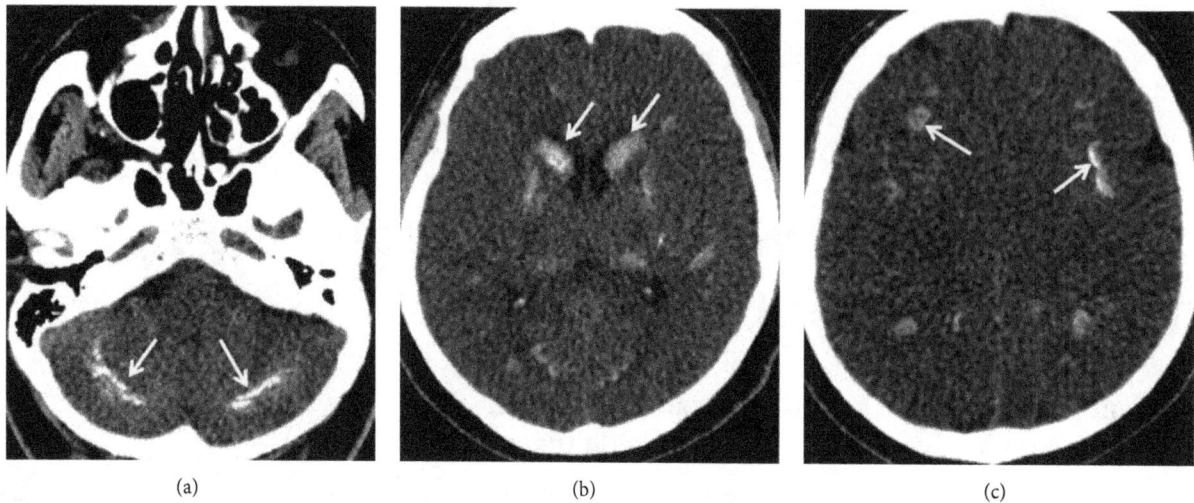

FIGURE 1: A large number of calcifications are observed in both cerebellar hemispheres (a), basal ganglions (b), and subcortical white matter (c) in axial CT sections (white arrows).

The patients with IBGC generally present with a clinical picture such as progressive mental damage, convulsion, Parkinson-like picture, and neuropsychiatric behavior disorders. However admission with impulse control disorder is not a frequently observed condition. In the present paper, a 43-year-old male patient who has been admitted to psychiatry policlinic with the complaints of aggressive behavior episodes and who has been diagnosed with impulse control disorder and idiopathic basal ganglia calcification was evaluated in the light of the literature.

2. Case Presentation

A 43-year-old male patient was evaluated in psychiatry policlinic due to the complaints of bursts of anger. From his medical history, it was learnt that his complaints have begun 5 years ago and have gradually increased within the last years. It was learnt that burst of anger has caused disturbance in social and professional life and important legal and financial problems and thus he wanted to have psychiatric support. The patient told that bursts of anger generally develop suddenly, continue for approximately half an hour, and include verbal, physical attacks and attacks against objects. He mentioned that he completely loses his control during burst of anger and it is not possible to oppose him and he is in a condition just like seizure and the severity of anger might be more or less independent of the stress causing the burst.

There was no feature in his medical and family history. As hypocalcemia was detected in laboratory examinations, he was consulted with the internal medicine department. On physical examination, general condition of the patient was normal; he was conscious and cooperated. Vital signs were normal (blood pressure 120/85 mm Hg, pulse 75 beat/min, respiratory rate 15/min, and body temperature: 36.8) and Chvostek test was (+) in his systemic and neurological examination. There was no additional pathology and the laboratory findings of the patient are summarized in Table 1.

TABLE 1: Laboratory findings of the patient.

Parameters	Values
Sodium (mEq)	143
WBC ($10^3/mm^3$)	7300
Hb (mg/dL)	13.85
Platelets (/μL)	240.000
Glucose (mg/dL)	65
BUN (mg/dL)	28
Creatinine (mg/dL)	0.82
ALT (U/L)	25
AST (U/L)	21
Folate (ng/mL)	9.63
Vitamin D (ng/mL)	43
Triglyceride (mg/dL)	494
Magnesium	1.64
Phosphor (U/L)	3.8
Albumin (gr/dL)	4.44
Calcium (mg/dL)	6.53
Ionized calcium (mg/dL)	2.86
PTH (pg/m)	21
fT3 (pmol/L)	4.96
fT4 (pmol/L)	16.62
TSH (μIU/m)	0.899
vitB12 (pg/mL)	229.2
Cholesterol (mg/dL)	222
VLDL (mg/dL)	99

On posterior-anterior chest X-ray there was no pathological finding. ECG was in normal sinus rhythm. Computerized cranial tomography was performed for both differential diagnosis of hypocalcemia and differentiation of the burst of anger from an organic cause (Figure 1). There were a great number of calcifications in both cerebellar hemispheres (Figure 1(a)), basal ganglions (Figure 1(b)), and subcortical white matter (Figure 1(c)) in axial sections of cranial tomography. In the light of the present findings, the patient was diagnosed with idiopathic basal ganglia calcification.

Some tests were performed to exclude other diagnoses and VDRL test was negative; TORCH group Ig M was negative and Ig G was positive. Anti-HIV antibody was negative. No pathology was observed in ultrasonography of thyroid and parathyroid glands. Thyroid function tests were normal and thus hyperthyroidism and hypothyroidism were excluded. Vitamin D level was normal. As there were no previous infection, previous thyroid surgery, drug use, and autoimmune disease in detailed medical history of the patient, the hypocalcemia was thought to be caused by an idiopathic etiology. On psychiatric evaluation which was performed according to DSM IV criteria, the patient was diagnosed with impulse control disorder. With the present findings, the patient was accepted as IBGC and impulse control disorder. Intravenous and oral calcium replacement therapy was administered and carbamazepine 200 mg/dy was started by the psychiatry department. After normalization of calcium values the patient was discharged to be followed up in the policlinic.

3. Discussion

IBGC which is named as bilateral striopallidodentate calcinosis is a disease with unknown etiology and characterized with neurodegenerative disturbances developing after almost always bilateral accumulation of especially calcium and phosphor in basal ganglions, cerebellar dentate nucleus, and thalamus [4]. Although there is no certain information related to how the intracerebral calcifications develop, they are thought to be possibly related to mainly infectious diseases, metabolic and genetic disturbances [5]. In postmortem examinations of the patients with idiopathic basal ganglia calcification, calcifications are observed most commonly in cerebral sulcus, basal ganglion (especially globus pallidus), dentate nucleus, and subthalamus. The calcifications in adventitia and media layers of the vessels might surround all lumen and also it might be related to the intimal fibrosis and obstruction. The variability in extent of neuronal degeneration and gliosis is possibly related to the severity of ischemia.

The disease is slowly progressive. It is observed twofold more in males when compared with females. Most the patients demonstrate symptoms at the fourth and sixth decades. However, it is known that although rarely present, there are also cases reported in children in the literature [6].

Although IBGC seems to be related to many clinical conditions, there is still no consensus related to its etiology. Although, today, the most accepted opinion is development of the disease due to disturbances in calcium and phosphor metabolism, it has been demonstrated that the disease could also develop as a result of genetic damage without any change in calcium metabolism. The disease is generally inherited in autosomal dominant pattern [7]. But genetic heterogeneity also comes into question, because sporadic, familial, and autosomal recessive forms have also been reported. In a study which was conducted in a family in which this syndrome is observed, it has been demonstrated that a defect in short arm

of 14th chromosome is important in development and progression of this disease [8].

The clinical symptoms have a wide range. Primarily neurological and psychiatric findings are observed in the patients. Among these the most common are Parkinsonism-like movement disorders and second common are cognitive disorders related to especially cerebellar involvement. While the conditions such as dystonia, tremor, chorea, ataxia, dementia, epilepsia, syncope, or stroke are frequently observed, behavioral disorders, personality changes, and several eye problems are observed at a lesser extent [9]. If the calcifications in the cranium are diffuse, other symptoms depending on the localization of the involved region could also develop. The most commonly involved basal ganglion is globus pallidus. The cause of many neuropsychiatric symptoms which could develop during the disease course is related to the anatomical localization of the globus pallidus and its relations.

In the literature it has been reported that neuropsychiatric symptoms are observed in patients with idiopathic basal ganglia calcification. There are reported cases which had been admitted with epilepsia, visual hallucinations, and sudden loss of consciousness. However, no case of IBGC accompanied with only impulse control disorder has been found in the literature review.

The most important parameter for diagnosis of IBGC is the presence of bilateral and symmetrical calcifications. An important part of these calcifications is accidentally recognized in computerized cranial tomography (CT) which is performed due to other causes. Among the radiological methods, as CT is more sensitive for calcifications, it is more valuable in diagnosis of IBGC when compared with magnetic resonance imaging (MR) [10]. In the presence of neuropsychiatric findings together with calcification in imaging methods as a supportive finding, idiopathic basal ganglia calcification should be considered in differential diagnosis if there is no other disease causing this clinical picture, because IBGC is an exclusion diagnosis.

Hypoparathyroidism and aged related physiological calcifications should be among the most commonly encountered differential diagnoses. Besides endocrinological causes such as pseudohypoparathyroidism, hypothyroidism, and D hypervitaminosis; infectious diseases such as toxoplasmosis, rubella, cytomegalovirus, HIV, and tuberculosis; vascular diseases such as Sturge-Weber disease; clinical situations related to toxic causes such as Wilson's disease, anoxia, carbon monoxide, and lead intoxication which are associated with calcifications in basal ganglions should also be considered [11].

There is no certain treatment method defined for FD in which the benefit has been demonstrated. Today the treatment is generally symptomatic. So the disease leads to progressive neurological impairment and death. However, calcium replacement therapy which is administered in the presence of hypocalcemia in addition to symptomatic treatment has been demonstrated to prevent the clinical progression of the disease. Because it has been demonstrated that long-term hypocalcemia increases the severity of calcifications in basal ganglions [12]. Furthermore, a calcium channel blocker, nimodipine which is specific to central nervous system, has been used together with regulation of calcium metabolism but successful results have not been obtained. It has been found that although disodium etidronate does not decrease calcifications, it provides symptomatic recovery [13]. Anticonvulsants have been used in cases accompanied with convulsions. Also cases have been reported in which ECT had beneficial effects on some psychotic symptoms.

4. Conclusion

Although IBGC has been known approximately for a century, it could be easily bypassed as it is rarely encountered in clinical practice.

IBGC should be considered in differential diagnosis of the patients admitted with the complaints of sudden impulse control disturbance who have calcium metabolism disturbance.

The cases with IBGC should be evaluated with laboratory tests assessing calcium metabolism and cranial CT.

References

[1] T. Fahr, "Idiopathische verkalkung der hirngefässe. Zentralblatt für allgemeine Pathologie und pathologische," *Anatomie*, vol. 50, pp. 129–133, 1930.

[2] P. J. Modrego, J. Mojonero, M. Serrano, and N. Fayed, "Fahr's syndrome presenting with pure and progressive presenile dementia," *Neurological Sciences*, vol. 26, no. 5, pp. 367–369, 2005.

[3] H. Deng, W. Zheng, and J. Jankovic, "Genetics and molecular biology of brain calcification," *Ageing Research Reviews*, vol. 22, pp. 20–38, 2015.

[4] Y. Baba, D. F. Broderick, R. J. Uitti, M. L. Hutton, and Z. K. Wszolek, "Heredofamilial brain calcinosis syndrome," *Mayo Clinic Proceedings*, vol. 80, no. 5, pp. 641–651, 2005.

[5] C. Ertan, E. Karaman, H. Oğuztürk, and D. Ertan, "Fahr's syndrome: a patient with idiopathic hypoparathyroidy in the emergency department," *Journal of Academic Emergency Medicine Case Reports*, vol. 4, no. 2, pp. 76–78, 2013.

[6] R. S. de Oliveira, M. C. M. Amato, M. V. Santos, G. N. Simão, and H. R. Machado, "Extradural arachnoid cysts in children," *Child's Nervous System*, vol. 23, no. 11, pp. 1233–1238, 2007.

[7] S. Koçac, E. Erdemir, A. Bayrak, H. Kara, and M. Gül, "Fahr's disease: two cases report," *Eurasian Journal of Emergency Medicine*, vol. 8, no. 4, pp. 46–49, 2009.

[8] C. Baydar, H. N. Güneş, T. H. Yoldaş, and A. Yılmaz, "Tension type headache and Fahr's disease," *Ankara Medical Journal*, vol. 14, no. 2, pp. 68–70, 2014.

[9] L. Cartier R, C. Passig V, A. Gormaz W, and J. López C, "Neuropsychological and neurophysiological features of Fahr's disease," *Revista Medica de Chile*, vol. 130, no. 12, pp. 1383–1390, 2002.

[10] R. H. Goodwin, "Computed tomographic image of Fahr disease mistaken for acute hemorrhagic cerebrovascular accident," *The American Journal of Emergency Medicine*, vol. 24, no. 3, article 378, 2006.

[11] J. R. Oliviera, E. Spiteri, M. J. Sobrido et al., "Genetic heterogeneity in familial IBGC (İdiopathic basal ganglia calcification)," *Neurology*, vol. 63, no. 11, pp. 2165–2167, 2004.

[12] M. Karimi, F. Habibzadeh, and V. De Sanctis, "Hypoparathyroidism with extensive intracerebral calcification in patients with β-thalassemia major," *Journal of Pediatric Endocrinology and Metabolism*, vol. 16, no. 6, pp. 883–886, 2003.

[13] B. V. Manyam, "What is and what is not 'Fahr's disease'," *Parkinsonism and Relat Disorders*, vol. 11, no. 2, pp. 73–80, 2005.

Paraganglioma Presenting as Postpartum Fever of Unknown Origin

Shraddha Narechania,[1] Amrita Bath,[1] Laleh Ghassemi,[1] Chetan Lokhande,[2] Abdo Haddad,[3] Ali Mir Yousuf,[4] Jessica Marquard,[5] and K. V. Gopalakrishna[1]

[1]*Internal Medicine Residency, Fairview Hospital, Cleveland, OH 44111, USA*
[2]*Anesthesia Department, Fairview Hospital, Cleveland, OH 44111, USA*
[3]*Cleveland Clinic Taussig Cancer Institute, Fairview Hospital, Cleveland, OH 44111, USA*
[4]*Strongsville Family Health and Surgery Center, 16761 Southpark Center, Strongsville, OH 44136, USA*
[5]*Genomic Medicine Institute, 9500 Euclid Avenue NE5, Cleveland, OH 44195, USA*

Correspondence should be addressed to Shraddha Narechania; drshraddhanarechania@gmail.com

Academic Editor: Toshihiro Kita

A young healthy postpartum mother presented with intermittent high fevers and tachycardia. Appropriate testing was done to rule out infectious causes including pan cultures but no identifiable infectious source was found. A CT of the abdomen showed a retroperitoneal mass with two small pulmonary nodules and a bony metastatic lesion. She was found to have stage 4 extra-adrenal paraganglioma with metastases to the lungs and spine. She underwent resection of the mass and is currently undergoing palliative radiation to the spine for pain control. Subsequent genetic testing identified a likely pathogenic variant in *SDHB*, confirming a diagnosis of Hereditary Paraganglioma-Pheochromocytoma syndrome.

1. Introduction

We report a rare and unique case of a young primigravida female patient who developed postpartum fever. After appropriate diagnostic testing, the patient was found to have a retroperitoneal paraganglioma. We report this case to emphasize that pheochromocytoma or paraganglioma should be considered in the differential diagnosis of postpartum fever especially with a history of preeclampsia during pregnancy.

2. Case Presentation

A 21-year-old primigravida at 37-week gestation presented to the outpatient clinic for a routine obstetrical examination. Her pregnancy course had been uneventful. Her blood pressure at this visit was 184/108. She was asymptomatic except for occasional mild headaches. A urine dipstick showed 3+ proteinuria. Patient was diagnosed with preeclampsia and was admitted to the hospital for emergency induction of labor. She was started on IV magnesium for preeclampsia and labor was induced with oxytocin. She underwent an emergency cesarean section due to fetal decelerations during induction. Subsequently, she delivered a healthy male infant by low transverse C section. Four days after partum, she started spiking high fevers up to 39.5 degrees Celsius and developed tachycardia with heart rate of 140 to 150/min. She was otherwise completely asymptomatic and clinical exam was negative for any localizing signs. Her cesarean section incision looked clean; she had no breast tenderness. Infectious work-up including blood and urine cultures was negative. Her chest X-ray was normal; EKG showed sinus tachycardia. She was empirically started on broad spectrum antibiotics. After 48 hours of IV antibiotics, patient continued to spike high fevers and was still tachycardic. The differential diagnosis of endometritis and septic thrombophlebitis was high on the list even though her abdominal exam was benign. Computerized tomography (CT) scan of the abdomen and pelvis with contrast (Figure 1) was ordered to rule out septic

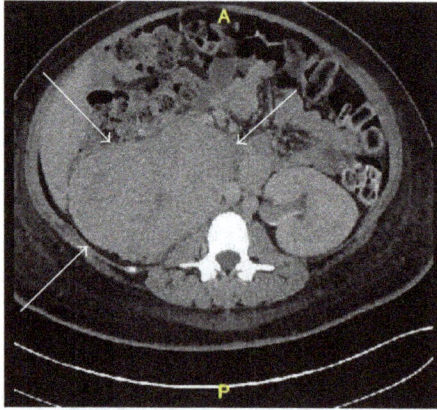

FIGURE 1: CT scan abdomen/pelvis with contrast showing large retroperitoneal mass.

thrombophlebitis, which showed a large right retroperitoneal 9.2 cm anteroposterior × 14 cm transverse × 12.5 cm craniocaudal mass with severe right renal hydronephrosis. Due to absence of any fat layer between the kidney and the mass, it was felt to be coming from the lower pole of the right kidney. The mass extended superiorly to the inferior vena cava (IVC) with a possible tumor thrombus in the IVC. The liver was mildly enlarged measuring 19.6 cm with fatty infiltration. The first segment of the sacrum showed a 3 cm × 2.1 cm × 2.6 cm lytic lesion. CT scan of the chest showed 2 pulmonary nodules measuring 7 mm and 11 mm in the left and right lower lobes of the lung, respectively. Due to the above imaging findings, suspicion was high for a stage 4 metastatic cancer arising from the kidney. Renal ultrasound confirmed a large retroperitoneal mass with hydronephrosis. MRI lumbar spine reported an abnormal marrow signal in the S1–S3 segments and an exophytic bony metastatic lesion in the dorsal aspect of S1 causing severe narrowing of the thecal sac. MRI abdomen/pelvis confirmed extension of the retroperitoneal mass into the inferior vena cava (IVC). MRI brain and CT brain were obtained showing calvarial lesions consistent with hemangiomas. A percutaneous CT guided right renal mass biopsy (Figure 2) revealed a cellular epithelioid proliferation arranged in nests and composed of round to ovoid cells with hyperchromatic nuclei, inconspicuous nucleoli, and granular amphophilic cytoplasm. Immunohistochemical staining was negative for HMB-45, S100, PAX-8, cytokeratin AE1/AE3, CD117, and DOG-1 but was positive for synaptophysin and chromogranin (Figure 3). The overall morphological and immunohistochemical findings were consistent with a diagnosis of paraganglioma. 24-hour urine testing revealed high levels of urinary nor epinephrine which was 862 mcg/24 hours (normal range 15 to 100 mcg/24 hours) and dopamine which was 902 mcg/24 hours (normal range 52 to 480 mcg/24 hours). Plasma-free metanephrine levels were also elevated at 1690 pg/mL (normal range 18 to 101 pg/mL). The patient continued to remain severely hypertensive after delivery and was started on combined alpha and beta blockade with doxazosin 8 mg daily and propranolol 40 mg twice daily. The patient underwent right sided nephrectomy, removal

of the retroperitoneal mass, and resection of the perirenal IVC. Her postoperative course was complicated by severe hypotension and extensive bilateral lower extremity deep venous thromboses in the external iliac and common femoral veins. She required vasopressors for two days and was started on therapeutic anticoagulation with enoxaparin for the DVTs. She was discharged home 2 weeks after her surgery. A metaiodobenzylguanidine (MIBG) whole body scan done later as an outpatient did not demonstrate any focal abnormal uptake. Whole body PET scan showed increased FDG uptake in 3 pulmonary nodules, a large lytic sacral lesion, and a T9 vertebral body lesion all consistent with metastases. The patient underwent gamma knife palliative radiation of the S1 lesion and was started on Zometa for her bony metastases. The tyrosine kinase receptor inhibitor Sunitinib was started to treat her systemic disease.

The patient underwent genetic counseling and pursued genetic testing for multiple hereditary paraganglioma syndromes. She had no known family history of paraganglioma, pheochromocytoma, kidney cancer, or thyroid cancer. Next generation sequencing of *MAX*, *NF1*, *RET*, *SDHA*, *SDHAF2*, *SDHB*, *SDHC*, *SDHD*, *TMEM127*, and *VHL* identified a likely pathogenic variant in *SDHB*, c.418G>T (p.Val140Phe). This result confirmed a diagnosis of Hereditary Paraganglioma-Pheochromocytoma syndrome, an autosomal dominant condition with reduced penetrance.

3. Discussion

Paragangliomas, also sometimes called extra-adrenal pheochromocytomas, are rare neuroendocrine tumors arising from sympathetic and parasympathetic paraganglia outside the adrenal medulla. They can occur at almost any site in the body including head, neck, thorax, and abdominal cavity. Most of the thoracic and abdominal paragangliomas arise from sympathetic ganglia and are secretory while head and neck paragangliomas are generally nonsecretory as they arise from parasympathetic ganglia [1, 2]. They are closely related to pheochromocytomas and are clinically undifferentiable from them causing symptoms attributable to excessive catecholamine secretion such as episodic hypertension, diaphoresis, headaches, and palpitations. Histologically, the main difference between these is that paragangliomas arise from extra-adrenal chromaffin tissue cells whereas pheochromocytomas arise from adrenal chromaffin tissue [3].

Most paragangliomas occur sporadically; however, up to 30% are due to a hereditary predisposition syndrome [4]. All individuals diagnosed with a paraganglioma or pheochromocytoma should be referred for genetic counseling. Factors that increase the likelihood of a hereditary cause include early age at diagnosis, extra-adrenal location, and positive family history. *SDHB*-associated paragangliomas are malignant in up to 37% of cases [5]. Individuals with Hereditary Paraganglioma-Pheochromocytoma syndrome should be followed with annual biochemical screening for functional paraganglioma and periodic imaging of the neck, chest, abdomen, and pelvis. Their first-degree relatives have a 50%

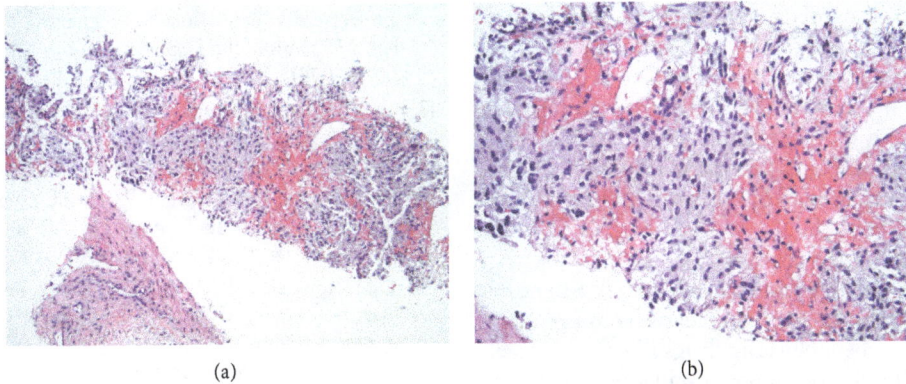

FIGURE 2: Microscopic examination of renal biopsy specimen in 100x view (a) and 200x view (b) showing cellular epithelioid proliferation arranged in nests and composed of round to ovoid cells with hyperchromatic nuclei, inconspicuous nucleoli, and granular amphophilic cytoplasm.

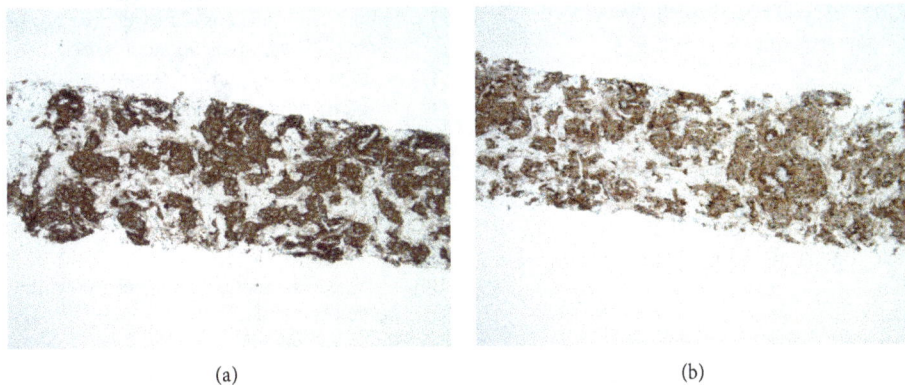

FIGURE 3: CT guided renal mass biopsy showing positive staining for synaptophysin (a) and chromogranin (b).

chance of having the familial pathogenic variant and should have genetic counseling and testing.

Paragangliomas are seen most commonly located in the inferior para-aortic region; however, they also occur in other regions like the urinary bladder, mediastinum, head, and neck [6]. Paragangliomas rarely produce epinephrine, majority of them producing norepinephrine or a combination of norepinephrine and dopamine and some rarely even producing dopamine alone. Most adrenal tumors on the other hand produce epinephrine and norepinephrine [7]. Majority of these tumours are benign and only up to 3% are malignant [8].

The occurrence of paragangliomas in pregnancy is extremely rare and has been reported to be about 5 per million pregnancies in some studies to 18.5 per million live births in others [6, 9, 10]. Paragangliomas have been reported to occur at various sites during pregnancy including bladder and heart [11, 12]. We report a rare and unique case of a paraganglioma presenting as postpartum fever and hypertension in a young female. Kleiner et al. had, in 1982, described a similar case of paraganglioma presenting as postpartum fever [13]. To the best of our knowledge, this is the first reported case of a paraganglioma causing IVC thrombosis with extensive lower extremity deep venous

thrombosis and the second reported case of paraganglioma presenting as postpartum fever.

Timely diagnosis and treatment are of paramount importance as the maternal and fetal mortality can be as high as 50% if this condition is undiagnosed and untreated [6]. A hypertensive crisis can be precipitated by uterine contractions during labor and vaginal delivery [10]. Data indicates that about 20% of patients pass through pregnancy undiagnosed due to the nonspecific nature of signs and symptoms and the much higher prevalence of gestational hypertension [14]. The best initial screening test recommended for diagnosis is the measurement of plasma-free metanephrines [15]. However, a general consensus has not been reached in regard to the diagnostic testing of pheochromocytoma or paraganglioma. It has been suggested that, for patients with a low pretest probability, testing with 24-hour urinary metanephrines and catecholamines is preferable as it can avoid high false positive rates seen with measurement of plasma-free metanephrines [16].

After biochemical confirmation, imaging is used to identify the location of the tumour. In pregnant females, the imaging modality of choice is Magnetic Resonance Imaging whose sensitivity can be as high as 90% in diagnosing paragangliomas and it minimizes fetal exposure to ionizing radiation [10, 14]. Ultrasound can also be used for detection but it is not the preferred modality as it is not as sensitive as MRI in detecting adrenal tumors [13]. The accuracy of ultrasound depends on the technical skill of the operator, the ultrasound quality, and the body habitus of the patient [17]. In a pregnant patient, the bulky uterus might preclude the detection of adrenal and retroperitoneal structures as might have happened in our case [13, 18].

Surgical resection is the mainstay of treatment during pregnancy [10]. Presurgical preparation of patients is done by initiating alpha blocking agents like phenoxybenzamine or doxazosin followed by beta blocking drugs like propranolol or atenolol to avoid unopposed alpha stimulation which can lead to a hypertensive crisis. In pregnant women the optimum time for removal of the tumor is either before 24 weeks if diagnosed that early or after delivery if diagnosed after 24 weeks. The second trimester is the safest for surgery due to the high risk of spontaneous abortion in the first trimester. Prolonged follow-up is necessary as these tumors have a high rate of recurrence.

4. Conclusion

Due to the extremely high mortality rate of this rare but treatable condition, it is essential to conduct a meticulous history taking and clinical examination so that early diagnosis and treatment can save maternal and fetal lives and improve clinical outcomes.

References

[1] L. Fishbein, R. Orlowski, and D. Cohen, "Pheochromocytoma/Paraganglioma: review of perioperative management of blood pressure and update on genetic mutations associated with pheochromocytoma," *Journal of Clinical Hypertension*, vol. 15, no. 6, pp. 428–434, 2013.

[2] K. E. Joynt, J. J. Moslehi, and K. L. Baughman, "Paragangliomas: etiology, presentation, and management," *Cardiology in Review*, vol. 17, no. 4, pp. 159–164, 2009.

[3] G. Eisenhofer, "Screening for pheochromocytomas and paragangliomas," *Current Hypertension Reports*, vol. 14, no. 2, pp. 130–137, 2012.

[4] M. Mannelli, M. Castellano, F. Schiavi et al., "Clinically guided genetic screening in a large cohort of Italian patients with pheochromocytomas and/or functional or nonfunctional paragangliomas," *Journal of Clinical Endocrinology and Metabolism*, vol. 94, no. 5, pp. 1541–1547, 2009.

[5] D. E. Benn, A.-P. Gimenez-Roqueplo, J. R. Reilly et al., "Clinical presentation and penetrance of pheochromocytoma/paraganglioma syndromes," *Journal of Clinical Endocrinology and Metabolism*, vol. 91, no. 3, pp. 827–836, 2006.

[6] F. J. Bosch, J. Goedhals, W. De Lange, M. Ackermann, and J. M. M. Koning, "A pelvic paraganglioma presenting as

a hypertensive emergency in pregnancy," *Journal of Endocrinology, Metabolism and Diabetes of South Africa*, vol. 17, no. 3, pp. 145–147, 2012.

[7] G. Eisenhofer and M. Peitzsch, "Laboratory evaluation of pheochromocytoma and paraganglioma," *Clinical Chemistry*, vol. 60, no. 12, pp. 1486–1499, 2014.

[8] A. Roberton and A. Ferro, "Metastatic paraganglioma: management of orthostatic hypotension—a case report," *JRSM Cardiovascular Disease*, vol. 1, no. 6, pp. 16–16, 2012.

[9] T. M. Koroscil, S. McDonald, S. Stutes, and R. J. Vila, "Use of fluorine-18-labelled deoxyglucose positron emission tomography with computed tomography to localize a paraganglioma in pregnancy," *Southern Medical Journal*, vol. 103, no. 12, pp. 1238–1242, 2010.

[10] A. Del Giudice, M. Bisceglia, M. D'Errico et al., "Extra-adrenal functional paraganglioma (phaeochromocytoma) associated with renal-artery stenosis in a pregnant woman," *Nephrology Dialysis Transplantation*, vol. 13, no. 11, pp. 2920–2923, 1998.

[11] O. Demirkesen, B. Cetinel, O. Yaycioglu, N. Uygun, and V. Solok, "Unusual cause of early preeclampsia: bladder paraganglioma," *Urology*, vol. 56, no. 1, article 154, 2000.

[12] T. G. Pickering, O. W. Isom, G. W. Bergman, and J. M. Barbieri, "Pheochromocytoma of the heart," *American Journal of Cardiology*, vol. 86, no. 11, pp. 1288–1289, 2000.

[13] G. J. Kleiner, W. M. Greston, P. T. Yang, J. L. Levy, and A. D. Newman, "Paraganglioma complicating pregnancy and the puerperium," *Obstetrics and Gynecology*, vol. 59, supplement 6, pp. 2S–6S, 1982.

[14] J. W. M. Lenders, "Pheochromocytoma and pregnancy: a deceptive connection," *European Journal of Endocrinology*, vol. 166, no. 2, pp. 143–150, 2012.

[15] J. W. M. Lenders, K. Pacak, M. M. Walther et al., "Biochemical diagnosis of pheochromocytoma: which test is best?" *The Journal of the American Medical Association*, vol. 287, no. 11, pp. 1427–1434, 2002.

[16] Y. C. Kudva, A. M. Sawka, and W. F. Young Jr., "The laboratory diagnosis of adrenal pheochromocytoma: the Mayo Clinic experience," *Journal of Clinical Endocrinology and Metabolism*, vol. 88, no. 10, pp. 4533–4539, 2003.

[17] Y.-L. Wan, "Ultrasonography of the adrenal gland," *Journal of Medical Ultrasound*, vol. 15, no. 4, pp. 213–227, 2007.

[18] S. Grodski, C. Jung, P. Kertes, M. Davies, and S. Banting, "Phaeochromocytoma in pregnancy," *Internal Medicine Journal*, vol. 36, no. 9, pp. 604–606, 2006.

3

A Case of Glucocorticoid Remediable Aldosteronism and Thoracoabdominal Aneurysms

Anahita Shahrrava,[1] Sunnan Moinuddin,[1] Prajwal Boddu,[1] and Rohan Shah[2]

[1]Department of Internal Medicine, Advocate Illinois Masonic Medical Center, 836 West Wellington Avenue, Chicago, IL 60657, USA
[2]Department of Radiology, Advocate Illinois Masonic Medical Center, 836 West Wellington Avenue, Chicago, IL 60657, USA

Correspondence should be addressed to Anahita Shahrrava; anahita.shahrrava@advocatehealth.com

Academic Editor: John Broom

Glucocorticoid remediable aldosteronism (GRA) is rare familial form of primary aldosteronism characterized by a normalization of hypertension with the administration of glucocorticoids. We present a case of GRA and thoracoabdominal aneurysm complicated by multiple aortic dissections requiring complex surgical and endovascular repairs. Registry studies have shown a high rate of intracranial aneurysms in GRA patients with high case fatality rates. The association of thoracoabdominal aneurysms with GRA has not been described, thus far, in literature. Studies have shown that high tissue aldosterone levels concomitant with salt intake have a significant role in the pathogenesis of aneurysms and this may explain the formation of aneurysms in the intracranial vasculature and aorta. The association of GRA with thoracic aortic aneurysms needs to be further studied to develop screening recommendations for early identification and optimal treatment. Also, the early use of mineralocorticoid antagonists may have a significant preventive and attenuating effect in aneurysm formation, an association which needs to be confirmed in future studies.

1. Introduction

Glucocorticoid remediable aldosteronism is rare familial form of primary aldosteronism characterized by a unique clinical response of hypertension and aldosterone production to the administration of glucocorticoids. First described in 1996 by Sutherland and colleagues in a family of father and son, it was observed that the clinical findings of mineralocorticoid excess including hypertension and hypokalemia reversed dramatically with administration of dexamethasone giving it the name dexamethasone remediable hyperaldosteronism, also referred to as Familial Hyperaldosteronism Type 1 [1]. GRA has been associated with early onset familial intracranial aneurysms, a potentially fatal complication carrying high fatality rates. The association of GRA with thoracoabdominal aneurysms has not been studied. Studies suggest that high aldosterone levels and high salt intake have a significant hypertension-independent effect in the pathogenesis of aneurysms [2].

2. Case Report

A 24-year-old male presented to our hospital with daily complaints of chest pain and palpitations for the past three months. He endorsed to not being compliant with his prednisone and antihypertensives in the recent past. His medical history was significant for glucocorticoid remediable hyperaldosteronism (GRA) diagnosed at the age of 18, HTN, depression, and anxiety. His cardiovascular history was notable for 3 aortic dissections, at ages of 10, 17, and 22, midthoracic aortic aneurysm requiring endovascular repair at the age of 18, and abdominal aortic aneurysm which required open surgical repair at the age of 22. Childhood history was remarkable for early onset hypertension discovered at the age of 10 after his first episode of dissection. He also had severe headaches during childhood which were attributed to hypertension by his treating physicians. He was started then on amlodipine, carvedilol, and clonidine for the management of his hypertension. 8 years later, he was diagnosed with

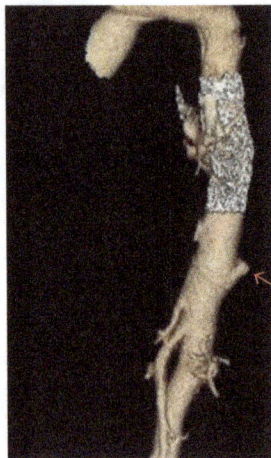

FIGURE 1

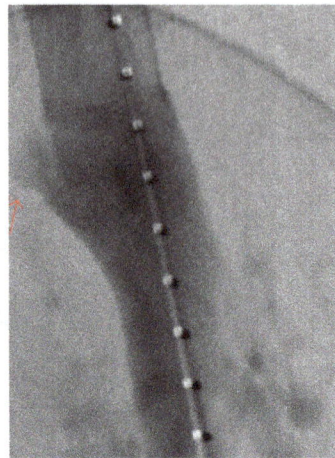

FIGURE 2

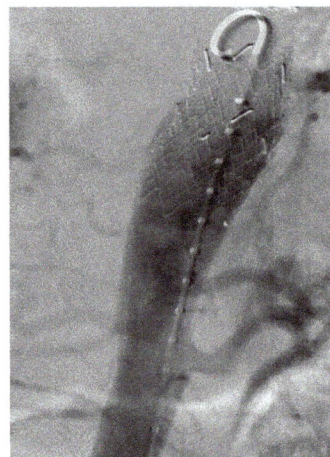

FIGURE 3

GRA by another physician and was started on prednisone and spironolactone. The biochemical data could not be obtained as it was done many years ago at an outside hospital, but diagnosis was confirmed by detecting the chimeric gene via PCR testing. Genetic testing was done on parents and the father was found to have abnormal gene. No family history of aortic aneurysms and negative gene testing ruled out familial thoracic aortic aneurysm and dissection. The patient's mother and father were not consanguineous, and both parents died of drug overdose. The patient's sister has Crohn's disease. The patient had a 4 pack-year smoking history.

On initial exam, patient was hypertensive with a blood pressure of 206/109. Physical exam was unremarkable except for a 4/6 systolic murmur most prominent in the aortic area with radiation to the apex. The patient did not have morphological features of related conditions like Marfan's syndrome, Ehlers-Danlos syndrome, or Loeys-Dietz syndrome. Labs either were within normal limits or were unremarkable. Transthoracic echocardiogram revealed concentric hypertrophy with an ejection fraction of 60% and an intimal flap suggestive of aortic dissection. There was no evidence of cardiac anomalies of bicuspid valve on echocardiograph. CT angiogram (Figure 1) demonstrated chronic dissection of the aortic arch (not shown in figure) terminating at thoracic stent and extending into the innominate and common carotid arteries and a pseudoaneurysm of the distal thoracic aorta just above the celiac artery (Figures 1 and 2). The patient was started on antihypertensives and prednisone with gradual improvement of blood pressure back to baseline. Review of past medical records confirms that the aortic dissection was chronic and it was decided not to operate upon the patient due to high risk of surgical complications. Interventional radiology was consulted and an endovascular repair of the pseudoaneurysm was planned. An endovascular aortic stent was placed successfully without complications (Figures 2 and 3) and the patient was transferred to ICU for close monitoring.

3. Discussion

Glucocorticoid remediable aldosteronism is a rare form of familial hyperaldosteronism characterized by an autosomal dominant pattern of inheritance [3]. GRA is the most common monogenetic form of hypertension. Molecular studies have characterized the genetic basis of GRA to be from the unequal crossing over between CYP11B1 (11β-hydroxylase) and CYP11B2 (aldosterone synthase) loci resulting in chimeric gene involving the 5$'$ ACTH-responsive promoter of the 11β-hydroxylase gene to the 3$'$ coding sequences of the aldosterone synthase [4, 5]. This results in ectopic expression of aldosterone synthase in zona fasciculata under the modulation of ACTH resulting in ACTH mediated aldosteronism [4, 6].

GRA is characterized by early onset severe hypertension starting in early childhood with up to 80% of the affected presenting before the age of 13 [7]. However, associated studies have observed a large variation in the expression of phenotype among affected family members with some having only mild hypertension and others being normotensive [8]. Most patients with GRA are normokalemic in salt restricted state making potassium levels an insensitive tool for evaluating GRA indicating PHA [9, 10]. GRA is a low renin hypertension characterized by high aldosterone/renin ratio, failure to suppress aldosterone with salt loading, and elevated 18-hydroxycortisol, 18-hydroxycorticosterone, and 18-oxocortisol levels [11, 12]. However, definitive diagnosis is best accomplished by genetic testing for the chimeric gene by PCR in the peripheral blood DNA [13]. Physicians should maintain a high degree of suspicion for GRA in children with early onset severe hypertension especially with a supporting family history of early onset hypertension [7].

Early cerebrovascular complications in GRA were systemically reviewed in a cohort of 376 patients from 27 GRA pedigrees which showed the presence of intracranial aneurysms in 48% of all GRA pedigrees and case fatality rates of up to 61% [14] leading to screening recommendations for intracranial aneurysms every 5 years after puberty [15]. However, the incidence of thoracoabdominal aneurysms in GRA has not been studied to date. Mineralocorticoid receptors are expressed not only in the kidneys but also in the heart and the aorta [16]. It has been proven that aldosterone exerts widespread cardiovascular effects including left ventricular hypertrophy, hypertension, and heart failure independent of changes in systemic blood pressure indicating a potential remodeling role for mineralocorticoid antagonists [17]. A case report of successful treatment of a pseudoaneurysm in a type 2 diabetes mellitus patient while treating primary aldosteronism with spironolactone has been described [18]. Mouse models of aortic aneurysms have identified a significant role of aldosterone in the pathogenesis of aortic aneurysms. High aldosterone concomitant with increased salt intake leads to age-dependent aneurysmal changes in the aorta which do not correlate with blood pressure increases and reduce in size with mineralocorticoid receptor antagonists like spironolactone [2]. The results of this study lend to the proposal that early use of mineralocorticoid antagonists may have a significant preventative and remodeling effect of aneurysm formation in GRA patients and that early diagnosis of GRA remains pivotal to allow for prompt screening and early initiation of these agents. Also, case studies of aortic dissection in hyperaldosteronism suggest that high aldosterone levels may exert structural alterations in the aorta beyond and independent of aldosteronism-induced hypertension [19, 20]. The combined risk factor profile of hypertension, smoking, and hyperaldosteronism may well explain early onset of dissection and aneurysms in our patient.

The first-line treatment of GRA is the nightly use of dexamethasone or prednisone in doses sufficient to suppress early morning surges in ACTH and normalize blood pressure [21]. The initiation of mineralocorticoid antagonists in the treatment regimen is less clear and is generally considered in patients whose blood pressure is not normalized on glucocorticoids or if there is coexisting essential hypertension [22]. As discussed above, early use of mineralocorticoid antagonists may have far reaching benefits in preventing and/or attenuating aneurysm formation and should be considered early in the course of therapy even in normotensives.

To our knowledge, thoracoabdominal aneurysms in GRA have not been described in literature. The association of GRA with thoracic aortic aneurysms needs to be further studied to inform screening recommendations for early detection and optimal management of aortic aneurysms in these select groups of patients. The early use of mineralocorticoid antagonists may have a significant preventive and attenuating effect in aneurysm formation, an effect which needs to be confirmed in future studies.

References

[1] V. M. Vehaskari, "Heritable forms of hypertension," *Pediatric Nephrology*, vol. 24, no. 10, pp. 1929–1937, 2009.

[2] S. Liu, Z. Xie, A. Daugherty et al., "Mineralocorticoid receptor agonists induce mouse aortic aneurysm formation and rupture in the presence of high salt," *Arteriosclerosis, Thrombosis, and Vascular Biology*, vol. 33, no. 7, pp. 1568–1579, 2013.

[3] D. J. Sutherland, J. L. Ruse, and J. C. Laidlaw, "Hypertension, increased aldosterone secretion and low plasma renin activity relieved by dexamethasone," *Canadian Medical Association Journal*, vol. 95, no. 22, pp. 1109–1119, 1966.

[4] R. V. Jackson, A. Lafferty, D. J. Torpy, and C. Stratakis, "New genetic insights in familial hyperaldosteronism," *Annals of the New York Academy of Sciences*, vol. 970, pp. 77–88, 2002.

[5] L. Pascoe, K. M. Curnow, L. Slutsker et al., "Glucocorticoid-suppressible hyperaldosteronism results from hybrid genes created by unequal crossovers between CYP11B1 and CYP11B2," *Proceedings of the National Academy of Sciences of the United States of America*, vol. 89, no. 17, pp. 8327–8331, 1992.

[6] R. P. Lifton, R. G. Dluhy, M. Powers, S. Ulick, and J. M. Lalouel, "The molecular basis of glucocorticoid-remediable aldosteronism, a mendelian cause of human hypertension," *Transactions of the Association of American Physicians*, vol. 105, pp. 64–71, 1992.

[7] R. G. Dluhy, B. Anderson, B. Harlin, J. Ingelfinger, and R. Lifton, "Glucocorticoid-remediable aldosteronism is associated with severe hypertension in early childhood," *The Journal of Pediatrics*, vol. 138, no. 5, pp. 715–720, 2001.

[8] F. Fallo, C. Pilon, T. A. Williams et al., "Coexistence of different phenotypes in a family with glucocorticoid-remediable aldosteronism," *Journal of Human Hypertension*, vol. 18, no. 1, pp. 47–51, 2004.

[9] G. M. Rich, S. Ulick, S. Cook, J. Z. Wang, R. P. Lifton, and R. G. Dluhy, "Glucocorticoid-remediable aldosteronism in a large kindred: cinical spectrum and diagnosis using a characteristic biochemical phenotype," *Annals of Internal Medicine*, vol. 116, no. 10, pp. 813–820, 1992.

[10] E. A. Espiner and R. A. Donald, "Aldosterone regulation in primary aldosteronism: influence of salt balance, posture and ACTH," *Clinical Endocrinology*, vol. 12, no. 3, pp. 277–286, 1980.

[11] O. Vonend, C. Altenhenne, N. J. Büchner et al., "A German family with glucocorticoid-remediable aldosteronism," *Nephrology Dialysis Transplantation*, vol. 22, no. 4, pp. 1123–1130, 2007.

[12] P. Mulatero, S. M. di Cella, S. Monticone et al., "18-Hydroxycorticosterone, 18-hydroxycortisol, and 18-oxocortisol in the diagnosis of primary aldosteronism and its subtypes," *Journal of Clinical Endocrinology and Metabolism*, vol. 97, no. 3, pp. 881–889, 2012.

[13] J. R. Jonsson, S. A. Klemm, T. J. Tunny, M. Stowasser, and R. D. Gordon, "A new genetic test for familial hyperaldosteronism type I AIDS in the detection of curable hypertension," *Biochemical and Biophysical Research Communications*, vol. 207, no. 2, pp. 565–571, 1995.

[14] W. R. Litchfield, B. F. Anderson, R. J. Weiss, R. P. Lifton, and R. G. Dluhy, "Intracranial aneurysm and hemorrhagic stroke in glucocorticoid- remediable aldosteronism," *Hypertension*, vol. 31, no. 1, pp. 445–450, 1998.

[15] F. Crawley, A. Clifton, and M. M. Brown, "Should we screen for familial intracranial aneurysm?" *Stroke*, vol. 30, no. 2, pp. 312–316, 1999.

[16] M. J. Young and A. J. Rickard, "Mechanisms of mineralocorticoid salt-induced hypertension and cardiac fibrosis," *Molecular and Cellular Endocrinology*, vol. 350, no. 2, pp. 248–255, 2012.

[17] H. V. Joffe and G. K. Adler, "Effect of aldosterone and mineralocorticoid receptor blockade on vascular inflammation," *Heart Failure Reviews*, vol. 10, no. 1, pp. 31–37, 2005.

[18] Y. Ito, K. Yoshimura, Y. Matsuzawa et al., "Successful treatment of a mycotic aortic pseudoaneurysm in a patient with type 2 diabetes mellitus while treating primary aldosteronism with spironolactone," *Journal of Atherosclerosis and Thrombosis*, vol. 17, no. 7, pp. 771–775, 2010.

[19] K. L. Harvey, C. V. Riga, M. O'Connor, M. S. Hamady, N. Chapman, and R. G. J. Gibbs, "A rare case of aortic dissection and primary hyperaldosteronism," *EJVES Extra*, vol. 20, no. 3, pp. e22–e24, 2010.

[20] J.-M. Tartière, L. Kesri, J.-J. Mourad, M. Safar, and J. Blacher, "Primary aldosteronism: a risk factor for aortic dissection?" *Journal des Maladies Vasculaires*, vol. 28, no. 4, pp. 185–189, 2003.

[21] M. Stowasser, A. W. Bachmann, P. R. Huggard, T. R. Rossetti, and R. D. Gordon, "Treatment of familial hyperaldosteronism type I: only partial suppression of adrenocorticotropin required to correct hypertension," *Journal of Clinical Endocrinology and Metabolism*, vol. 85, no. 9, pp. 3313–3318, 2000.

[22] F. Halperin and R. G. Dluhy, "Glucocorticoid-remediable Aldosteronism," *Endocrinology and Metabolism Clinics of North America*, vol. 40, no. 2, pp. 333–341, 2011.

4

Cerebral Malaria: An Unusual Cause of Central Diabetes Insipidus

Resmi Premji, Nira Roopnarinesingh, Joshua Cohen, and Sabyasachi Sen

Division of Endocrinology, Diabetes and Metabolism, George Washington University, Washington, DC 20037, USA

Correspondence should be addressed to Sabyasachi Sen; ssen1@gwu.edu

Academic Editor: Osamu Isozaki

Central diabetes insipidus is an uncommon feature of malaria. A previously healthy 72-year-old man presented with fever, rigors, and altered mental status after a recent trip to Liberia, a country known for endemic falciparum malaria. Investigations confirmed plasmodium falciparum parasitemia. Within one week after admission, the serum sodium rose to 166 mEq/L and the urine output increased to 7 liters/day. Other labs were notable for a high serum osmolality, low urine osmolality, and low urine specific gravity. The hypernatremia did not respond to hypotonic fluids. Diabetes insipidus was suspected and parenteral desmopressin was started with a prompt decrease in urinary output and improvement in mental status. Additional testing showed normal anterior pituitary hormones. The desmopressin was eventually tapered off with complete resolution of symptoms. Central diabetes insipidus occurred likely as a result of obstruction of the neurohypophyseal microvasculature. Other endocrinopathies that have been reported with malaria include hyponatremia, adrenal insufficiency, hypothyroidism, hypocalcemia, hypophosphatemia, hyper-, and hypoglycemia, but none manifested in our patient. Though diabetes insipidus is a rare complication of malaria, clinicians need to be aware of this manifestation, as failure to do so may lead to fatality particularly if the patient is dehydrated.

1. Introduction

Malaria remains a major public health challenge. As per WHO, there were about 198 million cases of malaria in 2013 with an estimated 584,000 deaths. Cerebral malaria is defined as an unexplained coma in a patient with malarial parasitemia. This is a life-threatening complication of malaria. Cytoadherence and sequestration of red blood cells in the microvasculature are thought to be the key pathophysiology. Here we present the case report of a 72-year-old patient who developed an unusual complication of cerebral malaria and central diabetes insipidus followed by a review on endocrine complications associated with malaria.

2. Case Presentation

A previously healthy 72-year-old man presented with a four-day history of fever, rigors, back pain, and altered mental status. He had returned from a trip to Liberia, a country with endemic chloroquine-resistant falciparum malaria, two weeks prior to presentation. He took doxycycline chemoprophylaxis during the trip however discontinued it prematurely upon return.

Investigations confirmed plasmodium falciparum parasitemia (greater than 10%) with acute kidney injury. He was started on parenteral quinidine followed by artesunate and exchange transfusion. The serum sodium was 132 mEq/L at admission. A head CT scan at admission did not reveal any acute findings. A brain MRI done 2 months prior as work up of an unexplained syncope was within normal limits.

Within a week after admission, there was rise in serum sodium and urine output as shown in Figure 1. Other studies were notable for high serum osmolality (354 mOsm/Kg), low urine osmolality (199 Osm/kg), and low urine specific gravity (1.010).

The hypernatremia did not respond to fluid therapy. Diabetes insipidus was suspected based on the above findings and parenteral desmopressin was started with a prompt decrease in serum sodium and urine output (Figure 1). This was accompanied by a significant improvement in

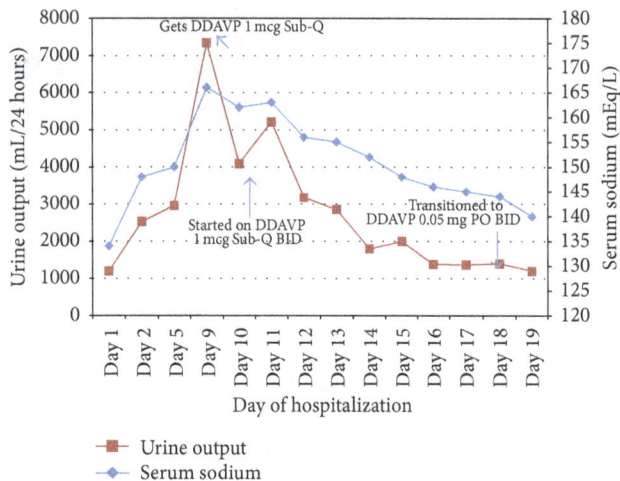

FIGURE 1: Graph of patient's serum sodium and urine output in response to desmopressin over hospital course. Sub-Q: subcutaneous; DDAVP: desmopressin; PO: per os; BID: twice daily.

mental status. Additional testing revealed morning cortisol 15.5 mcg/dL, free T4 1.3 ng/dL, and prolactin 34 ng/mL. These were done to exclude possibilities of adrenal and thyroid insufficiency. Acute kidney injury resolved with hydration and other electrolytes were found to be within normal limits as follows: calcium: 8.8 mg/dL, phosphorous: 3.2 mg/dL, and magnesium: 2.1 mg/dL. Fasting glucose ranged between 70 and 130 mg/dL during the hospital stay. Desmopressin was eventually changed to 0.05 mg twice daily orally on discharge and 0.05 mg at bedtime a week later. The serum sodium was 134 mEq/L on the day of discharge. Desmopressin was discontinued two weeks later with complete resolution of thirst and polyuria and serum sodium remained normal at 138 mEq/L during that time.

3. Discussion

We have described a patient who presented with cerebral malaria developing a very rare complication, central diabetes insipidus. The classic presentation of malaria with relapsing and remitting fevers occurs in only 50–70% of persons infected with plasmodium species [1] and the rest is accounted by atypical features.

3.1. Literature Review on Endocrine Abnormalities Associated with Malaria. Endocrine and metabolic abnormalities that have been reported in the literature with malaria include hyponatremia, diabetes insipidus, hypercortisolemia, adrenal insufficiency, primary and secondary hypothyroidism, hyper- and hypoglycemia, hyper- and hypokalemia, hypophosphatemia, hypocalcemia, and hypomagnesemia. Hyponatremia could result due to SIADH (syndrome of inappropriate antidiuretic hormone), cerebral salt wasting, or gastrointestinal and renal losses. Holst and his group [2] estimated antidiuretic hormone (ADH) concentrations along with serum and urine osmolality, serum, and urine sodium in 17 patients with falciparum malaria and found that the ADH concentrations

were raised inappropriately in relation to the serum osmolality in 6 patients. The high ADH might be a marker of decrease in the effective plasma volume suggesting TNF-alpha induced endothelial damage and leakage. However, dehydration more than SIADH was suggested as the cause of hyponatremia in severe childhood malaria according to English and colleagues [3]. In their study 47 children with cerebral malaria were prospectively recruited and serial indices of fluid/electrolyte balance and renal function were monitored during admission. 21% of patients had pronounced hyponatremia and in comparison to the eunatremic group, hyponatremic children gained less weight, had higher urea concentrations, and were more acidotic consistent with dehydration.

Diabetes insipidus as occurred in our patient could have resulted due to obstruction of neurohypophyseal microvasculature by the malarial parasites. Mature forms of the parasite, including trophozoites and the meronts, sequester in the microvasculature; nonparasitized RBCs adhere to the parasitized RBCs (rosetting) and parasitized RBCs adhere among each other (agglutination). As the parasites grow within the RBCs, they become less deformable causing mechanical obstruction and impaired microvascular circulation. A variety of proinflammatory cytokines, including TNF-alpha increases the cytoadherence [4]. Only a few case reports have described diabetes insipidus as a complication of cerebral malaria. In a study conducted by Grimwade et al. [5], in 411 patients with malaria, 37 of 175 patients with severe malaria had polyuria, and 10 patients had low urine osmolality and high serum osmolality consistent with diabetes insipidus. Another case report by Schubert et al. [6] described central diabetes insipidus in a patient with cerebral malaria, which responded to desmopressin. The microvascular obstruction gradually resolves with treatment of the parasitemia and hence the requirement of desmopressin is temporary as illustrated in our case. The mild hyperprolactinemia noted was likely secondary to the temporary cessation of the regulatory dopamine impulses reaching the anterior pituitary.

Both cortisol excess and adrenal insufficiencies have been reported as a complication of malaria. In a study conducted by Wilson et al. [7] it was shown that, in persons infected with malaria, there is inappropriate suppression of cortisol after one milligram dexamethasone suppression test. They proposed that this could be possibly due to proinflammatory cytokines activating the adrenal cortex in order to protect from complications such as hypoglycemia associated with the infection. On the other hand, Davis et al. [8] in a study of 9 patients with complicated malaria found that the rise in ACTH and cortisol after CRH stimulation was blunted. The primary and secondary adrenal insufficiency may be attenuated by increased circulating IL-6 and impaired cortisol metabolism. Authors also suggested that if hypoglycemia was present and/or if cortisol levels were within or below the normal range, stress dose steroids should be considered. Secondary adrenal insufficiency and central hypothyroidism leading to delayed anesthetic recovery have been reported in a patient with history of cerebral malaria [9]. Another interesting feature described in the literature includes cortisolemia leading to loss of immunity in pregnant women infected with falciparum malaria. In this study Adam et al. investigated 50 consecutive women with uncomplicated falciparum malaria and observed a positive correlation between cortisol levels and parasite count ($r = 0.332$, $P = 0.02$) [10]. In our patient, there was no evidence of either primary or secondary adrenal insufficiency depicted by normal fasting morning cortisol of 15.5 mcg/dL and normal blood pressure throughout his hospital stay.

Thyroid abnormalities previously published include primary and secondary hypothyroidism [11]. These changes may be an adaptation to the accelerated catabolism when infected with malaria; however, the role of thyroid replacement in such patients is uncertain. Wartofsky et al. [12] studied thyroid function in healthy volunteers who were inoculated with malaria; they found an initial decrease followed by a rebound rise in thyroid hormone release. Our patient had normal thyroid axis as illustrated by normal free T4 of 1.3 ng/dL.

Thien and coworkers studied gluconeogenesis in different populations of individuals affected with falciparum malaria to various degrees of severity and found an increased rate of gluconeogenesis in both complicated and uncomplicated cases. This finding was additionally supported by the presence of low levels of the gluconeogenic amino acid precursor, glutamine. The authors commented that prolonged fasting is an important risk factor for hypoglycemia and full recognition of this complication is especially critical in the most susceptible population, children and pregnant women [13]. Another study by Kawo and colleagues did not find any significant difference in the frequency of hypoglycemia between malarial and control patients (5.2% versus 11.2%) nor between the comatose (11.1% versus 18.8%) and conscious malarial and control (1.6% versus 7.0%) subgroups [14]. Similar to the Thien et al. study, the authors emphasized hypoglycemia as a consequence of prolonged fasting resulting from glycogen depletion. Hyperglycemia could also occur because of associated sepsis or due to the stress response with increased counterregulatory hormones [15, 16]. Our patient was, however, euglycemic throughout the course of hospital stay.

Hyperkalemia associated with severe malaria is thought to be due to a combination of acute renal failure and lactic acidosis. Increased extra cellular release of potassium could also occur in the context of hemolysis and rhabdomyolysis. Our patient, although presented with acute kidney injury, did not develop hyperkalemia and there was a prompt decrease in creatinine with hydration. Hypokalemia had been described in up to 40% of children [17] with severe malaria by Maitland et al. within a few hours of hospitalization. The authors suggested that it could be due to rapid correction of acidosis leading to intracellular shift of potassium and/because of renal potassium loss. A lower renal threshold for phosphorus could lead to hypophosphatemia. Screening for hypophosphatemia was especially important in our patient as low phosphorous can further worsen the neuro hypophyseal perfusion through platelet dysfunction and decreased 2,3-diphosphoglycerate. The main reason for hypocalcemia cited in the literature is a blunted response of parathyroid hormone to hypocalcemia, also called "sick euparathyroid state" [18]. Mild asymptomatic hypomagnesemia is also known to occur with malaria and this in turn alters the set point of parathyroid hormone

release with hypocalcemia. Throughout the hospital stay, our patient had normal potassium, phosphorous calcium, and magnesium levels.

In summary, central diabetes insipidus is a rare and atypical complication of malaria. Although uncommon, clinicians need to be aware of this manifestation since early diagnosis prevents serious outcomes. Particularly in hot, humid, and arid climates of sub-Saharan Africa and Indian subcontinent where parasitic infection and dehydration are common, dehydration compounded by diabetes insipidus can even lead to death if left unrecognized. Our patient did not have other metabolic or hormonal abnormalities that have been reported in the literature including hyponatremia, adrenal insufficiency, cortisol excess, thyroid dysfunction, hyper/hypoglycemia, or other electrolyte imbalances.

In our patient the diabetes insipidus symptoms lasted for around four weeks and desmopressin was eventually tapered off. It is important to carefully monitor other anterior pituitary hormone status along with electrolytes while caring for a patient with acute onset of central diabetes insipidus.

References

[1] P. J. Krause, "Malaria (Plasmodium)," in Nelson Textbook of Pediatrics, R. E. Behrman, R. M. Kliegman, and H. B. Jenson, Eds., pp. 1477–1485, WB Saunders, Philadelphia, Pa, USA, 18th edition, 2007.

[2] F. G. Holst, C. J. Hemmer, P. Kern, and M. Dietrich, "Inappropriate secretion of antidiuretic hormone and hyponatremia in severe falciparum malaria," The American Journal of Tropical Medicine and Hygiene, vol. 50, no. 5, pp. 602–607, 1994.

[3] M. C. English, C. Waruiru, C. Lightowler, S. A. Murphy, G. Kirigha, and K. Marsh, "Hyponatraemia and dehydration in severe malaria," Archives of Disease in Childhood, vol. 74, no. 3, pp. 201–205, 1996.

[4] F. Gimenez, S. B. Barraud de Lagerie, C. Fernandez, P. Pino, and D. Mazier, "Tumor necrosis factor α in the pathogenesis of cerebral malaria," Cellular and Molecular Life Sciences, vol. 60, no. 8, pp. 1623–1635, 2003.

[5] K. Grimwade, N. French, D. Mthembu, and C. Gilks, "Polyuria in association with Plasmodium falciparum malaria in a region of unstable transmission," Transactions of the Royal Society of Tropical Medicine and Hygiene, vol. 98, no. 4, pp. 255–260, 2004.

[6] S. Schubert, H. Achenbach, L. Engelmann, G. Borte, M. Stumvoll, and C. A. Koch, "Central diabetes insipidus in a patient with malaria tropica," Journal of Endocrinological Investigation, vol. 29, no. 3, pp. 265–266, 2006.

[7] M. Wilson, T. M. E. Davis, T. Q. Binh, T. T. A. Long, P. T. Danh, and K. Robertson, "Pituitary-adrenal function in uncomplicated falciparum malaria," Southeast Asian Journal of Tropical Medicine and Public Health, vol. 32, no. 4, pp. 689–695, 2001.

[8] T. M. Davis, T. A. Li, Q. B. Tran et al., "The hypothalamic-pituitary adrenocortical axis in severe falciparum malaria:

effects of cytokines," *The Journal of Clinical Endocrinology & Metabolism*, vol. 82, no. 9, pp. 3029–3033, 1997.

[9] V. Selvaraj, "Hypopituitarism: a rare sequel of cerebral malaria—presenting as delayed awakening from general anesthesia," *Anesthesia: Essays and Researches*, vol. 9, no. 2, pp. 287–289, 2015.

[10] I. Adam, B. Y. Nour, W. A. Almahi, E. S. M. Omer, and N. I. Ali, "Malaria susceptibility and cortisol levels in pregnant women of eastern Sudan," *International Journal of Gynecology and Obstetrics*, vol. 98, no. 3, pp. 260–261, 2007.

[11] T. M. E. Davis, W. Supanaranond, S. Pukrittayakamee et al., "The pituitary-thyroid axis in severe falciparum malaria: evidence for depressed thyrotroph and thyroid gland function," *Transactions of the Royal Society of Tropical Medicine and Hygiene*, vol. 84, no. 3, pp. 330–335, 1990.

[12] L. Wartofsky, K. D. Burman, R. C. Dimond, G. L. Noel, A. G. Frantz, and J. M. Earll, "Studies on the nature of thyroidal suppression during acute falciparum malaria: Integrity of pituitary response to TRH and alterations in serum T_3 and reverse T_3," *The Journal of Clinical Endocrinology & Metabolism*, vol. 44, no. 1, pp. 85–90, 1977.

[13] H. V. Thien, P. A. Kager, and H. P. Sauerwein, "Hypoglycemia in falciparum malaria: is fasting an unrecognized and insufficiently emphasized risk factor?" *Trends in Parasitology*, vol. 22, no. 9, pp. 410–415, 2006.

[14] N. G. Kawo, A. E. Msengi, A. B. M. Swai, L. M. Chuwa, K. G. M. M. Alberti, and D. G. McLarty, "Specificity of hypoglycaemia for cerebral malaria in children," *The Lancet*, vol. 336, no. 8713, pp. 454–457, 1990.

[15] M. Tombe, K. M. Bhatt, and A. O. Obel, "Clinical surprises and challenges of severe malaria at Kenyatta National Hospital, Kenya," *East African Medical Journal*, vol. 70, no. 2, pp. 117–119, 1993.

[16] R. Dass, H. Barman, S. G. Duwarah, N. M. Deka, P. Jain, and V. Choudhury, "Unusual presentations of malaria in children: an experience from a tertiary care centre in North East India," *Indian Journal of Pediatrics*, vol. 77, no. 6, pp. 655–660, 2010.

[17] K. Maitland, A. Pamba, C. R. J. C. Newton, B. Lowe, and M. Levin, "Hypokalemia in children with severe falciparum malaria," *Pediatric Critical Care Medicine*, vol. 5, no. 1, pp. 81–85, 2004.

[18] T. M. Davis, G. Q. Li, X. B. Guo, J. L. Spencer, and A. St John, "Serum ionized calcium, serum and intracellular phosphate, and serum parathormone concentrations in acute malaria," *Transactions of the Royal Society of Tropical Medicine and Hygiene*, vol. 87, no. 1, pp. 49–53, 1993.

5

46,XY Disorder of Sex Development Caused by 17α-Hydroxylase/17,20-Lyase Deficiency due to Homozygous Mutation of *CYP17A1* Gene: Consequences of Late Diagnosis

Giampaolo Papi [ID],[1,2] **Rosa Maria Paragliola** [ID],[2] **Paola Concolino,**[3] **Carlo Di Donato,**[1,4] **Alfredo Pontecorvi,**[2] **and Salvatore Maria Corsello**[2]

[1]*Endocrinology Unit of the Northern Area, Azienda USL di Modena, Modena, Italy*
[2]*Unit of Endocrinology, Università Cattolica del Sacro Cuore and Fondazione Policlinico Universitario Agostino Gemelli, Rome, Italy*
[3]*Laboratory of Molecular Biology, Institute of Biochemistry and Clinical Biochemistry, Catholic University of Sacred Heart, Rome, Italy*
[4]*Department of Internal Medicine, Azienda USL Modena, Modena, Italy*

Correspondence should be addressed to Giampaolo Papi; papigiampaolo@hotmail.com

Academic Editor: Eli Hershkovitz

Context. Congenital adrenal hyperplasia (CAH) is an autosomal recessive disease due to specific enzyme deficiencies in the adrenal steroidogenesis pathway. *Case Description.* A 40-year-old Chinese woman was referred to the Endocrine Unit for the work-up of a syndrome characterized by long-lasting and multidrug resistant high blood pressure, severe hypokalemia with metabolic alkalosis, and primary amenorrhea. The patient presented with sexual infantilism, lack of breast development, absence of axillary and pubic hair, tall stature, and slenderness. CT scan revealed enlarged adrenal glands bilaterally and the absence of the uterus, the ovaries, and the Fallopian tubes. Furthermore, diffuse osteopenia and osteoporosis and incomplete ossification of the growth plate cartilages were demonstrated. Chromosomal analysis showed a normal male 46,XY, karyotype, and on molecular analysis of the *CYP17A1* gene she resulted homozygous for the g.4869T>A; g.4871delC (p.Y329Kfs?) mutation in exon 6. Hydrocortisone and ethinyl-estradiol supplementation therapy led to incomplete withdrawal of antihypertensive drug and breast development progression to Tanner stage B2 and slight height increase, respectively. *Conclusions.* We describe a late-discovered case of CAH with 46,XY disorder of sex development. Deficiency of 17α-hydroxylase/17,20-lyase due to a homozygous CYP17A1 gene mutation was the underlying cause. Laboratory, imaging, and genetic features are herein reported and discussed.

1. Introduction

Congenital adrenal hyperplasia (CAH) is an autosomal recessive disease due to specific enzyme deficiencies in the adrenal steroidogenesis pathway [1]. Depending on either the type of enzyme mutation or the level of enzymatic activity, the clinical presentation of CAH is manifold [2]. Whatever be the underlying enzyme mutation, the biochemical result is characterized by the impairment in cortisol biosynthesis.

21-Hydroxylase deficiency is by far the most frequent cause of CAH, accounting for approximately 95% of CAH forms, and is caused by mutations in the gene encoding for a cytochrome P450 *(CYP21A2)* [3]. Mutations in the cytochrome P450 family 17 subfamily A member 1 *(CYP17A1)*

gene located on chromosome 10q24.3 lead to the rare deficiency of 17α-hydroxylase/17,20-lyase [4]. The clinical features of such a severe CAH subtype are the consequence of the enzymatic block at the level of the pregnenolone's and progesterone's conversion towards glucocorticoid and sex steroid production [5]. Indeed, this combined enzyme deficiency affects both the adrenal and the gonadal steroidogenesis. The accumulation of mineralocorticoid precursors (mainly, deoxycorticosterone and corticosterone) causes hypokalemic alkalosis and hypertension. The impaired gonadal steroidogenesis causes a lack of androgens in males and, then, a 46,XY disorder of sex development with variable phenotypes including a completely female phenotype. Also, a lack of estrogen in both males and females occurs, provoking a primary amenorrhea in 46,XX and a low bone mineral density in both sexes.

To date, several mutations in the *CYP17A1* gene have been reported in the literature [5–11]. The most severe deficiency affects both steps (17α-hydroxylase and 17,20-lyase) of the enzyme's activity, whereas, in even the rarest cases of mild deficiency, 17α-hydroxylase activity can be preserved leading to isolated 17,20-lyase deficiency with only gonadal deficiency.

Here, we describe the peculiar clinical, laboratory, imaging, and genetic features of a Chinese patient affected by 17α-hydroxylase/17,20-lyase deficiency.

2. Case Report

A 40-year-old Chinese woman was admitted to the Emergency Room because of a serious car crash. She had received concussion, traumatic rupture of the aortic isthmus, and multiple fractures to left femur, left elbow, right leg, and pelvis. She underwent endovascular aortic stent graft and fractures' closed reduction and immobilization in a plaster cast. Although the head computed tomography (CT) revealed a tentorial blood suffusion, the patient did not experience neurologic damage. Lab-analysis showed the following: normal renal, hepatic, and thyroid function; normal coagulation tests; normal white cell and platelet count; mild normocytic anemia (Hb = 10 g/dl); metabolic alkalosis associated with severe hypokalemia.

Patient's past history consisted of long-lasting high blood pressure and primary amenorrhea. She was born in China (Zhejiang), where she had been living for 28 years; later, she was married and moved to Carpi (Modena), Italy, where she was employed in a textile factory. Since her twenties, she was taking a multidrug antihypertensive and potassium replacement therapy, which on admission included doxazosin 8 mg/day, lisinopril 20 mg/day, hydrochlorothiazide 25 mg/day, amlodipine 10 mg/day, canrenone 100 mg/day, bisoprolol 5 mg/day, and potassium chloride 1800 mg/day. Furthermore, owing to the recent implantation of aortic stent graft, she was given acetylsalicylic acid 100 mg/day. The patient declared that all attempts to get pregnant failed and, therefore, she had adopted a male kid. She stated that she was the eldest of three siblings: a 36-year-old sister, who was taking antihypertensive drugs, suffered of primary amenorrhea, and was sterile; a 34-year-old sister, who was mother of 3 kids and was doing well. Her father had died because of lung carcinoma (maybe due to heavy smoking), whilst her mother was alive and was doing well. The two sisters and the mother still live in China.

Once the patient's clinical conditions improved, she was referred to the Endocrine Unit, Department of Internal Medicine, for the endocrine work-up.

The patient presented with sexual infantilism, lack of breast development, complete absence of axillary and pubic hair, tall stature, and slenderness. The external genitalia were phenotypically female, the height was 175 cm, the weight was 64 Kg, and the body mass index (BMI) was 20.9. On admission, the blood pressure (BP) was persistently high throughout the day: mean systolic BP values were 170 mmHg; mean diastolic BP values were 110 mmHg. The patient received biochemical and endocrine lab tests. The results—which are

summarized in Table 1—showed the following: low-undetectable levels of testosterone, DHEA-S, androstenedione, 17-OH-progesterone, estradiol and active renin; low-normal 24-h urinary cortisol and serum aldosterone; high ACTH, progesterone, LH and FSH concentrations; metabolic alkalosis with severe hypokalemia. The clinical evidence and laboratory results both suggested the diagnosis of the rarest forms of CAH rather than the commonest 21-hydroxylase deficiency. Chromosomal analysis demonstrated a normal male 46,XY, karyotype. Interestingly, when the patient's sex life was examined, despite the prepuberal condition, she acknowledged having weekly—albeit unsatisfying (i.e., anorgasmic)—intercourses.

A computed tomography of the abdomen and pelvis showed enlarged adrenal glands bilaterally (Figure 1(a)); the absence of the uterus, the ovaries, and the Fallopian tubes was shown, too (Figure 1(b)). Furthermore, the radiography of the left hand and wrist revealed that the ossification of the epiphysial cartilage of distal end of radius and ulna, 1st metacarpus, and phalanxes was not yet complete (Figure 2). To investigate the possible negative impact of chronic hypoestrogenic state, the bone mineral density (BMD) was checked at the lumbar spine and the femoral neck, and it was consistent with osteoporosis and osteopenia, respectively. In particular, the T-score and the Z-score at L1–L4 level were reduced at −3.6 SD and −3.4 SD, respectively; they were equal to −2.4 SD and − 2.2 SD at the femur, respectively.

Overall, the clinical, laboratory, and imaging features were consistent with CAH caused by combined 17α-hydroxylase and 17,20-lyase deficiency, as suggested by very high progesterone levels and low 17-OH-progesterone and sex steroids values (Figure 3). To confirm this diagnosis, the molecular analysis of the *CYP17A1* gene was performed as previously reported [12].

Mutation analysis by direct DNA sequencing demonstrated the base change from T to A at position 4869 (g.4869T>A) and the deletion of the g.4871 nucleotide (g.4871delC): such genetic alterations lead to the substitution from tyrosine to lysine at aminoacidic position 329 producing a frameshift (p.Y329Kfs?). The patient resulted homozygous for the most prevalent *CYP17A1* mutation in Chinese patients [13]. A possible loss of heterozygosity (LOH) was excluded using the SALSA MLPA probemix P334-A3 Gonadal Development Disorder (MRC Holland) in a MLPA (Multiplex Ligation-dependent Probe Amplification) assay.

Treatment with oral hydrocortisone 20 mg/day and ethinyl-estradiol 1 mg was started. One month later, step by step, all the antihypertensive drugs—with the only exception of amlodipine—and potassium supplements could be stopped, since blood pressure values constantly were in the normal range. Six months after estradiol supplementation, the patient's breast development progressed to Tanner stage B2 and her stature grew to 177 cm.

Table 1 summarizes the results of biochemical and endocrine analysis performed before patient's discharge from the hospital.

The patient signed the written informed consent for both genetic examinations and use of personal data in the current study.

TABLE 1: Results of biochemical and endocrine tests in the patient reported, before and after the administration of estradiol and glucocorticoid therapy.

Lab test	Results		Normal range
	Before treatment	After therapy	
TSH (mcIU/ml)	2.4	NA	0.35–4
ACTH (pg/ml)	655.7	19.3	4.3–52
Active renin (mcIU/ml)	<0.5	<0.5	4.4–46.1
Aldosterone (pg/ml)	23.1	26	30–150
24-h urinary cortisol (mcg/24 h)	60	304	58–403
FSH (mIU/ml)	40.8	0.8	1.5–12.4
LH (mIU/ml)	23.7	0.7	1.8–12
Estradiol (pg/ml)	<10	NA	10–40
DHEA-S (mcg/ml)	0.04	0.05	0.48–2.44
Progesterone (ng/ml)	6.5	NA	0.2–1.4
17-OH-progesterone (ng/ml)	0.2	NA	0.2–1.3
Androstenedione (ng/dl)	<10	<10	85–275
Testosterone (ng/ml)	<0.1	<0.1	2.4–9.5
pH (venous sample)	7.56	7.4	7.37–7.45
Na+ (mEq/L)	140	136	136–146
K+ (mEq/L)	2.1	4.1	3.5–5.3

ACTH = adrenocorticotrophic hormone; DHEA-S = dehydroepiandrosterone sulfate; FSH = follicle-stimulating hormone; LH = luteinizing hormone; NA = not available; TSH = thyroid stimulating hormone.

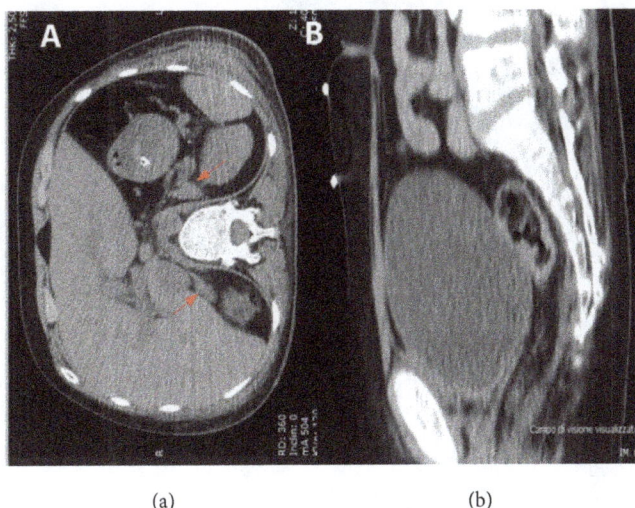

(a) (b)

FIGURE 1: Abdomen and pelvis CT scan. (a) The adrenal glands are enlarged bilaterally (red arrow); (b) gonads are not detectable.

3. Discussion

The present report describes a CAH patient with 46,XY disorder of sex development due to cytochrome P450c17 deficiency caused by the homozygous g.4869T>A; g.4871delC (p.Y329Kfs?) mutation in exon 6 of CYP17A1 gene. The P450c17 deficiency is very rare per se, representing almost 1% of all CAH cases, with an estimated incidence of 1 in 50,000–100,000 individuals [13, 14]. What is peculiar to this case and makes it unique lies on the following: (i) the remarkable delay in the diagnosis of CAH and, nonetheless, the possibility of investigating the long-term consequences of P450c17 enzyme deficiency on the clinical point of view;

(ii) the combined loss of 17α-hydroxylase and 17,20-lyase action; (iii) the homozygous mutation in CYP17A1 gene associated with male XY karyotype.

P450c17 is a cytochrome that plays a crucial role in the adrenal and gonadal steroid biosynthetic pathway (Figure 3). Indeed, it carries out two enzymatic activities: the 17-hydroxylase and the 17,20-lyase activity. The first one acts by converting pregnenolone in to 17OH-pregnenolone and progesterone into 17OH-progesterone; the 17,20-lyase activity converts 17OH-pregnenolone into dehydroepiandrosterone and, to a lesser extent, 17OH-progesterone into androstenedione [15–17]. The final result is the block of production of cortisol and sex steroids and the accumulation of

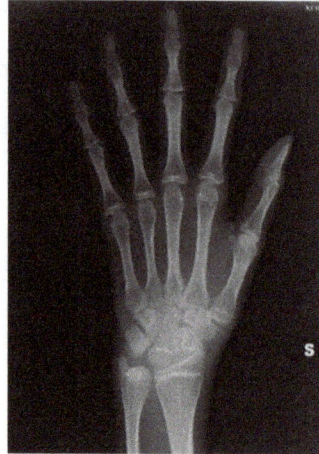

FIGURE 2: Left hand and wrist X-ray. The ossification of the epiphysial cartilage of distal end of radius and ulna, 1st metacarpus, and phalanxes is not yet complete.

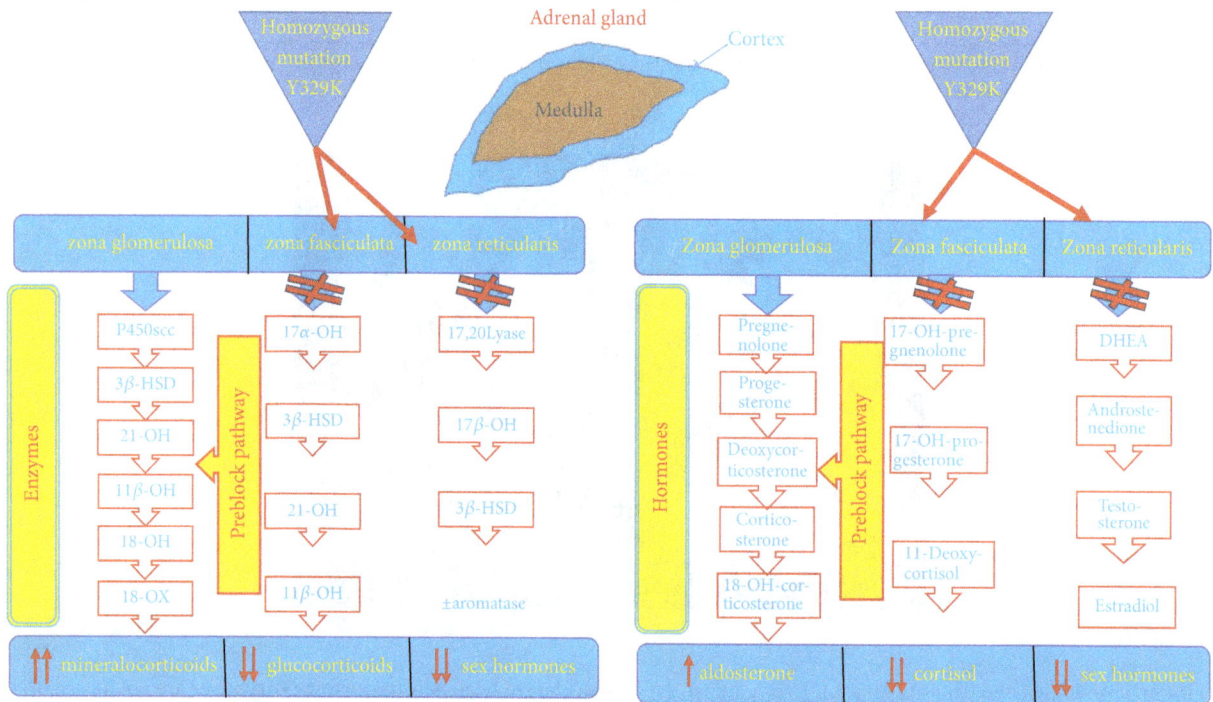

FIGURE 3: The adrenal steroid biosynthetic pathway: involved enzymes, hormones, and precursors. The "block" sites of hormone production in patients affected by 17α-hydroxylase/17,20-lyase deficiency are highlighted by the red stop signs.

preblock metabolites of the mineralocorticoid pathway (mainly, 11-deoxycorticosterone, corticosterone, and 18-OH-corticosterone), overstimulated by ACTH hypersecretion due to the attempt by the hypophysis gland to solve the cortisol deficiency. In this context, severe hypokalemic alkalosis and high blood pressure develop, owing to the potent mineralocorticoid effects of aldosterone precursors, which induce on the one hand sodium and fluid retention and on the other hand loss of potassium and hydrogen. Thus, the renin-angiotensin-aldosterone system is shut down, and laboratory analyses detect suppressed renin and low-normal aldosterone values. It should be noted that the low cortisol production is balanced by the high concentrations of corticosterone, which exhibits a mild glucocorticoid effect [18, 19].

The same attempt made by the corticotroph cells to overcome cortisol deficiency is (unsuccessfully) performed by the gonadotroph cells, which produce high amounts of luteinizing (LH) and follicle-stimulating (FSH) hormone in response to undetectable sex hormone levels. The impairment of sex hormone production leads to a manifold spectrum of clinical manifestations, ranging from mildest forms—characterized by infertility with phenotype corresponding to karyotype—to severe forms presenting with ambiguous genitalia or disorders of sex development [20]. In our patient, the altered biosynthetic process manifested clinically with lack of secondary sexual characteristics (including complete absence of axillary and pubic hair, primary amenorrhea, and no breast development), tall stature, and high blood pressure. Besides obvious hyperplasia of the adrenal cortex, imaging exams did detect neither the female (uterus, the ovaries, and the Fallopian tubes) nor the male (prostate, seminal vesicles, and vas deferens) genitalia. This picture confirms that both the 17-hydroxylase and the 17,20-lyase activity are essential for gonadal steroidogenesis [21].

With respect to high blood pressure values detected on admission, the glucocorticoid substitution therapy allowed the partial discontinuation of antihypertensive drugs. In most patients suffering from 17-hydroxylase/17,20-lyase deficiency reported in the literature [5, 8], the glucocorticoid supplementation was able to maintain normal blood pressure values after complete discontinuation of antihypertensive drugs. We suppose that, in our patient, long-standing hypertension caused irreversible damage of the cardiovascular system. This hypothesis was supported by echocardiophic exam, showing left ventricle hypertrophy (data not shown).

A further interesting finding in this case was the lack of ossification of the epiphysial cartilages, as demonstrated by X-ray of the wrist. Such a feature is the consequence of lacking action of sex hormones on cartilage and bone maturation. The same mechanism explains the important reduction in bone mineral density found in our patient. Thus, a double repercussion occurs on the clinical side: the patient presents with a tall stature and is still growing up; she has a significantly fragile and osteoporotic bone. Actually, except anecdotal cases [10], most Chinese subjects affected by 17-hydroxylase/17,20-lyase deficiency are unusually tall with respect to their ethnicity. The bone mineral density in our patient was frankly low compared to subjects of the same age; probably, both an earlier diagnosis of the underlying disease and the prompt sex hormone substitution therapy would have prevented the development of osteopenia or, at least, of osteoporosis. With regard to the best sex hormone substitution therapy, since our patient was assigned the female sex and had always considered herself as female, we suggested her taking estradiol. Of interest, according to previous observations [5], at 6-month follow-up she experienced breast development and she was satisfied and grateful for this. Moreover, she was 2 cm taller than before starting therapy.

In conclusion, we report a case of 17α-hydroxylase/17,20-lyase deficiency causing CAH with 46,XY disorder of sex development. Although further research occurs, this work sheds new light on role of cytochrome P450c17 in the steroidogenesis at both the adrenal and the gonadal level and on the harmful consequences of its deficiency in the short and long term, respectively.

Acknowledgments

The authors acknowledge Dr. Raffaele Sansone and Dr. Sonia Ferraresi, Department of Radiology, Azienda USL Modena, Modena, Italy, for their invaluable contribution to this work.

References

[1] D. El-Maouche, W. Arlt, and D. P. Merke, "Congenital adrenal hyperplasia," The Lancet, vol. 390, no. 10108, pp. 2194–2210, 2017.

[2] S. F. Witchel and R. Azziz, "Congenital adrenal hyperplasia," Journal of Pediatric & Adolescent Gynecology, vol. 24, no. 3, pp. 116–126, 2011.

[3] B. Wilcken, "Congenital adrenal hyperplasia: one hundred years of data," The Lancet Diabetes & Endocrinology, vol. 1, no. 1, pp. 4-5, 2013.

[4] R. J. Auchus, "The genetics, pathophysiology, and management of human deficiencies of P450c17," Endocrinology and Metabolism Clinics of North America, vol. 30, no. 1, pp. 101–119, 2001.

[5] S. Xu, S. Hu, X. Yu, M. Zhang, and Y. Yang, "17α-hydroxylase/17,20-lyase deficiency in congenital adrenal hyperplasia: a case report," Molecular Medicine Reports, vol. 15, no. 1, pp. 339–344, 2017.

[6] M. Fernández-Cancio, E. García-García, C. González-Cejudo et al., "Discordant genotypic sex and phenotype variations in two Spanish siblings with 17α-hydroxylase/17,20-lyase deficiency carrying the most prevalent mutated CYP17A1 alleles of Brazilian patients," Sexual Development, vol. 11, no. 2, pp. 70–77, 2017.

[7] A. F. Turcu and R. J. Auchus, "The next 150 years of congenital adrenal hyperplasia," The Journal of Steroid Biochemistry and Molecular Biology, vol. 153, article no. 4423, pp. 63–71, 2015.

[8] C. Wu, S. Fan, Y. Qian et al., "17α-hydroxylase/17, 20-lyase deficiency: clinical and molecular characterization of eight Chinese patients," Endocrine Practice, vol. 23, no. 5, pp. 576–582, 2017.

[9] P. H. D. M. Bianchi, G. R. F. C. A. Gouveia, E. M. F. Costa et al., "Successful live birth in a woman with 17α-hydroxylase deficiency through IVF frozen-thawed embryo transfer," The Journal of Clinical Endocrinology & Metabolism, vol. 101, no. 2, pp. 345–348, 2016.

[10] L. Ma, F. Peng, L. Yu et al., "Combined 17α-hydroxylase/17,20-lyase deficiency with short stature: case study," Gynecological Endocrinology, vol. 32, no. 4, pp. 264–266, 2015.

[11] A. Deeb, H. Al Suwaidi, S. Attia, and A. Al Ameri, "17-hydroxylase/17,20-lyase deficiency due to a R96Q mutation causing hypertension and poor breast development," Endocrinology, Diabetes & Metabolism Case Reports, 2015.

[12] J. Yang, B. Cui, S. Sun et al., "Phenotype-genotype correlation in eight Chinese 17α-hydroxylase/17,20 lyase-deficiency patients with five novel mutations of CYP17A1 gene," The Journal of Clinical Endocrinology & Metabolism, vol. 91, no. 9, pp. 3619–3625, 2006.

[13] M. Zhang, S. Sun, Y. Liu et al., "New, recurrent, and prevalent mutations: clinical and molecular characterization of 26 Chinese patients with 17alpha-hydroxylase/17,20-lyase deficiency," The Journal of Steroid Biochemistry and Molecular Biology, vol. 150, article no. 4372, pp. 11–16, 2015.

[14] Y. K. Oh, U. Ryoo, D. Kim et al., "17α-hydroxlyase/17, 20-lyase deficiency in three siblings with primary amenorrhea and absence of secondary sexual development," Journal of Pediatric & Adolescent Gynecology, vol. 25, no. 5, pp. e103–e105, 2012.

[15] W. L. Miller, "Congenital adrenal hyperplasias," *Endocrinology Metabolism Clinics of North America*, vol. 20, pp. 721–749, 1991.

[16] W. L. Miller and C. E. Flück, "Adrenal cortex and its disorders," in *Pediatric Endocrinology*, M. A. Sperling, Ed., pp. 471–532, Elsevier, USA, 4th edition, 2014.

[17] C. A. Marsh and R. J. Auchus, "Fertility in patients with genetic deficiencies of cytochrome P450c17 (CYP17A1): combined 17-hydroxylase/17,20-lyase deficiency and isolated 17,20-lyase deficiency," *Fertility and Sterility*, vol. 101, no. 2, pp. 317–322, 2014.

[18] C. E. Flück, W. L. Miller, and R. J. Auchus, "The 17, 20-lyase activity of cytochrome P450c17 from human fetal testis favors the $\Delta 5$ steroidogenic pathway," *The Journal of Clinical Endocrinology & Metabolism*, vol. 88, no. 8, pp. 3762–3766, 2003.

[19] W. L. Miller, "Disorders in the initial steps of steroid hormone synthesis," *The Journal of Steroid Biochemistry and Molecular Biology*, vol. 165, pp. 18–37, 2017.

[20] K. Chapman, M. Holmes, and J. Seckl, "11β-hydroxysteroid dehydrogenases intracellular gate-keepers of tissue glucocorticoid action," *Physiological Reviews*, vol. 93, no. 3, pp. 1139–1206, 2013.

[21] V. Gomez-Lobo and A.-M. Amies Oelschlager, "Disorders of sexual development in adult women," *Obstetrics & Gynecology*, vol. 128, no. 5, pp. 1162–1173, 2016.

Pegvisomant-Induced Cholestatic Hepatitis in an Acromegalic Patient with UGT1A1*28 Mutation

Maria Susana Mallea-Gil,[1] Ignacio Bernabeu,[2] Adriana Spiraquis,[3] Alejandra Avangina,[4] Lourdes Loidi,[2] and Carolina Ballarino[1]

[1] Servicio de Endocrinologıa, Hospital Militar Central, 726 Luis María Campos Avenue, 1425 Buenos Aires, Argentina
[2] Endocrinology Division and Fundacion Publica Galega de Medicina Xenomica (Unidad de Medicina Molecular), Complejo Hospitalario Universitario de Santiago de Compostela, Universidad de Santiago de Compostela, Travesia Choupana s/n, Santiago de Compostela, 15706 La Coruña, Spain
[3] Servicio de Gastroenterologıa, Hospital Militar Central, 726 Luis María Campos Avenue, 1425 Buenos Aires, Argentina
[4] Departamento de Anatomıa Patologica, Hospital de Clínicas, Universidad de Buenos Aires, 2351 Córdoba Avenue, 1120 Buenos Aires, Argentina

Correspondence should be addressed to Maria Susana Mallea-Gil; smalleagil@gmail.com

Academic Editor: Osamu Isozaki

Pegvisomant (PEGv) is a growth hormone receptor antagonist approved for the treatment of acromegaly; one of its documented adverse effects is reversible elevation of hepatic enzymes. We report a 39-year-old male acromegalic patient with a pituitary macroadenoma who underwent transsphenoidal surgery. The patient's condition improved but GH and IGF-I levels did not normalize; as a consequence, we first administered dopamine agonists and then somatostatin receptor ligands (SRLs) with poor response. PEGv 15 mg every other day was added to lanreotide 120 mg monthly. The patient developed a severe hepatitis five months after starting the combination therapy. Elevated ferritin, iron, and transferrin saturation suggested probable hepatitis due to haemochromatosis. We performed a liver biopsy which showed an acute cholestatic hepatitis consistent with toxic etiology. A heterozygous genotype UGT1A1*28 polymorphism associated with Gilbert's syndrome was also found in this Argentine patient. The predominant clinical presentation resembled an acute cholestatic hepatitis associated with severe hemosiderosis, a different and new pattern of PEGv hepatotoxicity.

1. Introduction

Acromegaly is a rare disease usually derived from a GH-secreting pituitary tumor.

The increased mortality among persons with acromegaly includes higher prevalence of hypertension, hyperglycemia or overt diabetes, cardiomyopathy, and sleep apnea [1].

Currently, surgery is the primary approach for treating most patients. If cure is not achieved with this treatment, pharmacotherapy should be considered. Somatostatin receptor ligands (SRLs) are usually the first line therapy for treating active acromegaly. Pegvisomant (PEGv), a pegylated GH receptor antagonist, is another effective therapeutic option that could be administered alone or in combination with SRLs [2–4]. PEGv is usually well-tolerated; however, it

might cause adverse events such as drug-induced liver injury [3].

Bernabeu et al. found that the UGT1A1*28 genotype associated with Gilbert's syndrome predicts an increased incidence of liver abnormalities during PEGv therapy in Spanish acromegalic patients [4].

We report here clinical, biochemical, genotype, and histological findings in an Argentine acromegalic patient who developed a severe cholestatic hepatitis during PEGv therapy.

2. Case Report

In 1996 a 39-year-old man was referred to the Endocrinology Service of the Hospital Militar Central of Buenos Aires City because he presented arterial hypertension and acromegalic

TABLE 1: Chronological development and values of alkaline phosphatase (APh), γ-glutamyltranspeptidase (GGT), total bilirubin (T. Bil), ferritin, transferrin saturation (TSAT), and iron during the combination therapy with PEGv and after stopping this treatment.

	During combination therapy		After stopping combination therapy				
	2 Months	5 Months	10 Days	1 Month	2 Months	3 Months	4 Months
APh (40–120 UI/L)	136	272	242	99	99	92	80
GGT (8–61 UI/L)			549	166	166	77	17
T. Bil (0.1–1 mg/dL)	0.4	2.5	1.9	0.64	0.64	0.61	0.61
Ferritin (30–400 ng/mL)			4836	763	595	374	191
Transferrin (200–360 ug/dL)			212	198	194	210	244
TSAT (15–50%)			104	72			50
Iron (59–158 ug/dL)			180	180			154

features. He had a two-year history of headaches, sweating, feet and hands enlargement, weight gain, erectile dysfunction, and hyperglycemia. His lab tests showed an elevated IGF-I level: >5.4 U/mL (NR: 0.6–5.4) and nonsuppressible GH postoral glucose tolerance test (OGTT) (GH nadir: 78 ng/mL). He underwent a magnetic resonance imaging (MRI) which showed a pituitary macroadenoma of 18 × 15 mm with suprasellar extension. The patient was operated on by transsphenoidal approach. The pathology report informed a diffuse eosinophilic pituitary adenoma. At that time we could not perform immunochemistry.

The symptoms and hormonal test improved; however, GH and IGF-I levels were persistently elevated.

In December 1996 bromocriptine 3.75 mg/day was indicated without normalization of IGF-I. Two years later, he was medicated with cabergoline 0.5 mg/week with poor tolerance and response; therefore, he returned to bromocriptine 5 mg/day. He stopped treatment and was lost to follow-up for five years. When the patient returned in 2003, an MRI showed no tumor but his IGF-I level was elevated; therefore, cabergoline was indicated. He was not consistent with the treatment because he presented poor tolerance to this drug. In 2005 he was started on octreotide 30 mg/month with partial response.

Due to severe coronary heart disease, in October 2007 the patient underwent a coronary bypass surgery. In December 2008, as he presented glucose intolerance, a more sensible diet and metformin (1,700 mg/day) were indicated.

In 2010 a cholecystectomy was performed because of the development of gallstones. In 2011 two benign polyps and a villous adenoma were removed during a colonoscopy.

In 2012 octreotide was switched to lanreotide 120 mg/month. Because of increased IGF-I levels, in March 2013 PEGv 15 mg every other day was added. Up to that moment the patient's liver function tests had always been normal. It is important to note that he did not drink alcohol. He was also medicated with atenolol 25 mg/day and enalapril 10 mg/day and continued metformin treatment. In May 2013 he presented transient symptoms of flu and a slight increase of transaminases, less than 3 times above the upper limit of normal (×ULN). In August 2013 the patient, under treatment with lanreotide and PEGv, had a normal IGF-I level, 154 ng/mL (81–225), but he unexpectedly experienced abdominal pain, severe asthenia, decreased appetite, and presented choluria the day before the visit to the hospital.

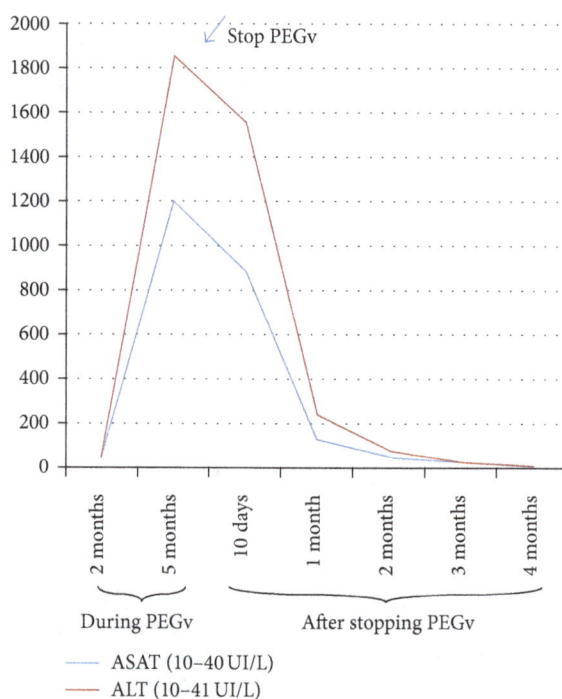

FIGURE 1: Chronological development of ASAT and ALT transaminases during the combination therapy with PEGv and after stopping this treatment.

Liver tests results showed elevated levels of aspartate aminotransferase (ASAT) 29.9 ×ULN, alanine aminotransferase (ALT) 45.3 ×ULN, alkaline phosphatase (APh) 2.26 ×ULN, and total bilirubin 2.5 ×ULN. Prothrombin time (PT) and activated partial thromboplastin time (aPTT) were both normal (PT: 85% (70–120) and aPTT: 39 seconds (27–42)). Blood cell count was normal: hematocrit 45%, hemoglobin: 15 grams/dL, and white blood cell count: 7100 cells/mcL with no eosinophilia. There were no changes in the normal pattern of coagulation tests and blood cell count during the course of the hepatic disease. The tests for viral and autoimmune hepatitis were negative. Elevated ferritin, iron, and transferring saturation (TSAT) suggested probable hepatitis due to haemochromatosis. Liver and iron tests are shown in Table 1 and in Figure 1. The abdominal ultrasonography was normal. We decided to stop treatment with both lanreotide and PEGv.

(a)

(b)

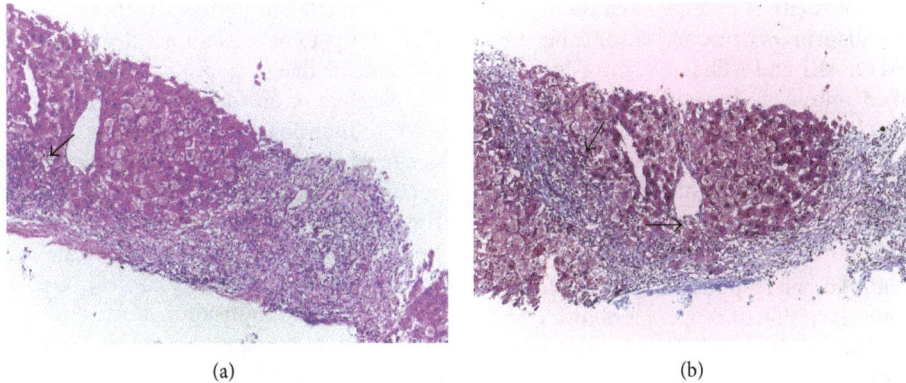

FIGURE 2: (a and b) Bridging periportal collapse with a mild number of inflammatory cells, HE, and Masson's trichrome, 100x, respectively. See arrows.

We performed a liver biopsy which showed an acute cholestatic hepatitis with confluent necrosis, which formed portocentral bridges of parenchymal collapse (Figures 2(a) and 2(b)). There were deposits of iron predominantly in reticuloendothelial cells, a pattern which does not correspond to genetic haemochromatosis (Figure 3). Inflammatory cells included eosinophils (Figure 4). These findings were consistent with a severe acute hepatitis of toxic etiology.

Haemochromatosis was also ruled out through a negative result of C282Y and H63D genotypes of haemochromatosis HFE.

The genotype UGT1A1*28 associated with Gilbert's syndrome was performed and a heterozygous genotype UGT1A1*28 polymorphism was found. The UGT1A1*28 genotyping was performed by PCR amplification of a fragment of the UGT1A1 gene promoter, which included the TATA box, and Sanger sequencing of the amplification product.

Liver function tests returned to normal four months after PEGv discontinuation and they have been normal since then.

Without combination therapy, IGF-I levels increased to 367 ng/mL (NR: 81–225) (1.63 ×ULN). In January 2014 lanreotide 120 mg monthly and cabergoline 0.5 mg/week were indicated with good tolerance and thus IGF-I levels normalized: 205 ng/mL.

3. Discussion

The association of PEGv therapy with drug-induced hepatic events is well-documented; however, the mechanisms responsible for its toxicity remain unclear [3].

In the German Pegvisomant Observational Study, PEGv administration was associated with an increase in liver enzymes in 9% of patients [5]. ACROSTUDY reported that 30 (2.5%) of 1178 patients had elevated aspartate aminotransferase or alanine aminotransferase greater than three times the upper level of normal during PEGv therapy; a spontaneous recovery of transaminases frequently occurred despite continuation of PEGv [6].

According to Bernabeu et al., the UGT1A1*28 genotype associated with Gilbert's syndrome predicts an increased incidence of liver abnormalities during PEGv therapy in Spanish

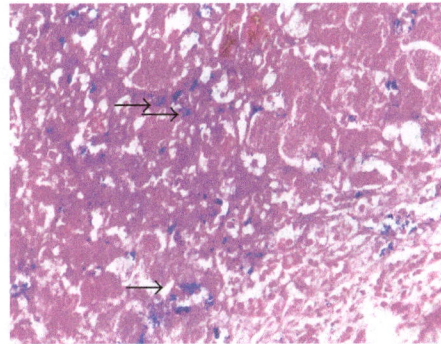

FIGURE 3: Moderate hemosiderosis: iron stores in reticuloendothelial cells, Perls stain, 400x. See arrows.

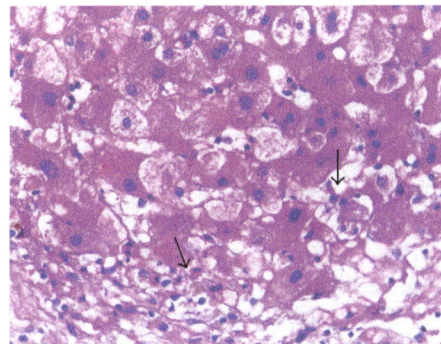

FIGURE 4: Focal acinar collapse. Sinusoidal inflammatory foci with some eosinophils. Hepatocyte cytoplasmic cholestasis, HE, 400x. See arrows.

patients. The excretion pathways of PEGv are unknown; in humans <0.6% of unchanged PEGv is excreted in urine. Nothing is known about the hepatic metabolism of PEGv and whether it requires UGT1A1-mediated glucuronidation [4, 5]. Although our patient had never shown increased bilirubin in order for us to be able to diagnose Gilbert's syndrome, we found a heterozygous genotype UGT1A1*28 [7].

Drug-induced hepatotoxicity is a frequent cause of liver disease and can mimic all forms of acute and chronic hepatobiliary diseases. Based on ALT and APh levels, drug-induced liver injury is classified into acute hepatitis, cholestasis, or mixed patterns. This classification was established by the Council for International Organization of Medical Sciences and modified by US FDA Drug Hepatotoxicity Steering Committee [8]. Establishing its diagnosis requires exclusion of other causes of liver injury.

The liver is the central organ responsible for the selective uptake, metabolism, and excretion of drugs, xenobiotics, and environmental toxins. This essential function predisposes the liver to drug toxicity [9].

Adverse hepatic events caused by drugs can be considered to be either predictable (high incidence) or unpredictable (low incidence). The most common example of a drug causing predictable drug-induced liver injury (DILI) is acetaminophen. This type of drug injury has a short latency period, is dose-related, and is the most common form of DILI. On the contrary, idiosyncratic DILI is unpredictable, has longer/variable latency, and is less common [10].

The pathogenesis of drug-induced liver injury usually involves the participation of a toxic drug or a metabolite that either elicits an immune response or directly affects the biochemistry of the cell. Most adverse drug-induced hepatic events are unpredictable and are either immune-mediated hypersensitivity reactions or idiosyncratic ones [11].

The liver removes lipophilic chemicals from blood, including drugs, and biotransforms them into water-soluble metabolites which are excreted. This process involves cytochrome P450 (phase 1), conjugation (phase 2), and transport (phase 3). The expression of the enzymes and transporters involved in the hepatic handling of drugs are under the control of transcriptions factors (nuclear hormone receptors). In humans, polymorphisms of the genes that regulate each phase and transcription factors affect their activities and expression in response to environmental factors. So it is likely that the level of exposure to the toxic moiety (reactive metabolite or the parent drug) is the most upstream determinant of DILI [12].

Acromegaly by itself is correlated with a high prevalence of gallbladder stones and the long-term treatment with SRLs increases the incidence of cholelithiasis [13]. Our patient underwent a cholecystectomy, probably related to octreotide treatment. Five years later, at the onset of symptoms of hepatitis, his abdominal ultrasound was normal; that is why liver or biliary diseases were excluded.

Laboratory tests showed elevated ferritin and transferrin saturation suggesting probable hepatitis due to haemochromatosis, which was ruled out through a negative of C282Y and H63D genotypes and the liver biopsy. It is known that both ferritin and TSAT can also be elevated in many inflammatory conditions such as viral hepatitis, regular alcohol consumption, and fatty liver disease [14].

Filopanti et al. showed that in acromegalic patients treated with PEGv, multitherapies and previous episodes of liver disease were associated with increased risk of hepatotoxicity; however, they did not find any increased risk of liver toxicity in Italian patients with UGT1A1*28 polymorphism [15]. Our patient was not medicated with any other probable hepatotoxic drug.

Neggers et al. found only 13.5% of transiently elevated liver transaminases (TET) above 3 ×ULN, of which 83% occurred within the first year of combination treatment with somatostatin analogs and PEGv. In their study, they detected the UGT1A1*28 polymorphism in 54.2% of their patients; however, they could not confirm any association between this polymorphism and TET [16]. Our patient presented a slight increase of transaminases two months after starting the combination therapy and developed a severe hepatitis five months afterwards.

The presence of the UGT1A1*28 genotype in our Argentine patient might be related to his Spanish ancestry (he had three Spanish grandparents). This finding is in accordance with Bernabeu et al. study in Spanish acromegalic population. Besides there is another coincidence with their study: our patient is male [4].

The mechanism of pegvisomant-induced liver injury remains the subject of conjecture. We report a patient with acromegaly who developed a severe drug-induced hepatitis during treatment with PEGv. When PEGv was discontinued, his laboratory tests normalized in four months.

Although in this case we might assume that it was an idiosyncratic drug toxicity, to the best of our knowledge, it is the first case described in which its predominant clinical presentation resembles an acute cholestatic hepatitis associated with severe hemosiderosis, a different pattern of PEGv hepatotoxicity.

Acknowledgment

The authors are grateful to Ms. Claudia Muschitiello for her assistance in the English version.

References

[1] S. Melmed, "Acromegaly," New England Journal of Medicine, vol. 355, no. 24, pp. 2558–2573, 2006.

[2] A. Ben-Shlomo and S. Melmed, "Acromegaly," Endocrinology Metabolism Clinics of North America, vol. 37, no. 1, pp. 101–122, 2008.

[3] H. Biering, B. Saller, J. Bauditz et al., "Elevated transaminases during medical treatment of acromegaly: a review of the German pegvisomant surveillance experience and a report of a patient with histologically proven chronic mild active hepatitis," European Journal of Endocrinology, vol. 154, no. 2, pp. 213–220, 2006.

[4] I. Bernabeu, M. Marazuela, T. Lucas et al., "Pegvisomant-induced liver injury is related to the UGT1A1*28 polymorphism of Gilbert's syndrome," Journal of Clinical Endocrinology and Metabolism, vol. 95, no. 5, pp. 2147–2154, 2010.

[5] I. Schreiber, M. Buchfelder, M. Droste et al., "Treatment of acromegaly with the GH receptor antagonist pegvisomant in clinical practice: safety and efficacy evaluation from the German Pegvisomant Observational Study," *European Journal of Endocrinology*, vol. 156, no. 1, pp. 75–82, 2007.

[6] A. J. van der Lely, B. M. K. Biller, T. Brue et al., "Long-term safety of pegvisomant in patients with acromegaly: comprehensive review of 1288 subjects in ACROSTUDY," *Journal of Clinical Endocrinology and Metabolism*, vol. 97, no. 5, pp. 1589–1597, 2012.

[7] I. Bernabeu, J. Cameselle-Teijeiro, F. F. Casanueva, and M. Marazuela, "Pegvisomant-induced cholestatic hepatitis with jaundice in a patient with Gilbert's syndrome," *European Journal of Endocrinology*, vol. 160, no. 5, pp. 869–872, 2009.

[8] C. Benichou, J. P. Benhamou, and G. Danan, "Criteria of drug-induced liver disorders. Report of an international consensus meeting," *Journal of Hepatology*, vol. 11, no. 2, pp. 272–276, 1990.

[9] M. S. Padda, M. Sanchez, A. J. Akhtar, and J. L. Boyer, "Drug-induced cholestasis," *Hepatology*, vol. 53, no. 4, pp. 1377–1387, 2011.

[10] M. D. Leise, J. J. Poterucha, and J. A. Talwalkar, "Drug-induced liver injury," *Mayo Clinic Proceedings*, vol. 89, no. 1, pp. 95–106, 2014.

[11] N. Kaplowitz, "Drug-induced liver injury," *Clinical Infectious Diseases*, vol. 1, no. 38, supplement 2, pp. s44–s48, 2004.

[12] S. Verma and N. Kaplowitz, "Diagnosis, management and prevention of drug-induced liver injury," *Gut*, vol. 58, no. 11, pp. 1555–1564, 2009.

[13] M. Montini, D. Gianola, M. D. Pagani et al., "Cholelithiasis and acromegaly: therapeutic strategies," *Clinical Endocrinology*, vol. 40, no. 3, pp. 401–406, 1994.

[14] K. Wong and P. C. Adams, "The diversity of liver diseases among outpatient referrals for elevated serum ferritin," *Canadian Journal of Gastroenterology*, vol. 20, no. 7, pp. 467–470, 2006.

[15] M. Filopanti, A. M. Barbieri, G. Mantovani et al., "Role of UGT1A1 and ADH gene polymorphisms in pegvisomant-induced liver toxicity in acromegalic patients," *European Journal of Endocrinology*, vol. 170, no. 2, pp. 247–254, 2014.

[16] S. J. C. M. M. Neggers, S. E. Franck, F. W. M. de Rooij et al., "Long-term efficacy and safety of pegvisomant in combination with long-acting somatostatin analogs in acromegaly," *The Journal of Clinical Endocrinology & Metabolism*, vol. 99, no. 10, pp. 3644–3652, 2014.

7

Treatment of Ipilimumab Induced Graves' Disease in a Patient with Metastatic Melanoma

Umal Azmat,[1] David Liebner,[2] Amy Joehlin-Price,[3] Amit Agrawal,[4] and Fadi Nabhan[1]

[1]*Division of Endocrinology, Diabetes, and Metabolism, The Ohio State University, Columbus, OH, USA*
[2]*Division of Medical Oncology and Department of Biomedical Informatics, The Ohio State University, Columbus, OH, USA*
[3]*Department of Pathology, The Ohio State University, Columbus, OH, USA*
[4]*Department of Otolaryngology, Head and Neck Surgery, The Ohio State University, Columbus, OH, USA*

Correspondence should be addressed to Fadi Nabhan; fadi.nabhan@osumc.edu

Academic Editor: Yuji Moriwaki

Objective. Thyroid disease has been reported among the endocrinopathies that can occur after treatment with ipilimumab. Graves' disease, however, has been rarely reported with this medication. Here we report a case of Graves' disease diagnosed after initiation of ipilimumab in a patient with melanoma. *Methods.* We present the clinical presentation and management course of this patient followed by a related literature review. *Results.* A 67-year-old male with metastatic melanoma was started on ipilimumab. He developed hyperthyroidism after two doses of ipilimumab. The cause of hyperthyroidism was determined to be Graves' disease. Ipilimumab was held and the patient was started on methimazole with return to euthyroid status. Ipilimumab was resumed and the patient continued methimazole during the course of ipilimumab therapy, with controlled hyperthyroidism. Restaging studies following four cycles of ipilimumab showed complete response in the lungs, with residual melanoma in the neck. The patient then underwent total thyroidectomy and left neck dissection as a definitive treatment for both hyperthyroidism and residual melanoma. *Conclusion.* Graves' disease can develop after starting ipilimumab and methimazole can be an effective treatment. For patients whose hyperthyroidism is well-controlled on methimazole, ipilimumab may be resumed with close monitoring.

1. Introduction

Ipilimumab is an FDA-approved human monoclonal antibody that blocks an immune checkpoint molecule called cytotoxic T-lymphocyte-associated antigen 4 (CTLA-4) leading to increased antitumor activity of tumor-specific T-cells and improved survival in patients with melanoma [1]. However, it is associated with risk of autoimmune toxicities, including endocrinopathies such as hypophysitis, hypothyroidism, and thyroiditis [2, 3]. Graves' disease also has been rarely reported with this medication [4–7]. We present a case in which Graves' disease was diagnosed after starting a patient with metastatic melanoma on ipilimumab and discuss the clinical presentation and therapeutic interventions.

2. Case Report

The patient is a 67-year-old male with metastatic melanoma involving cervical lymph nodes and lungs. He had normal thyroid function tests before initiation of ipilimumab and he has no previous history of thyroid disease. Ipilimumab was started at a dose of 3 mg/kg every three weeks. After receiving two of four planned cycles of therapy, he developed clinical and biochemical hyperthyroidism (Table 1). There was no thyroid tenderness on exam and no palpable thyroid nodules. There were also no signs of ophthalmopathy. Laboratories revealed an elevated thyroid stimulation immunoglobulin level and I-123 scan revealed diffuse homogeneous uptake that was elevated at 6 hours at 30.4% (normal is 5–15%) and at 24 hours at 47.4% (normal 10–33%), consistent with Graves' disease. Ipilimumab was held, and the patient was started on methimazole at a dose of 30 mg/day with titration to control the thyroid hormone levels (Table 1). The highest dose of methimazole used was a total of 35 mg a day. Restaging CT scans showed persistent cervical adenopathy, but resolution of his lung nodules consistent with an immune response to ipilimumab. Given the excellent early clinical response to ipilimumab and the desire to achieve the greatest

TABLE 1: Thyroid function tests changes during treatments.

	Before ipilimumab	1 month after ipilimumab	Ipilimumab held, methimazole started	2 months after ipilimumab	Ipilimumab restarted	1 month after restarting ipilimumab	1 month after total thyroidectomy
TSH (0.55–4.78 mUJ/mL)	1.561	0.009	<0.008	0.015	0.015	0.071	0.892
Free T4 (0.89–1.76 ng/dL)	1.42	3.38	3.64	1.36	1.31	1.01	1.47
Free T3 (2/3–4.2 pg/mL)		8.8	9.8	4.1	4.1	3.6	
TSI (thyroid stimulating immunoglobulin) (<140%)		368					

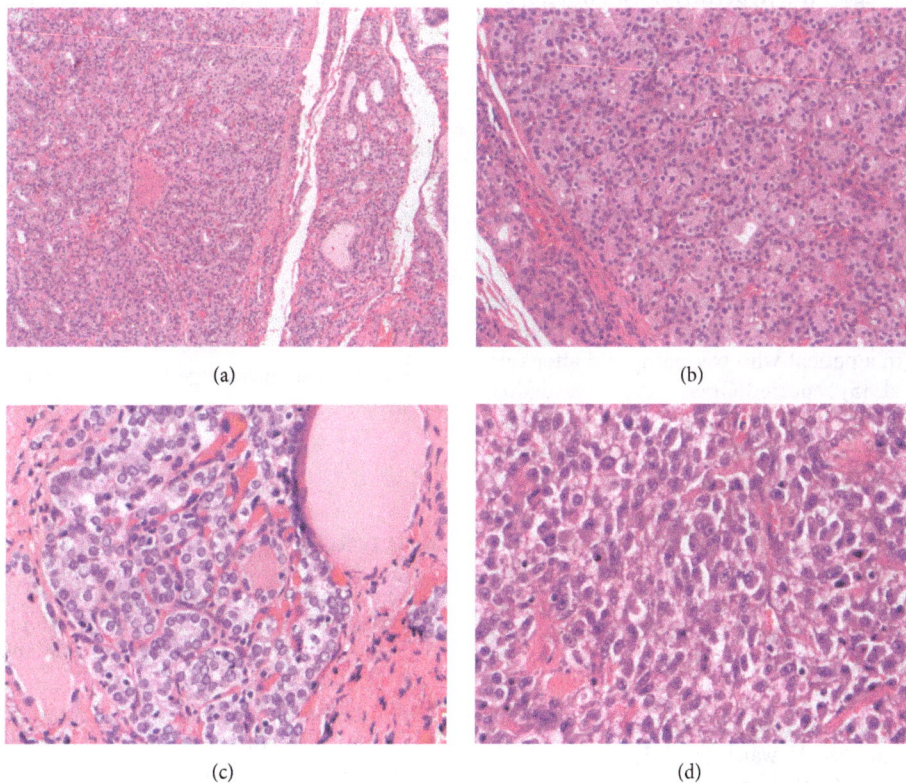

FIGURE 1: Nodular hyperplasia of the thyroid (a) secondary to the patient's Graves' disease, demonstrating abundant follicular structures with scant colloid (b); high power view of patient's papillary thyroid microcarcinoma demonstrating vesicular nuclei, nuclear grooves, and nuclear crowding (c); and representative discohesive, high grade malignant cells of the patient's malignant melanoma requiring ipilimumab therapy (d).

presurgical response, it was recommended that he complete all 4 cycles of ipilimumab if his hyperthyroidism could be safely controlled. He subsequently received two additional cycles of ipilimumab on methimazole to complete the treatment plan for the melanoma. Methimazole was continued during this time and hyperthyroidism remained controlled (Table 1). He subsequently underwent a left neck dissection for residual metastatic melanoma along with total thyroidectomy. Pathology (Figure 1) revealed nodular and papillary hyperplasia of the thyroid, common findings in Graves' disease, along with an incidental papillary thyroid microcarcinoma. The patient was started on levothyroxine after surgery and his thyroid function tests normalized (Table 1).

3. Discussion

Ipilimumab is an immune therapy that has been shown to increase survival in patients with melanoma [1]. Ipilimumab works by blocking CTLA-4, which is an immune checkpoint receptor expressed on the surface of helper T-cells. CTLA-4 normally functions to impair the costimulatory activation of T-cells by CD28, leading to downregulation of T-cell activity. By blocking CTLA-4, ipilimumab removes this negative regulation and induces immune responses that can lead to antitumor activity.

Ipilimumab has been associated with the development of new autoimmune endocrinopathies, likely related directly to its mechanism of action. The most common endocrine side effect is hypophysitis with an incidence rate of 11% in one study [8] and 8% in another [2]. Ipilimumab can lead to autoimmune thyroid disease, with the most common manifestation being hypothyroidism in about 6% followed by thyroiditis characterized by hyperthyroid and hypothyroid phases [2]. Hyperthyroidism resulting from overproduction of thyroid hormone as seen in Graves's disease has been more rarely reported. One case of thyroid storm was reported by Yu et al. [9] in a patient receiving ipilimumab, which occurred after two doses of ipilimumab and subsequently responded to antithyroid medication. Other studies reported eye disease typical of Graves's disease after using ipilimumab [4–7]. In one of these cases [6], hyperthyroidism developed in addition to the eye disease. The diagnosis of Graves' disease was confirmed in our patient given his elevated thyroid stimulating immunoglobulin, which has very high specificity for diagnosis of Graves' disease [10]. This was also supported by elevated iodine uptake and a homogenous scan, which further confirmed Graves's disease [11]. Pathologically, the nodular hyperplasia noted at the time of resection was supportive of the diagnosis as well.

It is difficult to characterize a typical time-course for the development of ipilimumab-related Graves' disease due to the small number of cases. McElnea et al. [4] reported the case of ophthalmopathy in a patient who was euthyroid after two doses while Min et al. [5] reported Graves' eye disease after four doses of ipilimumab. These are similar to the present case in which the disease developed after two doses of ipilimumab.

The pathogenesis of Graves' disease is due to the development of activating antibodies directed against the TSH receptor, which results in hyperthyroidism. This antibody formation involves activation of T2 helper cells. Therefore it is plausible to hypothesize that blocking CTLA-4 results in the development of activating antibodies against the TSH receptor thereby causing Graves' disease in susceptible individuals.

There are several points that support this relation between CTLA-4 and Graves' disease. Heward et al. [12] showed allelic association between the G allele of the CTLA-4 gene and Graves' disease. Furthermore in the same study [12] there was a relationship between allelic variation of the CTLA-4 gene and circulating free T4 concentration at the time of diagnosis suggesting a link between the gene and the severity of Graves' disease. Daroszewski et al. [13] showed that serum levels of a transcript of CTLA-4 were increased in patients with Graves' disease.

Management of patients with Graves's disease in patients being treated with ipilimumab is not well described. It is recommended that ipilimumab be stopped for any endocrinopathy that is not controlled [14]. In our case, ipilimumab was initially held and hyperthyroidism was controlled with methimazole. Then ipilimumab was restarted with successful control of thyroid hormone levels throughout the remainder of the treatment course with methimazole. The choice to perform surgery in this patient was influenced by the fact that radical neck surgery was already indicated for treatment of his melanoma. Other treatment options such as radioactive iodine treatment or continuation of methimazole were also valid choices for our patient. It is also possible that

Graves' disease would remit over time after completion of the ipilimumab therapy. Following TSH receptor antibodies to undetectable levels after taking methimazole can help in predicting Graves' disease remission [11].

It has not yet been determined whether it is possible to predict the development of Graves' disease after starting ipilimumab. Measuring thyroid stimulating immunoglobulins may be helpful; however these may not be elevated unless the patient develops hyperthyroidism. Given the challenge in predicting Graves' disease, it is important to monitor all patients receiving this medication by measuring thyroid function regularly.

In summary Graves's disease can develop after starting ipilimumab. Managing these patients can be challenging, especially if further doses of ipilimumab are recommended, and this management has not been well described in the literature. As in our case, methimazole appears to be efficacious in this treatment, as it would be in the more commonplace cases of Graves's disease developing without the use of ipilimumab.

Acknowledgment

The authors acknowledge Dr. Matthew Ringel for his critical review of this paper.

References

[1] F. S. Hodi, S. J. O'Day, D. F. McDermott et al., "Improved survival with ipilimumab in patients with metastatic melanoma," *The New England Journal of Medicine*, vol. 363, no. 8, pp. 711–723, 2010.

[2] M. Ryder, M. Callahan, M. A. Postow, J. Wolchok, and J. A. Fagin, "Endocrine-related adverse events following ipilimumab in patients with advanced melanoma: a comprehensive retrospective review from a single institution," *Endocrine-Related Cancer*, vol. 21, no. 2, pp. 371–381, 2014.

[3] S. M. Corsello, A. Barnabei, P. Marchetti, L. De Vecchis, R. Salvatori, and F. Torino, "Endocrine side effects induced by immune checkpoint inhibitors," *The Journal of Clinical Endocrinology & Metabolism*, vol. 98, no. 4, pp. 1361–1375, 2013.

[4] E. McElnea, Á. Ní Mhéalóid, S. Moran, R. Kelly, and T. Fulcher, "Thyroid-like ophthalmopathy in a euthyroid patient receiving ipilimumab," *Orbit*, vol. 33, no. 6, pp. 424–427, 2014.

[5] L. Min, A. Vaidya, and C. Becker, "Thyroid autoimmunity and ophthalmopathy related to melanoma biological therapy," *European Journal of Endocrinology*, vol. 164, no. 2, pp. 303–307, 2011.

[6] G. E. Borodic and D. Hinkle, "Ipilimumab-induced orbital inflammation resembling graves disease with subsequent development of systemic hyperthyroidism from CTLA-4 receptor suppression," *Ophthalmic Plastic & Reconstructive Surgery*, vol. 30, no. 1, article 83, 2014.

[7] M. A. Sohrab, R. U. Desai, C. B. Chambers, and G. S. Lissner, "Re:'drug-induced graves disease from CTLA-4 receptor suppression," *Ophthalmic Plastic & Reconstructive Surgery*, vol. 29, no. 3, pp. 239–240, 2013.

[8] A. T. Faje, R. Sullivan, D. Lawrence et al., "Ipilimumab-induced hypophysitis: a detailed longitudinal analysis in a large cohort of patients with metastatic melanoma," *The Journal of Clinical Endocrinology & Metabolism*, vol. 99, no. 11, pp. 4078–4085, 2014.

[9] C. Yu, I. J. Chopra, and E. Ha, "A novel melanoma therapy stirs up a storm: ipilimumab-induced thyrotoxicosis," *Endocrinology, Diabetes & Metabolism Case Reports*, vol. 2015, Article ID 140092, 2015.

[10] G. Barbesino and Y. Tomer, "Clinical utility of TSH receptor antibodies," *The Journal of Clinical Endocrinology & Metabolism*, vol. 98, no. 6, pp. 2247–2255, 2013.

[11] R. S. Bahn, H. B. Burch, D. S. Cooper et al., "Hyperthyroidism and other causes of thyrotoxicosis: management guidelines of the American Thyroid Association and American Association of Clinical Endocrinologists," *Thyroid*, vol. 21, no. 6, pp. 593–646, 2011.

[12] J. M. Heward, A. Allahabadia, M. Armitage et al., "The development of Graves' disease and the CTLA-4 gene on chromosome 2q33," *The Journal of Clinical Endocrinology and Metabolism*, vol. 84, no. 7, pp. 2398–2401, 1999.

[13] J. Daroszewski, E. Pawlak, L. Karabon et al., "Soluble CTLA-4 receptor an immunological marker of Graves' disease and severity of ophthalmopathy is associated with CTLA-4 Jo31 and CT60 gene polymorphisms," *European Journal of Endocrinology*, vol. 161, no. 5, pp. 787–793, 2009.

[14] L. A. Fecher, S. S. Agarwala, F. Stephen Hodi, and J. S. Weber, "Ipilimumab and its toxicities: a multidisciplinary approach," *The Oncologist*, vol. 18, no. 6, pp. 733–743, 2013.

8

Posaconazole-Induced Adrenal Insufficiency in a Case of Chronic Myelomonocytic Leukemia

Ann Miller [iD],[1] Lauren K. Brooks,[2] Silpa Poola-Kella,[2] and Rana Malek [iD][2]

[1]Department of Medicine, University of Maryland Medical Center, Baltimore, MD, USA
[2]Department of Medicine, Division of Endocrinology, Diabetes and Nutrition, University of Maryland Medical Center, Baltimore, MD, USA

Correspondence should be addressed to Rana Malek; rmalek@som.umaryland.edu

Academic Editor: Osamu Isozaki

Introduction. Posaconazole is an azole used in treatment and prophylaxis of a broad spectrum of fungal infections. Antifungals such as ketoconazole have been shown to cause primary adrenal insufficiency (AI) as a result of direct inhibition on the steroidogenesis pathway. There is only one reported case of primary AI induced by posaconazole in a patient with mucormycosis. We report a case of posaconazole-related primary AI. *Case.* A 63-year-old man with chronic myelomonocytic leukemia was admitted for fatigue and intermittent nausea and vomiting. He had recently discontinued prophylactic posaconazole 300 mg daily. He was assessed for AI with a morning cortisol of 1.9 mcg/dL followed by a failed cosyntropin stimulation (CS) test. Adrenocorticotropic hormone (ACTH) level was 154.6 pg/mL with negative 21-hydroxylase antibodies. The patient's symptoms improved with initiation of hydrocortisone and fludrocortisone. One year after discontinuation of posaconazole, he underwent a repeat CS test which showed normal adrenal function with normal ACTH at 34.1 pg/mL. *Conclusion.* In this case, we demonstrate that prolonged use of posaconazole is associated with primary AI. As use of posaconazole increases, knowledge of the potential risk of AI is important and must be included in the differential diagnosis when these patients present with hypotension, hypoglycemia, and failure to thrive.

1. Introduction

Adrenal insufficiency occurs when there is inadequate secretion of cortisol from the adrenal glands due to either failure of the adrenal glands or other causes such as critical illness or pituitary adrenocorticotropic hormone (ACTH) deficiency. Primary adrenal insufficiency is rare and is caused by insufficient cortisol production from the adrenal glands. Lab abnormalities include very low cortisol and significantly elevated ACTH. This is in contrast to secondary adrenal insufficiency in which there is an abnormality at the level of the pituitary gland, resulting in insufficient secretion of ACTH to stimulate cortisol production. Patients will concomitantly have low or inappropriately normal ACTH levels and low cortisol levels. The cosyntropin test can help distinguish between primary and secondary adrenal insufficiency. A normal adrenal gland will secrete cortisol in response to the administration of cosyntropin and reach a peak of >500 nmol/L thirty minutes later. Primary adrenal insufficiency will result in little or no increase in cortisol production. Measurement of ACTH can further help delineate primary versus secondary adrenal insufficiency [1].

The clinical presentation of adrenal insufficiency depends on disease chronicity and the presence of physical stressors. Manifestations of adrenal crisis include shock, hypotension, fever, nausea, vomiting, abdominal pain, tachycardia, and death. Causes of primary adrenal insufficiency include autoimmune adrenalitis, infections such as tuberculosis, disseminated fungal infections, human immunodeficiency virus, hemorrhagic infarction, or metastatic cancerous infiltration of the adrenal glands, and drugs.

Ketoconazole and posaconazole are both members of the azole antifungal family. They are primarily used as antifungal agents. Azole antifungals work by inhibiting the cytochrome P450 dependent enzyme lanosterol 14 alpha-demethylase, an enzyme necessary for the conversion of lanosterol to ergosterol, a vital component of the cell membrane in fungi. This enzyme is not present in mammalian cells.

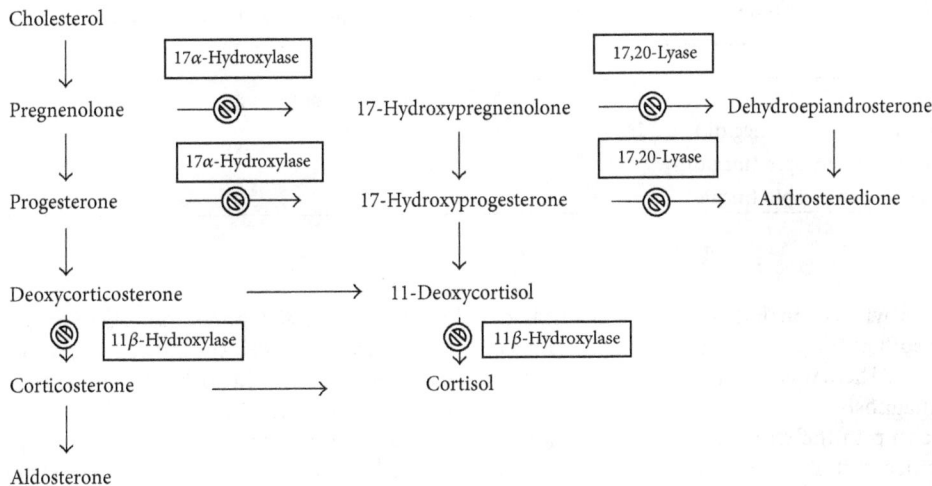

FIGURE 1: Diagram of the steroid synthesis pathway showing the steps where ketoconazole inhibits synthesis.

Ketoconazole is known to inhibit human steroidogenesis [2]. It impedes human steroid production by inhibiting human cytochrome P450 enzymes including the cholesterol side-chain cleavage complex 17,20-lyase, 11β-hydroxylase, and 17α-hydroxylase [3] (Figure 1). Due to its steroidogenesis inhibitory effects, ketoconazole can be used as a treatment for Cushing's syndrome. While its use has been shown to effectively reduce urinary free cortisol in patients with Cushing's syndrome, adrenal insufficiency is a known side effect of therapy [4, 5]. In 2013, the US Food and Drug Administration (FDA) limited the use of Nizoral (ketoconazole) oral tablets due to the side effects of hepatotoxicity and adrenal insufficiency [6].

Ketoconazole is an imidazole derivative, meaning that there are 2 nitrogen atoms in the azole ring. Triazoles are members of the azole class that have 3 nitrogen atoms in the azole ring. First-generation triazoles include fluconazole and itraconazole and second-generation triazoles include posaconazole and voriconazole. The most recent azole to be approved for use against invasive aspergillosis and invasive mucormycosis infections is isavuconazole. It was approved by the FDA in 2015.

Posaconazole has been FDA approved for the prophylaxis and treatment of refractory invasive fungal infections. During phase I, II, and III clinical trials, posaconazole was found to be safe and well tolerated. During phase I studies, the most common side effects included gastrointestinal symptoms, headache, dry mouth, somnolence, dizziness, and constipation. These side effects were mild and transient in nature [7]. Here we present a case in which posaconazole is theorized to be the cause of primary adrenal insufficiency.

2. Case

A 63-year-old African-American male with type 2 diabetes on metformin, rheumatoid arthritis not on oral corticosteroid therapy, chronic low back pain alleviated with intermittent epidural steroid injections, hepatitis C, and chronic myelomonocytic leukemia (CMML) who was on decitabine

for chemotherapy presented to the hospital on 6/25/16 for hematemesis and poor oral intake. Prior to arrival, he had been feeling weak and his weakness acutely worsened in the two to three weeks before admission. His other symptoms included nausea and poor appetite. He had vomited at least twice. Two days prior to his admission, he was seen in his outpatient oncologist's office. He told his oncologist that he had not been feeling well and had been experiencing dehydration and fatigue. He said his symptoms started around the time the posaconazole 300 mg daily was started in April of 2016 for fungal prophylaxis. His oncologist held his posaconazole at that visit on 6/23/16. The only relevant steroid exposure was intermittent steroid injections into his spine for low back pain. His last injection had been in March of 2016. It was estimated that he had received a total of five steroid injections into his back prior to admission. The time interval between and the time course of injections are not specified. His full medication list included potassium supplementation, hydroxychloroquine, indomethacin, tramadol, docusate, acyclovir, levofloxacin, decitabine, allopurinol, gabapentin, aspirin, lisinopril, and metformin.

Blood pressure on admission was within normal limits at 125/60 mmHg. Labs on admission showed hypokalemia (3.1 mmol/L) and hypocalcemia (8.5 mg/dL) but normal sodium and glucose. To evaluate his adrenal function, the primary team sent a morning cortisol on 6/26/16 which resulted as 1.9 mcg/dL at 5:39 AM. To further evaluate his adrenal function, he underwent a cosyntropin stimulation test. On the morning of 6/27/16, his cortisol at 5:28 AM was 2.2 mcg/dL. He was then given one dose of cosyntropin 250 mcg IV at 8:00 AM with repeat cortisol measurements resulting in 3.7 mcg/dL at 30 minutes and 4.1 mcg/dL at 60 minutes. A CT scan of the abdomen and pelvis without contrast was done on 6/26/16 and showed bilateral thickened adrenal glands consistent with hyperplasia. During that admission, he was started on hydrocortisone 15 mg by mouth in the morning and 10 mg by mouth in the evening. ACTH measured on 6/27/16 was 154.6 pg/mL. After the ACTH results returned, he was started on fludrocortisone 0.1 mg by

Table 1: Comparison of labs just after discontinuation of posaconazole and a year later.

Labs	2016	2017
ACTH (7–69 pg/mL)	154.6 (7–69 pg/mL)	34.1 (7–69 pg/mL)
Cortisol, morning baseline (4.4–22.7 mcg/dL)	2.2	5 mcg/dL
Cortisol, 30 minutes after cosyntropin (mcg/dL)	3.7	n/a
Cortisol, 60 minutes after cosyntropin (mcg/dL)	4.1	18.5 mcg/dL

mouth daily as the providers concluded that the patient had primary adrenal insufficiency given his elevated ACTH and failed cosyntropin test. There was no renin value measured at the time of initial diagnosis.

He was followed up in the endocrine clinic one month later. During the office visit, it was documented that he had hyperpigmentation of the skin but the patient stated that this had been present for years. After starting hydrocortisone and fludrocortisone, his symptoms improved including increased appetite and resolution of headache and nausea. He was rehospitalized in September 2016 for a stem cell transplant for his CMML. 21-OH antibodies were tested during that admission and were negative (<0.1). On discharge, he was prescribed hydrocortisone 10 mg by mouth in the morning and 5 mg by mouth in the afternoon. He tolerated this regimen well. He re-presented to the endocrine clinic in July of 2017 (one year after discontinuation of posaconazole) for repeat cosyntropin testing. Cosyntropin 250 mcg IV was given after measurement of a baseline cortisol of 5 mcg/dL. One hour after the cosyntropin was given, it rose to 18.5 mcg/dL. Pretesting ACTH was 34.1 pg/mL (7–69 pg/mL) and renin was 0.176 ng/mL/hr (0.167–5.380 ng/mL/hr). Based on his improved cosyntropin testing (Table 1), he discontinued the hydrocortisone and fludrocortisone.

3. Discussion

This case report describes a patient presenting with nausea and vomiting in the setting of recently taking posaconazole who was found to have failed a cosyntropin test with simultaneous elevated ACTH suggesting posaconazole-induced primary adrenal insufficiency that resolved after discontinuation of the medication.

There are several case reports of azoles causing adrenal insufficiency. These generally have been in the setting of drug-drug interactions when azoles are taken concomitantly with steroids. With regard to the first-generation triazoles, there are three documented cases of fluconazole-induced adrenal insufficiency in the critically ill [8, 9], two case reports of fluconazole-induced adrenal insufficiency due to drug interactions leading to synergistic inhibition of the adrenal gland [10, 11], and only one documented case report of fluconazole-induced acute primary adrenal insufficiency when it was used as a prophylactic measure against fungal infections in a patient undergoing high dose cytotoxic chemotherapy [12]. What many of these cases share is the inhibition of CYP3A4 which results in supraphysiologic levels of corticosteroids (inhaled, intranasal, intra-articular, or oral) leading to iatrogenic Cushing's syndrome with resultant adrenal suppression. There are also case reports of itraconazole-induced central adrenal insufficiency, but in all cases, it was thought to be due to a drug interaction with inhaled corticosteroids [13, 14]. The etiology of itraconazole-induced adrenal insufficiency due to drug interactions with inhaled corticosteroids was further evaluated by Skov et al. in 2002 [15]. The researchers from Denmark evaluated adrenal function in patients with cystic fibrosis or chronic granulomatous disease who were treated for allergic bronchopulmonary aspergillosis with itraconazole either alone ($N = 12$) or with inhaled budesonide ($N = 25$). Eleven of 25 patients who were treated with combination itraconazole and inhaled budesonide did not respond to ACTH stimulation testing. These were the only patients who experienced any evidence of adrenal insufficiency. Of these patients, 8 were also found to have low plasma ACTH levels. These findings suggest that itraconazole decreases the CYP3A4 metabolism of budesonide causing increased systemic levels of the steroid leading to central adrenal insufficiency.

With regard to incidences of adrenal insufficiency in second-generation triazoles, there is only one case report of voriconazole induced central adrenal insufficiency, again with the thought being the adrenal insufficiency was due to a drug interaction with inhaled corticosteroids [16]. There is only one documented case of posaconazole-induced adrenal insufficiency [17]. The patient had a past medical history significant for type 1 diabetes and was hospitalized for diabetic ketoacidosis and developed rhino-orbital mucormycosis. The patient was treated with posaconazole, starting on day 10, and it was continued on discharge, day 55. She was noted to develop falling insulin requirements and progressive hypotension. Further work-up revealed a failed cosyntropin stimulation test and negative anti-adrenal antibody testing which led the authors to conclude that posaconazole was the cause of the patient's adrenal insufficiency. We present a similar case where posaconazole was thought to be the cause of adrenal insufficiency but we were able to follow the ACTH and repeat the cosyntropin test and show resolution of the adrenal function after discontinuation of the posaconazole. There have been no case reports of isavuconazole induced adrenal insufficiency.

We argue that our patient experienced primary adrenal insufficiency given his lab findings of elevated ACTH and failed cosyntropin testing. Further information to support this diagnosis is the bilateral adrenal hyperplasia found on his abdominal CT scan. The pathophysiology of our patient's adrenal hyperplasia could be similar to that of congenital adrenal hyperplasia where cortisol synthesis is also impaired, although in most cases due to the deficiency of

21-hydroxylase. The decreased cortisol production in both cases leads to increased ACTH secretion causing hyperplasia of the adrenal glands [18]. The difference in the two clinical scenarios is the mechanism of inability for cortisol production.

Our patient's potassium and sodium levels were not suggestive of primary adrenal insufficiency as it usually presents with hyponatremia and hyperkalemia. However, these lab abnormalities could be explained by his vomiting and infusions. The vomiting caused hypokalemia due to gastrointestinal losses and his sodium may have been normal due to recent boluses of normal saline outpatient, the most recent on 6/24/16, the day prior to admission.

With respect to other etiologies of the patient's primary adrenal insufficiency, autoimmune disease was ruled out by his negative 21-OH antibodies and adrenal hemorrhage was not present on his imaging. Finally, his facial hyperpigmentation predated his acute adrenal insufficiency and was unlikely to be related to his short standing elevation of ACTH.

While we argue that this patient experienced primary adrenal insufficiency from posaconazole inhibition of steroidogenesis, there are weaknesses in our case that we must consider. Most importantly, the patient had been receiving corticosteroid injections for his back pain throughout this time, the timing of which is not well documented. Steroids can cause adrenal insufficiency due to their negative feedback on corticotropin releasing hormone and ACTH. This leads to adrenal atrophy and decreased cortisol secretion from the adrenal gland. However, his CT results showing adrenal hyperplasia and his elevated ACTH argue strongly for primary adrenal insufficiency.

4. Conclusion

Here we present a case of primary adrenal insufficiency attributed to long-term posaconazole use. As posaconazole use for the prophylaxis against and treatment of invasive fungal infections increases, clinicians should be aware of this possible long-term side effect. Clinicians should caution against its use in patients at risk of developing adrenal insufficiency. Clinical signs or symptoms of adrenal insufficiency, such as weight loss, hypotension, or hypoglycemia, may be clues suggesting the development of this side effect. Awareness of this side effect may also be warranted with the newest approved azole, isavuconazole.

Disclosure

This case report was presented on April 2, 2017, at the Endocrine Society's 99th Annual Meeting and Expo (Endo 2017) in Orlando, Florida.

References

[1] W. Arlt, "The approach to the adult with newly diagnosed adrenal insufficiency," *The Journal of Clinical Endocrinology & Metabolism*, vol. 94, no. 4, pp. 1059–1067, 2009.

[2] N. Sonino, "The use of ketoconazole as an inhibitor of steroid production," *The New England Journal of Medicine*, vol. 317, no. 13, pp. 812–818, 1987.

[3] R. Pivonello, M. De Leo, A. Cozzolino, and A. Colao, "The treatment of Cushing's disease," *Endocrine Reviews*, vol. 36, no. 4, pp. 385–486, 2015.

[4] F. Castinetti, L. Guignat, P. Giraud et al., "Ketoconazole in Cushing's disease: is it worth a try?" *The Journal of Clinical Endocrinology & Metabolism*, vol. 99, no. 5, pp. 1623–1630, 2014.

[5] D. Moncet, D. J. Morando, F. Pitoia, S. B. Katz, M. A. Rossi, and O. D. Bruno, "Ketoconazole therapy: An efficacaious alternative to achieve eucortisolism in patients with Cushing's syndrome," *Medicina*, vol. 67, no. 1, pp. 26–31, 2007.

[6] FDA Drug Safety Communication, "FDA limits usage of Nizoral (ketoconazole) oral tablets due to potentially fatal liver injury and risk of drug interactions and adrenal gland problems," 2017(4/15), 2013.

[7] S. Langner, P. B. Staber, and P. Neumeister, "Posaconazole in the management of refractory invasive fungal infections," *Therapeutics and Clinical Risk Management*, vol. 4, no. 4, pp. 747–757, 2008.

[8] S. G. Albert, M. J. DeLeon, and A. B. Silverberg, "Possible association between high-dose fluconazole and adrenal insufficiency in critically ill patients," *Critical Care Medicine*, vol. 29, no. 3, pp. 668–670, 2001.

[9] S. G. Santhana Krishnan and R. K. Cobbs, "Reversible acute adrenal insufficiency caused by fluconazole in a critically ill patient.," *Postgraduate Medical Journal*, vol. 82, no. 971, p. e23, 2006.

[10] W. C. Hoover, L. J. Britton, J. Gardner, T. Jackson, and H. Gutierrez, "Rapid onset of iatrogenic adrenal insufficiency in a patient with cystic fibrosis-related liver disease treated with inhaled corticosteroids and a moderate CYP3a4 inhibitor," *Annals of Pharmacotherapy*, vol. 45, no. 7-8, 2011.

[11] K. St Clair and J. D. Maguire, "Role of fluconazole in a case of rapid onset ritonavir and inhaled fluticasone-associated secondary adrenal insufficiency," *International Journal of STD & AIDS*, vol. 23, no. 5, pp. 371–372, 2012.

[12] S. Shibata, M. Kami, Y. Kanda et al., "Acute adrenal failure associated with fluconazole after administration of high-dose cyclophosphamide," *American Journal of Hematology*, vol. 66, no. 4, pp. 303–305, 2001.

[13] M.-C. Blondin, H. Beauregard, and O. Serri, "Iatrogenic cushing syndrome in patients receiving inhaled budesonide and itraconazole or ritonavir: Two cases and literature review," *Endocrine Practice*, vol. 19, no. 6, pp. e138–e141, 2013.

[14] M. J. Bolland, W. Bagg, M. G. Thomas, J. A. Lucas, R. Ticehurst, and P. N. Black, "Cushing's Syndrome Due to Interaction between Inhaled Corticosteroids and Itraconazole," *Annals of Pharmacotherapy*, vol. 38, no. 1, pp. 46–49, 2004.

[15] M. Skov, K. M. Main, I. B. Sillesen, J. Müller, C. Koch, and S. Lanng, "Iatrogenic adrenal insufficiency as a side-effect of combined treatment of itraconazole and budesonide," *European Respiratory Journal*, vol. 20, no. 1, pp. 127–133, 2002.

9

Adrenal Insufficiency under Standard Dosage of Glucocorticoid Replacement after Unilateral Adrenalectomy for Cushing's Syndrome

Kentaro Fujii,[1] Kazutoshi Miyashita,[1] Isao Kurihara,[1] Ken Hiratsuka,[1] Seiji Sato,[1] Kenichi Yokota,[1] Sakiko Kobayashi,[1] Hirotaka Shibata,[2] and Hiroshi Itoh[1]

[1]Department of Internal Medicine, School of Medicine, Keio University, 35 Shinanomachi, Shinjuku-ku, Tokyo 160-8582, Japan
[2]Department of Endocrinology, Metabolism, Rheumatology and Nephrology, Faculty of Medicine, Oita University, 700 Dannoharu, Oita 870-1192, Japan

Correspondence should be addressed to Kazutoshi Miyashita; miyakaz@z6.keio.jp

Academic Editor: Yuji Moriwaki

Glucocorticoid replacement is needed for patients after adrenal surgery for Cushing's syndrome; however, the adequate dosage is not easily determined. The patient was a 62-year-old woman who has had hypertension for 5 years and presented with heart failure due to hypertrophic cardiomyopathy. She consulted with us because of general fatigue, facial edema, and muscle weakness and was diagnosed with Cushing's syndrome. A laparoscopic left adrenalectomy was performed, standard dosage of postoperative replacement was administered, and she was discharged with 30 mg/day of hydrocortisone (cortisol). However, she suffered from loss of appetite and was transferred to an emergency unit with the symptoms of adrenal insufficiency on postoperative day 15. After initial hydrocortisone replacement with 200 mg/day, the dosage was gradually decreased during hospitalization; however, reduction of hydrocortisone dosage lower than 60 mg/day was difficult because of nausea and fatigue. Her circadian cortisol profile after hydrocortisone administration showed delayed and lowered peaks, which suggested that hydrocortisone absorption in the intestine was impaired. Therefore, complicated heart failure may have led to the adrenal insufficiency in the patient. In such cases, we should consider postoperative administration of more than the standard dosage of hydrocortisone to avoid adrenal insufficiency after surgery for Cushing's syndrome.

1. Introduction

The patients who have undergone a unilateral adrenalectomy for Cushing's syndrome become steroid-dependent. Therefore, sufficient replacement of glucocorticoid is needed during the postoperative period [1, 2]. Although a standard protocol for postoperative replacement has not been developed yet, the dosage was empirically suggested by some previous reports. For example, a 200 mg dose of hydrocortisone was administered within the first 24 hours after surgery; thereafter, 100 mg every 8 hours for a day, 100 mg every 12 hours for a day, and 50 mg every 12 hours for a day were applied during the following three days, respectively. On the fourth day, an oral dose of 25 mg hydrocortisone was subsequently used instead of intravenous agents, followed by

a reduction of 5 mg every 3 days until a maintenance dose (15–20 mg/day) [3].

Previous reports indicate that patients with Cushing's syndrome who undergo a unilateral adrenalectomy can usually be tapered off of all steroids within 6 months to 2 years; however, the adequate dosage and duration are not easily determined [4–6]. Moreover, some patients suffer from glucocorticoid withdrawal symptoms and need an increase in the glucocorticoid dose. Recently, the dosage of postoperative glucocorticoid replacement has a trend to be reduced to help the recovery of adrenal function after adrenalectomy [1]. However, it should not be always the case. Here we show an instructive case of a patient who suffered from symptoms of adrenal insufficiency after a unilateral adrenalectomy for Cushing's syndrome, which

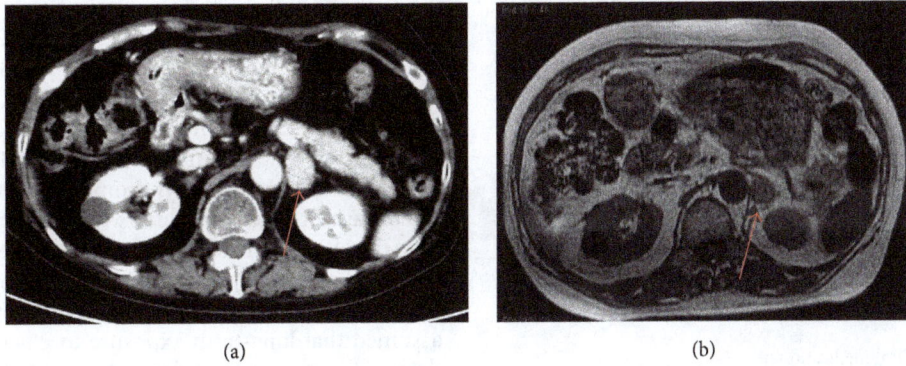

FIGURE 1: A 62-year-old woman with Cushing's syndrome: (a) computed tomography and (b) magnetic resonance imaging showed an adrenal tumor (29 × 22 mm, red arrow).

occurred despite treatment with more than 30 mg/day of hydrocortisone.

2. Case Presentation

A 62-year-old Japanese woman consulted with us because of progressively worsening general fatigue, facial edema, and muscle weakness. She has suffered from hypertension for 5 years and recognized the easy bruising, edematous face, and loss of muscle strength. Past medical history showed heart failure due to hypertrophic cardiomyopathy and hepatitis B virus (HBV) infection. Her medications included furosemide, spironolactone, bisoprolol, verapamil, cibenzoline, lovastatin, and entecavir. No family history of hypertension was recorded.

Physical examination showed normal vital signs with a blood pressure of 127/86 mmHg and a pulse rate of 74 bpm. Her BMI was 23.2 kg/m^2. Heart sounds were clear and regular without murmurs. Breath sounds were also clear. Pitting edema was observed in the lower extremities. Moon-shaped face and buffalo hump were also present. Laboratory findings revealed mild renal dysfunction [creatinine 1.03 mg/dL (0.60–1.20 mg/dL), blood urea nitrogen 34.4 mg/dL (7–20 mg/dL)] and fluid retention [brain natriuretic peptide (BNP) 547.6 pg/mL (<18.4 pg/mL)]. Serum electrolytes were within normal limits [potassium 4.7 mmol/L (3.6–5.0 mmol/L), sodium 144.9 mmol/L (136–146 mmol/L), and chloride 105 mmol/L (97–107 mmol/L)]. Electrocardiogram (ECG) and ultrasound cardiography (UCG) revealed that hypertrophic cardiomyopathy was present in the left ventricle but it did not obstruct the ventricular outflow tract. The inferior vena cava was not distended.

Endocrinological evaluations revealed elevated urinary free cortisol (114 μg/day), without suppression of serum cortisol at midnight (18.1 μg/day) and with suppression of ACTH (<1.0 pg/mL) in the morning. After an overnight 8 mg dexamethasone challenge, the serum cortisol level was maintained at 34.4 μg/dL and ACTH was <1.0 pg/mL in the next morning. Abdominal computed tomography (CT) and magnetic resonance imaging (MRI) detected a 30 mm left adrenal mass (Figure 1) and 131I-adosterol scintigraphy revealed unilateral uptake in the left adrenal mass. Under a diagnosis of Cushing's syndrome caused by an adrenal

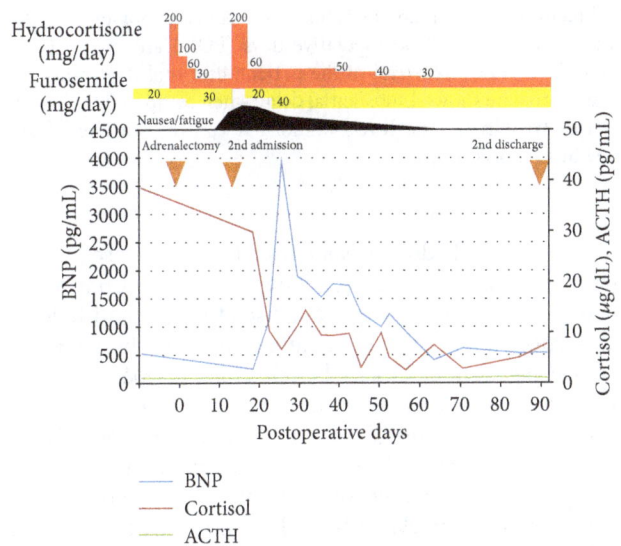

FIGURE 2: Clinical course of the patient after the operation. The brain natriuretic peptide (BNP) level (blue line) is shown on the left side. The levels of cortisol (red line) and ACTH (green line) are shown on the right side. The dosages of hydrocortisone and furosemide are demonstrated on the upper side.

adenoma, a laparoscopic left adrenalectomy was performed and 200 mg/day of hydrocortisone was started postoperatively. The dose was reduced gradually and she was discharged on postoperative day 14 with 30 mg/day of oral hydrocortisone.

However, she felt severe nausea and fatigue just after discharge and was transferred to an emergency unit on postoperative day 15 (Figure 2). Her blood pressure had declined to 95/64 mmHg, hyponatremia [sodium 138.6 mmol/L (136–146 mmol/L)] was observed, and ACTH was undetectable. From these facts, she was diagnosed with adrenal insufficiency. The symptoms immediately disappeared by an intravenous infusion of 200 mg hydrocortisone. After the initial treatment, she felt dyspnea and her BNP level was remarkably increased to 3934.5 pg/mL (<18.4 pg/mL). Under the diagnosis of acute exacerbation of heart failure, furosemide was increased to treat the fluid retention and the BNP level gradually decreased. The signs and symptoms of acute coronary syndrome were not observed.

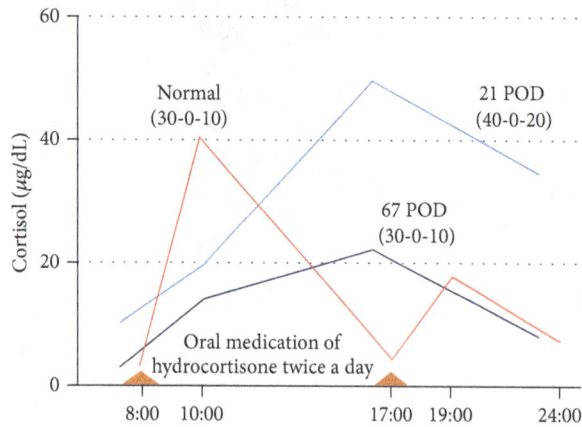

FIGURE 3: Delayed and lowered peaks of serum cortisol level after oral medications of hydrocortisone. The serum cortisol levels of the patient on 21 and 67 postoperative days (POD) are shown (blue lines). The peak of cortisol of the patient after oral medication of hydrocortisone showed substantial delay when compared to normal control (red line). The levels of normal control are cited from previous reports [15].

The dose of hydrocortisone was slowly decreased under hospitalization; however, reduction of hydrocortisone lower than 60 mg/day was difficult because of nausea and fatigue. We suspected that the heart failure caused malabsorption of the hydrocortisone, because her circadian profile of cortisol showed delayed and lowered peaks after hydrocortisone administration (Figure 3). The daily dose of hydrocortisone was carefully decreased from 60 mg/day, in accordance with her symptoms. However, she presented fatigue and loss of appetite which correlated with the dose of hydrocortisone and it was difficult to reduce the dosage until the standard maintenance dose (15–20 mg/day). Finally, she was discharged on postoperative day 92 at a dose of 30 mg/day, because the nausea and fatigue had disappeared and she resumed daily life activities. Three years after the operation, her hypothalamus-pituitary-adrenal (HPA) axis has completely recovered.

3. Discussion

Cushing's syndrome was first described by Cushing in 1932 [7] and it is currently classified as ACTH dependent or independent. The syndrome is defined as an endocrine disorder with a constitutively elevated level of glucocorticoids. The patients present with central obesity, diabetes mellitus, osteoporosis, and other metabolic symptoms. In general, patients who have undergone a unilateral adrenalectomy for Cushing's syndrome become steroid deficient; therefore, they absolutely need postoperative replacement therapy [2]. A clinical practice guideline stated that glucocorticoid replacement after surgery is required until the HPA axis recovers and the mean period of replacement is eighteen months after a unilateral adrenalectomy [1].

Although the standardized protocol for glucocorticoid replacement during the perioperative period was not mentioned in the guideline, some previous reports showed recommended protocols. For example, Orth and Kovaks stated that 200 mg of hydrocortisone should be given within the first 24 hours after surgery, and then 100 mg, 75 mg, and 50 mg/day on the following days with a gradual reduction of hydrocortisone to a maintenance dose (15–25 mg/day) [8]. Since steroid withdrawal syndrome (SWS) may happen when the dosage of glucocorticoid is decreased too quickly, even after the HPA axis has begun to recover, the dosage should be tapered down slowly or a temporary increase may be needed [1]. The mechanism of SWS is still unknown; however, it is assumed that long-term exposure to glucocorticoids causes the patients to develop a dependence on glucocorticoids [9].

In our case, a standard steroid replacement with 30 mg/day of hydrocortisone was not enough to avoid adrenal insufficiency after a unilateral adrenalectomy for Cushing's syndrome. The patient had presented with the typical clinical features of Cushing's syndrome for five years and was exposed to excessive cortisol for a long time. Chronic exposure to excessive glucocorticoids is known to impair biological effects due to downregulation of the receptor [10]. Therefore, decreased glucocorticoid receptors may have caused her to need more hydrocortisone than the standard dose. However, it does not explain the delayed cortisol level peaks after hydrocortisone administration (Figure 3).

We considered that "worsening of heart failure due to adrenal insufficiency" after the second admission would be an important factor for the increase in the required amount of glucocorticoids. Hemodynamic impairment, caused by volume depletion and low cardiac output, is a common problem in adrenal insufficiency [11]. Several reports have shown structural myocardial changes during adrenal insufficiency, such as stress cardiomyopathy, as well as a rapid recovery under steroid therapy [12, 13]. An excessive amount of crystalloid solutions, which was used for fluid resuscitation against volume depletion and lower blood pressure in adrenal insufficiency, might be an exacerbating factor for the heart failure. Since the patient had hypertrophic cardiomyopathy and a higher baseline BNP level before surgery, the heart failure might be much easier to exacerbate for the above reasons. Furthermore, intestinal edema and reduced absorption of intestinal contents are well known problems in patients with heart failure [14]. In this case, the delayed and lowered peaks of cortisol level after hydrocortisone administration suggested malabsorption in the intestine. In these contexts, we judged that adrenal insufficiency of the patient on second admission triggered the exacerbation of heart failure which led to malabsorption of hydrocortisone. That is, adrenal insufficiency after surgery made heart failure and malabsorption more serious and formed a vicious cycle. In such cases with heart failure, a hydrocortisone replacement of more than a 30 mg/day dose should be considered after a unilateral adrenalectomy for Cushing's syndrome.

4. Conclusion

We presented a case of a patient with adrenal insufficiency after a unilateral adrenalectomy for Cushing's syndrome who was resistant to a reduction in glucocorticoid replacement. The glucocorticoid receptors would have been downregulated due to the long-term exposure of excessive cortisol before surgery. It was suggested that complicated heart failure reduced the absorption of hydrocortisone in the intestine. We judged that adrenal insufficiency after surgery exacerbated the heart failure and malabsorption of hydrocortisone which formed a vicious cycle. In cases with heart failure, enough hydrocortisone replacement with a dose of more than 30 mg/day should be considered to avoid adrenal insufficiency after a unilateral adrenalectomy for Cushing's syndrome.

References

[1] L. K. Nieman, B. M. K. Biller, J. W. Findling et al., "Treatment of Cushing's syndrome: an endocrine society clinical practice guideline," *The Journal of Clinical Endocrinology & Metabolism*, vol. 100, no. 8, pp. 2807–2831, 2015.

[2] W. T. Shen, J. Lee, E. Kebebew, O. H. Clark, and Q.-Y. Duh, "Selective use of steroid replacement after adrenalectomy: lessons from 331 consecutive cases," *Archives of Surgery*, vol. 141, no. 8, pp. 771–774, 2006.

[3] X. Cui, L. Yang, J. Li et al., "Perioperative endocrine therapy for patients with cushing's syndrome undergoing retroperitoneal laparoscopic adrenalectomy," *International Journal of Endocrinology*, vol. 2012, Article ID 983965, 6 pages, 2012.

[4] M. A. Zeiger, D. L. Fraker, H. I. Pass et al., "Effective reversibility of the signs and symptoms of hypercortisolism by bilateral adrenalectomy," *Surgery*, vol. 114, no. 6, pp. 1138–1143, 1993.

[5] A. Meyer and M. Behrend, "Cushing's syndrome: adrenalectomy and long-term results. Digestive surgery," *Digestive Surgery*, vol. 21, no. 5-6, pp. 363–370, 2004.

[6] G. M. Doherty, L. K. Nieman, G. B. Cutler Jr., G. P. Chrousos, and J. A. Norton, "Time to recovery of the hypothalamic-pituitary-adrenal axis after curative resection of adrenal tumors in patients with Cushing's syndrome," *Surgery*, vol. 108, no. 6, pp. 1085–1090, 1990.

[7] H. Cushing, "The basophil adenomas of the pituitary body and their clinical manifestations (pituitary basophilism)," *Johns Hopkins Hospital Bulletin*, vol. 50, pp. 137–195, 1932.

[8] D. N. Orth and W. J. Kovaks, "The adrenal cortex," in *Williams Textbook of Endocrinology*, pp. 517–664, W. B. Saunders, Philadelphia, Pa, USA, 1998.

[9] Z. Hochberg, K. Pacak, and G. P. Chrousos, "Endocrine withdrawal syndromes," *Endocrine Reviews*, vol. 24, no. 4, pp. 523–538, 2003.

[10] M. J. M. Schaaf and J. A. Cidlowski, "Molecular mechanisms of glucocorticoid action and resistance," *The Journal of Steroid Biochemistry and Molecular Biology*, vol. 83, no. 1–5, pp. 37–48, 2002.

[11] G. Bouachour, P. Tirot, N. Varache, J. P. Gouello, P. Harry, and P. Alquier, "Hemodynamic changes in acute adrenal insufficiency," *Intensive Care Medicine*, vol. 20, no. 2, pp. 138–141, 1994.

[12] B. Wolff, K. Machill, I. Schulzki, D. Schumacher, and D. Werner, "Acute reversible cardiomyopathy with cardiogenic shock in a patient with Addisonian crisis: a case report," *International Journal of Cardiology*, vol. 116, no. 2, pp. e71–e73, 2007.

[13] C. Ukita, H. Miyazaki, N. Toyoda, A. Kosaki, M. Nishikawa, and T. Iwasaka, "Takotsubo cardiomyopathy during acute adrenal crisis due to isolated adrenocorticotropin deficiency," *Internal Medicine*, vol. 48, no. 5, pp. 347–352, 2009.

[14] A. Sandek, J. Bauditz, A. Swidsinski et al., "Altered intestinal function in patients with chronic heart failure," *Journal of the American College of Cardiology*, vol. 50, no. 16, pp. 1561–1569, 2007.

[15] N. Simon, F. Castinetti, F. Ouliac, N. Lesavre, T. Brue, and C. Oliver, "Pharmacokinetic evidence for suboptimal treatment of adrenal insufficiency with currently available hydrocortisone tablets," *Clinical Pharmacokinetics*, vol. 49, no. 7, pp. 455–463, 2010.

Acute Primary Adrenal Insufficiency after Hip Replacement in a Patient with Acute Intermittent Porphyria

Adele Latina ⓘ,[1] **Massimo Terzolo,**[2] **Anna Pia,**[2] **Giuseppe Reimondo,**[2] **Elena Castellano,**[1] **Micaela Pellegrino,**[1] **and Giorgio Borretta**[1]

[1]*Division of Endocrinology, Diabetology and Metabolism, Santa Croce e Carle Hospital, Via M. Coppino 26, 12100 Cuneo, Italy*
[2]*Internal Medicine 1, Department of Clinical and Biological Sciences, University of Turin, San Luigi Gonzaga Hospital, Regione Gonzole 10, Orbassano, 10043 Turin, Italy*

Correspondence should be addressed to Adele Latina; adelelatina@hotmail.it

Academic Editor: Wayne V. Moore

Adrenal insufficiency is a potentially life-threatening condition when it occurs acutely, as in adrenal hemorrhage. Generally it is not reversible and requires chronic replacement therapy. Acute intermittent porphyria (AIP) is a rare genetic disease characterized by alterations in heme biosynthesis that result in accumulation of precursors in tissues. A crisis can be triggered by many conditions such as surgery and infections. Symptoms are similar to those of acute hypoadrenalism. Moreover, both conditions are characterized by hyponatremia. We describe the case of a postmenopausal woman known to be affected by AIP who developed after surgery a primary adrenal insufficiency associated with adrenal enlargement; the latter completely reverted in six months.

1. Introduction

Adrenal insufficiency is an infrequent endocrine disorder mostly due to autoimmune adrenalitis; less common causes are infections, trauma, and metastatic cancer. Adrenal insufficiency is a potentially life-threatening condition when acute, as in adrenal hemorrhage, necrosis or thrombosis. Generally, adrenal damage is not reversible and requires chronic replacement therapy.

Transient adrenal insufficiency has been described as a manifestation of viral, parasitic, or mycotic infection, in particular in premature newborn infants or immunocompromised patients.

Acute intermittent porphyria (AIP) is a rare genetic disease characterized by alterations in heme biosynthesis which result in the accumulation of precursors in tissues. An AIP crisis can be triggered by many conditions such as surgery, infections, fasting, and the use of many drugs including anesthetics. The symptoms of a crisis are abdominal pain, nausea, and vomiting, similar to those of acute hypoadrenalism. Both conditions are also characterized by the development of hyponatremia and, in biochemically active AIP, cortisol levels have been reported to be reduced; thus the diagnosis may be challenging.

We describe the case of a postmenopausal woman known to be affected by AIP who after surgery developed a primary adrenal insufficiency associated with adrenal enlargement, which completely reverted in six months. She was initially treated with replacement therapy which was subsequently reduced in dose, obtaining basal adrenocorticotrophic hormone (ACTH) and cortisol normalization, while maintaining an inadequate cortisol response to the ACTH test.

2. Case Presentation

A 65-year-old woman was referred to the intensive care unit under suspicion of a postoperative AIP crisis.

She had a history of previous surgery for breast fibroadenoma and was chronically affected by colonic diverticulosis, chronic gastritis, hypertension, and mild depressive syndrome. She was treated with a proton-pump inhibitor, metoprolol, enalapril, acetylsalicylic acid, and trazodone.

Porphyria had been diagnosed one year previously, after demonstration of porphobilinogen and aminolevulinic acid

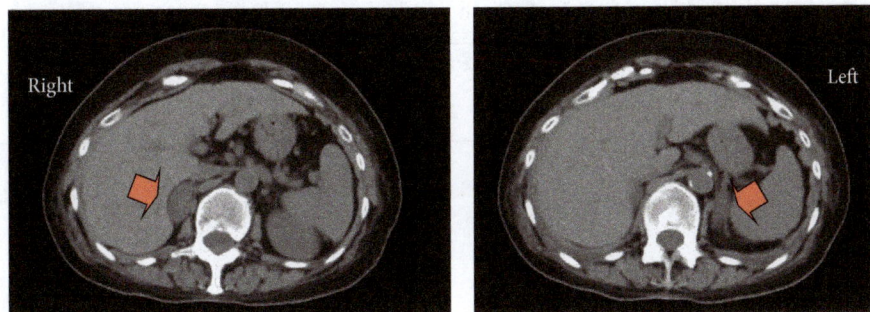

FIGURE 1: Abdomen CT showing bilateral adrenal enlargement, highlighted by red arrows, with a hyperdense central area of 2 cm of maximum diameter (HU 25–35) in right adrenal gland.

TABLE 1: Biochemical data nine days after hip replacement.

		Reference values
RBC ($\times10^6$/uL)	2.96	4.2–5.4
Hb (g/dL)	9.0	12.0–16.0
MCV (fl)	88.9	77–94
PLT ($\times10^3$/uL)	150	150–400
aPTT (sec.)	47.2	25–40
CRP (mg/L)	215	<10
PCT (ng/mL)	0.305	<0.046
Na (mmol/L)	132.6	137–145
K (mmol/L)	3.0	3.6–5.0

increase during an episode of abdominal pain, vomiting, and hyponatremia. During the same hospitalization, because of the onset of chest pain, ECG alterations, and troponin increase, the patient underwent a coronary angiography which was negative for stenosis. Thus takotsubo, a stress cardiomyopathy simulating an acute coronary syndrome, was diagnosed. In this critical care context, an ACTH and cortisol assay were performed, resulting in 4.0 pM/L (n.v. 2–14) and 998.8 nM/L (n.v. 165.5–507.7), respectively.

Nine days after a right hip replacement surgery due to severe arthrosis, the patient developed nausea and vomiting, abdominal pain with paralytic ileus, urinary retention, and upper limb paresthesia.

Laboratory analysis (see Table 1) showed normochromic anemia, a platelet count in the lower range, prolonged partial thromboplastin time, elevated C-reactive protein and procalcitonin, hypokalemia, and hyponatremia. Thus, considering the symptoms, an acute AIP crisis was suspected.

A chest X-ray was taken, which showed focal pneumonia with bilateral pleural effusion.

The patient started treatment for AIP with hemin and glucose solution, in addition to antibiotic treatment.

Due to the persistence of severe hyponatremia (123.8 mmol/L) and symptoms such as asthenia and nausea 19 days later, hypoadrenalism was suspected. The ACTH was 43 pM/L and cortisol 163.3 nM/L (data confirmed by a second sample) with PRA 0.3 μg/L/h (normal values: 0,60–4,18; RIA Immunotech Beckman Coulter), aldosterone 47.2 pmol/L (normal values: 48,3–270,0; RIA Immunotech Beckman Coulter), and DHEA-S < 0.4 umol/L (CLIA, Centaur XPT, Siemens). The patient was treated with no drug interfering with adrenal function. The ACTH test 250 μg iv showed no response of cortisol (see Table 2).

An abdominal computed tomography (CT) showed bilateral adrenal enlargement, with a hyperdense central area of 2 cm maximum diameter (HU 25–35) in the right adrenal gland (Figure 1). No suspicious lesion was identified.

Anti-adrenal antibodies were undetectable, as were anti-cardiolipin antibodies.

A tuberculin test was negative and so were tests on candida and aspergillus antigens. CMV DNA was undetectable. Anti-HIV and anti-treponema antibodies were also negative. Other mycosis infections (cryptococcosis, histoplasmosis, and coccidioidomycosis) and parasitoses (trypanosomiasis) were ruled out through appropriate serological tests.

The patient was initially treated with oral cortisone acetate, 25 mg in the morning and 12.5 mg in the afternoon, with rapid improvement of symptoms and normalization of sodium levels. The patient was then discharged on glucocorticoid replacement therapy (cortisone acetate 12.5 mg twice a day). Diagnosis of primary hypoadrenalism of uncertain etiology associated with bilateral adrenal enlargement was confirmed.

Three months later, the basal cortisol was 149.0 nM/L which did not increase (see Table 2) after the ACTH test (24 h after cortisone acetate withdrawal). Basal ACTH was 71 pM/L, PRA 1.0 μg/L/h, aldosterone 322.2 pmol/L, and DHEA-S < 0.4 umol/L.

In a CT repeated 6 months later, adrenal glands presented with normalized volume (Figure 2), and, in particular, the right lesion was no longer detected.

One year later, after gradual reduction in the dose of cortisone acetate (6.25 mg twice a day and then 6.25 mg once a day), ACTH and basal cortisol had normalized (see Table 2). However the cortisol remained nonresponsive after ACTH, with PRA and aldosterone always normal and DHEA-S unchanged.

At present (30 months after diagnosis) the patient is continuing a minimal dose of cortisone acetate (6.25 mg once a day) without symptoms. The last ACTH was 18 pM/L with normal PRA and aldosterone. Cortisol basal levels remain in the normal range and are progressively increasing

TABLE 2: Adrenal function before hip replacement and during follow-up.

	Time with respect to hip replacement					
	One year before	19 days after	21 days after	3 months after	12 months after	30 months after
ACTH (pM/L) n.v. 2–14	4	43		71	11	18
Basal cortisol (nM/L) n.v. 165.5–507.7	998.8	163.3	278.7	149.0	366.9	477.3
Cortisol 30' after ACTH 250 μg iv			278.7	162.8	366.9	460.8
Cortisol 60' after ACTH 250 μg iv			264.9	154.5	331.1	502.1

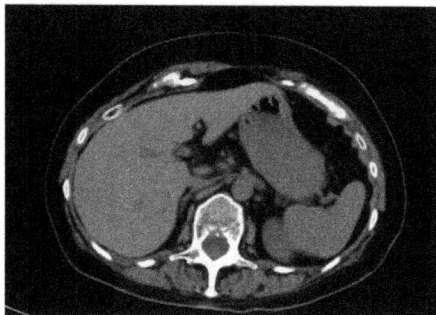

FIGURE 2: Abdomen CT showing adrenal glands normalized in volume 6 months later.

(see Table 2), although there has still been no response of the cortisol to the ACTH test. At CT examination the left adrenal gland was of normal volume, while the right one showed an apparent reduction in size with an inhomogeneous structure. These recent data support the progressive recovery of the glucocorticoid secretion, although with an incomplete functional normalization. Subsequent follow-up will assess whether the partial deficit is persistent or if definitive recovery is possible.

3. Discussion

Adrenal insufficiency is a rare condition mostly due to autoimmune disease but potentially developing after trauma, infections, neoplastic infiltration, or vascular damage, which generally requires chronic replacement therapy.

Transient adrenal insufficiency on the other hand is infrequent and is reported in the literature in premature newborn, in infective diseases, in survivors of critical illness [1], or, rarely, following acute adrenal hemorrhage [2]. Such a hemorrhage is a severe potentially life-threatening or even lethal condition when massive and bilateral. The clinical diagnosis is challenging. This is particularly the case in critically ill patients, due to nonspecific symptoms and signs such as abdominal pain, vomiting, fever, hypotension, and altered conscious state. Moreover a limited adrenal hemorrhage may give nonspecific symptoms. Hemorrhage has been described after surgery, such as cholecystectomy, total knee arthroplasty, duodenopancreatectomy, and vertebral surgery,

in sepsis, and is rarely reported as a spontaneous event, mostly in pregnancy and in particular conditions such as polycythemia vera and antiphospholipid syndrome.

In our patient, who experienced an acute primary hypoadrenalism with bilateral glandular enlargement, the CT appearance and subsequent partial normalization of the adrenal function could be consistent with a bilateral congestion leading to a hemorrhage, more evident in the right adrenal gland, which had presumably occurred 1-2 weeks before the imaging.

The history of AIP delayed the diagnosis of hypoadrenalism due to the development of symptoms suggesting a postoperative crisis. This delay may explain the CT appearance of the adrenals, which was not typical of a hemorrhage [3], though the hyperdense central area could be due to the outbreak where the greatest concentrations of hemoglobin were localized.

In our patient adrenal insufficiency seems to be a consequence of recent surgery, which can potentially induce adrenal hemorrhage, by itself but in particular due to the heparin treatment, which is routinely used in the postoperative period. The cortisol increase which had been observed during a critical stress condition (takotsubo cardiomyopathy) presumably indicates normal adrenal function, at least one year before. Autoimmune and infective hypoadrenalism were ruled out. Risk factors for adrenal hemorrhage were present such as postsurgery heparin treatment (which could explain the platelet count in the lower range and the prolonged partial thromboplastin time) and the occurrence of septic condition, which may have worsened the clinical status. Undetectable anticardiolipin antibodies, which are the most sensitive in diagnosing antiphospholipid syndrome [4], allow reasonably excluding this cause of adrenal failure.

The hypothesis of transient adrenal insufficiency related to a poor entity hemorrhage is consistent with the clinical evolution of the patient who reverted to normal adrenal CT presentation in 6 months and to almost normal basal function in 12 months. However, the lack of cortisol response to ACTH test suggests that cortisol secretion could not be further stimulated and therefore that the adrenal functional recovery was partial.

AIP patients present similar symptoms to those of acute hypoadrenalism (abdominal pain, nausea, and vomiting) thus resulting in a potential confounder for clinicians. To the best of our knowledge only two cases of acute hypoad-renalism have been reported after hip replacement. The first was subsequent to enoxaparin-induced thrombocytopenia [5], and the second was in a 75-year-old woman treated after surgery with dabigatran who underwent thrombolysis for massive pulmonary embolism [6]. In both cases, adrenal insufficiency was definitive.

Our case highlights how difficult the differential diagnosis is in AIP patients, in whom adrenal insufficiency can be misdiagnosed because of similar manifestations. A cause-effect relationship between AIP, major surgery, and hypoa-drenalism is conceivable but it cannot be proved: these conditions could be coincident even if independent.

However, acute hypoadrenalism represents a potential life-threatening condition which needs to be taken into account, especially when severe and persistent hyponatremia is observed.

Disclosure

This research was not supported by any specific grant from any funding agency in the public, commercial, or nonprofit sector.

References

[1] E. S. Nylen and B. Muller, "Endocrine changes in critical illness," *Journal of Intensive Care Medicine*, vol. 19, no. 2, pp. 67–82, 2004.

[2] A. Vella, T. B. Nippoldt, and J. C. Morris III, "Adrenal hemorrhage: a 25-year experience at the Mayo Clinic," *Mayo Clinic Proceedings*, vol. 76, no. 2, pp. 161–168, 2001.

[3] M. G. Lykissas, S. H. Galanis, A. C. Borodimos, and S. G. Pakos, "CT diagnosis of acute adrenal insufficiency due to bilateral adrenal haemorrhage," *European Journal of Radiology Extra*, vol. 57, no. 1, pp. 31–33, 2006.

[4] F. Presotto, F. Fornasini, C. Betterle, G. Federspil, and M. Rossato, "Acute adrenal failure as the heralding symptom of primary antiphospholipid syndrome: report of a case and review of the literature," *European Journal of Endocrinology*, vol. 153, no. 4, pp. 507–514, 2005.

[5] F. Reverdy, M. Freichet, J.-M. Grozel, C. Tassin, and V. Piriou, "Bilateral adrenal hemorrhage after heparin-induced thrombocytopenia, a rare cause of shock," *Annales Françaises d'Anesthésie et de Réanimation*, vol. 32, no. 3, pp. 206-207, 2013.

[6] M. Best, K. Palmer, Q. C. Jones, and C. G. Wathen, "Acute adrenal failure following anticoagulation with dabigatran after hip replacement and thrombolysis for massive pulmonary embolism," *BMJ Case Reports*, vol. 2013, no. 11, 2013.

11

A Large PROP1 Gene Deletion in a Turkish Pedigree

Suheyla Gorar ⓘ,[1] **Doga Turkkahraman** ⓘ,[2] **and Kanay Yararbas**[3]

[1]*Department of Endocrinology and Metabolism, Antalya Education and Research Hospital, 07100 Antalya, Turkey*
[2]*Department of Pediatric Endocrinology, Antalya Education and Research Hospital, 07100 Antalya, Turkey*
[3]*Department of Medical Genetics, Acibadem Mehmet Ali Aydinlar University, 34752 Istanbul, Turkey*

Correspondence should be addressed to Suheyla Gorar; sgorar@hotmail.com

Academic Editor: J. Paul Frindik

Pituitary-specific paired-like homeodomain transcription factor, PROP1, is associated with multiple pituitary hormone deficiency. Alteration of the gene encoding the PROP1 may affect somatotropes, thyrotropes, and lactotropes, as well as gonadotropes and corticotropes. We performed genetic analysis of PROP1 gene in a Turkish pedigree with three siblings who presented with short stature. Parents were first degree cousins. Index case, a boy, had somatotrope, gonadotrope, thyrotrope, and corticotrope deficiency. However, two elder sisters had somatotroph, gonadotroph, and thyrotroph deficiency and no corticotroph deficiency. On pituitary magnetic resonance, partial empty sella was detected with normal bright spot in all siblings. In genetic analysis, we found a gross deletion involving PROP1 coding region. In conclusion, we report three Turkish siblings with a gross deletion in PROP1 gene. Interestingly, although little boy with combined pituitary hormone deficiency has adrenocorticotropic hormone (ACTH) deficiency, his elder sisters with the same gross PROP1 deletion have no ACTH deficiency. This finding is in line with the fact that patients with PROP1 mutations may have different phenotype/genotype correlation.

1. Introduction

The anatomical development of hypothalamic-pituitary-thyroid axis is completed during the first gestational trimester. Transcription factor genes playing a role in the development of hypothalamus and pituitary are pituitary transcription factor 1 (PIT1), Prophet of Pit-1 (PROP1), LIM Homeobox 3 (LHX3), LIM Homeobox 4 (LHX4), and HESX Homeobox 1 (HESX1) which all are known to be important for organ commitment and embryonic pituitary cell differentiation. In case of incomplete differentiation of anterior pituitary gland, one or more of these hormones may be affected, causing combined pituitary hormone deficiency (CPHD) [1]. This condition is mainly sporadic in occurrence, but familial forms have also been described with autosomal recessive, autosomal dominant, and X-linked recessive modes of inheritance. In familial or sporadic CPHD cases, the most common causes are PIT1 and PROP1 gene defects [2].

PROP1 gene is located on chromosome 5q35. Inactivating mutations in PROP1 perturb ontogenesis of pituitary gonadotrophs, somatotrophs, lactotrophs, and thyrotrophs. Somatotropic, thyrotropic, and gonadotropic function impairments manifests clinically as short stature, neonatal hypoglycemia, sequential loss of anterior pituitary tropic hormones [3].

Index case admitted to pediatric endocrinology clinic with complaint of short stature. His family history revealed presence of similar symptoms in his two siblings. Following hormonal examination of the cases, we conducted genetic analyses. PROP1 mutation screening detected a homozygous deletion of the entire PROP1 in three patients.

2. Case Presentation

2.1. Case 1: Index Case. A 12.3-year-old male patient was referred to our pediatric endocrinology clinic for evaluation of short stature. He has been using levothyroxine (LT4) for hypothyroidism for more than 2 years. In medical history, he was born at term weighing 3500 g with uneventful gestation and delivery. His parents were first degree cousins. The height of the mother and the father was 165.5 and 172 cm, respectively. He had three sisters and one brother. His brother and one of the elder sisters were healthy and 175 cm and 165 cm tall, respectively. On physical examination, height was 129 cm (SDS: −3.2) and weight was 28 kg (body mass index, BMI: 16.8, −1.0 SDS).

Target height was 175.2 cm (SDS: −0.2). Testicular volume was 2 ml bilaterally with a 3 cm penile length. Bone age was 9 years. Laboratory findings revealed that free thyroxine (FT4) is 1.2 ng/dl (N: 0.61–1.57), thyroid stimulating hormone (TSH) is 0.01 μIU/ml (N: 0.37–5), thyroid autoantibodies were negative, prolactin (PRL) is 4.5 ng/ml (N: 2.6–13.1), adrenocorticotropic hormone (ACTH) is 21.3 pg/ml (N: 4.7–48.8), cortisol is 6.8 μg/dl (N: 6.7–22.6), and insulin-like growth factor 1 (IGF-1) is 12.8 ng/ml (N: 85.2–248.8). Thyroid ultrasonography revealed a hypoplasic thyroid gland (1.7 ml) with normal parenchyma. On pituitary magnetic resonance (MRI), partial empty sella was detected with normal bright spot (pituitary height was 2.8 mm). Clonidine and L.DOPA stimulated peak serum growth hormone (GH) levels were 2.1 ng/ml and 1.9 ng/ml, respectively. With these results diagnosis of GH deficiency was confirmed, and recombinant growth hormone (rGH) was initiated. On follow-up, low dose (1 μg) ACTH stimulation test was performed, and adrenal deficiency was confirmed (peak cortisol: 12.1 μg/dl). Then, oral hydrocortisone replacement therapy was initiated (10 mg/m^2/day).

At 14.3 years, he was still prepubertal with testicular volume of 3 ml bilaterally. Basal level of testosterone was <0.01 ng/ml. Then, LHRH stimulation test was performed, and central hypogonadism was confirmed (peak luteinizing hormone, LH; 0.62 mIU/ml, and peak follicle stimulating hormone, FSH; 0.85 mIU/ml). Intramuscular depot form of testosterone was initiated, 50 mg/monthly.

2.2. Case 2: 3-Sister Siblings of Index Case. The 22- and 24-year-old females who are sisters of index case were referred to our endocrinology outpatient clinic. In their delivery history, they were delivered via spontaneous vaginal birth with uneventful gestation and delivery. They did not present hypoglycemia or respiratory distress during the neonatal period.

At the age of 13, junior sister was diagnosed with GH deficiency and received rGH and LT4 replacement therapy for 8 years but the hormonal examination resulting from that period could not be retrieved. Her height and weight measurements were 145 cm (−2.83 SDS) and 37 kg (BMI: 17.6, −1.7 SDS), respectively. She was 12 years old at the onset of menarche and was having irregular menstrual cycles with long periods of amenorrhea/oligomenorrhea. There was no axillary/pubic hair, and breast development was Tanner stage II. Her mental function was normal. Bone age was adult, and epiphyseal lines were closed. The ovaries were atrophic on pelvic USG. On pituitary MRI, partial empty sella was detected with normal bright spot (pituitary height was 1.5 mm). Her basal hormone levels are shown in Table 1. The patient did not respond to LHRH test (basal FSH was 0.01 mIU/ml and LH was 0.11 mIU/ml; peak FSH was 0.01 mIU/ml and peak LH was 0.12 mIU/ml). There was no response to thyrotropin releasing hormone (TRH) stimulation test (basal TSH 0.04 mU/L; peak TSH 0.03 mU/L). Although sufficient cortisol response was obtained in insulin-induced hypoglycemia test, no sufficient GH response was obtained. During hypoglycemia, peak cortisol level was 26 μg/dL, while peak GH level was 0.01 ng/mL. The patient

TABLE 1: Baseline hormone levels of sister siblings.

Hormone (normal range)	Sibling 1	Sibling 2
ACTH (4,5–48 pg/ml)	12,5	7,5
Kortizol (6,7–22,6 ug/dl)	9,82	2,34
FSH (1,2–19,1 mIU/ml)	0,01	0,08
LH (1,24–8,6 mIU/ml)	0,01	0,04
TSH (0,34–5,86 ulU/ml)	0,01	0,03
FT4 (0,61–1,12 ng/dl)	1,10	0,99
Prolactin (2–15 ng/ml)	9,12	4,43
GH (0,003–0,971 ng/ml)	0,02	0,01
IGF-1 (135–449 ng/ml)	4,11	10,62

ACTH: adrenocorticotropic hormone; FSH: follicle stimulating hormone; LH: luteinizing hormone; TSH: thyroid stimulating hormone; FT4: free thyroxine; GH: growth hormone; IGF-1: insulin-like growth factor 1.

was put on LT4, conjugated estrogen, and adult-dose of rGH replacement therapy.

At the age of 15, elder sister was diagnosed with GH deficiency and central hypothyroidism and has received rGH and LT4 replacement therapy for 9 years. The hormonal evaluation results from that period could not be retrieved. Height was 154 cm (−1.43 SDS) and weight was 49 kg (BMI: 20.6, −0.3 SDS). Her age at onset of menarche was 12 years and her menstruation history was similar to that of her sister. Upon psychiatric evaluation, she had hard time in social interaction and self-expression, and she was found to have borderline intelligence with an Intelligence Quotient Test (IQT) score of 80. Her bone age was adult, and epiphyseal lines were closed. Ovaries were atrophic on pelvic USG. On pituitary MRI, partial empty sella was detected with normal bright spot (pituitary height was 2.5 mm). Basal hormone levels are given Table 1. The patient did not respond to the LHRH test (basal FSH 0.08 mIU/ml and LH 0.09 mIU/ml; peak FSH 0.09 mIU/ml and LH 0.11 mIU/ml). Additionally, there was no response to TRH stimulation test (basal TSH 0.01 mU/L; peak TSH 0.01 mU/L). During insulin-induced hypoglycemia test, maximum cortisol level was measured as 19.5 mg/dL, and growth hormone level was 0.01 ng/mL. With these findings, the case was put on LT4, conjugated estrogen, and adult doses of rGH replacement therapy.

2.3. Genetic Analysis. Genomic DNA of the family members was extracted according to the manufacturer's standard procedure using the QIAamp DNA Blood Midi Kit (Qiagen, Hilden, Germany). The DNA samples were quantified with a nanophotometer (Implen, Germany) and used at a concentration of 50 ng/μL. PROP1 gene was amplified using PCR primers: Forward (5′ ACCTACACACACATTCAGAGAC 3′), Reverse (5′ TGGAGCCTATGCTTTCAGC 3′), Forward (5′ AAAGACTGGAGCAGCACAGG3′), Reverse (5′ GGTGGTGAGATGAGGCCTGT 3′), and Forward (5′ GCCTTGTGGAAGAGCTTTACTCC 3′), Reverse (5′ CACCATGCATCTGCTTCACCC 3′). PCRs were validated by using 2% agarose gel electrophoresis (Fermentas, Lituenia). PCRs for each individual were mixed to obtain PCR pools, purified and quantified.

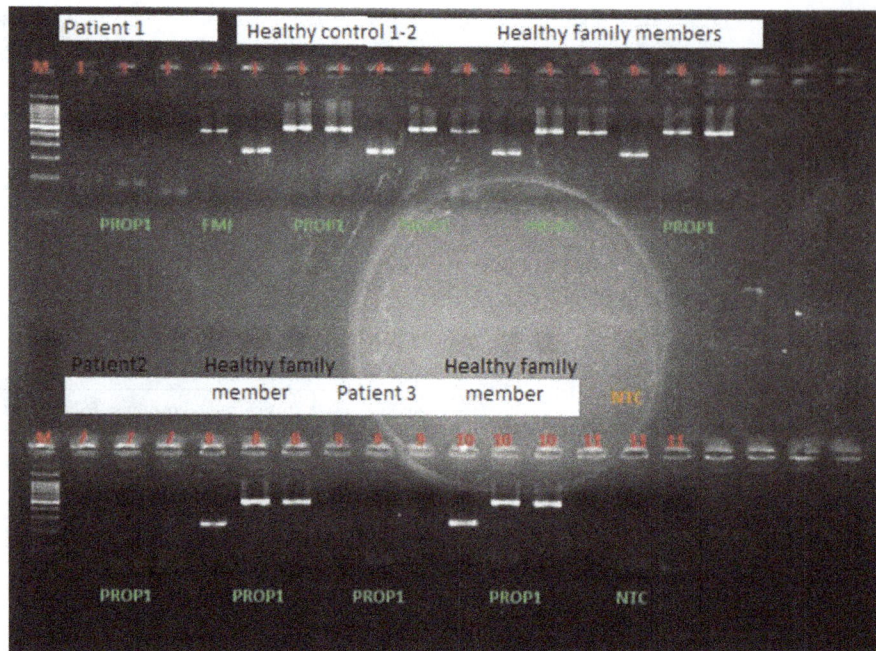

FIGURE 1: Three patients showed no amplification in PROP1 locus, whereas reference gene (Mediterranean fever-MEFV) was amplified. Healthy controls and healthy family members showed successful amplifications either.

Purifications were done by using exosap purification program (ExoSAP-IT, Affymetrix Inc., USA). Second Sephadex column (Sigma, Germany) was used for the PCR purification. Gel electrophoresis revealed no amplification of the gene, so in order confirm a possible gross deletion, healthy controls were tested for the same gene, as well as healthy family members. In addition Mediterranean fever (MEFV) gene amplification was performed simultaneously as reference amplification. MEFV amplification was successful in all patients. On behalf of these results, gross deletion involving PROP1 coding region was concluded as disease causing mutation in these patients (Figure 1).

3. Discussion

Genetic aetiologies of isolated pituitary hormone deficiency or CPHD have been researched for many years. CPHD occurs due to recognized mutations of transcription factors such as HESX1, PROP1, POU1F1, LHX3, and LHX4. PROP1 mutations represent the most common known genetic defect of both familial and sporadic CPHD. Phenotypic characteristics may be variable in CPHD result from these transcription factors' mutations, including PROP1. Published case reports, population studies, and reviews on genetic analysis of CPHD have shown new genetic variations, differences in the severity of the hormonal deficits, and the time of onset. As a result from clinical and hormonal phenotype highly variable [4–6], general properties of PROP1 mutation are a clinical disorder where GH deficiency is observed together with one or more anterior pituitary hormone deficiencies. The main clinical symptom is growth retardation with an onset during infancy or early childhood. Hypothyroidism is often mild and develops during late infancy or childhood. The affected individuals

are not expected to be infertile, but their secondary sexual development can be delayed and incomplete. Untreated men generally have smaller testes and penis. Some of the affected women have menstrual bleeding, but may often require hormone replacement therapy afterwards. ACTH deficiency is less common but may also be seen, which usually develops during adolescence or adulthood [6]. PROP1 deficiency was first discovered among Ames mice which clinically results in dwarf mice with CPHD. The most common pituitary hormone deficiencies are of GH, TSH, FSH, LH, and PRL, while ACTH deficiency is also observed, though rarely [3].

It was shown that deletion of PROP1 in mice causes severe pituitary hypoplasia with failure of the entire PIT1 lineage and delayed gonadotrope development. Pituitary hormone deficiencies caused secondary endocrine problems and a high rate of perinatal mortality due to respiratory distress. Lung atelectasis in mutants correlated with reduced levels of NKX2.1 (TITF1; 600635) and surfactant (SFTPA1; 178630). Lethality of mice homozygous for either the null allele or a spontaneous hypomorphic allele was strongly influenced by genetic background [7]. As further human studies included familial total deletions of the gene all causing CPHD phenotype, gross deletions became well characterized in Human Gene Mutation Database (HGMD) as disease causing mutations [2, 8–11]. PROP1 spans less than 4 kb of genomic DNA; no benign copy number or deletion variations are defined in Decipher or Genomic Variant Database (DGV). The extent of the reported deletions was variable but all totally covered the PROP1 gene. This is the sixth report of gross PROP1 deletion worldwide. No further information about the deletion is available in this family since high resolution array was not performed. Deletions were detected by PCR gel electrophoresis. Amplification was obtained in obligate heterozygote carriers and since the reactions were performed with reference genes and healthy controls, no further confirmatory test was performed.

In this study, we presented the hormonal and genetic evaluations of three siblings having PROP1 deletion. Interestingly, although little boy with CPHD has ACTH deficiency, her elder sisters with the same gross PROP1 deletion have no ACTH deficiency. Peak cortisol levels of elder sisters were considered adequate in insulin-induced hypoglycemia test [12, 13]. Also, they were stable in terms of clinical and biochemical status. But, clinical and hormonal evaluations of cases were continued follow-up because of possible adrenal insufficiency in adulthood period. This finding is in line with the fact that patients with PROP1 mutations definitely may have different phenotype/genotype correlation. Deladoëy et al. [14] studied 36 families with a total of 73 affected patients with CPHD. They demonstrated, based on a great variability in phenotype, the secretion of pituitary-derived hormones (GH, TSH, LH, and FSH) decline gradually with age, following a different pattern and time scale in each individual. On the other hand, seven patients presented low basal levels of cortisol and ACTH, but stimulated levels after insulin-induced hypoglycemia revealed no abnormality. None of the patients were on cortisol replacement therapy. Similarly, et al. [15] showed that two siblings with PROP1 mutation who presented with short stature have not corticotropin deficiency. In a multicentric study conducted by Vallette-Kasic et al. [16] in France, 27 unrelated families originated from five different countries screened for PROP1 gene anomalies. Patients were included on the basis of GH deficiency associated with at least one other pituitary hormone deficiency. Cortisol was initially found normal in all patients, but late onset ACTH deficiency was observed in four patients. In insulin-induced hypoglycemia test, two patients were blunted cortisol response and given cortisol replacement therapy. As a result, they emphasized that corticotroph deficiency was frequently observed in association with GH, TSH, and gonadotropin deficiency in PROP1 gene alteration and should be carefully sought during follow-up. In another study, discussed by Reynaud et al. [17], genetic screening was performed in 195 patients with combined pituitary hormone deficiency. In 109 patients without extrapituitary abnormalities, 20 had PROP1 mutations, including eight patients with a family history of CPHD. Eighteen of 20 patients carried PROP1 mutations had gonadotroph and somatotroph deficiency at postpubertal age, while two patients had corticotroph, thyrotroph, and somatotroph deficiency at pubertal age.

In conclusion, PROP1 gene has maintenance role in five types of principal anterior pituitary hormone-secreting cells, which are somatotroph, lactotroph, thyrotroph, gonadotroph, and corticotroph, basis, and their differentiation progress. But, in human trials different mutations that cause CPHD in the PROP1 gene have been shown [2, 5]. Variability of mutations and deletions in PROP1 gene can cause different types of hormone deficiency. This state is very important for therapy and follow-up of the patients.

Disclosure

Suheyla Gorar is the corresponding and primary author of this report.

Authors' Contributions

Index case and his siblings were evaluated, diagnosed, and treated by Doga Turkkahraman and Suheyla Gorar, respectively. Kanay Yararbas analyzed and interpreted the patient's genetic data. All authors read and approved the final paper.

References

[1] D. Kelberman and M. T. Dattani, "Hypopituitarism oddities: congenital causes.," *Hormone Research*, vol. 68, pp. 138–144, 2007.

[2] M. G. Abrão, M. V. Leite, L. R. Carvalho et al., "Combined pituitary hormone deficiency (CPHD) due to a complete PROP1 deletion," *Clinical Endocrinology*, vol. 65, no. 3, pp. 294–300, 2006.

[3] C. Asteria, J. H. A. Oliveira, J. Abucham, and P. Beck-Peccoz, "Central hypocortisolism as part of combined pituitary hormone deficiency due to mutations of PROP-1 gene," *European Journal of Endocrinology*, vol. 143, no. 3, pp. 347–352, 2000.

[4] L. Brunerova, I. Cermakova, B. Kalvachova, J. Skrenkova, R. Poncova, and P. Sedlak, "Therapy-induced growth and sexual maturation in a developmentally infantile adult patient with a PROP1 Mutation," *Frontiers in Endocrinology*, vol. 8, 2017.

[5] M. Elizabeth, A. C. S. Hokken-Koelega, J. Schuilwerve et al., "Genetic screening of regulatory regions of pituitary transcription factors in patients with idiopathic pituitary hormone deficiencies," *Pituitary*, vol. 21, pp. 76–83, 2018.

[6] M. Giordano, "Genetic causes of isolated and combined pituitary hormone deficiency," *Best Practice & Research Clinical Endocrinology & Metabolism*, vol. 30, no. 6, pp. 679–691, 2016.

[7] I. O. Nasonkin, R. D. Ward, L. T. Raetzman et al., "Pituitary hypoplasia and respiratory distress syndrome in Prop1 knockout mice," *Human Molecular Genetics*, vol. 13, no. 22, pp. 2727–2735, 2004.

[8] D. Kelberman, J. P. G. Turton, K. S. Woods et al., "Molecular analysis of novel PROP1 mutations associated with combined pituitary hormone deficiency (CPHD)," *Clinical Endocrinology*, vol. 70, no. 1, pp. 96–103, 2009.

[9] A. Akcay, K. Ulucan, N. Taskin et al., "Suprasellar mass mimicking a hypothalamic glioma in a patient with a complete PROP1 deletion," *European Journal of Medical Genetics*, vol. 56, no. 8, pp. 445–451, 2013.

[10] K. Hemchand, K. Anuradha, S. Neeti et al., "Entire prophet of Pit-1 (PROP-1) gene deletion in an Indian girl with combined pituitary hormone deficiencies," *Journal of Pediatric Endocrinology and Metabolism*, vol. 24, no. 7-8, pp. 579–580, 2011.

[11] H. Zhang, Y. Wang, L. Han, X. Gu, and D. Shi, "A large deletion of PROP1 gene in patients with combined pituitary hormone deficiency from two unrelated Chinese pedigrees," *Hormone Research in Paediatrics*, vol. 74, no. 2, pp. 98–105, 2010.

[12] S. R. Bornstein, B. Allolio, W. Arlt et al., "Diagnosis and treatment of primary adrenal insufficiency: an endocrine society clinical practice guideline," *The Journal of Clinical Endocrinology & Metabolism*, vol. 101, no. 2, pp. 364–389, 2016.

[13] Y. Simsek, Z. Karaca, F. Tanriverdi, K. Unluhizarci, A. Selcuklu, and F. Kelestimur, "A comparison of low-dose ACTH, glucagon stimulation and insulin tolerance test in patients with pituitary disorders," *Clinical Endocrinology*, vol. 82, no. 1, pp. 45–52, 2015.

[14] J. Deladoëy, C. Flück, A. Büyükgebiz et al., "Hot spot in the PROP1 gene responsible for combined pituitary hormone deficiency," *The Journal of Clinical Endocrinology & Metabolism*, vol. 84, no. 5, pp. 1645–1650, 1999.

[15] T. C. Vieira, M. R. Dias da Silva, J. M. Cerutti et al., "Familial combined pituitary hormone deficiency due to a novel mutation R99Q in the hot spot region of Prophet of Pit-1 presenting as constitutional growth delay," *The Journal of Clinical Endocrinology & Metabolism*, vol. 88, no. 1, pp. 38–44, 2003.

[16] S. Vallette-Kasic, A. Barlier, C. Teinturier et al., "PROP1 gene screening in patients with multiple pituitary hormone deficiency reveals two sites of hypermutability and a high incidence of corticotroph deficiency," *The Journal of Clinical Endocrinology & Metabolism*, vol. 86, no. 9, pp. 4529–4535, 2001.

[17] R. Reynaud, M. Gueydan, A. Saveanu et al., "Genetic screening of combined pituitary hormone deficiency: Experience in 195 patients," *The Journal of Clinical Endocrinology & Metabolism*, vol. 91, no. 9, pp. 3329–3336, 2006.

12

A Rapid Biochemical and Radiological Response to the Concomitant Therapy with Temozolomide and Radiotherapy in an Aggressive ACTH Pituitary Adenoma

Ana Misir Krpan,[1] **Tina Dusek,**[2] **Zoran Rakusic,**[1] **Mirsala Solak,**[3] **Ivana Kraljevic,**[3] **Vesna Bisof,**[4] **David Ozretic,**[5] **and Darko Kastelan**[2]

[1]*Department of Oncology, University Hospital Center Zagreb, Kispaticeva 12, 10000 Zagreb, Croatia*
[2]*Zagreb University School of Medicine, Department of Endocrinology, University Hospital Center Zagreb, Kispaticeva 12, 10000 Zagreb, Croatia*
[3]*Department of Endocrinology, University Hospital Center Zagreb, Kispaticeva 12, 10000 Zagreb, Croatia*
[4]*Osijek University School of Medicine, Department of Oncology, University Hospital Center Zagreb, Kispaticeva 12, 10000 Zagreb, Croatia*
[5]*Department of Radiology, University Hospital Center Zagreb, Kispaticeva 12, 10000 Zagreb, Croatia*

Correspondence should be addressed to Ana Misir Krpan; anamisirkrpan@yahoo.com

Academic Editor: Takeshi Usui

Background and Importance. In the last eight years temozolomide (TMZ) has been used as the last-line treatment modality for aggressive pituitary tumors to be applied after the failure of surgery, medical therapy, and radiotherapy. The objective was to achieve a rapid control of tumor growth and hormone normalization with concurrent chemoradiotherapy in a patient with very aggressive ACTH pituitary adenoma. *Clinical Presentation.* We describe a patient with an aggressive ACTH-producing adenoma treated with concurrent temozolomide and radiotherapy. The patient suffered from an aggressive ACTH adenoma resistant to surgical and medical treatment. After two months of concurrent temozolomide and radiotherapy, cortisol normalization and significant tumor shrinkage were observed. After 22 months of follow-up, there is still no evidence of tumor recurrence. *Conclusion.* Concurrent treatment with temozolomide and irradiation appears to be highly effective in the achievement of the tumor volume control as well as in the control of ACTH secretion in aggressive ACTH adenoma.

1. Background and Importance

Pituitary adenomas are common, mostly benign tumors that are rarely subject to oncological treatment. In symptomatic or secretory pituitary adenomas the first-line treatment is the surgical removal of the tumor, which may be followed by medical therapy if no satisfactory results are achieved by surgery. Radiation therapy is often part of a multidisciplinary treatment of functional and nonfunctional tumors, usually as a third-line treatment after the failure of surgical and/or medical treatment. Radiotherapy is indicated for recurrent or progressive tumors after surgery, surgically inaccessible tumors (e.g., tumors extending to cavernous sinus), and biochemically uncontrolled tumors after maximal surgical and medical therapy, and it is also used as the treatment of choice for patients who are not candidates for surgery.

In the last eight years, temozolomide (TMZ) has increasingly been used as the last-line treatment for aggressive pituitary tumors resistant to conventional therapy [1–12]. TMZ is an oral alkylating agent approved for the treatment of glioblastoma. When used for aggressive pituitary tumors, TMZ is usually given in the conventional scheme including up to 12 cycles of therapy [13]. We report a case of an aggressive ACTH-producing pituitary adenoma in which a combination of radiotherapy and TMZ led to rapid biochemical, radiological, and clinical response.

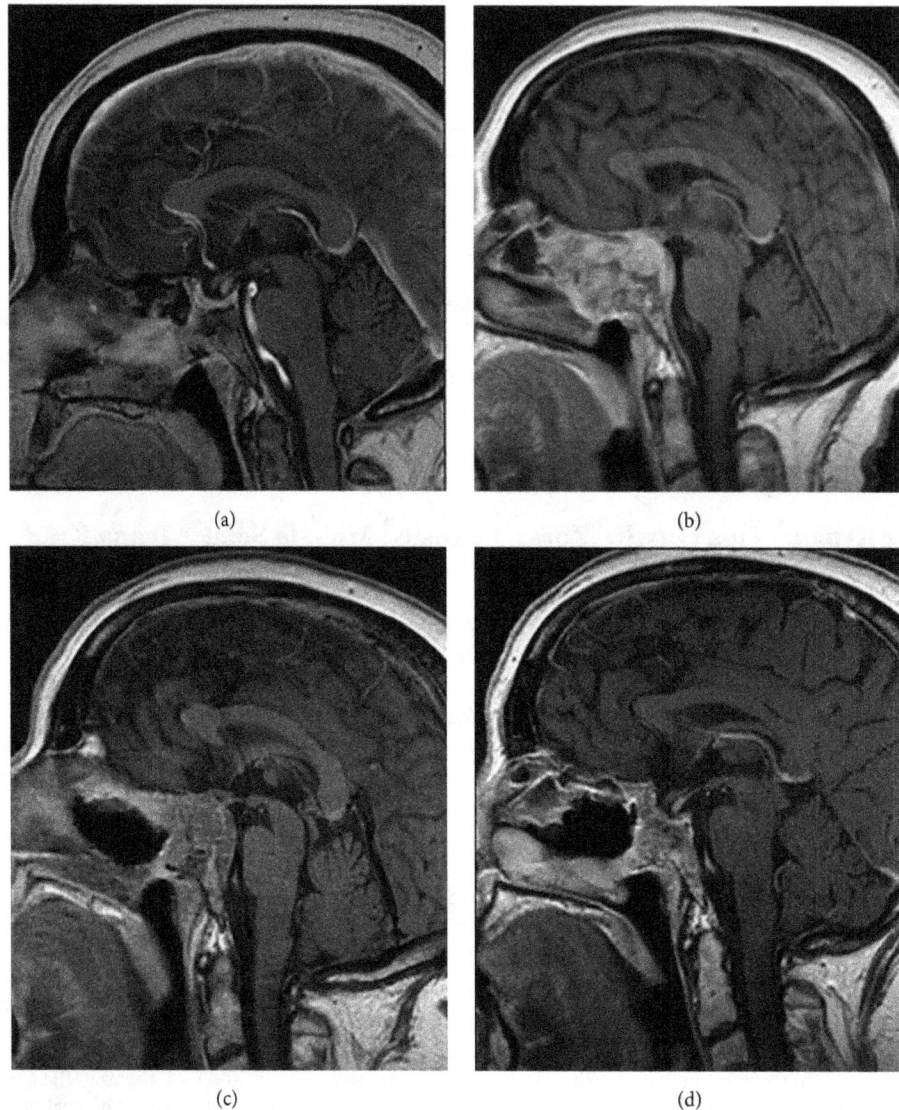

FIGURE 1: Pituitary MRI appearances (T1 postgadolinium weighted sagittal images). (a) After the first transsphenoidal operation for macrocorticotropinoma in 2010 with a small tumor remnant. (b) Three years after the first operation. Pituitary adenoma with destruction of the floor of the sella and invasion into sphenoid sinus and both cavernous sinuses. (c) Three months after the initiation of the concurrent therapy with TMZ and radiotherapy. (d) After the 6 cycles of TMZ. Stable pituitary remnant and biochemical control of the disease.

2. Clinical Presentation

We report a 64-year-old female with Cushing's disease (CD). In April 2010, the patient first had a transsphenoidal surgery of a 15 mm large macrocorticotropinoma. The surgery led to biochemical remission with a presence of a small tumor remnant (Figure 1(a)). The tumor histology was consistent with atypical adenoma (Ki-67 20%, no mitoses, p53 not tested). Two years after the operation, tumor regrowth and biochemical relapse were observed. Urinary free cortisol and ACTH levels were 3,400 nmol/dU (NV < 369 nmol/dU) and 65.3 pmol/l (NV < 16 pmol/L), respectively. MRI confirmed tumor progression in sphenoid and ethmoid sinuses, both cavernous sinuses, with infiltration of the sellar wall, clivus, and chiasmal compression (Figure 1(b)). The patient

suffered from headaches, visual field deficit, diplopia, ophthalmoplegia, and decreased visual acuity. The ketoconazole treatment was started. Transsphenoidal tumor reduction was performed, but severe hypercortisolism and ophthalmoplegia persisted. Postoperative MRI confirmed a large tumor remnant with infiltrative growth pattern destructing the bone (Figure 1(c)). The tumor tissue was positive for AE1/AE3, chromogranin, adrenocorticotropic hormone (ACTH), and growth hormone in some cells. Ki-67 was 10–20% and p53 positivity was present in less than 5% of cells (Figure 2). The repair enzyme O6-methylguanine-DNA methyltransferase (MGMT) was not determined. No distant metastases were found. The patient's general condition worsened with the right-side blepharoptosis, progressive visual impairment, and metabolic disturbances due to severe hypercortisolism.

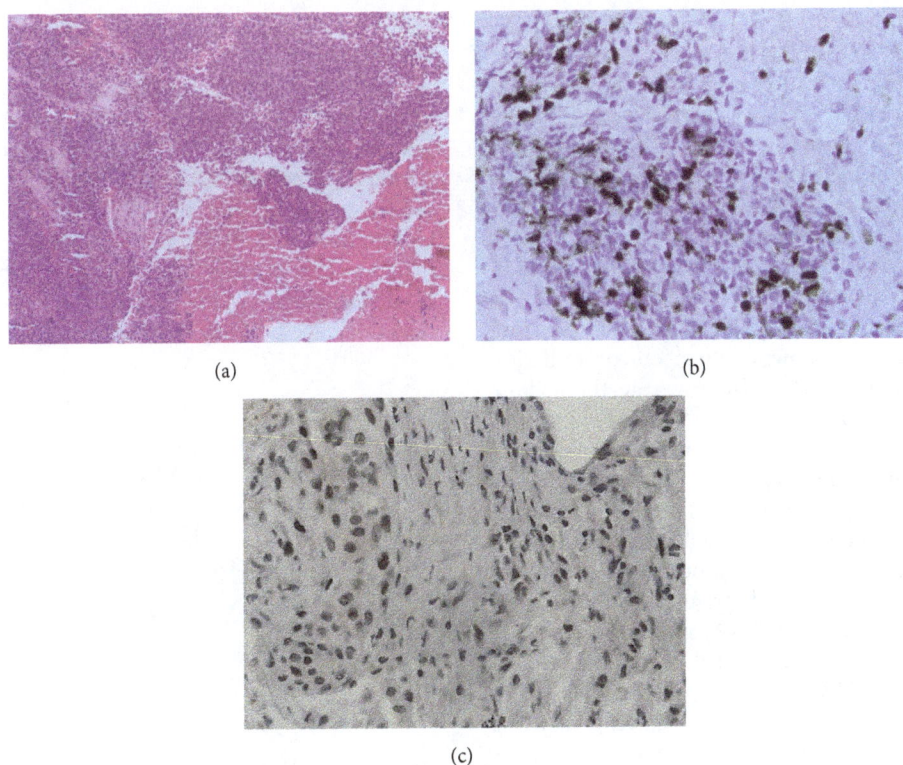

(a)

(b)

(c)

FIGURE 2: (a) HE staining of the pituitary macroadenoma tissue confirming atypical pituitary adenoma (magnification ×100). (b) Ki-67 positivity in tumor tissue of 10–20% (magnification ×400). (c) p53 positivity in less than 5% of cells (magnification ×400).

Due to the rapid growth of the tumor remnant and the high value of the proliferation marker Ki-67, we decided not to wait for the effect of radiotherapy, but to immediately proceed with concurrent chemoradiotherapy (daily radiotherapy fractions of 2.0 Gy to a total dosage of TD 54 Gy concurrent with TMZ 75 mg/m^2 per day). Radiotherapy was delivered by the linear accelerator and two opposed fields of 6/18 MV. Gross tumor volume (GTV) was 38.5 cm^3 and planning target volume (PTV) 137.7 cm^3. After two weeks, the patient's vision improved significantly with the recovery of the blepharoptosis and ophthalmoplegia, but she started to complain of weakness, dizziness, and fatigue. Low levels of morning cortisol (55 nmol/L (NR > 330 nmol/L)) were observed indicating biochemical remission of Cushing's disease and adrenocortical insufficiency. Ketoconazole was taken off and replacement therapy with hydrocortisone was started. The first follow-up MRI performed after 2 months of chemoradiotherapy showed the reduction of tumor volume of about 70%. We preceded with adjuvant TMZ in the dosage of 150 mg/m^2 in the first cycle (from day 1 to 5) and 200 mg/m^2 in the following five cycles (from day 1 to 5 every 28 days). The patient was in a significantly better clinical condition, on hydrocortisone replacement therapy and without major complaints or adverse events. The MRI after 3 and 6 months of therapy showed further tumor regression (Figure 1(d)). We decided to stop the treatment after 6 cycles and continued with a close follow- up. The last chemotherapy cycle was administered in January 2015. The patient tolerated the treatment very well, except for the fatigue reported from the beginning. Twenty-two months after the cessation of the TMZ treatment, the patient is still in remission of CD, with a stationary volume of the tumor remnant.

3. Discussion

ACTH-producing pituitary adenomas are generally benign tumors that are usually successfully treated with surgery. Medical therapy and radiotherapy are used in the case of surgical failure. In patients with CD, the overall tumor and hormone control rates in the reported studies are 97% and 74%, respectively, after a median follow-up of 8 years [14]. Fifty percent reduction in the urinary free cortisol level is usually observed 6 to 12 months after radiotherapy. It is estimated that the normalization of the serum cortisol level in patients with CD occurs about 24 months after radiotherapy [15]. The delay in the therapeutic response to radiotherapy is often unacceptable for some secretory, drug refractory tumors, as well as for aggressive tumors showing expansive growth.

Temozolomide is an orally available monofunctional DNA alkylating agent of the imidazotetrazine class. After spontaneous activation, it preferentially methylates DNA at N7 positions of guanine in guanine rich regions but also methylates N3 adenine and O6 guanine. There is a narrow pH window close to physiological pH at which the whole process of TMZ prodrug activation can occur. Brain tumors possess a more alkaline pH compared to surrounding healthy tissue, a situation which favors prodrug activation preferentially within tumor tissue. Methylation results in persistent DNA strand breaks, causing replication fork collapse. G2/M cell cycle arrest is triggered, occurring in the second cell cycle following treatment [16]. Both MGMT activity and mismatch repair (MMR) status of the tumor are important parameters that determine sensitivity to temozolomide [17].

In concomitant chemoradiotherapy, temozolomide reduces the number of cells in tumors undergoing radiation therapy by their independent cytotoxic action and by rendering tumor cells more susceptible to killing by ionizing radiation. Such drugs are potent enhancers of radiation response and thus might further improve the therapeutic outcome of chemoradiation therapy. The strategy of chemoradiation is to exploit the ability of chemotherapeutic agents to enhance tumor radioresponse. The enhancement denotes the existence of some type of interaction between drug and radiation at the molecular, cellular, or pathophysiologic level resulting in an antitumor effect greater than would be expected on the basis of additive actions. Temozolomide makes damaged DNA more susceptible to radiation damage resulting in enhanced cell killing [18]. In recent years the use of TMZ has been reported in aggressive pituitary tumors [1–12]. Raverot et al. reported 18 patients with ACTH tumors treated with TMZ. After 9.1 ± 4.7 cycles of therapy, biochemical response, defined as a 50% decrease in ACTH secretion, was observed in 67% of patients. In the same study, a reduction in tumor volume, defined as a 20% decrease in maximal tumor size, was observed in 56% of patients. According to the results of different studies, tumor shrinkage or hormonal response to temozolomide treatment is usually observed within weeks after treatment initiation in responding patients [19]. Treatment regimens with TMZ in pituitary tumors are variable, but the one most frequently used is the conventional regimen with 150–200 mg/m^2/day from days 1 to 5 every 28 days [20].

In the majority of the reported cases, TMZ has been used after the exhaustion of all the three treatment modalities (surgery, medical therapy, and radiotherapy). However, due to the rapid tumor growth resulting in the mass effect and uncontrolled hypercortisolism, we decided to apply a more aggressive therapeutic strategy using TMZ together with radiotherapy. Such a treatment regimen is usually applied in the treatment of high-grade glioma [21], which was the rationale for the choice of the treatment in the case of the aggressive pituitary adenoma in question. Besides the expected synergistic effects of the two different treatment modalities (TMZ and radiotherapy), a possible disadvantage of concurrent chemoradiotherapy is that it bears the risk of increased toxicity and side effects.

In our patient the effect of the combination of TMZ and radiotherapy was unexpectedly fast and led to rapid tumor shrinkage as well as to rapid control of hypercortisolism. The excellent therapeutic response could probably be attributed to the tumor histology consistent with atypical adenoma characterized by high proliferative indices and rapid cell division. Until now, there has only been one published case report on the use of the concurrent radiotherapy and TMZ in an aggressive nonfunctional adenoma, also showing good therapeutic

results [22]. Therefore, we might speculate about the possible potentiation of the radiation effect by TMZ in aggressive pituitary adenoma as reported in relation to glioblastomas [23]. We might also hypothesize that concurrent chemoradiotherapy has a promising role in the treatment of selected cases of rapidly growing, aggressive pituitary corticotropinoma with high proliferation indices. Since temozolomide has low toxicity, good tolerability, and two decades of proven efficacy in other brain tumors, the concurrent chemoradiotherapy should be considered earlier in the course of the disease.

4. Conclusion

The concurrent use of TMZ and radiotherapy appears to be a helpful alternative for the treatment of rapidly growing, aggressive pituitary ACTH-producing adenomas resistant to conventional treatment.

References

[1] L. V. Syro, H. Uribe, L. C. Penagos et al., "Antitumour effects of temozolomide in a man with a large, invasive prolactin-producing pituitary neoplasm," *Clinical Endocrinology*, vol. 65, no. 4, pp. 552–553, 2006.

[2] T. H. Dillard, S. H. Gultekin, J. B. Delashaw Jr., C. G. Yedinak, E. A. Neuwelt, and M. Fleseriu, "Temozolomide for corticotroph pituitary adenomas refractory to standard therapy," *Pituitary*, vol. 14, no. 1, pp. 80–91, 2011.

[3] A. K. Annamalai, A. F. Dean, N. Kandasamy et al., "Temozolomide responsiveness in aggressive corticotroph tumours: a case report and review of the literature," *Pituitary*, vol. 15, no. 3, pp. 276–287, 2012.

[4] Z. M. Bush, J. A. Longtine, T. Cunningham et al., "Temozolomide treatment for aggressive pituitary tumors: correlation of clinical outcome with O6-methylguanine methyltransferase (MGMT) promoter methylation and expression," *Journal of Clinical Endocrinology and Metabolism*, vol. 95, no. 11, pp. E280–E290, 2010.

[5] M. Losa, E. Mazza, M. R. Terreni et al., "Salvage therapy with temozolomide in patients with aggressive or metastatic pituitary adenomas: experience in six cases," *European Journal of Endocrinology*, vol. 163, no. 6, pp. 843–851, 2010.

[6] V. J. Moyes, G. Alusi, H. I. Sabin et al., "Treatment of Nelson's syndrome with temozolomide," *European Journal of Endocrinology*, vol. 160, no. 1, pp. 115–119, 2009.

[7] S. Mohammed, K. Kovacs, W. Mason, H. Smyth, and M. D. Cusimano, "Use of temozolomide in aggressive pituitary tumors: case report," *Neurosurgery*, vol. 64, no. 4, pp. E773–E774, 2009.

[8] D. Bengtsson, H. D. Schrøder, M. Andersen et al., "Long-term outcome and MGMT as a predictive marker in 24 patients with atypical pituitary adenomas and pituitary carcinomas given treatment with temozolomide," *Journal of Clinical Endocrinology and Metabolism*, vol. 100, no. 4, pp. 1689–1698, 2015.

[9] C. E. Fadul, A. L. Kominsky, L. P. Meyer et al., "Long-term response of pituitary carcinoma to temozolomide. Report of

two cases," *Journal of Neurosurgery*, vol. 105, no. 4, pp. 621–626, 2006.

[10] B. C. Whitelaw, D. Dworakowska, N. W. Thomas et al., "Temozolomide in the management of dopamine agonist-resistant prolactinomas," *Clinical Endocrinology*, vol. 76, no. 6, pp. 877–886, 2012.

[11] M. Campderá, N. Palacios, J. Aller et al., "Temozolomide for aggressive ACTH pituitary tumors: failure of a second course of treatment," *Pituitary*, vol. 19, no. 2, pp. 158–166, 2016.

[12] I. Zemmoura, A. Wierinckx, A. Vasiljevic, M. Jan, J. Trouillas, and P. François, "Aggressive and malignant prolactin pituitary tumors: pathological diagnosis and patient management," *Pituitary*, vol. 16, no. 4, pp. 515–522, 2013.

[13] G. Raverot, N. Sturm, F. De Fraipont et al., "Temozolomide treatment in aggressive pituitary tumors and pituitary carcinomas: a French multicenter experience," *Journal of Clinical Endocrinology and Metabolism*, vol. 95, no. 10, pp. 4592–4599, 2010.

[14] T. Ajithkumar and M. Brada, "Pituitary radiotherapy," in *Oxford Textbook of Endocrinology and Diabetes*, J. A. Wass, S. A. Amiel, and M. C. Davies, Eds., Oxford University Press, Oxford, UK, 2011.

[15] G. Minniti, M. Osti, M. L. Jaffrain-Rea, V. Esposito, G. Cantore, and R. Maurizi Enrici, "Long-term follow-up results of postoperative radiation therapy for Cushing's disease," *Journal of Neuro-Oncology*, vol. 84, no. 1, pp. 79–84, 2007.

[16] J. Zhang, M. F. G. Stevens, and T. D. Bradshaw, "Temozolomide: mechanisms of action, repair and resistance," *Current Molecular Pharmacology*, vol. 5, no. 1, pp. 102–114, 2012.

[17] A. Thomas, M. Tanaka, J. Trepel, W. C. Reinhold, V. N. Rajapakse, and Y. Pommier, "Temozolomide in the era of precision medicine," *Cancer Research*, vol. 77, no. 4, pp. 823–826, 2017.

[18] H. Choy, R. Macre, and L. Milas, "Basic concepts of chemotherapy and irradiation interaction," in *Principles and Practice of Radiation Oncology*, A. Perez, L. W. Brady, E. C. Halperin, and R. K. Schmidt-Ullrich, Eds., pp. 736–756, Lippincot Williams and Wilkins, Philadelphia, Pa, USA, 2004.

[19] G. Raverot, F. Castinetti, E. Jouanneau et al., "Pituitary carcinomas and aggressive pituitary tumours: merits and pitfalls of temozolomide treatment," *Clinical Endocrinology*, vol. 76, no. 6, pp. 769–775, 2012.

[20] M. Bower, E. S. Newlands, N. M. Bleehen et al., "Multicentre CRC phase II trial of temozolomide in recurrent or progressive high-grade glioma," *Cancer Chemotherapy and Pharmacology*, vol. 40, no. 6, pp. 484–488, 1997.

[21] R. Stupp, W. P. Mason, M. J. Van Den Bent et al., "Radiotherapy plus concomitant and adjuvant temozolomide for glioblastoma," *New England Journal of Medicine*, vol. 352, no. 10, pp. 987–996, 2005.

[22] C. Zhong, S. Yin, P. Zhou, and S. Jiang, "Pituitary atypical adenoma or carcinoma sensitive to temozolomide combined with radiation therapy: a case report of early identification and management," *Turkish Neurosurgery*, vol. 24, no. 6, pp. 963–966, 2014.

[23] D. J. Sher, J. W. Henson, B. Avutu et al., "The added value of concurrently administered temozolomide versus adjuvant temozolomide alone in newly diagnosed glioblastoma," *Journal of Neuro-Oncology*, vol. 88, no. 1, pp. 43–50, 2008.

13

Hypercalcemia of Malignancy in Thymic Carcinoma: Evolving Mechanisms of Hypercalcemia and Targeted Therapies

Cheng Cheng, Jose Kuzhively, and Sanford Baim

Division of Endocrinology and Metabolism, Rush University Medical Center, Chicago, IL, USA

Correspondence should be addressed to Sanford Baim; sanford_baim@rush.edu

Academic Editor: Lucy Mastrandrea

Here we describe, to our knowledge, the first case where an evolution of mechanisms responsible for hypercalcemia occurred in undifferentiated thymic carcinoma and discuss specific management strategies for hypercalcemia of malignancy (HCM). *Case Description.* We report a 26-year-old male with newly diagnosed undifferentiated thymic carcinoma associated with HCM. Osteolytic metastasis-related hypercalcemia was presumed to be the etiology of hypercalcemia that responded to intravenous hydration and bisphosphonate therapy. Subsequently, refractory hypercalcemia persisted despite the administration of bisphosphonates and denosumab indicative of refractory hypercalcemia. Elevated 1,25-dihydroxyvitamin D was noted from the second admission with hypercalcemia responding to glucocorticoid administration. A subsequent PTHrP was also elevated, further supporting multiple mechanistic evolution of HCM. The different mechanisms of HCM are summarized with the role of tailoring therapies based on the particular mechanism underlying hypercalcemia discussed. *Conclusion.* Our case illustrates the importance of a comprehensive initial evaluation and reevaluation of all identifiable mechanisms of HCM, especially in the setting of recurrent and refractory hypercalcemia. Knowledge of the known and possible evolution of the underlying mechanisms for HCM is important for application of specific therapies that target those mechanisms. Specific targeting therapies to the underlying mechanisms for HCM could positively affect patient outcomes.

1. Clinical Presentation

A 26-year-old African American male, with no significant past medical history, presented to the emergency department in early November 2016 with complaints of fever, malaise, 18 lb weight loss over 2 weeks, and multiple neck masses. Medications prior to admission consisted of cyclobenzaprine, meloxicam, tramadol, and recreational use of marijuana. Initial imaging revealed an anterior mediastinal mass with intrathoracic lymphadenopathy, bilateral pulmonary nodules, and spine lesions on CT.

Physical exam demonstrated bilateral supraclavicular lymphadenopathy that was tender to palpation, pain on palpation of the cervical and lumbar spine, and normal neurological exam.

Labs on admission were notable for corrected total calcium (Calc) of 15.1 mg/dL, ionized calcium (iCa) of 1.59 mg/dL (ref: 0.95–1.32 mg/dL), PTH of 4.8 pg/mL (ref: 8–85 pg/mL), phosphorus (Phos) of 2 mg/dL (ref: 2/5–4.6 mg/dL), creatinine of 1.16 mg/dL (ref: 0.75–1.2 mg/dL), and blood count

with no atypical cells seen on the differential. Aggressive IV hydration with normal saline at a rate of 250 cc/hr was promptly started and maintained throughout this admission with administration of pamidronate 90 mg on hospital day 2. Additional studies included supraclavicular lymph node and bone marrow biopsies consistent with Epstein-Barr virus positive metastatic undifferentiated, non-keratinizing, lymphoepithelioma-like carcinoma of thymic origin. After undergoing staging with additional imaging, the patient completed his first cycle of chemotherapy with cisplatin, doxorubicin, and cytoxan in the next 2 weeks. His Calc decreased to 10.5 mg/dL at the time of discharge.

Approximately 2 weeks after discharge, the patient was readmitted for a second admission with increasing somnolence. Laboratory analysis disclosed Calc of 15.4 mg/dL and iCa of 1.72 mg/dL for which IV hydration with normal saline at 250 cc/hr was initiated followed by pamidronate 90 mg and calcitonin 300 U with improvement of iCa to as low as 1.16 mg/dL. PTH-related peptide (PTHrP) and 1,25-dihydroxyvitamin D (calcitriol) were sent during this

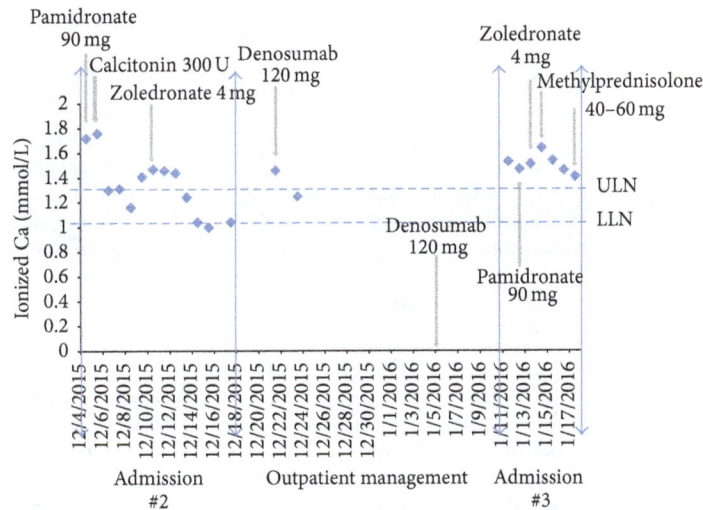

FIGURE 1: Evolution of hypercalcemia in relation to medical therapies instituted. Please note that majority of ionized calcium data from first admission are unavailable. Also, ionized calcium levels are unavailable on 1/5/2016 when denosumab was administered.

admission but results were not available. Repeat MRI of the entire spine noted new hyperintense metastatic lesions. Over the ensuing 3 days, iCa slowly increased to 1.46 mg/dL and required administration of zoledronate 4 mg resulting in normalization of iCa between 1 and 1.1 mg/dL for the rest of the admission (Figure 1). The patient subsequently began cycle 2 of cisplatin, doxorubicin, and cytoxan which was completed prior to discharge with a plan to initiate denosumab as an outpatient.

During outpatient follow-up and 5 days after discharge, a rapid rebound in hypercalcemia occurred with Calc of 12.6 mg/dL and iCa of 1.46 mg/dL, requiring administration of denosumab 120 mg which decreased iCa to 1.25 mg/dL (Figure 1). A second dose of denosumab 120 mg was given 1 week later with concurrent Calc of 12.7 mg/dL.

One month later, the patient was readmitted with altered mental status with Calc of 13.6 mg/dL, iCa of 1.53 mg/dL, Phos of 1.6 mg/dL, and normal renal function. The patient received prompt administration of IV hydration with normal saline and pamidronate 90 mg. Although iCa level decreased to 1.3–1.4 mg/dL within 2 days, it rebounded over the next 24–48 hours to 1.64 mg/dL, requiring further administration of zoledronate 4 mg (Figure 1).

At this time, it was noted that his 1,25-dihydroxyvitamin D level from the previous admission was elevated at 131 pg/mL (ref: 18–64 pg/mL) and PTHrP at 27 pg/mL (ref: 14–27 pg/mL). Methylprednisolone 60 mg per day was subsequently instituted over the next 2 days with decrease in iCa level to 1.3–1.4 mg/dL (Figure 1).

However, the patient continued to clinically deteriorate, despite iCa being maintained at 1.3–1.4 mg/dL (Figure 1) with development of multiorgan failure, and he expired shortly after. It is noteworthy that the third admission repeated PTHrP and calcitriol levels that returned to the medical record posthumously were 58 pg/mL and 499 pg/mL, respectively.

2. Introduction

Hypercalcemia of malignancy (HCM) commonly presents as the initial manifestation of undiagnosed cancer. HCM is a paraneoplastic syndrome with poor prognosis and up to 50% mortality within the first 2 months of the diagnosis [1, 2]. HCM may be caused by either humoral factors (humoral hypercalcemia of malignancy, HHM) which indirectly enhances bone resorption or direct skeletal invasion by malignant cells (osteolytic metastasis-related hypercalcemia, OMRH). Humoral factors responsible for hypercalcemia are usually PTHrP in 80% of HCM [3] followed by excessive 1,25-dihydroxyvitamin D production by tumor cells or macrophages (calcitriol-induced hypercalcemia, HHM-CIH) in less than 1% [3] and excessive ectopic parathyroid hormone (PTH) producing tumors being rare. Another rare humoral cause is the production of excessive systemic cytokine and/or chemokine induced bone resorption (HHM-SCCBR) with normal PTHrP, calcitriol, and PTH levels and no evidence of OMRH [4]. Usually HCM has a single etiology. Rarely interplay of multiple mechanisms can be the cause [5–8].

The currently elucidated five known mechanisms for HCM and their respective associated cancers are summarized in Table 1. Here we present a case of severe hypercalcemia due to undifferentiated thymic carcinoma involving several hypercalcemia inducing mechanisms that evolved over the course of three admissions. The response of serum calcium to the institution of different therapies based on the identification of the underlying mechanisms is additionally described.

3. Discussion

Bisphosphonates, namely, pamidronate and zoledronate, have essentially become the standard therapy following aggressive fluid resuscitation in the management of HCM. The mechanism of action of bisphosphonates in the treatment

TABLE 1: Respective cancers associated with mechanisms of hypercalcemia of malignancy [4, 9–30].

	Hematologic malignancy	Solid organ malignancy
Calcitriol-induced hypercalcemia	(i) Non-Hodgkin's lymphoma (ii) Hodgkin's lymphoma (iii) Chronic lymphocytic leukemia	(i) Gastrointestinal stromal tumor (ii) Glioblastoma multiforme (iii) Metastatic squamous cell carcinoma of tongue (iv) Non-small cell lung carcinoma (v) Metastatic carcinoma of unknown primary (vi) Ovarian dysgerminoma (vii) Renal cell carcinoma (viii) Seminoma
PTHrP-related hypercalcemia	(i) Non-Hodgkin's lymphoma (ii) Chronic myelogenous leukemia (iii) Chronic lymphocytic leukemia (iv) Hodgkin's lymphoma (v) Multiple myeloma (vi) Plasma cell leukemia (vii) Waldenstrom's macroglobulinemia	(i) Squamous cell carcinoma[a](ii) Adenocarcinoma[b](iii) Benign congenital mesoblastic nephroma (iv) Bladder cancer (v) Epithelioid hemangioendothelioma (vi) Melanoma (vii) Merkel cell carcinoma (viii) Myxoid sarcoma (ix) Neuroendocrine tumor (x) Seminoma (xi) Uterine leiomyoma
Local osteolysis	(i) Acute lymphocytic leukemia (ii) Multiple myeloma (iii) Non-Hodgkin's lymphoma	(i) Breast cancer (ii) Lung cancer
Ectopic PTH secretion	(i) Acute myelogenous leukemia	(i) Gastric carcinoma (ii) Lung cancer 　(a) Small cell 　(b) Squamous cell (iii) Neuroendocrine cancer of pancreas (iv) Thyroid cancer 　(a) Medullary 　(b) Papillary adenocarcinoma (v) Ovarian carcinoma (vi) Thymoma (vii) Rhabdomyosarcoma
Cytokine-induced hypercalcemia	(i) Acute lymphocytic leukemia (ii) Multiple myeloma (iii) Non-Hodgkin's lymphoma 　(a) Diffuse large B-cell lymphoma 　(b) Follicular lymphoma 　(c) Adult T-cell leukemia/lymphoma	(i) Squamous cell carcinoma of hand

[a]Anus, esophagus, head and neck cancer, lung, manubrium, parotid, penis, skin, scrotum, and vulva [9].

[b]Breast, cholangiocarcinoma, colon, duodenum, endometrium, lung, ovary, pancreas, renal cell, and stomach [9].

of HCM is the inhibition of osteoclast-mediated bone resorption, increased osteoclast apoptosis, and decreased osteoblast apoptosis [25, 31]. The rapid rebound of hypercalcemia despite the additional administration of bisphosphonate therapy in our patient, even after his second admission (Figure 1), is consistent with incomplete inhibition of bone resorption [32]. This is often observed with progression of tumor by means of the specific underlying mechanism for HCM whether it be OMRH, PTHrP, or HHM-SCCBR.

The implementation of the novel antiresorptive agent denosumab, a RANKL antibody that inhibits osteoclastic activity, was followed by improvement of iCal to the upper limit of the normal range which persisted until the third admission (Figure 1). This course of action is consistent with findings from recent studies in which the introduction of denosumab is of particular benefit in HCM refractory to bisphosphonates [33]. The recurrent hypercalcemia that prompted our patient's last admission was indicative of both bisphosphonate and denosumab failure but demonstrated dramatic response to glucocorticoid therapy (Figure 1) which is consistent with a different mechanism of HCM or HHM-CIH

The elevated 1,25-dihydroxyvitamin D, as noted in our case, did trigger the prompt administration of prednisone therapy which led to rapid improvement in calcium levels (Figure 1). Although HHM-CIH is widely recognized and studied extensively in granulomatous diseases, increased expression and activity of 1-α hydroxylase resulting in overproduction of serum 1,25-dihydroxyvitamin D have also been demonstrated in in vivo studies investigating hypercalcemia associated with dysgerminomas [34] and B-cell lymphoma [35]. The treatment of HHM-CIH is glucocorticoid therapy that inhibits 1-α hydroxylase activity, blocking conversion of calcidiol to calcitriol, resulting in decreased absorption of calcium from the intestine, reabsorption of calcium in the renal tubules, and decreased bone resorption [2]. The optimal glucocorticoid treatment dose and duration of therapy remain undefined, with doses ranging from 20 to 400 mg of prednisone or its equivalent administered daily [9, 36].

Hypercalcemia resulting from multiple mechanisms, HHM-CIH and HHM-PTHrP, has been described in rare cases of HTLV-1 positive ATLL [5], neuroendocrine tumors of the pancreas [6], seminoma [7], and ovarian carcinoma [8]. The mechanism elucidated to cause HHM-SCCBR has been described in conjunction with HHM-PTHrP or OMRH, as observed in multiple myeloma and breast cancer [37, 38]. None of these cases illustrated the simultaneous or independent development of multiple mechanisms underlying HCM over time.

Our case is novel in several aspects from other case reports. The first two admissions were presumed to be associated with OMRH, evidenced by extensive bone metastases. The discovery of a progressive elevation of calcitriol over time, refractoriness of treatment with bisphosphonates and denosumab (Figure 1), and significant response to glucocorticoids therapy is consistent with evolution of an alternative mechanism for HCM. The subsequent discovery of a progressive elevation of PTHrP supports an additional mechanism for HCM in this case.

Our case is also unique given the observation of malignancy associated hypercalcemia in undifferentiated thymic carcinoma. To our knowledge, paraneoplastic hypercalcemia has been previously described in only two cases of squamous cell carcinoma of the thymus [10, 11]. The etiology of hypercalcemia, in one of the aforementioned cases, was believed to be secondary to HHM [11].

4. Conclusion

Our patient represents the first reported case of the progressive evolution of HCM mechanisms as demonstrated by the findings of refractory and recurrent hypercalcemia associated with discovery of an additional specific mechanism that subsequently responded to the targeted treatment.

In patients presenting with paraneoplastic hypercalcemia, especially in the setting of recurrent or refractory hypercalcemia, it is prudent to evaluate all potential mechanisms

of HCM by obtaining measurement of PTH, PTHrP, and calcitriol levels.

Acknowledgments

The authors thank Dr. Brian W Kim and Dr. Ambika Amblee for their invaluable comments on the article. This work was funded by Department of Endocrinology and Metabolism at Rush University Medical Center.

References

[1] S. H. Ralston, S. J. Gallacher, U. Patel, J. Campbell, and I. T. Boyle, "Cancer-associated hypercalcemia: morbidity and mortality—clinical experience in 126 treated patients," *Annals of Internal Medicine*, vol. 112, no. 7, pp. 499–504, 1990.

[2] S.-J. Zhang, Y. Hu, J. Cao et al., "Analysis on survival and prognostic factors for cancer patients with malignancy-associated hypercalcemia," *Asian Pacific Journal of Cancer Prevention*, vol. 14, no. 11, pp. 6715–6719, 2013.

[3] A. F. Stewart, "Clinical practice. Hypercalcemia associated with cancer," *The New England journal of medicine*, vol. 352, no. 4, pp. 373–379, 2005.

[4] P. Martens, B. Addissie, and R. Kumar, "Follicular lymphoma presenting with hypercalcaemia: an unusual mechanism of hypercalcaemia," *Acta Clinica Belgica*, vol. 70, no. 3, pp. 200–203, 2015.

[5] S. R. D. Johnston and P. J. Hammond, "Elevated serum parathyroid hormone related protein and 1,25-dihydroxycholecalciferol in hypercalcaemia associated with adult T-cell leukaemia-lymphoma," *Postgraduate Medical Journal*, vol. 68, no. 803, pp. 753–755, 1992.

[6] G. G. Van den Eynden, A. Neyret, G. Fumey et al., "PTHrP, calcitonin and calcitriol in a case of severe, protracted and refractory hypercalcemia due to a pancreatic neuroendocrine tumor," *Bone*, vol. 40, no. 4, pp. 1166–1171, 2007.

[7] R. Rodríguez-Gutiérrez, M. A. Zapata-Rivera, D. L. Quintanilla-Flores et al., "1,25-dihydroxyvitamin D and PTHrP mediated malignant hypercalcemia in a seminoma," *BMC Endocrine Disorders*, vol. 14, article no. 32, 2014.

[8] K. Hoekman, Y. I. Tjandra, and S. E. Papapoulos, "The role of 1,25-dihydroxyvitamin D in the maintenance of hypercalcemia in a patient with an ovarian carcinoma producing parathyroid hormone-related protein," *Cancer*, vol. 68, no. 3, pp. 642–647, 1991.

[9] P. J. Donovan, L. Sundac, C. J. Pretorius, M. C. D'Emden, and D. S. A. McLeod, "Calcitriol-mediated hypercalcemia: causes and course in 101 patients," *Journal of Clinical Endocrinology and Metabolism*, vol. 98, no. 10, pp. 4023–4029, 2013.

[10] J. M. Negron-Soto and P. N. Cascade, "Squamous cell carcinoma of the thymus with paraneoplastic hypercalcemia," *Clinical Imaging*, vol. 19, no. 2, pp. 122–124, 1995.

[11] K. Suzuki, H. Tanaka, T. Shibusa et al., "Parathyroid-hormone-related-protein-producing thymic carcinoma presenting as a giant extrathoracic mass," *Respiration*, vol. 65, no. 1, pp. 83–85, 1998.

[12] M. Demura, T. Yoneda, F. Wang et al., "Ectopic production of parathyroid hormone in a patient with sporadic medullary thyroid cancer," *Endocrine Journal*, vol. 57, no. 2, pp. 161–170, 2010.

[13] I. J. Diel, J. J. Body, A. T. Stopeck et al., "The role of denosumab in the prevention of hypercalcaemia of malignancy in cancer patients with metastatic bone disease," *European Journal of Cancer*, vol. 51, no. 11, pp. 1467–1475, 2015.

[14] P. J. Donovan, N. Achong, K. Griffin, J. Galligan, C. J. Pretorius, and D. S. A. McLeod, "PTHrP-mediated hypercalcemia: causes and survival in 138 patients," *Journal of Clinical Endocrinology and Metabolism*, vol. 100, no. 5, pp. 2024–2029, 2015.

[15] F. Firkin, H. Schneider, and V. Grill, "Parathyroid hormone-related protein in hypercalcemia associated with hematological malignancy," *Leukemia and Lymphoma*, vol. 29, no. 5-6, pp. 499–506, 1998.

[16] H. Fukasawa, A. Kato, Y. Fujigaki, K. Yonemura, R. Furuya, and A. Hishida, "Hypercalcemia in a patient with B-cell acute lymphoblastic leukemia: a role of proinflammatory cytokine," *The American Journal of the Medical Sciences*, vol. 322, no. 2, pp. 109–112, 2001.

[17] H. Iguchi, C. Miyagi, K. Tomita et al., "Hypercalcemia caused by ectopic production of parathyroid hormone in a patient with papillary adenocarcinoma of the thyroid gland," *Journal of Clinical Endocrinology and Metabolism*, vol. 83, no. 8, pp. 2653–2657, 1998.

[18] P. Jasti, V. T. Lakhani, A. Woodworth, and K. M. Dahir, "Hypercalcemia secondary to gastrointestinal stromal tumors: parathyroid hormone-related protein independent mechanism?" *Endocrine Practice*, vol. 19, no. 6, pp. e158–e162, 2013.

[19] G. Kaiafa, V. Perifanis, N. Kakaletsis, K. Chalvatzi, and A. I. Hatzitolios, "Hypercalcemia and multiple osteolytic lesions in an adult patient with relapsed pre-B acute lymphoblastic leukemia: a case report," *Hippokratia*, vol. 19, no. 1, pp. 78–81, 2015.

[20] H. Mori, K. Aoki, I. Katayama, K. Nishioka, and T. Umeda, "Humoral hypercalcemia of malignancy with elevated plasma PTHrP, TNFα and IL-6 in cutaneous squamous cell carcinoma," *Journal of Dermatology*, vol. 23, no. 7, pp. 460–462, 1996.

[21] K. Nakajima, M. Tamai, S. Okaniwa et al., "Humoral hypercalcemia associated with gastric carcinoma secreting parathyroid hormone: a case report and review of the literature," *Endocrine Journal*, vol. 60, no. 5, pp. 557–562, 2013.

[22] S. Nakayama-Ichiyama, T. Yokote, K. Iwaki et al., "Hypercalcaemia induced by tumour-derived parathyroid hormone-related protein and multiple cytokines in diffuse large B cell lymphoma, not otherwise specified," *Pathology*, vol. 43, no. 7, pp. 742–745, 2011.

[23] P. K. Nielsen, Å. K. Rasmussen, U. Feldt-Rasmussen, M. Brandt, L. Christensen, and K. Olgaard, "Ectopic production of intact parathyroid hormone by a squamous cell lung carcinoma in vivo and in vitro," *Journal of Clinical Endocrinology and Metabolism*, vol. 81, no. 10, pp. 3793–3796, 1996.

[24] S. R. Nussbaum, R. D. Gaz, and A. Arnold, "Hypercalcemia and ectopic secretion of parathyroid hormone by an ovarian carcinoma with rearrangement of the gene for parathyroid hormone," *New England Journal of Medicine*, vol. 323, no. 19, pp. 1324–1328, 1990.

[25] R. G. G. Russell, Z. Xia, J. E. Dunford et al., "Bisphosphonates: an update on mechanisms of action and how these relate to clinical efficacy," *Annals of the New York Academy of Sciences*, vol. 1117, pp. 209–257, 2007.

[26] T. Srivastava, A. Kats, T. J. Martin, S. Pompolo, and U. S. Alon, "Parathyroid-hormone-related protein-mediated hypercalcemia in benign congenital mesoblastic nephroma," *Pediatric Nephrology*, vol. 26, no. 5, pp. 799–803, 2011.

[27] G. J. Strewler, A. A. Budayr, O. H. Clark, and R. A. Nissenson, "Production of parathyroid hormone by a malignant nonparathyroid tumor in a hypercalcemic patient," *Journal of Clinical Endocrinology and Metabolism*, vol. 76, no. 5, pp. 1373–1375, 1993.

[28] E. Tarnawa, S. Sullivan, P. Underwood, M. Richardson, and L. Spruill, "Severe hypercalcemia associated with uterine leiomyoma in pregnancy," *Obstetrics and Gynecology*, vol. 117, no. 2, part 2, pp. 473–476, 2011.

[29] H. Vacher-Coponat, A. Opris, A. Denizot, B. Dussol, and Y. Berland, "Hypercalcaemia induced by excessive parathyroid hormone secretion in a patient with a neuroendocrine tumour," *Nephrology Dialysis Transplantation*, vol. 20, no. 12, pp. 2832–2835, 2005.

[30] K. Wong, S. Tsuda, R. Mukai, K. Sumida, and R. Arakaki, "Parathyroid hormone expression in a patient with metastatic nasopharyngeal rhabdomyosarcoma and hypercalcemia," *Endocrine*, vol. 27, no. 1, pp. 83–86, 2005.

[31] X.-L. Xu, W.-L. Gou, A.-Y. Wang et al., "Basic research and clinical applications of bisphosphonates in bone disease: what have we learned over the last 40 years?" *Journal of Translational Medicine*, vol. 11, no. 1, article no. 303, 2013.

[32] M. I. Hu, I. G. Glezerman, S. Leboulleux et al., "Denosumab for treatment of hypercalcemia of malignancy," *The Journal of Clinical Endocrinology & Metabolism*, vol. 99, no. 9, pp. 3144–3152, 2014.

[33] N. A. Breslau, J. L. McGuire, J. E. Zerwekh, E. P. Frenkel, and C. Y. Pak, "Hypercalcemia associated with increased serum calcitriol levels in three patients with lymphoma," *Annals of Internal Medicine*, vol. 100, no. 1, pp. 1–6, 1984.

[34] K. N. Evans, H. Taylor, D. Zehnder et al., "Increased expression of 25-hydroxyvitamin D-1α-hydroxylase in dysgerminomas: a novel form of humoral hypercalcemia of malignancy," *The American Journal of Pathology*, vol. 165, no. 3, pp. 807–813, 2004.

[35] M. Hewison, V. Kantorovich, H. R. Liker et al., "Vitamin D-mediated hypercalcemia in lymphoma: evidence for hormone production by tumor-adjacent macrophages," *Journal of Bone and Mineral Research*, vol. 18, no. 3, pp. 579–582, 2003.

[36] H. Sternlicht and I. G. Glezerman, "Hypercalcemia of malignancy and new treatment options," *Therapeutics and Clinical Risk Management*, vol. 11, pp. 1779–1788, 2015.

[37] T. A. Guise and G. R. Mundy, "Cancer and bone," *Endocrine Reviews*, vol. 19, no. 1, pp. 18–54, 1998.

[38] G. A. Clines and T. A. Guise, "Hypercalcaemia of malignancy and basic research on mechanisms responsible for osteolytic and osteoblastic metastasis to bone," *Endocrine-Related Cancer*, vol. 12, no. 3, pp. 549–583, 2005.

14

A Novel T55A Variant of $G_s\alpha$ Associated with Impaired cAMP Production, Bone Fragility, and Osteolysis

Kelly Wentworth,[1] Alyssa Hsing,[1] Ashley Urrutia,[1] Yan Zhu,[2] Andrew E. Horvai,[3] Murat Bastepe,[2] and Edward C. Hsiao[1]

[1]*Division of Endocrinology, Diabetes, and Metabolism and The Institute for Human Genetics, Department of Medicine, University of California, San Francisco, San Francisco, CA 94143, USA*
[2]*Endocrine Unit, Massachusetts General Hospital and Harvard Medical School, Boston, MA 02114, USA*
[3]*Departments of Pathology and Laboratory Medicine, University of California, San Francisco, San Francisco, CA 94143, USA*

Correspondence should be addressed to Edward C. Hsiao; edward.hsiao@ucsf.edu

Academic Editor: Hidetoshi Ikeda

G-protein coupled receptors (GPCRs) mediate a wide spectrum of biological activities. The GNAS complex locus encodes the stimulatory alpha subunit of the guanine nucleotide binding protein ($G_s\alpha$) and regulates production of the second messenger cyclic AMP (cAMP). Loss-of-function GNAS mutations classically lead to Albright's Hereditary Osteodystrophy (AHO) and pseudohypoparathyroidism, often with significant effects on bone formation and mineral metabolism. We present the case of a child who exhibits clinical features of osteolysis, multiple childhood fractures, and neonatal SIADH. Exome sequencing revealed a novel *de novo* heterozygous missense mutation of GNAS (c.163A<G, p.T55A) affecting the p-loop of the catalytic $G_s\alpha$ GTPase domain. In order to further assess whether this unique mutation resulted in a gain or loss of function of $G_s\alpha$, we introduced the mutation into a rat GNAS plasmid and performed functional studies to assess the level of cAMP activity associated with this mutation. We identified a 64% decrease in isoproterenol-induced cAMP production *in vitro*, compared to wild type, consistent with loss of $G_s\alpha$ activity. Despite a significant decrease in isoproterenol-induced cAMP production *in vitro*, this mutation did not produce a classical AHO phenotype in our patient; however, it may account for her presentation with childhood fractures and osteolysis.

1. Introduction

Mutations affecting the GNAS complex locus can lead to either activation or inhibition of $G_s\alpha$ [1, 2]. Several diseases result from GNAS mutations, including those that activate $G_s\alpha$ (McCune-Albright Syndrome and fibrous dysplasia of the bone) [3] and those that inhibit $G_s\alpha$, such as AHO and pseudohypoparathyroidism [1, 4–7].

GNAS is a highly complex locus encoding multiple products with exclusively maternal or paternal expression. While $G_s\alpha$ expression is biallelic in most tissues, the paternal $G_s\alpha$ promoter is silenced in the proximal renal tubules, pituitary, thyroid, and gonads. Consequently, the phenotype of patients with inactivating GNAS mutations differs depending on which parental allele is affected.

Patients with AHO exhibit characteristic features including obesity, brachydactyly, shortened fourth metacarpals, short stature, subcutaneous ossification, and occasionally cognitive impairment [1]. AHO has two common subtypes: pseudo-hypoparathyroidism (PHP-Type-Ia) and pseudopseudohypoparathyroidism (PPHP). PHP-Type-Ia occurs when the maternal allele harbors the mutation and causes classical AHO features and end-organ resistance to PTH in the proximal tubule. These patients often show resistance to growth-hormone-releasing hormone, thyroid-stimulating hormone, and gonadotropins. In contrast, when the paternal GNAS allele is affected, patients exhibit AHO features without PTH resistance (PPHP), since the paternal allele is silenced in the proximal tubule. This is distinct from patients with activating GNAS mutations as seen with McCune-Albright

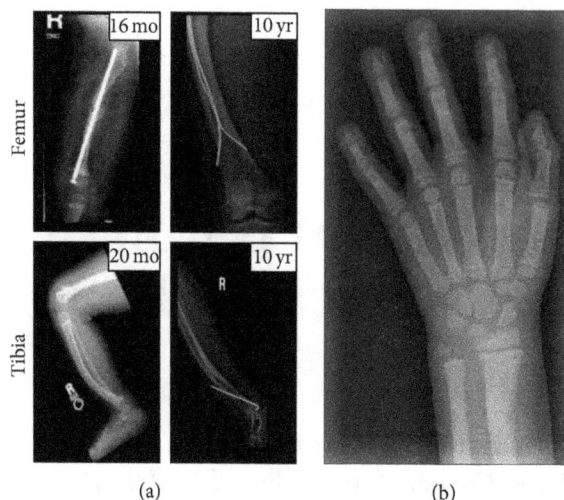

FIGURE 1: (a) Right femoral diaphysis rod and bowing of the tibia at 16 months of age, 20 months, and 10 years. (b) Arrow depicting acroosteolysis of the L hand (age: 6).

Syndrome (MAS), who typically present with the classic triad of polyostotic fibrous dysplasia of the bone, café-au-lait skin hyperpigmentation, and precocious puberty. MAS is also a mosaic disease, and, depending on the degree of mosaicism, patients can present with other endocrinopathies including hyperthyroidism, acromegaly, and Cushing's syndrome. Here, we present a young female with osteolysis, multiple fractures, and a history of SIADH, who harbors a novel inactivating GNAS mutation.

2. Case Presentation

Our patient was born to nonconsanguineous parents of Asian descent. Pregnancy was complicated by oligohydramnios and prematurity at 34-3/7 weeks. She developed respiratory distress syndrome requiring intubation for the first 24 hours. She was severely hyponatremic (Na^+ = 116 mmol/L) and did not respond to sodium chloride or glucocorticoids. No hypoaldosteronism or ADH receptor gene mutations were found. She was diagnosed with neonatal SIADH and successfully treated with fluid restriction. She also had a congenital fracture of her right femoral diaphysis. A bone survey at two days of age showed skeletal hypomineralization.

During early childhood, she developed bowing of her femora, tibiae, and fibulae and a two-centimeter leg length discrepancy. At age 16 months, she sustained a closed fragility fracture of her right femoral diaphysis requiring fixation with a Bailey-Dubow rod (Figure 1). A bone survey at 16 months of age demonstrated possible acro-osteolysis with a metaphyseal corner fracture of her right tibia. At 20 months, a repeat bone survey showed osteolysis of the distal phalanges, metacarpals, and metatarsals and bowing of the femora, tibiae, and fibulae.

She was evaluated by a medical geneticist who felt her clinical picture was consistent with an unspecified osteolytic syndrome. A bone biopsy showed increased bone resorption and mild hypomineralization without collagen defects. She received IV pamidronate from ages two to four for fracture prevention with a subsequent Z-score of −1.1 on DEXA and stabilization of osteolysis. At the age of four, she was transitioned to 35 mg of oral alendronate weekly but sustained right fibular and bilateral wrist fractures in the setting of minimal trauma. At the age of six, the alendronate was increased to 70 mg weekly. This was discontinued one year later when she had achieved a normal BMD for her age (Z-score: +0.4).

At the age of seven, she developed right ankle pain and X-ray imaging confirmed pseudarthrosis of her distal fibula. She underwent excision, bone grafting, and intramedullary nail placement. Bone pathology showed pseudarthrosis of the right fibula and presence of cortical-type bone without increased turnover or resorption (estimated osteoclast activity <5%). We could not assess the degree of hypomineralization due to the decalcification used to process and section the bone tissue (Figure 2). At the age of nine, she sustained another right femoral fracture requiring intramedullary nail placement, which was complicated by delayed healing. Intraoperative bone biopsy demonstrated fibroosseous proliferation of the lesion and scant normal-appearing bone, thought to be related to the intramedullary nail. Again, hypomineralization could not be assessed as the samples were decalcified. A subsequent DEXA confirmed stable BMD (Z-score: +0.5). At the age of 10, she refractured her fibula around the hardware.

In addition to her bony abnormalities, she was diagnosed with probable Asperger's syndrome and attention deficit hyperactivity disorder. She underwent menarche at the age of nine. Due to concern for possible precocious puberty, she was evaluated by a pediatric endocrinologist, who determined that the age of nine was consistent with normal menarche. She otherwise developed normally. Her prior diagnosis of SIADH has been managed successfully with fluid restriction.

Physical examination revealed normal vital signs and no abnormal facies except bilateral iris hypopigmentation. She has four small (0.5–1.2 cm) hyperpigmented spots on her right flank and multiple keloids from orthopedic procedures.

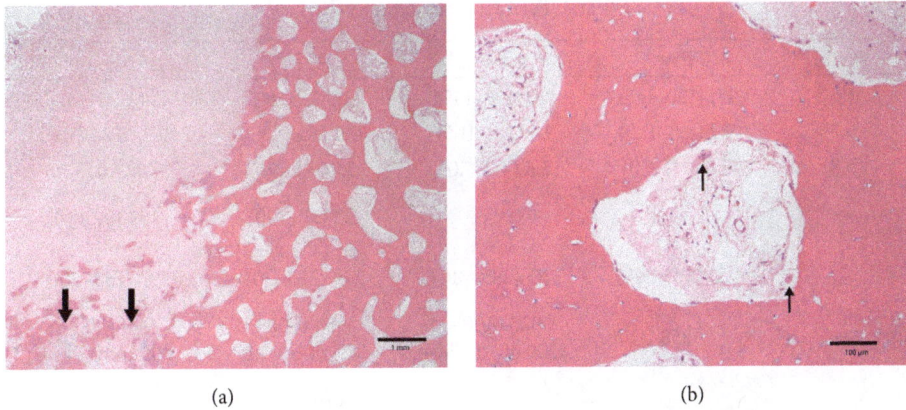

(a)   (b)

FIGURE 2: (a) The R fibula pseudarthrosis biopsy from 2011 demonstrated a fibroosseous lesion (top left) contiguous with fracture callus-type changes (arrows) buttressed on lamellar bone (right); H&E stain; scale bar: 1 mm. (b) Bone resorption of native bone was not increased as osteoclasts were inconspicuous and uncommon (arrows); H&E stain; scale bar: 100 microns.

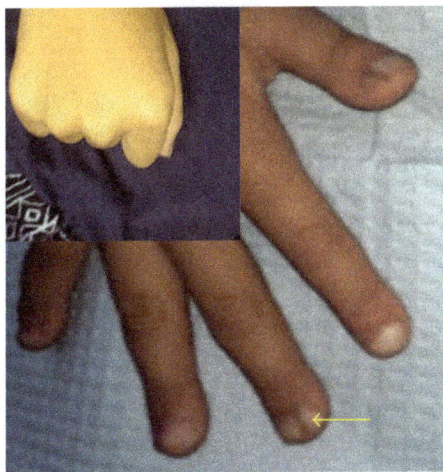

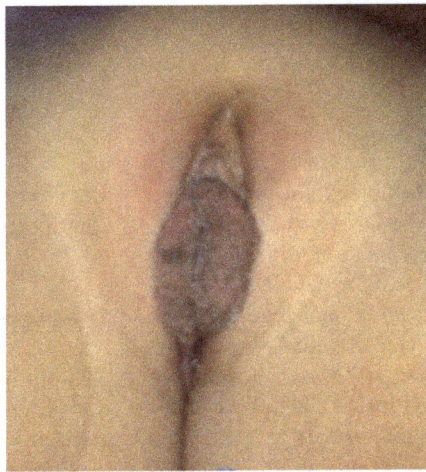

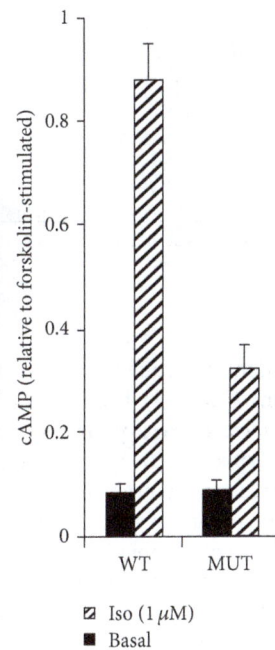

(a)   (b)   (c)

FIGURE 3: (a) Shortened distal phalanges with arrow depicting Bonde's lines. Insert shows no evidence of shortened fourth metacarpal. (b) Labia minora hyperplasia without clitoromegaly. (c) $G_s\alpha$-null mouse embryonic fibroblasts transfected with cDNA encoding the c.163A>G mutant showed a 64% reduction in isoproterenol-induced cAMP production compared to WT $G_s\alpha$. The difference between the WT and mutant isoproterenol-induced cAMP accumulations is statistically significant ($p < 0.01$).

She has mild bowing of both legs without tenderness, bony clubbing of her fingertips, shortened distal phalanges, and hyperpigmented nail lines. She has labia minora hyperplasia and hyperpigmentation without clitoromegaly (Figure 3). The remainder of her examination was normal. Notably, she does not have the short stature, shortened fourth metacarpals, obesity, or subcutaneous ossifications classically seen in AHO. Her laboratory evaluation, including calcium, PTH, and vitamin D, was unremarkable except for mild hyperphosphatemia (Table 1).

Comparative genomic hybridization (CGH) array analysis showed no deleterious deletions or duplications in either the patient or her parents. The CGH was performed through Sunquest Laboratories (#M14494; SignatureChipOS v2 12-plex; 134829 Oligo Probes) on a DNA sample from the patient's blood. The microarray covered 3397 loci across the whole genome including subtelomeric regions and pericentromeric regions. No clinically significant abnormalities were identified in these studies. Since microarray analysis could miss a small deletion and is insensitive for sequence variants,

TABLE 1: Pertinent laboratory values.

Laboratory values	Birth	7 days*	5 months*	Age 10	Age 11	Age 11.5
Na$^+$ (mmol/L)	116	131 (130–145)	120 (135–145)	137 (135–145)	137 (135–145)	—
Ca^{++} (mg/dL)	9.3	9.2 (8.0–11.5)	9.6 (8.0–11.5)	10.1 (8.8–10.3)	9.6 (8.8–10.3)	10.0 (8.8–10.3)
Phos (mg/dL)	5.8	5.0 (4.2–7.0)	5.8 (4.2–7.0)	5.7 (3.0–5.7)	6.8 (3.0–5.7)	4.9 (3.0–5.7)
Vit D 25-OH (ng/mL)	—	—	—	22 (30–100)	25 (30–100)	30 (30–100)
Serum osmolarity (mmol/kg)	—	281 (285–310)	262 (285–310)	299 (283–301)	293 (283–301)	—
Urine osmolarity	—	258	825 (300–1200 mosm/kg)	984 (300–900 mmol/kg)	947 (300–900 mmol/kg)	—
Urine cAMP (nmol/L)	—	—	—	7.4 (0.5–10.0)	—	—
PTH (ng/L)	27	—	—	—	57 (12–65)	20 (12–65)
Alkaline phosphatase	106 (<400 units/L)	—	—	—	—	92.7 (24.2–154.2 mcg/L)
Plasma renin activity (mg/mL/hr)	—	—	<20 (200–3500)	0.80 (0.25–5.82)	—	—
Aldosterone	—	29 (5–175)	4.4 (5–90)	—	—	—
Cortisol (mcg/dL) before and after stimulation	—	2.67 → 31.9 (4–26)	—	—	—	—
TSH	—	2.13 (mIU/mL)	—	—	—	0.76 (0.45–4.12 mIU/L)

Laboratory values at different points during childhood. * indicates values obtained while receiving oral sodium chloride supplementation.

the patient subsequently underwent whole exome sequencing (Ambry Genetics) from lymphocyte DNA which revealed a *de novo*, heterozygous missense mutation within GNAS exon 2 affecting the G$_s\alpha$ transcript (c.163A>G, p.T55A). The sequence read depth was 7x. Thirty additional gene variants were identified in addition to the GNAS c.163A>G variant (Supplemental Table 1 in Supplementary Material available online at http://dx.doi.org/10.1155/2016/2691385). Two were characterized as autosomal dominant variants that did not have any phenotypic correlation to our patient. The remaining variants were novel autosomal dominant and autosomal recessive variants with minor phenotypic overlap and were felt to be unlikely to produce clinically significant findings. Cosegregation analysis revealed that the unaffected parents do not carry the GNAS c.163G>A alteration, indicating that this likely represents a *de novo* mutation. No additional high-probability pathogenic variants were identified.

The GNAS c.163A>G missense mutation has not been reported previously in healthy cohorts. This mutation was not observed among any of the 6,502 individuals in the NHLBI Exome Sequencing Project. There are no data available for the allele frequency of this nucleotide change in the 1000 Genomes Project, and the mutation is not listed in the Database of Single Nucleotide Polymorphisms (dbSNP). This suggests that the GNAS c.163A>G mutation is exceedingly rare in healthy populations. The patient is of mixed heritage (Asian descent) and there is no data on the rate of this mutation in an ethnically matched population. A thorough literature search at the time of the original diagnosis did not identify any other patients who harbor this mutation.

3. cAMP Assay Methods and Results

This study was performed in accordance with the UCSF Committee on Human Research. A rat G$_s\alpha$-HA cDNA plasmid [12] was modified using QuikChange mutagenesis (Invitrogen) with primers AU058 5′ GTCTGGCAAAAG-CGCCATTGTGAAGCAG 3′ and AU059 5′ CTGCTT-CACAATGGCGCTTTTCCAGAC 3′. Wild-type (WT) and mutant G$_s\alpha$-HA plasmids were cotransfected with GloSensor plasmid (Promega, Madison, WI) using Lipofectamine® LTX with Plus™ Reagent (Life Technologies, Grand Island, NY) into 2B2 cells [12] grown adherently in high glucose DMEM (SH30022.01, HyClone, Logan, UT, USA), 10% FBS (HyClone, South Logan, UT), and 1% penicillin/streptomycin (Corning Cellgro Mediatech, Manassas, VA) at 37°C in 5% CO$_2$ and 95% O$_2$ for cAMP analysis using an EnVision 2104 Multilabel Reader (PerkinElmer, Waltham, MA) [13]. The basal, unstimulated cAMP accumulation in the presence of 1 mM 3-isobutyl-1-methylxanthine (Sigma, St. Louis, MO) was comparable between cells expressing the WT or mutant G$_s\alpha$. In contrast, the mutant G$_s\alpha$-HA construct produced 64% less cAMP after isoproterenol stimulation compared to WT G$_s\alpha$, when normalized to 10 μM forskolin-stimulated cAMP levels (Figure 3).

TABLE 2: Reported GNAS mutations in exon 2.

Nucleotide position	Protein position	Mutation type	Observed phenotype	Reference
c.144dupT	p.(Gly49Trpfs*5)	Frameshift	AHO	[7]
c.150dupA	p.(Ser51IIefs*3)	Frameshift	PHPIa, PPHP	[8]
c.188_189delTG	p.(Ser51IIefs*3)	Frameshift	PHPIa, PPHP	[9]
c.191A>T	p.(His64Leu)	Missense	PHPIa	[10]
c.163A>G	p.(Thr55Ala)	Missense	Osteolysis, low BMD, frequent fractures	This case

Published GNAS mutations affecting exon 2. Adapted from Lemos and Thakker Human Mutation, 2015 [11].

4. Discussion

Our patient harbors a novel loss-of-function GNAS mutation and a phenotype of osteolysis, bone fragility, and fractures. Exome sequencing revealed a *de novo* missense mutation (c.163A>G, p.T55A) on exon 2 of GNAS. This mutation occurs within the p-loop of the GTPase domain of $G_s\alpha$ and may change its catalytic properties. We used the Ensemble Variant Effect Predictor model to determine if this variant might produce deleterious effects. The variant was considered "damaging" by SIFT, "probably damaging" by PolyPhen, and "deleterious" by both ConDel and Mutation Taster. Although this SNP was recently reported to be associated with MAS (rs797044895) [14], our data suggest otherwise since transfection of $G_s\alpha$-null mouse embryonic fibroblasts with cDNA encoding the T55A mutant caused a 64% reduction in isoproterenol-induced cAMP production compared to wild-type $G_s\alpha$. This strongly suggests that this mutation is associated with loss of $G_s\alpha$ activity. Interestingly, several other loss-of-function GNAS mutations that are associated with AHO also affect exon 2 (Table 2) [11]. This further supports our hypothesis that our patient's novel GNAS mutation lies in a biologically important region for $G_s\alpha$ activity.

Surprisingly, our patient lacks many classical features of AHO or PHP, such as obesity, subcutaneous calcifications, and major mineral ion metabolism abnormalities. This might reflect the partial loss of cAMP production from a hypomorphic allele. $G_s\alpha$ expression is typically biallelic in bone; thus, it is surprising that a 64% decrease in activity on one allele confers such dramatic bone fragility and osteolysis, given that we would anticipate 100% activity of the wild-type allele. We were unable to identify whether the GNAS mutation affected the maternal or paternal allele, since exome sequencing analysis does not have the ability to determine this. The absence of hormone resistance may suggest that the *de novo* somatic mutation occurred on the paternally inherited allele; however, we were unable to perform endocrine stimulation tests on the parents to exclude subclinical hormone resistance as the family was unavailable for detailed follow-up. An alternative possibility is that this mutation affects $G_s\alpha$ splicing, which could produce full loss of $G_s\alpha$ function. Furthermore, other GNAS transcripts utilize exon 2, and it is possible that our patient's phenotype reflects disrupted activity of another GNAS product, particularly one with monoallelic expression, such as XLαS. It is also possible that this amino acid substitution produces a dominant negative effect, accounting for the 64% decrease in cAMP

accumulation. The mutation is in the alpha-1 helix and is facing out towards Arg201, a region considered to be within the p-loop. The mutation may weaken GTP binding since Thr55 is one of the 20 residues that are in contact with GTP and cause a loss of function through this mechanism. When we modeled the T55A protein using Swiss-Model, we confirmed that the GTP binding site was not conserved and did not fit the GTP into the ribbon model [15]. Finally, exome sequencing only detects mutations that occur in the coding portion of the genome; therefore, we cannot exclude the possibility that there are additional genetic mutations that occur in noncoding or regulatory sequences that could be contributing to this patient's phenotype. Further studies would be needed to elucidate these potential mechanisms.

We do not have a clear explanation for the prior history of hyponatremia; however, it is intriguing to hypothesize that there could be tissue-specific effects of this mutation because of the imprinting of the GNAS locus. There are 2 case reports in the literature describing 2 boys who harbor $G_s\alpha$ mutations (A366S) that caused both testotoxicosis and PHP. The A366S $G_s\alpha$ mutation constitutively activates cAMP *in vitro*, which explains the testotoxicosis, but the A366S protein is rapidly degraded at body temperature (37°C) resulting in functional loss of GNAS in other tissues and thus explaining the PHP phenotype. This is thought to be due to the lower temperature of the testes, which permits stability of the A366S $G_s\alpha$ mutation. A similar mechanism has been described with a $G_s\alpha$ mutation that led to neonatal diabetes due to hyperactivity but also caused PHP [16].

Our patient's comorbid diagnosis of early childhood SIADH suggests that this mutation could affect extraskeletal GPCR pathways, but the evaluation is confounded by the pulmonary complications at birth. While SIADH and bony abnormalities are not clinically linked, GPCRs are key mediators of both pathways. The mechanism of any link remains unclear, and the persistence of the SIADH remains unknown as she continues on self-imposed fluid restriction. How this GNAS mutation results in this pathology remains to be elucidated.

In summary, this case describes a patient with a unique phenotype of decreased BMD, osteolysis, and childhood fractures and identifies a novel exon 2 GNAS mutation which causes a decrease in cellular cAMP production.

Authors' Contributions

Alyssa Hsing and Ashley Urrutia identified the mutation and performed the cloning for the expression constructs. Murat Bastepe and Yan Zhu performed the cAMP assays. Andrew E. Horvai analyzed the histological specimens. Kelly Wentworth and Edward C. Hsiao cared for the patient and provided detailed medical history. Kelly Wentworth, Alyssa Hsing, Edward C. Hsiao, and Murat Bastepe wrote the paper. All authors assisted with editing, approved the final version of the paper, and take responsibility for the integrity of the data analysis and presentation.

Acknowledgments

The authors gratefully acknowledge the funding support for this project. Kelly Wentworth is supported by an NIH T32 training grant (5T32DK007418-34; Michael S. German, MD, Program Director, Division of Diabetes, Endocrinology, and Metabolism) and by the Wilsey Family Fellowship to the UCSF Endocrinology, Diabetes, and Metabolism Training Program. Edward C. Hsiao receives research grant support from the Doris Duke Charitable Fund (2014099) and the March of Dimes (1-FY14-211). Edward C. Hsiao also receives research support from Clementia Pharmaceuticals for unrelated clinical research studies. Murat Bastepe receives funding from the NIH/NIDDK RO1 DK 073911.

References

[1] S. Turan and M. Bastepe, "GNAS spectrum of disorders," *Current Osteoporosis Reports*, vol. 13, no. 3, pp. 146–158, 2015.

[2] C. Blatt, P. Eversole-Cire, V. H. Cohn et al., "Chromosomal localization of genes encoding guanine nucleotide-binding protein subunits in mouse and human," *Proceedings of the National Academy of Sciences of the United States of America*, vol. 85, no. 20, pp. 7642–7646, 1988.

[3] L. S. Weinstein, A. Shenker, P. V. Gejman, M. J. Merino, E. Friedman, and A. M. Spiegel, "Activating mutations of the stimulatory G protein in the McCune-Albright syndrome," *The New England Journal of Medicine*, vol. 325, no. 24, pp. 1688–1695, 1991.

[4] J. L. Patten, D. R. Johns, D. Valle et al., "Mutation in the gene encoding the stimulatory G protein of adenylate cyclase in Albright's hereditary osteodystrophy," *The New England Journal of Medicine*, vol. 322, no. 20, pp. 1412–1419, 1990.

[5] L. S. Weinstein, P. V. Gejman, E. Friedman et al., "Mutations of the Gs α-subunit gene in Albright hereditary osteodystrophy detected by denaturing gradient gel electrophoresis," *Proceedings of the National Academy of Sciences of the United States of America*, vol. 87, no. 21, pp. 8287–8290, 1990.

[6] L. S. Weinstein, M. Chen, and J. Liu, "Gsα mutations and imprinting defects in human disease," *Annals of the New York Academy of Sciences*, vol. 968, pp. 173–197, 2002.

[7] M. A. Aldred and R. C. Trembath, "Activating and inactivating mutations in the human GNAS1 gene," *Human Mutation*, vol. 16, no. 3, pp. 183–189, 2000.

[8] W. Ahrens, O. Hiort, P. Staedt, T. Kirschner, C. Marschke, and K. Kruse, "Analysis of the GNAS1 gene in albright's hereditary osteodystrophy," *Journal of Clinical Endocrinology and Metabolism*, vol. 86, no. 10, pp. 4630–4634, 2001.

[9] M. C. Lemos and R. V. Thakker, "GNAS mutations in Pseudohypoparathyroidism type 1a and related disorders," *Human Mutation*, vol. 36, no. 1, pp. 11–19, 2015.

[10] D. N. Long, S. McGuire, M. A. Levine, L. S. Weinstein, and E. L. Germain-Lee, "Body mass index differences in pseudohypoparathyroidism type 1a versus pseudopseudohypoparathyroidism may implicate paternal imprinting of Gαs in the development of human obesity," *Journal of Clinical Endocrinology and Metabolism*, vol. 92, no. 3, pp. 1073–1079, 2007.

[11] M. C. Lemos and R. V. Thakker, "GNAS mutations in pseudohypoparathyroidism type 1a and related disorders," *Human Mutation*, vol. 36, no. 1, pp. 11–19, 2015.

[12] M. Bastepe, Y. Gunes, B. Perez-Villamil, J. Hunzelman, L. S. Weinstein, and H. Jüppner, "Receptor-mediated adenylyl cyclase activation through XLαs, the extra-large variant of the stimulatory G protein α-subunit," *Molecular Endocrinology*, vol. 16, no. 8, pp. 1912–1919, 2002.

[13] A. Maeda, M. Okazaki, D. M. Baron et al., "Critical role of parathyroid hormone (PTH) receptor-1 phosphorylation in regulating acute responses to PTH," *Proceedings of the National Academy of Sciences of the United States of America*, vol. 110, no. 15, pp. 5864–5869, 2013.

[14] V. N. Rykalina, A. A. Shadrin, V. S. Amstislavskiy, E. I. Rogaev, H. Lehrach, and T. A. Borodina, "Exome sequencing from nanogram amounts of starting DNA: comparing three approaches," *PLoS ONE*, vol. 9, no. 7, Article ID e101154, 2014.

[15] J. J. G. Tesmer, R. K. Sunahara, R. A. Johnson, G. Gosselin, A. G. Gilman, and S. R. Sprang, "Two-metal-ion catalysis in adenylyl cyclase," *Science*, vol. 285, no. 5428, pp. 756–760, 1999.

[16] N. Makita, J. Sato, P. Rondard et al., "Human $G_{s\alpha}$ mutant causes pseudohypoparathyroidism type Ia/neonatal diarrhea, a potential cell-specific role of the palmitoylation cycle," *Proceedings of the National Academy of Sciences of the United States of America*, vol. 104, no. 44, pp. 17424–17429, 2007.

Isolated Liver Metastasis in Hürthle Cell Thyroid Cancer Treated with Microwave Ablation

Konstantinos Segkos,[1] Carl Schmidt,[2] and Fadi Nabhan[1]

[1]Endocrinology, Diabetes and Metabolism, The Ohio State University Wexner Medical Center, 5th Floor McCampbell Hall, 1581 Dodd Drive, Columbus, OH 43210, USA
[2]Surgical Oncology, The Ohio State University Wexner Medical Center, N-924 Doan Hall, 410 W. 10th Avenue, Columbus, OH 43210, USA

Correspondence should be addressed to Fadi Nabhan; fadi.nabhan@osumc.edu

Academic Editor: Osamu Isozaki

Hürthle cell thyroid cancer (HCTC) is a less common form of differentiated thyroid cancer. It rarely metastasizes to the liver, and when it does, the metastasis is almost never isolated. Here we report a 62-year-old male with widely invasive Hürthle cell thyroid cancer, who underwent total thyroidectomy and received adjuvant treatment with I-131 with posttreatment scan showing no evidence of metastatic disease. His thyroglobulin however continued to rise after that and eventually an isolated liver metastasis was identified. He underwent laparoscopic microwave ablation of the liver metastasis, with dramatic decline in thyroglobulin and no structural disease identified to date. This case highlights the rare occurrence of isolated liver metastasis from HCTC and also illustrates the utility of thermoablation as an alternative to surgical resection in the treatment of small isolated liver metastases from HCTC.

1. Introduction

Hürthle cell thyroid carcinoma (HCTC) accounts for 3% of all thyroid malignancies. If distant metastases develop, then the most common site is the lung, followed by bone, with other sites being much rarer [1]. When liver metastases are present, they are almost always multiple or diffuse and are usually accompanied by metastases at other sites. We present a rare case of HCTC, with an isolated liver metastasis, treated with intraoperative microwave ablation (MWA).

2. Case Presentation

A 62-year-old male presented with dysphagia for 6 months and a palpable neck mass. A neck ultrasound (US) showed a 5.3 cm solid hypoechoic mass. He underwent an ultrasound-guided thyroid fine needle aspiration (FNA). The cytology was suspicious but not diagnostic for anaplastic thyroid cancer. He underwent total thyroidectomy with final pathology demonstrating a 7.4 cm HCTC, with breached capsule,

no extrathyroidal extension, and vascular space invasion (6 vessels). His postoperative thyroglobulin (Tg) level was at 40 ng/mL (Table 1). He received 152 mCi I-131 with recombinant TSH stimulation. A posttreatment scan only showed persistent radioiodine activity in the right thyroid bed.

Over the following 7 months, his Tg gradually increased to 318.1 ng/mL (Table 1). A neck US, neck computed tomography (CT), chest CT, and brain magnetic resonance imaging (MRI) were unremarkable. A positron emission tomography-computed tomography (PET-CT) at 4 months postoperatively was unremarkable (Figure 1(a)). A CT abdomen and pelvis at 8 months postoperatively demonstrated a new isolated hypodense lesion in the posterior lobe of the liver. PET scan was repeated and this lesion was fluorodeoxyglucose (FDG) avid (Figure 1(b)), and it was also confirmed with an abdominal MRI (Figure 2(a)). Overall, the lesion was consistent with a metastatic deposit.

The metastasis was deep in the right lobe of the liver. In order to remove it surgically, it would have required a major open liver resection. Given the possibility that other

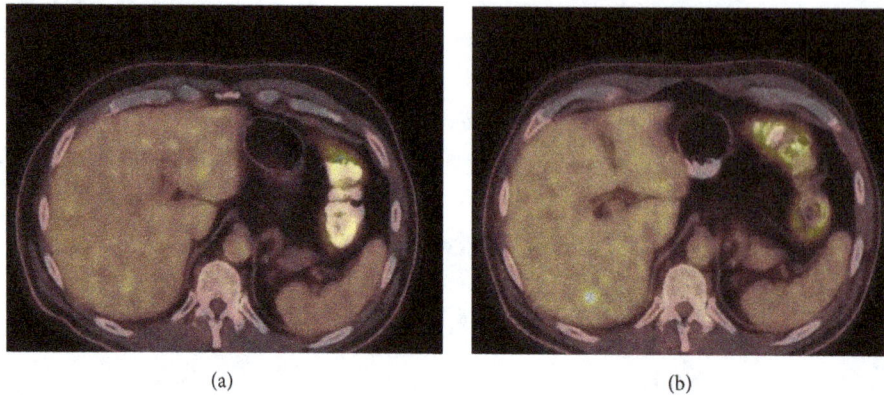

FIGURE 1: PET/CT at 4 months (a) and 8 months (b) after total thyroidectomy. There is new focal uptake within the posterior right lobe of the liver, measuring a maximum SUV of 5.4, consistent with metastatic disease. This was not evident on the initial PET/CT.

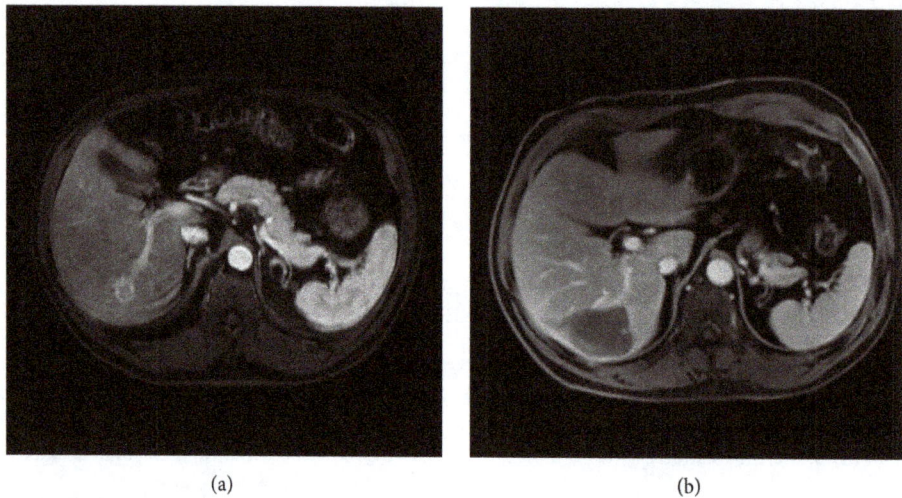

FIGURE 2: Abdominal MRI before microwave ablation shows a rounded lesion in liver segment 6, measuring 2.1 × 2.1 cm, which demonstrates T2 hyperintensity with heterogeneous internal enhancement or restricted diffusion on MRI (a). 2 months after microwave ablation of the liver, there is evidence of postoperative and postmicrowave changes in the liver, with no suspicious enhancement in the ablation bed to suggest definite residual or recurrent tumor, and no new focal liver lesions (b).

TABLE 1

Months after thyroidectomy	TSH (0.55–4.78 μIU/mL)	Tg (1.6–50 ng/mL)
1	9.661	40
2	216.12	62 (stimulated)
8	0.332	318.1
10	Liver metastasis ablation	
11	0.036	0.6
19	0.159	1.3
22	0.033	1.9

metastases would arise in the future and in order to avoid the morbidity of this procedure, the patient underwent simultaneous laparoscopic core biopsy and MWA of the liver mass, with intraoperative ultrasound guidance. The liver biopsy confirmed carcinoma metastatic to the liver, compatible with thyroid gland origin.

One month later, Tg dropped to 0.6 ng/mL. Abdominal MRI did not reveal residual or recurrent tumor (Figure 2(b)). His Tg has slowly increased to 1.3 ng/mL at 9-month follow-up and 1.9 ng/mL at 12-month follow-up after the ablation of the liver metastasis (Table 1). The Tg antibodies have remained undetectable. Up to date, with 12-month follow-up, no evidence of structural disease has been found with negative neck ultrasound, neck and chest CT, and abdominal MRI.

3. Discussion

HCTC has traditionally been considered as a variant of follicular thyroid cancer (FTC) [1, 2]. However, other data suggest that it is a distinct thyroid malignancy and accounts for 3% of all thyroid malignancies [1, 3, 4]. Nagar et al. performed a retrospective review of the Surveillance, Epidemiology, and

End Results (SEER) database and concluded that although in the past HCTC had worse prognosis than FTC, the survival rate of patients with HCTC has improved over the years and is now the same as the survival rate for FTC [5].

HCTC also has a greater propensity for distant metastases. A review of 108 patients with HCTC by Besic et al. identified 32 patients with distant metastatic disease either at presentation or during clinical follow-up. The most common site of distant metastases was the lung, followed by bone. Other sites were much less common, with liver being only one of them, and it was also accompanied by lung metastases [1]. This distribution of distant metastatic disease sites is similar to PTC and FTC [6]. Other metastatic sites in patients with differentiated thyroid cancer (DTC) are considered rare (frequency < 1%) and include brain, liver, renal, adrenal, parapharyngeal, parotid, breast, muscle, ovarian, pancreatic, and cutaneous metastases [6, 7]. Isolated liver metastases are extremely rare, with very few cases reported with PTC and FTC [8–13] and only one case with HCTC [14].

Detection of distant metastatic disease at less common sites can be challenging in patients with HCTC. There have been various reports regarding the radioactive iodine (RAI) avidity of HCTC metastases, with RAI uptake 22.5–69% in different studies [1, 15–17]. In contrast, FDG-PET has a sensitivity of 92–96% and specificity of 80–95% [18], which would make it a more preferable option for detection of metastases when suspected based on Tg level. Other cross sectional imaging modalities such as CT and/or MRI are also helpful when the above imaging techniques are negative. This was particularly evident in our patient, as the initial PET-CT did not show evidence of metastatic disease, but subsequent abdominal CT 4 months later demonstrated the liver metastasis. However, a repeat PET/CT 1 month after the abdominal CT did show this lesion, which, along with the rising Tg, suggests that there was interval growth of the liver lesion allowing detectable FDG uptake.

The preferable treatment for most types of isolated liver metastases is surgical resection; however this may not be always feasible due to patient or tumor characteristics. In the past years, there have been significant breakthroughs in the treatment of liver metastatic disease, and multiple nonresection methods have been introduced. These include the thermal ablation techniques of radiofrequency ablation (RFA) and microwave ablation, which have replaced the older method of cryotherapy, and irreversible electroporation, which is a newer method and not as widely used [19]. Compared to RFA, MWA can heat the liver tissue more effectively, and when it is close to blood vessels, the temperature does not drop as much [19]. Both methods of thermal ablation have shown good results in the treatment of hepatic metastasis based on studies performed in patients with colorectal cancer. Hof et al. demonstrated that percutaneous RFA can be used as an alternative to surgical resection of liver metastases from colorectal cancer, with comparable overall survival [20]. Shibata et al. demonstrated that MWA is comparable to surgical resection in colorectal cancer [21]. Less data are available for noncolorectal cancers, but it seems that the rate of local recurrence is higher and the MWA procedure is most successful in tumors <3 cm [22].

There are scarce published data regarding thermal ablation of liver metastases of thyroid cancer origin. These are almost exclusively related to medullary thyroid cancer except for a case of rapidly progressive FTC metastasis, with RFA used mainly for cytoreduction and palliation [23, 24]. In addition, to our knowledge, there are no available published data regarding treatment of any distal thyroid cancer metastases with MWA. The reported patients with thyroid cancer and isolated liver metastases have been treated with surgical resection [8–10, 12] and radioactive iodine [11].

Laparoscopic MWA was chosen for this patient because the tumor was <3 cm, surgical resection would have required a major open procedure with significant morbidity, and there was a possibility that other metastases would arise in the future that may require additional procedures. For unresectable metastatic disease in patients with HCTC, tyrosine kinase inhibitors have also been used [25], but we believe that for this patient, given the absence of other metastases, MWA has the likelihood of cure with less potential toxicity. The patient's Tg is still detectable in the months following the procedure, which either enhances our original suspicion for microscopic disease at other sites or suggests local recurrence and requires close clinical follow-up. However, at this time, he has a biochemical incomplete response to therapy, which has increased his projected overall survival compared to his previous structural incomplete response to therapy.

In summary, we present a rare case of HCTC with isolated liver metastasis. To our knowledge, there has only been one case with HCTC with isolated liver metastasis described in the literature but none treated with microwave ablation. Endocrinologists and other physicians caring for patients with solitary or low volume liver metastatic disease should be aware of thermoablation, whether done by MWA or RFA and through either a percutaneous or a laparoscopic approach, as an alternative treatment to surgical resection for these patients.

References

[1] N. Besic, A. Schwarzbartl-Pevec, B. Vidergar-Kralj, T. Crnic, B. Gazic, and M. Marolt Music, "Treatment and outcome of 32 patients with distant metastases of Hürthle cell thyroid carcinoma: a single-institution experience," *BMC Cancer*, vol. 16, no. 1, article 162, 2016.

[2] Y. Kushchayeva, Q.-Y. Duh, E. Kebebew, and O. H. Clark, "Prognostic indications for Hürthle cell cancer," *World Journal of Surgery*, vol. 28, no. 12, pp. 1266–1270, 2004.

[3] N. Bhattacharyya, "Survival and prognosis in Hürthle cell carcinoma of the thyroid gland," *Archives of Otolaryngology—Head and Neck Surgery*, vol. 129, no. 2, pp. 207–210, 2003.

[4] I. Ganly, J. R. Filho, S. Eng et al., "Genomic dissection of hurthle cell carcinoma reveals a unique class of thyroid malignancy," *Journal of Clinical Endocrinology and Metabolism*, vol. 98, no. 5, pp. E962–E972, 2013.

[5] S. Nagar, B. Aschebrook-Kilfoy, E. L. Kaplan, P. Angelos, and R. H. Grogan, "Hurthle cell carcinoma: an update on survival over the last 35 years," *Surgery*, vol. 154, no. 6, pp. 1263–1271, 2013.

[6] H.-J. Song, Y.-L. Xue, Y.-H. Xu, Z.-L. Qiu, and Q.-Y. Luo, "Rare metastases of differentiated thyroid carcinoma: pictorial review," *Endocrine-Related Cancer*, vol. 18, no. 5, pp. R165–R174, 2011.

[7] E. Farina, F. Monari, G. Tallini et al., "Unusual thyroid carcinoma metastases: a case series and literature review," *Endocrine Pathology*, vol. 27, no. 1, pp. 55–64, 2016.

[8] B. Djenic, D. Duick, J. O. Newell, and M. J. Demeure, "Solitary liver metastasis from follicular variant papillary thyroid carcinoma: a case report and literature review," *International Journal of Surgery Case Reports*, vol. 6, pp. 146–149, 2015.

[9] H. Kouso, T. Ikegami, T. Ezaki et al., "Liver metastasis from thyroid carcinoma 32 years after resection of the primary tumor: report of a case," *Surgery Today*, vol. 35, no. 6, pp. 480–482, 2005.

[10] T. Kondo, R. Katoh, K. Omata, T. Oyama, A. Yagawa, and A. Kawaoi, "Incidentally detected liver metastasis of well-differentiated follicular carcinoma of the thyroid, mimicking ectopic thyroid," *Pathology International*, vol. 50, no. 6, pp. 509–513, 2000.

[11] M. W. Graves, B. Zukerberg, K. Walace, D. Duncan, and A. Scheff, "Isolated liver metastases from follicular thyroid cancer," *Clinical Nuclear Medicine*, vol. 21, no. 2, pp. 147–148, 1996.

[12] S. Ohwada, Y. Iino, Y. Kawashima et al., "Solitary metastasis from papillary thyroid carcinoma in cirrhotic liver with hepatocellular carcinoma," *Japanese Journal of Clinical Oncology*, vol. 23, no. 5, pp. 309–312, 1993.

[13] H. Studer, P. Veraguth, and F. Wyss, "Thyrotoxicosis due to a solitary hepatic metastasis of thyroid carcinoma," *Journal of Clinical Endocrinology and Metabolism*, vol. 21, pp. 1334–1338, 1961.

[14] M. Salvatori, G. Perotti, V. Rufini et al., "Solitary liver metastasis from Hürthle cell thyroid cancer: a case report and review of the literature," *Journal of Endocrinological Investigation*, vol. 27, no. 1, pp. 52–56, 2004.

[15] N. Besic, B. Vidergar-Kralj, S. Frkovic-Grazio, T. Movrin-Stanovnik, and M. Auersperg, "The role of radioactive iodine in the treatment of Hürthle cell carcinoma of the thyroid," *Thyroid*, vol. 13, no. 6, pp. 577–584, 2003.

[16] L. Lopez-Penabad, A. C. Chiu, A. O. Hoff et al., "Prognostic factors in patients with Hürthle cell neoplasms of the thyroid," *Cancer*, vol. 97, no. 5, pp. 1186–1194, 2003.

[17] A. M. Chindris, J. D. Casler, V. J. Bernet et al., "Clinical and molecular features of Hürthle cell carcinoma of the thyroid," *Journal of Clinical Endocrinology & Metabolism*, vol. 100, no. 1, pp. 55–62, 2015.

[18] G. Treglia, S. Annunziata, B. Muoio, M. Salvatori, L. Ceriani, and L. Giovanella, "The role of fluorine-18-fluorodeoxyglucose positron emission tomography in aggressive histological subtypes of thyroid cancer: an overview," *International Journal of Endocrinology*, vol. 2013, Article ID 856189, 6 pages, 2013.

[19] J. Wong and A. Cooper, "Local ablation for solid tumor liver metastases: techniques and treatment efficacy," *Cancer Control*, vol. 23, no. 1, pp. 30–35, 2016.

[20] J. Hof, M. W. J. L. A. E. Wertenbroek, P. M. J. G. Peeters, J. Widder, E. Sieders, and K. P. De Jong, "Outcomes after resection and/or radiofrequency ablation for recurrence after treatment of colorectal liver metastases," *British Journal of Surgery*, vol. 103, no. 8, pp. 1055–1062, 2016.

[21] T. Shibata, T. Niinobu, N. Ogata, and M. Takami, "Microwave coagulation therapy for multiple hepatic metastases from colorectal carcinoma," *Cancer*, vol. 89, no. 2, pp. 276–284, 2000.

[22] U. Leung, D. Kuk, M. I. D'Angelica et al., "Long-term outcomes following microwave ablation for liver malignancies," *British Journal of Surgery*, vol. 102, no. 1, pp. 85–91, 2015.

[23] H. Mohan, P. Nicholson, D. C. Winter et al., "Radiofrequency ablation for neuroendocrine liver metastases: a systematic review," *Journal of Vascular and Interventional Radiology*, vol. 26, no. 7, pp. 935–942.e1, 2015.

[24] M. W. J. L. A. E. Wertenbroek, T. P. Links, T. R. Prins, J. T. M. Plukker, E. J. Van Der Jagt, and K. P. De Jong, "Radiofrequency ablation of hepatic metastases from thyroid carcinoma," *Thyroid*, vol. 18, no. 10, pp. 1105–1110, 2008.

[25] M.-H. Massicotte, M. Brassard, M. Claude-Desroches et al., "Tyrosine kinase inhibitor treatments in patients with metastatic thyroid carcinomas: a retrospective study of the TUTHYREF network," *European Journal of Endocrinology*, vol. 170, no. 4, pp. 575–582, 2014.

Does the Intensity of IGG4 Immunostaining Have a Correlation with the Clinical Presentation of Riedel's Thyroiditis?

**C. A. Simões ⓘD, M. R. Tavares ⓘD, N. M. M. Andrade, T. M. Uehara,
R. A. Dedivitis, and C. R. Cernea**

Department of Head and Neck Surgery, Hospital das Clínicas, School of Medicine, University of São Paulo, São Paulo, SP, Brazil

Correspondence should be addressed to C. A. Simões; simoesccp@terra.com.br

Academic Editor: Osamu Isozaki

Riedel's thyroiditis (RT) represents one type of IgG4-related thyroid disease (IgG4RTD) and the diagnosis involves quantitative immunohistochemistry showing dense lymphoplasmacellular inflammatory infiltrate consisting of IgG4-positive plasma cells with storiform fibrosis and obliterative phlebitis. We report a case of RT with progressive enlargement of the anterior neck, severe dysphagia, odynophagia, and dyspnea. The patient underwent surgical decompression of the airway, protection tracheotomy, and gastrostomy for nutritional intake 6 months after first symptoms. Complete resolution occurred after surgical treatment combined with prednisolone. Immunostaining revealed IgG4-positive plasma cells 12/HPF (high-power field) and the IgG4/IgG ratio 25%, values that were disproportionate to the intensity of the patient's symptoms. As to this case and the few cases described and analyzed in the literature, our impression is that there is no relation between the intensity of symptoms in RT with the total number of IgG4-positive plasma cells and the IgG4/IgG ratio, but more studies are needed.

1. Introduction

The German surgeon Bernhard Moritz Carl Ludwig Riedel first described Riedel's thyroiditis in 1883, as a rare disease which changes the thyroid parenchyma texture into an extremely hard lesion with adhesion to the trachea and obstructive symptoms [1]. It is a chronic inflammatory condition which destroys the gland and affects the surrounding structures [1, 2]. The more evident etiology is autoimmune [1, 3, 4].

The differential diagnosis should consider malignant thyroid tumors [5], including the undifferentiated carcinoma. If performed by an experienced team, the fine needle aspirative biopsy (FNAB) suggests the diagnosis of Riedel's thyroiditis. However, a definitive diagnosis depends on an open incisional biopsy of the gland [6]. The conservative treatment is well established [5], whereas the surgical approach has both diagnostic and decompression roles.

Riedel's thyroiditis shows several features that justify its inclusion into the spectrum of IgG4 related disease (IgG4-RD). Foremost among them are the fibroinflammatory nature of the infiltrate, the presence of obliterative phlebitis, and

its association with other forms of fibrosclerosis including sclerosing cholangitis, as well as retroperitoneal fibrosis, among others. One-third of patients with Riedel's thyroiditis develop fibrosing disorders in other organs. This inclusion was supported by the fact that RT showed elevated numbers of IgG4 positive plasma cells as well as the morphologic features of IgG4 related disease [7]. Glucocorticoids are the primary form of therapy in IgG4RD. However, their role in IgG4RTD needs to be evaluated [8, 9].

Today RT, the fibrosing variant of Hashimoto's thyroiditis, and a few patients of Graves' orbitopathy represent the types of IgG4-related thyroid disease (IgG4RTD). The diagnosis involves establishing high circulating levels of IgG4 > 135 mg/dL, increased serum IgG4 to IgG ratio of >8%, immunohistochemistry showing dense lymphoplasmacellular inflammatory infiltrate consisting of IgG4-positive plasma cells with storiform fibrosis and obliterative phlebitis, and increased IgG4 positive plasma cell > 10 cells per high-power field when at least three fields are evaluated and the IgG4/IgG ratio of RT is increased by varying degrees [7, 10].

One question not explained in the literature is the relation between the intensity of the thyroiditis, the total

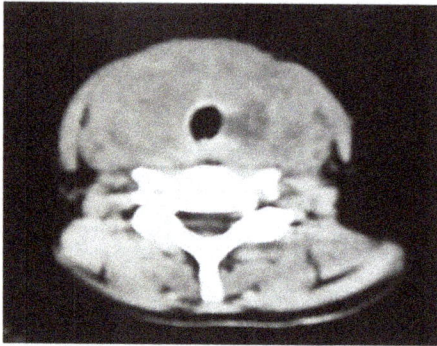

FIGURE 1: Axial computed tomography showing diffuse infiltrate with no precise boundaries around the thyroid.

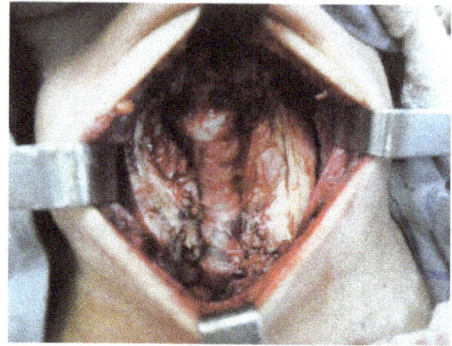

FIGURE 3: Intraoperative aspect of the tracheal decompression under an intense fibrotic thyroiditis.

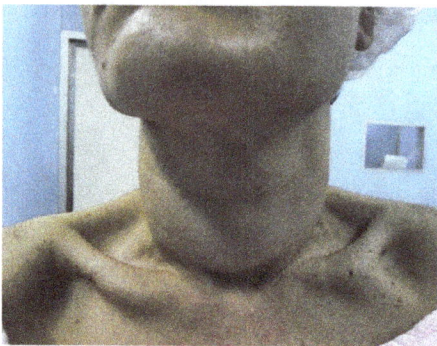

FIGURE 2: Increase of the anterior cervical volume during 4 months of evolution. Note the weight loss.

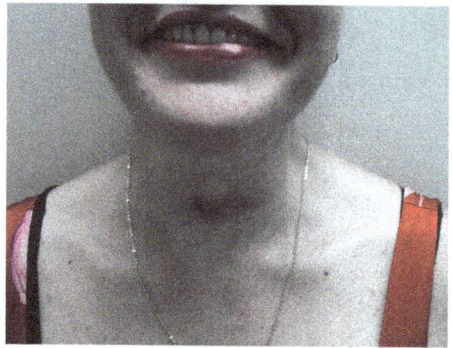

FIGURE 4: Aspect 2 years after surgery.

number of IgG4-positive plasma cells, and the IgG4/IgG ratio. Immunohistochemistry can show whether IgG-4 plasma cells are increased which could lead to fibrosis in other organs [11].

We present the case of an exuberant manifestation of the disease with dysphagia and dyspnea without a large quantitative manifestation in the immunohistochemical analysis.

2. Case Report

We describe a 40-year-old woman complaining of a progressive painless enlargement of the anterior neck, dyspnea, dysphagia, odynophagia, and weight loss of 7 Kg in 4 months. The thyroid gland was hard and the ultrasound exam calculated a volume of 70 g. The patient had hypothyroidism and was undergoing hormonal replacement. Fine needle aspiration was suggestive of Riedel's thyroiditis. The CT scan confirmed a large thyroid lesion with esophageal invasion and decreased tracheal lumen of about 50% (Figure 1). Bilateral vocal fold paresis was verified by means of a laryngoscopy. The dysphagia and dyspnea worsened progressively and the weight loss reached 21 Kg in 6 months after the first symptoms, so she needed a surgical approach for diagnosis and treatment (Figure 2).

The patient underwent surgical decompression of the airway (Figure 3), protection tracheotomy, and gastrostomy for nutritional intake. An extremely fibrotic and hard gland with

tracheal infiltration was found. The intraoperative frozen section exam confirmed the diagnosis of Riedel's thyroiditis.

The follow-up was satisfactory using prednisolone 40 mg/day. Her symptoms improved 5 months after surgery and the feeding intake was exclusively oral. Her weight recovered and the tracheal cannula was removed 5 months after the tracheotomy due to the improvement of the vocal folds motion. The prednisolone was discontinued after 2 years and the evolution has been excellent, nowadays only using levothyroxine (Figure 4).

We were unable to perform the blood dosage of IgG4 and IgG at the time of the active disease. The hematoxylin and eosin staining of the thyroid lesions revealed lymphoplasmacytic infiltration, severe fibrosis, and phlebitis (Figure 5). The IgG4 immunostaining revealed the total number of IgG4-positive plasma cells 12/HPF (Figure 6), and the IgG4/IgG ratio was 25%.

3. Discussion

Riedel's thyroiditis is a fibrosclerosing disease whose anatomopathologic aspect is a lymphocytic, plasmocytic, and histiocytic cell infiltration [1, 3]. This is a typical autoimmune response, with mature and hyalinizing fibrosis, similar to that found in Hashimoto's thyroiditis in its final or fibrotic status. The gland is extremely hard and infiltrates into the surrounding tissues. As a result, this condition can be mistaken for malignant neoplasm.

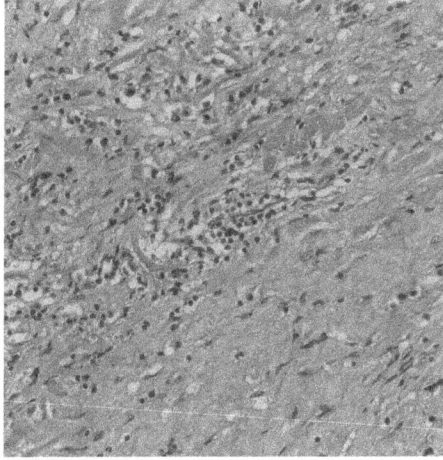

FIGURE 5: Hematoxylin and eosin staining of the thyroid lesions revealed lymphoplasmacytic infiltration, severe fibrosis, and phlebitis.

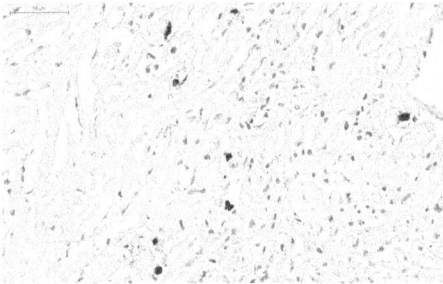

FIGURE 6: IgG4 immunostaining revealed the presence of IgG4-positive plasma cells.

Dyspnea and hoarseness can be found due to tracheal compression or recurrent laryngeal nerve involvement. Furthermore, dysphagia can be the result of pharyngoesophageal involvement and compression [6]. The thyroid function depends on the extension of the replacement of normal tissue by fibrosis. Thus, 64% of the patients present hypothyroidism, whereas 32% are euthyroidism and 4% hyperthyroidism [1]. Hypoparathyroidism can be observed. However, it is reversible under the administration of prednisolone. Anyway, it was not found in our case.

Open surgical biopsy during the cervicotomy is mandatory in order to confirm the diagnosis. Isthmusectomy is enough in order to perform the diagnosis. Broad resections should be avoided due to the risk of injuring the surrounding structures.

An exuberant clinical status with consumption and fast evolution can suggest the undifferentiated carcinoma, such as in the present case reported. The hypothesis of Riedel's thyroiditis was considered because of the FNAB exam. The operation was technically hard to perform, since there was a lack of dissection plane between the thyroid and the trachea, with high risk of injuries to tissues. The patient's weight recovered fast, after starting the use of corticoid. If this treatment is not efficient, other drugs could be employed, such as

tamoxifen [2]. Low doses of external beam radiotherapy are also an alternative approach. Spontaneous resolution has also been described [1].

In spite of being uncommon, Riedel's thyroiditis should be considered a differential diagnosis among the anterior neck masses with fast growth. Severe dysphagia has not been reported as a main symptom.

In order to characterize the relationship between RT and IgG4, we performed IgG4 and IgG staining. The total number of IgG4-positive plasma cells was more than 10/HPF, but the IgG4/IgG ratio was less than 40%. IgG4 immunostaining is important for the diagnosis, especially when serum IgG4 is not elevated. Although IgG4 plasma cells per high-power field has an acceptable specificity, an IgG4/IgG plasma cell ratio of greater than 40% is considered more valuable, as some inflammatory lesions have high IgG4 plasma cells [12]. For this case with exuberant symptoms, our expectation would be a larger number of IgG4-positive plasma cells and a larger IgG4/IgG ratio.

There is no study associating intensity of the symptoms with the count of inflammatory plasma cells in Riedel's thyroiditis, but in the spectrum of IgG4 related diseases Deshpande et al. [13] studied a group of patients with Fibrous Variant of a Hashimoto Thyroiditis (FVHT) and compared them with typical Hashimoto Thyroiditis (HT) patients, finding that FVHT patients have more hypothyroidism, a higher mean IgG4-positive cell count in affected thyroid tissue, and a higher IgG4/IgG ratio than typical HT patients.

As to this case, our impression is that there is no relation between the intensity of the thyroiditis, the total number of IgG4-positive plasma cells and the IgG4/IgG ratio. The guidelines proposed do not supplant careful clinicopathological correlation and sound clinical judgment [10].

Since RT is such a rare disease, immunohistochemical analyses have only been performed in limited cases and long-term investigations are further needed.

References

[1] J. M. Viel Martínez, M. Á. Agut Fuster, E. Grau Alario et al., "Riedel's thyroiditis: Report of one case with a lethal outcome," *Acta Otorrinolaringologica Española*, vol. 54, no. 6, pp. 465–469, 2003.

[2] M. De, A. Jaap, and J. Dempster, "Tamoxifen therapy in steroid resistant reidel's thyroiditis," *Scottish Medical Journal*, vol. 46, no. 2, pp. 56-57, 2001.

[3] T. Zimmermann-Belsing and U. Feldt-Rasmussen, "Riedel's thyroiditis: an autoimmune or primary fibrotic disease?" *Journal of Internal Medicine*, vol. 235, no. 3, pp. 271–274, 1994.

[4] S. M. Schwaegerle, T. W. Bauer, and C. B. Esselstyn Jr., "Riedel's thyroiditis," *American Journal of Clinical Pathology*, vol. 90, no. 6, pp. 715–722, 1988.

[5] K. Sato, H. Hanazawa, J. Watanabe, and S. Takahashi, "Differential diagnosis and management of airway obstruction in Riedel's thyroiditis: A case report," *Auris Nasus Larynx*, vol. 32, no. 4, pp. 439–443, 2005.

[6] R. Chong Xi, W. Hong Qiao, and L. Yan, "Severe trachea compression caused by Riedel's thyroiditis: A case report and review of the literature," *Annals of Medicine and Surgery*, vol. 12, pp. 18–20, 2016.

[7] V. Deshpande, "IgG4 related disease of the head and neck," *Head and Neck Pathology*, vol. 9, no. 1, pp. 24–31, 2015.

[8] D. Dutta, A. Ahuja, and C. Selvan, "Immunoglobulin G4-related thyroid disorders - Diagnostic challenges and clinical outcomes," *Endokrynologia Polska*, vol. 67, no. 5, pp. 520–524, 2016.

[9] S. Wang, Y. F. Luo, J. L. Cao et al., "IgG4 immunohistochemistry in riedel thyroiditis," *Zhonghua Bing Li Xue Za Zhi*, vol. 46, no. 3, pp. 166–169, 2017.

[10] V. Deshpande, Y. Zen, and J. K. Chan, "Consensus statement on the pathology of IgG4-related disease," *Modern Pathology*, vol. 25, no. 9, pp. 1181–1192, 2012.

[11] H. Falhammar, C. C. Juhlin, C. Barner, S. Catrina, C. Karefylakis, and J. Calissendorff, "Riedel's thyroiditis: clinical presentation, treatment and outcomes," *Endocrine Journal*, vol. 60, no. 1, pp. 185–192, 2018.

[12] D. Kottahachchi and D. J. Topliss, "Immunoglobulin G4-related thyroid diseases," *European Thyroid Journal*, vol. 5, no. 4, pp. 231–239, 2016.

[13] V. Deshpande, A. Huck, E. Ooi, J. H. Stone, W. C. Faquin, and G. P. Nielsen, "Fibrosing variant of hashimoto thyroiditis is an IgG4 related disease," *Journal of Clinical Pathology*, vol. 65, no. 8, pp. 725–728, 2012.

Vasopressin Bolus Protocol Compared to Desmopressin (DDAVP) for Managing Acute, Postoperative Central Diabetes Insipidus and Hypovolemic Shock

Anukrati Shukla,[1] **Syeda Alqadri,**[1] **Ashley Ausmus,**[2] **Robert Bell,**[3]
Premkumar Nattanmai,[1] **and Christopher R. Newey**[1]

[1]*Department of Neurology, University of Missouri, Columbia, MO, USA*
[2]*Department of Pharmacy, University of Missouri, Columbia, MO, USA*
[3]*Department of Neurosurgery, University of Missouri, Columbia, MO, USA*

Correspondence should be addressed to Christopher R. Newey; neweyc@health.missouri.edu

Academic Editor: Osamu Isozaki

Introduction. Management of postoperative central diabetes insipidus (DI) can be challenging from changes in volume status and serum sodium levels. We report a case successfully using a dilute vasopressin bolus protocol in managing hypovolemic shock in acute, postoperative, central DI. *Case Report.* Patient presented after bifrontal decompressive craniotomy for severe traumatic brain injury. He developed increased urine output resulting in hypovolemia and hypernatremia. He was resuscitated with intravenous fluids including a dilute vasopressin bolus protocol. This protocol consisted of 1 unit of vasopressin in 1 liter of 0.45% normal saline. This protocol was given in boluses based on the formula: urine output minus one hundred. Initial serum sodium was 148 mmol/L, and one-hour urine output was 1 liter. After 48 hours, he transitioned to 1-desamino-8-D-arginine vasopressin (DDAVP). Pre-DDAVP serum sodium was 149 mmol/L and one-hour urine output 320 cc. Comparing the bolus protocol to the DDAVP protocol, the average sodium was 143.8 ± 3.2 and 149.6 ± 3.2 mmol/L ($p = 0.0001$), average urine output was 433.2 ± 354.4 and 422.3 ± 276.0 cc/hr ($p = 0.90$), and average specific gravity was 1.019 ± 0.009 and 1.016 ± 0.01 ($p = 0.42$), respectively. *Conclusion.* A protocol using dilute vasopressin bolus can be an alternative for managing acute, central DI postoperatively, particularly in setting of hypovolemic shock resulting in a consistent control of serum sodium.

1. Introduction

Brain surgery and head trauma are two common causes of central diabetes insipidus (DI) [1–3]. DI can manifest either transiently, permanently, or in a triphasic pattern [1–3]. The three phases of the triphasic pattern are polyuric lasting for 4-5 days, antidiuretic lasting for 5-6 days, and then DI again [1–3]. 1-Desamino-8-D-arginine vasopressin (DDAVP) is a synthetic form of arginine vasopressin and is a primary treatment of central DI [1–3]. Owing to its prolonged duration of action, easy oral/nasal dosing, and beneficial side effect profile, it is the preferred medication in the long-term management of central DI [1–3]. The use of DDAVP, however, in the critically ill patient who develops DI is more challenging. Sodium changes during the triphasic

response of central DI in these patients can often be severe [1–3]. Additionally, the critically ill patient may also be fluid underresuscitated and/or hypotensive [4, 5]. Thus, the rationale behind the use of DDAVP in the acute management of critically ill patients with central DI is not clear.

Ralston and Butt showed that the use of continuous vasopressin infusion in the acute management of DI in the traumatically brain injured patient was associated with a steady decrease in serum sodium, ease of titration, and a huge benefit of physiological adaptation to change in fluid and electrolyte status [6]. Furthermore, the vasopressor effect of vasopressin can be beneficial in the critically ill patient [1, 6]. These physiological homeostatic benefits of vasopressin are advantageous particularly in the critically ill neurological patient. We present a case report comparing two regimens

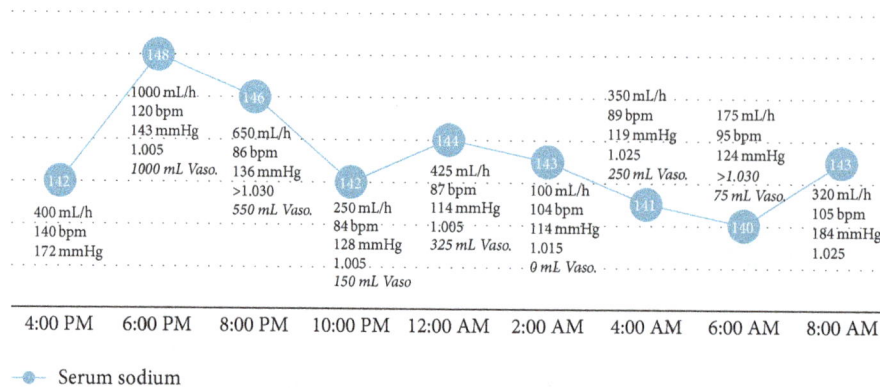

FIGURE 1: Day 1 vasopressin bolus curve. Sodium (mmol/L; blue circles), urine output (mL/h), heart rate (bpm), systolic blood pressure (mmHg), and urine specific gravity on day 1 of vasopressin/0.45% fluid replacement. Bolus doses of vasopressin replacement are noted to be italic. mL: milliliters; h: hour; bpm: beats per minute; mmHg: millimeters of mercury; vaso: vasopressin.

used to manage acute central DI status after neurosurgery in a single patient. The patient was initially treated with dilute vasopressin bolus regimen followed by DDAVP regimen. We compared the efficacy and safety profile of the two regimens by trending the serum sodium, urine output, urine specific gravity, and vitals hourly over the period of institution of the two regimens.

2. Case Presentation

A young, adult male was brought to the emergency department (ED) in a comatose state after he sustained self-inflicted gunshot wound injuries on both his temples and orbits. He was intubated and resuscitated. On arrival, he had a score of 6 on Glasgow coma scale (GCS) and absent pupillary and gag reflexes. Computed tomography (CT) scan showed bifrontal intracerebral contusions, uncal herniation, cerebral edema, and bilateral orbital floor fractures. Emergency bifrontal craniectomy with external ventricular drain (EVD) placement was successfully performed.

Postoperatively, his condition was monitored in the Trauma Unit for four days during the course of which his GCS improved from 6 to 10. Despite the procedure, his intracranial pressure (ICP) recordings continued to peak requiring continued cerebrospinal fluid (CSF) drainage via the EVD. Repeat CT head showed evidence of left parietal extradural hemorrhage. He subsequently had a left parietal craniectomy for clot evacuation. Postoperatively, he was transferred to the neurosciences intensive care unit (NSICU) for further critical care management of his cerebral edema and refractory ICP elevation. On arrival to the NSICU, he was in hypovolemic shock (overall 3.4 L negative fluid balance in past few hours) from clear polyuria. He had tachycardia and hypotension. His sodium was 154 mmol/L. His urine specific gravity was <1.005 and urine osmolality was 123 mOsm/Kg. Given the correlation between his urine osmolality and specific gravity, his DI was subsequently monitored using only urine specific gravity. There was no administration of mannitol or need for corticosteroid replacement.

Given the significant shock state, he was aggressively resuscitated using dilute vasopressin boluses for his DI. This dilute mixture consisted of 1 U of vasopressin in 1 L of 0.45% saline solution. This was given in boluses based on the formula, urine output minus one hundred milliliters.

After starting the dilute vasopressin bolus protocol, the polyuria quickly resolved within 6 hours and sodium decreased. The serum sodium and urine input and output were monitored carefully over the following days. The serum sodium remained in the desired range of 140–145 mmol/L while on vasopressin bolus protocol. Once resuscitated and stabilized, IV DDAVP was started.

Statistical analyses were performed on serum sodium, urine specific gravity, and urine output using student t-test with a $p \leq 0.05$ being considered significant.

Comparing the bolus protocol to the DDAVP protocol, the average sodium was 143.8 ± 3.2 and 149.6 ± 3.2 mmol/L ($p = 0.0001$), average urine output was 433.2 ± 354.4 and 422.3 ± 276.0 cc/hr ($p = 0.90$), and average specific gravity was 1.019 ± 0.009 and 1.016 ± 0.01 ($p = 0.42$), respectively. The serum sodium, urine output, heart rate, systolic blood pressure, and urine specific gravity (if available) are charted for days 1 and 2 of vasopressin bolus protocol (Figures 1 and 2) and for DDAVP regimen (Figure 3).

3. Discussion

Our case shows that the use of a dilute vasopressin urine replacement formula can safely and smoothly treat patients in DI and hypovolemic shock. This protocol provided a consistent serum sodium level compared to the use of DDAVP.

Diabetes insipidus is an endocrinological disorder characterized by polyuria, that is, urine output greater than $2 l/m^2/24$ h or 40–50 mL/Kg/24 h in adults, caused as a result of either vasopressin deficiency (central DI), vasopressin resistance (nephrogenic DI), or excessive water intake (primary polydipsia) [3]. The diagnosis of DI involves first confirming the polyuria (i.e., hypotonic urine) by recording urine output and urine osmolality (or specific gravity) and also

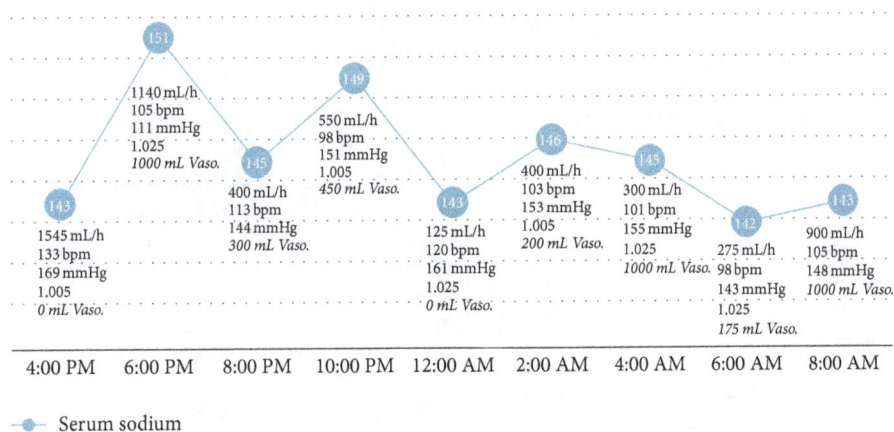

FIGURE 2: Day 2 vasopressin bolus curve. Sodium (mmol/L; blue circles), urine output (mL/h), heart rate (bpm), systolic blood pressure (mmHg), and urine specific gravity on day 2 of vasopressin/0.45% fluid replacement. Bolus doses of vasopressin replacement are noted to be italic. 1-Desamino-8-D-arginine vasopressin: DDAVP; mL: milliliters; h: hour; bpm: beats per minute; mmHg: millimeters of mercury; vaso: vasopressin.

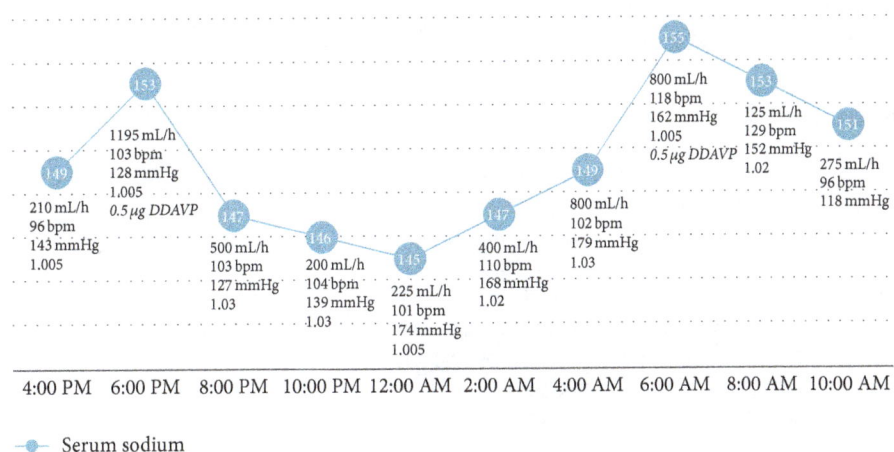

FIGURE 3: DDAVP curve. Sodium (mmol/L; blue circles), urine output (mL/h), heart rate (bpm), systolic blood pressure (mmHg), and urine specific gravity with DDAVP administrations. DDAVP doses noted to be italic. 1-Desamino-8-D-arginine vasopressin: DDAVP; mL: milliliters; h: hour; bpm: beats per minute; mmHg: millimeters of mercury.

the serum sodium [2, 3]. Postoperative DI can typically be managed with drinking to thirst. Water deprivation test is the confirmatory as well as the differentiating test [7]. In patients with normal neurohypophyseal function and patients with primary polydipsia, urine osmolality at the end of period of deprivation was greater than plasma osmolality and failed to increase by more than 5% after 5 units of aqueous vasopressin [7]. In patients with severe ADH deficiency urine osmolality prior to ADH administration was much less than plasma osmolality after it when the urine osmolality was increased by more than 50% [8]. However, in the neurocritical care patient, this thirst mechanism may be impaired or unable to monitor secondary to the critical illness. Management of DI with a defective thirst mechanism demands closer monitoring and observation.

The treatment of DI is targeted towards fluid resuscitation and maintaining normal electrolyte balance status. Hence,

volume replenishment is the mainstay of treatment irrespective of the cause. Underlying cause, if identified, must be treated. The primary pharmacological treatment of central DI is with the vasopressin analogue DDAVP. Removal of amine from position 1 of vasopressin increases the half-life of DDAVP and changing 1-arginine to d-arginine at position 8 reduces the vasopressor action [8–10]. DDAVP is available as oral tablets, nasal spray, and a solution [8–10]. For these reasons, it is deemed as a safe and efficacious treatment option for the management of DI [8–10]. In the critical care patient with DI and hypovolemic shock, these features may not be desirable and may result in underresuscitation and/or extreme fluctuation of serum sodium level. The use of dilute vasopressin bolus to replace urine loss may be more desirable.

Vasopressin in continuous infusion has been previously shown to result in a steady decrease in serum sodium with ease of titration resulting in an improvement in fluid and electrolyte status [6]. Furthermore, the vasopressor effect of vasopressin can be beneficial in the critically ill patient who may be in shock as we demonstrate in this case report [1, 6]. Additional studies are needed to assess the efficacy in a larger sample.

4. Conclusion

Our case demonstrates that in the acute management of a critically ill patient in DI and hypovolemic shock, dilute vasopressin bolus emerged as a better alternative over DDAVP. Steadier decrease in serum sodium levels, convenience of titration in inpatient setting, and a self-regulating dose modulation in accordance with the body's fluid status conferred a distinct advantage, especially in volume-depleted patients with poor neurological function. Therefore, in critically ill patients, the use of dilute vasopressin should be considered an option.

Disclosure

An earlier version of this work was presented as a poster at 14th Annual Neurocritical Care Society Meeting, 2016.

Authors' Contributions

Syeda Alqadri contributed to concept, design, and data acquisition. Anukrati Shukla contributed to concept and design and data acquisition. Ashley Ausmus contributed to concept and design and data acquisition. Robert Bell contributed to concept and design and data acquisition. Premkumar Nattanmai contributed to concept and design, supervision, and critical revision of manuscript for intellectual content. Christopher Newey contributed to concept and design, supervision, and critical revision of manuscript for intellectual content.

References

[1] A. A. Abla, S. D. Wait, J. A. Forbes et al., "Syndrome of alternating hypernatremia and hyponatremia after hypothalamic hamartoma surgery," *Neurosurgical Focus*, vol. 30, no. 2, article no. E6, 2011.

[2] S. G. Achinger, A. I. S. Arieff, K. Kalantar-Zadeh, and J. C. A. Ayus, "Desmopressin acetate (DDAVP)-associated hyponatremia and brain damage: a case series," *Nephrology, Dialysis, Transplantation*, vol. 29, no. 12, pp. 2310–2315, 2014.

[3] N. Di Iorgi, F. Napoli, A. E. M. Allegri et al., "Diabetes insipidus—diagnosis and management," *Hormone Research in Paediatrics*, vol. 77, no. 2, pp. 69–84, 2012.

[4] E. J. Hoorn and R. Zietse, "Water balance disorders after neurosurgery: the triphasic response revisited," *NDT Plus*, vol. 3, no. 1, pp. 42–44, 2010.

[5] K. Katz, J. Lawler, J. Wax, R. O'Connor, and V. Nadkarni, "Vasopressin pressor effects in critically ill children during

[6] evaluation for brain death and organ recovery," *Resuscitation*, vol. 47, no. 1, pp. 33–40, 2000.

[6] C. Ralston and W. Butt, "Continuous vasopressin replacement in diabetes insipidus," *Archives of Disease in Childhood*, vol. 65, no. 8, pp. 896–897, 1990.

[7] G. L. Robertson, "Disorders of the neurohypophysis," in *Harrison's Principles of Internal Medicine*, D. Kasper, A. Fauci, S. Hauser, D. Longo, J. L. Jameson, and J. Loscalzo, Eds., McGraw-Hill Education, New York, NY, USA, 19th edition, 2015.

[8] M. Miller, T. Dalakos, A. M. Moses, H. Fellerman, and D. H. Streeten, "Recognition of partial defects in antidiuretic hormone secretion," *Annals of Internal Medicine*, vol. 73, no. 5, pp. 721–729, 1970.

[9] C. R. W. Edwards, M. J. Kitau, T. Chard, and G. M. Besser, "Vasopressin analogue DDAVP in diabetes insipidus: clinical and laboratory studies," *British Medical Journal*, vol. 3, no. 5876, pp. 375–378, 1973.

[10] S. M. Seif, T. V. Zenser, F. F. Ciarochi, B. B. Davis, and A. G. Robinson, "DDAVP (1-desamino-8-D-arginine-vasopressin) treatment of central diabetes insipidus—mechanism of prolonged antidiuresis," *The Journal of Clinical Endocrinology & Metabolism*, vol. 46, no. 3, pp. 381–388, 1978.

Gigantomastia and Macroprolactinemia Responding to Cabergoline Treatment: A Case Report and Minireview of the Literature

Fatma Dilek Dellal,[1] **Didem Ozdemir,**[2] **Cevdet Aydin,**[2] **Gulfem Kaya,**[1]
Reyhan Ersoy,[2] **and Bekir Cakir**[2]

[1]*Department of Endocrinology and Metabolism, Ataturk Training and Research Hospital, 06800 Ankara, Turkey*
[2]*Department of Endocrinology and Metabolism, Faculty of Medicine, Yildirim Beyazit University, 06800 Ankara, Turkey*

Correspondence should be addressed to Fatma Dilek Dellal; drdellal@yahoo.com

Academic Editor: John Broom

Background. Macroprolactinemia is defined as predominance of high molecular weight prolactin forms in the circulation. Although macroprolactin is considered as a biologically inactive molecule, some authorities suggest treatment in symptomatic cases. Gigantomastia is defined as excess breast tissue and most cases in the literature were treated by surgical intervention. *Case.* A 44-year-old woman was admitted to our clinic with gigantomastia and galactorrhea. The patient had a demand for surgical therapy. In laboratory examination, she had hyperprolactinemia and macroprolactinemia. Pituitary imaging revealed 6 mm microadenoma in right side of the hypophysis. Since she was symptomatic, cabergolin treatment was started. Macroprolactin became negative, breast circumference decreased significantly, and galactorrhea resolved after treatment. *Conclusion.* Gigantomastia might be the presenting symptom in patients with macroprolactinemia. In these patients medical treatment with cabergoline may be used initially as an alternative to surgical approach.

1. Introduction

Prolactin (PRL) which is secreted from the pituitary gland is an essential hormone for lactation and has an important role in the development of breast tissue. It regulates lobular and acinar development by binding to cellular receptors on breast tissue and induces production of milk. Hyperprolactinemia secondary to pregnancy or dopamine antagonist treatment causes growth of breast [1]. It was shown that addition of PRL to breast tissue culture stimulates budding structures [2].

Macroprolactinemia is defined as predominance of high molecular weight PRL forms (big-big PRL, MW > 150 kDa) which occurs when PRL monomers form complex with anti-PRL autoantibodies [3]. There are controversies about the clinical importance of macroprolactinemia, the indications for macroprolactin measurement, and the need for treatment in patients with macroprolactinemia. There is not any clinical sign that can help to differentiate macroprolactinemic patients from real hyperprolactinemic ones. Although

oligomenorrhea and galactorhea are observed with less frequency in patients with macroprolactinemia, at least one of these symptoms might be seen in many patients [4]. Despite lack of any consensus about routine measurement of macroprolactin, it is recommended to determine its level in patients with asymptomatic hyperprolactinemia [5, 6]. It is thought that macroprolactin is a biologically inactive molecule [7–9]; however some authorities suggest treatment in symptomatic cases [3, 10].

Gigantomastia, macromastia, and breast hypertrophy are terms used as synonym. Although there is no clear definition for gigantomastia, it is generally defined as excess breast tissue. There are various causes of gigantomastia and it can be seen in 10–25% of patients with hyperprolactinemia [11]. Patients present with gigantomastia associated physical and pshycological problems. Physical symptoms and signs are usually related to increased weight of breast tissue such as pain in shoulders, back, neck, and breast. Irritation, erythema, and ulceration under the submammarian fold secondary to hygienic problems might be observed [12]. Surgical interventions, hormonal therapy, or combination of these may be used for treatment. However, it is concluded by many authors that gigantomastia can not be treated medically and surgical intervention is the only option [13]. Here, we report significant clinical improvement with cabergoline treatment in a patient with gigantomastia, macroprolactinemia, and pituitary microadenoma.

2. Case Presentation

A 44-year-old women applied to our clinic with enlargement of breast tissue, galactorrhea, and pain in breast and back for 6 months. The patient had normal menstrual cycles and the last pregnancy was 20 years ago. She did not have any history of chronic disease, drug use, or excess weight gain. Family history was negative for breast hypertrophy. The patient had a demand for surgical therapy. In physical examination, weight was 82 kg, height was 162 cm, and body mass index was 31.2 kg/m^2.

Both breasts were hard and there was not any mass by palpation. Breast skin was tense; superficial veins were prominent and dilated. The patient did not have fever and there was not any erythema, warmth, or ulceration on breast skin. Bilateral galactorrhea was observed. The widest horizontal line passing from the areola was determined as the circumference of breast and it was 116 cm. Serum prolactin level was 91.38 ng/mL (15–65 ng/mL) and polyethylene glycol (PEG) preciptation for macroprolactin was positive (22.37%). Prolactin levels before and after PEG precipitation and macroprolactin levels were shown in Figures 1 and 2, respectively. Biochemical analysis and other anterior pituitary hormone levels were normal (Table 1). Basal serum cortisol was 16.07 μg/dL and it was suppressed to 1.4 μg/dL after 1 mg overnight dexamethasone suppression test. Serum was diluted by 1/100 for prolactin measurement to exclude "hook effect" and the result was 87.36 ng/mL. In pituitary magnetic resonance imaging, a nodular lesion suggestive of a 6 mm microadenoma deviating the infindibulum to the left was detected in the right side of the hypophysis. Bilateral breast ultrasonography and mammography were normal.

Since the patient had galactorrhea, cabergoline treatment was started at a dose of 0.5 mg/week. One month after the treatment, macroprolactin was negative and prolactin level was in normal limits. Breast circumference measurements made by the same clinician at the 1st, 2nd, 3rd, and 5th months were 110, 108, 106, and 105 cm, respectively. During follow-up galactorrhea resolved, tenderness recovered, and breast became relaxed. The patient was satisfied with the medical treatment.

3. Discussion

The clinical importance of macroprolactinemia is a controversial issue for years. While it is associated with hyperprolactinemic symptoms in some studies [4, 14–16], it is reported not to cause any signs or symptoms in others [8, 11]. This contradiction in the literature may be explained by heterogeneity

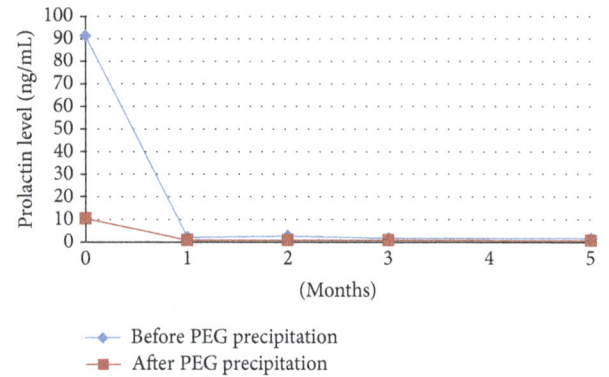

FIGURE 1: Prolactin levels before and after polyethylene glycol (PEG) precipitation.

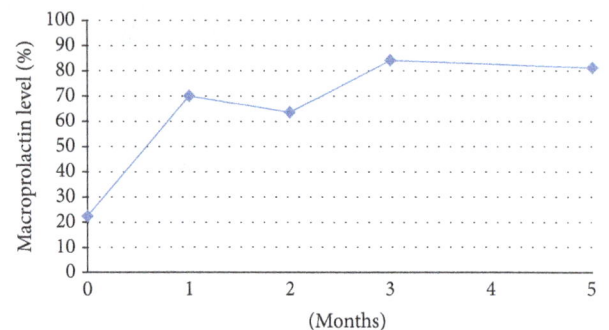

FIGURE 2: Macroprolactin levels.

in the structure of macroprolactin. Anti-PRL antibodies complexed with PRL are in the form of IgG in majority of cases; however antibodies in the form of IgA and IgM were also observed rarely [10].

Macroprolactin synthesis is generally believed to be a peripheral phenomenon. On the other hand, detection of pituitary adenoma in 20% of patients with macroprolactinemia has suggested that its origin might also be the pituitary gland. In addition, it was reported that 20% of patients with macroprolactinemia have galactorrhea and 45% have oligo/amenorrhea [5]. However, coincidental finding of pituitary nonfunctioning adenoma and macroprolactinemia may be a cause of the oligosymptomatic clinical presentation in these patients.

There is no consensus about the definition and classification of gigantomastia and macromastia yet. These two terms are generally used for each other. In general, they are defined as development of excess breast tissue compared to normal population resulting with physical and psychological pathologies. Surgically, enlargement of breast tissue which requires 1500 g reduction per breast may also be described as gigantomastia [17]. In the literature, there are studies reporting different values ranging from 300 to 2000 g for this amount [13]. According to another definition, if the resected breast tissue is under 300 g it is mild, if it is between 300 and 800 g it is moderate, and if it is over 800 gr it is severe macromastia [18]. Gigantomastia is classified etiologically into three main groups: idiopathic (Group 1), imbalance

TABLE 1: Biochemical and hormonal profile of the patient.

	Basal	1st month	2nd month	3rd month	5th month
Glucose (mg/dL)	74		79	72	71
Creatinine (mg/dL)	0.74		0.74	0.78	
ALT (U/L)	16	11	11	11	16
TSH (μIU/mL)	1.57	1.53	2.83	3.03	2.85
Free T4 (ng/dL)				1.04	1
Prolactin before PEG precipitation (ng/mL)	**91.38**	2.08	2.58	1.64	1.6
Prolactin after PEG precipitation (ng/mL)	10.22	0.78	0.82	0.69	0.65
Macroprolactin (%)	**22.37**	70	63.57	84.15	81.25
FSH (mIU/mL)	4.04			22.74	
LH (mIU/mL)	4.54			12.69	
Estradiol (pg/mL)	117.8			99.83	
Progesterone (ng/mL)				0.55	
GH (ng/mL)	0.03				
IGF-1 (ng/mL)	115.3				
Cortisol (μg/dL)	16.07				
ACTH (pg/mL)	13.64				
β-HCG (mIU/mL)	0.1			0.1	

Glucose (74–106 mg/dL), creatinine (0.5–1.2 mg/dL), ALT (0–33 U/L), TSH (0.27–4.2 μIU/mL), free T4 (0.9–1.7 ng/dL), prolactin (6–29.9 ng/mL), macroprolactin (0–40% positive, 40–60% borderline, and >60% negative; FSH (1.7–21.5 mIU/mL), LH (1–96 mIU/mL), estradiol (12.5–498 pg/mL), progesterone (0.1–3 ng/mL), GH (0–5 ng/mL), IGF-1 (94–252 ng/mL), cortisol (6.2–19.4 μg/dL), ACTH (0–60 pg/mL), and β-HCG (0–5 mIU/mL).

in endogenous hormone production (Group 2), and drug induced (Group 3) group. Group 1 is further devided into two: Group 1a includes obese patients, while Group 1b includes nonobese patients. Gigantomastia cases related to pubertal period and pregnancy are classifed as Group 2a and Group 2b, respectively. Idiopathic gigantomastia has unknown etiology and insidious onset. Suggested mechanisms in Group 2a (pubertal) are increased estrogen receptors in mammary gland and hypersensitivity of receptors to estrogen and progesterone. These patients have sudden disease onset, unilateral or bilateral gigantomastia, and family history. In Group 2b (pregnancy related), possible mechanism of gigantomastia is increased sensitivity to prolactin in mammary gland. Incidence is 1/28000–1/100000 of pregnancies, it has sudden onset and high rate of recurrence. Although possible mechanism in drug induced gigantomastia is unknown, it is commonly associated with other autoimmune diseases [13].

Generally, the first-line treatment of gigantomastia is surgery. Losing weight in Group 1a and withdrawal of medicine in Group 3 are the first treatment steps before surgery. Breast reduction surgery is the most frequently used surgical approach. However, recurrent surgery is required in most cases due to spontaneously continuing breast enlargement or hormonal impulses like pregnancy. In this situation total mastectomy might be an option. Hormonal treatment is generally applied before surgery, but not as a standalone option. Hormonal treatment alternatives present in the literature are bromocriptine, medroxyprogesterone, didrogesterone, tamoxifen, and danazol. Bromocriptine is effective particularly in Group 2b, while tamoxifen, medroxyprogesterone, and didrogesterone are used in Group 2a [13]. There exist no data in the literature about cabergoline treatment for gigantomastia.

In our case, coexistence of macroprolactinemia, gigantomastia, and pituitary adenoma was detected. Macroprolactinemia in the patient may be explained by three possiblities. Firstly, nonfunctioning pituitary adenoma and macroprolactinemia may be just a coincidental finding in this patient. Secondly, pituitary adenoma itself might be the origin of macroprolactin and, lastly, macroprolactin might be synthesized peripherally from breast-derived PRL. In the literature, there is evidence that supports the first two possibilities. Leslie et al. showed monomeric PRL isoform in pituitary adenoma tissue samples of patients with macroprolactinemia. This result is supportive of the peripheral synthesis of macroprolactin [19]. Conversely, there are two studies demonstrating higher macroprolactin concentrations in adenomatous prolactinoma tissue compared to normal pituitary tissue [20]. Additionally, Lakatos et al. reported 80-year-old male patient with intra- and parasellar pituitary mass and hyperprolactinemia largely in the form of macroprolactin [21]. These cases support the tumoral origin of macroprolactinemia. Although PRL is mainly secreted from the pituitary, studies have shown that bioactive PRL is also synthesized and secreted from adipose and glandular breast tissue [22]. In animal studies, breast-derived PRL was shown to play an important role particularly in postpartum secretory activity [23]. Breast-derived PRL production in our patient may also be considered an etiologic factor.

Cabergoline is an ergot derivative which has a selective, prolonged, and dose-dependent inhibitory effect on PRL. Its biological effect is regulated through dopamine, noradrenaline, and serotonin receptors. Stimulation of dopamine-2 receptors in lactotrop cells causes a decline in adenylate cyclase activity by decreasing the intracellular cAMP levels. PRL exerts its proliferative effect on breast tissue via RANKL and IGF-2 [23]. The fact that serum PRL levels are positively correlated with breast density on mammography in postmenopausal women is put forward as an evidence of mitogenic effect of PRL on breast tissue [24]. Cabergoline causes a reduction in cell volume in prolactinoma by early inhibition of secretory mechanisms and late inhibition of gene transcription and PRL synthesis. It also reduces prolactinoma size through perivascular fibrosis and partial cell necrosis [25, 26]. With a similar mechanism, it might cause a decrease in mitogenic activity in breast tissue and consequent reduction in size.

While coexistence of macroprolactinemia and gigantomastia was not reported in the literature previously, Oladele et al. presented 3 cases with hyperprolactinemia and gigantomastia [27]. In the first case, gigantomastia has started in pregnancy and PRL level was minimally increased. The second case was a 25-year-old nulliparous woman with minimally increased PRL levels. These two cases were not treated by dopamine agonists and underwent surgery for gigantomastia. The third patient was a 41-year-old, infertile woman who had a previous history of bromocriptine treatment. Her serum PRL level was high, other pituitary hormone levels were normal, and estradiol and progesterone levels were low. This patient was initially treated with bromocriptine and then a follow-up surgery was performed. PRL levels after surgery were not reported in all three patients. In the literature, other gigantomastia cases treated with cabergoline are all associated with pregnancy. All these patients underwent surgery after bromocriptine treatment [27]. In our case, the recovery of gigantomastia and macroprolactinemia with cabergoline treatment may be suggestive of possible role of macroprolactinemia in the etiology of gigantomastia. Whether the origin of macroprolactinemia was pituitary gland or peripheral tissue could not be identified because there was not any indication for pituitary surgery and histopathological evaluation was not made.

In conclusion, cabergoline seems to be reliable and effective option for the treatment of coexistant gigantomastia and macroprolactinemia, and it can be used as an alternative to surgery. Long term follow-up studies are required to evaluate the possibility of recurrence after withdrawal of cabergoline treatment. Although gigantomastia and macroprolactinemia are generally considered to be benign conditions, pituitary imaging, treatment with a dopamine agonist, and follow-up might be helpful in some cases.

References

[1] B. M. J. Stringer, J. Rowson, and E. D. Williams, "Effect of raised serum prolactin on breast development," *Journal of Anatomy*, vol. 162, pp. 249–261, 1989.

[2] L. Speroni, G. S. Whitt, J. Xylas et al., "Hormonal regulation of epithelial organization in a three-dimensional breast tissue culture model," *Tissue Engineering—Part C: Methods*, vol. 20, no. 1, pp. 42–51, 2014.

[3] M. Kasum, S. Oreskovic, I. Zec et al., "Macroprolactinemia: new insights in hyperprolactinemia," *Biochemia Medica*, vol. 22, no. 2, pp. 171–179, 2012.

[4] A. Alfonso, K. I. Rieniets, and R. A. Vigersky, "Incidence and clinical significance of elevated macroprolactin levels in patients with hyperprolactinemia," *Endocrine Practice*, vol. 12, no. 3, pp. 275–280, 2006.

[5] S. Melmed, F. F. Casanueva, A. R. Hoffman et al., "Diagnosis and treatment of hyperprolactinemia: an endocrine society clinical practice guideline," *Journal of Clinical Endocrinology and Metabolism*, vol. 96, no. 2, pp. 273–288, 2011.

[6] L. Vilar, M. Fleseriu, and M. D. Bronstein, "Challenges and pitfalls in the diagnosis of hyperprolactinemia," *Arquivos Brasileiros de Endocrinologia e Metabologia*, vol. 58, no. 1, pp. 9–22, 2014.

[7] F. A. Jamaluddin, P. Sthaneshwar, Z. Hussein, N. Othman, and S. P. Chan, "Importance of screening for macroprolactin in all hyperprolactinaemic sera," *Malaysian Journal of Pathology*, vol. 35, no. 1, pp. 59–63, 2013.

[8] R. Vaishya, R. Gupta, and S. Arora, "Macroprolactin; a frequent cause of misdiagnosed hyperprolactinemia in clinical practice," *Journal of Reproduction & Infertility*, vol. 11, no. 3, pp. 161–167, 2010.

[9] F. A. Cattaneo and M. N. Fahie-Wilson, "Concomitant occurrence of macroprolactin, exercise-induced amenorrhea, and a pituitary lesion: a diagnostic pitfall. Case report," *Journal of Neurosurgery*, vol. 95, no. 2, pp. 334–337, 2001.

[10] A. Elenkova, Z. Abadzhieva, N. Genov, V. Vasilev, G. Kirilov, and S. Zacharieva, "Macroprolactinemia in a patient with invasive macroprolactinoma: a case report and minireview," *Case Reports in Endocrinology*, vol. 2013, Article ID 634349, 5 pages, 2013.

[11] A. Shimatsu and N. Hattori, "Macroprolactinemia: diagnostic, clinical, and pathogenic significance," *Clinical and Developmental Immunology*, vol. 2012, Article ID 167132, 7 pages, 2012.

[12] G. A. Rahman, I. A. Adigun, and I. F. Yusuf, "Macromastia: a review of presentation and management," *The Nigerian Postgraduate Medical Journal*, vol. 17, no. 1, pp. 45–49, 2010.

[13] A. Dancey, M. Khan, J. Dawson, and F. Peart, "Gigantomastia—a classification and review of the literature," *Journal of Plastic, Reconstructive and Aesthetic Surgery*, vol. 61, no. 5, pp. 493–502, 2008.

[14] S. Vallette-Kasic, I. Morange-Ramos, A. Selim et al., "Macroprolactinemia revisited: a study on 106 patients," *Journal of Clinical Endocrinology and Metabolism*, vol. 87, no. 2, pp. 581–588, 2002.

[15] J. Gibney, T. P. Smith, and T. J. McKenna, "The impact on clinical practice of routine screening for macroprolactin," *Journal of Clinical Endocrinology and Metabolism*, vol. 90, no. 7, pp. 3927–3932, 2005.

[16] M. Taghavi and F. Sedigheh, "Macroprolactinemia in patients presenting with hyperandrogenic symptoms and hyperprolactinemia," *International Journal of Endocrinology and Metabolism*, vol. 6, no. 3, pp. 140–143, 2008.

[17] A. Gliosci and F. Presutti, "Virginal gigantomastia: validity of combined surgical and hormonal treatments," *Aesthetic Plastic Surgery*, vol. 17, no. 1, pp. 61–65, 1993.

[18] F. R. Grippaudo, D. C. Kennedy, P. Tiwari, F. Talavera, S. M. Shenaq, and N. G. Slenkovich, "Liposuction only breast reduction," eMedicine.com, July 2009, http://emedicine.medscape.com/article/1276259.

[19] H. Leslie, C. H. Courtney, P. M. Bell et al., "Laboratory and clinical experience in 55 patients with macroprolactinemia identified by a simple polyethylene glycol precipitation method,"

Journal of Clinical Endocrinology and Metabolism, vol. 86, no. 6, pp. 2743–2746, 2001.

[20] C. Mounier, J. Trouillas, B. Claustrat, R. Duthel, and B. Estour, "Macroprolactinaemia associated with prolactin adenoma," *Human Reproduction*, vol. 18, no. 4, pp. 853–857, 2003.

[21] G. Lakatos, N. Szücs, Z. Kender, S. Czirják, and K. Rácz, "Macroprolactinemia associated with pituitary macroadenoma: treatment with quinagolide," *Orvosi Hetilap*, vol. 151, no. 26, pp. 1072–1075, 2010.

[22] M. Zinger, M. McFarland, and N. Ben-Jonathan, "Prolactin expression and secretion by human breast glandular and adipose tissue explants," *Journal of Clinical Endocrinology and Metabolism*, vol. 88, no. 2, pp. 689–696, 2003.

[23] N. D. Horseman and K. A. Gregerson, "Prolactin actions," *Journal of Molecular Endocrinology*, vol. 52, no. 1, pp. R95–R106, 2013.

[24] G. A. Greendale, M.-H. Huang, G. Ursin et al., "Serum prolactin levels are positively associated with mammographic density in postmenopausal women," *Breast Cancer Research and Treatment*, vol. 105, no. 3, pp. 337–346, 2007.

[25] J. S. Bevan, J. Webster, C. W. Burke, and M. F. Scanlon, "Dopamine agonists and pituitary tumor shrinkage," *Endocrine Reviews*, vol. 13, no. 2, pp. 220–240, 1992.

[26] P. G. Crosignani and C. Ferrari, "2 Dopaminergic treatments for hyperprolactinaemia," *Bailliere's Clinical Obstetrics and Gynaecology*, vol. 4, no. 3, pp. 441–455, 1990.

[27] A. O. Oladele, J. K. Olabanji, and G. H. Alabi, "Reduction mammoplasty: the experience in Ile-Ife, Nigeria," *Nigerian Journal of Medicine*, vol. 16, no. 3, pp. 261–267, 2007.

19

Hypocalciuric Hypercalcemia due to Impaired Renal Tubular Calcium Excretion in a Type 2 Diabetic Patient

Sihao Yang,[1,2] Yan Ren,[1] Xi Li,[1] Haoming Tian,[1] Zhenmei An,[1] and Tao Chen[1]

[1]*Department of Endocrinology and Metabolism, West China Hospital of Sichuan University, Chengdu, China*
[2]*Department of Chinese Traditional Medicine, The Second People's Hospital of Yibin, Yibin, China*

Correspondence should be addressed to Zhenmei An; 848948343@qq.com and Tao Chen; dr.chentao@qq.com

Academic Editor: Wayne V. Moore

The case we presented here was a 73-year-old gentleman, who was admitted to endocrinology department due to recurrent fatigue for 1 year. He had medical histories of type 2 diabetes for 18 years and developed CKD 4 years ago. He also suffered from dilated cardiomyopathy, and coronary heart disease, moderate sleep apnea syndrome, primary hypothyroidism, and gout. His treatment regimen was complicated which included Caltrate D and compound α-keto acid (1200 mg calcium/d). Laboratory examination revealed that his serum calcium level elevated, 24-hour urine calcium output decreased, PTH level was suppressed, and 25-hydroxyvitamin D was in normal low range. No other specific abnormalities were found in serum bone turnover markers, ultrasonography, computed tomography, and bone scintigraphy. The diagnosis was suggested to be hypocalciuric hypercalcemia but was different from familial or acquired hypocalciuric hypercalcemia which were featured by elevated PTH level. The patient was asked to restrict calcium intake and to take diuretics; then his serum calcium level gradually lowered. In brief, patients with CKD could present with hypocalciuric hypercalcemia due to impaired renal calcium excretion. In this case, calcium restriction should be applied for treatment.

1. Introduction

Hypercalcemia related to PTH, malignancy diseases (PTHrP or destruction), and vitamin D metabolites usually could be easily diagnosed according to clinical setting [1]. However, in other cases, especially in cases with PTH independent hypercalcemia, the etiology is often difficult to identify. A published review summarized the rare causes of hypercalcemia and showed the potential mechanisms including calcitriol overdosage, occult milk-alkali syndrome, some medications (e.g., omeprazole, theophylline toxicity, and growth hormone), and other diversity causes [2]. Other recent studies showed that sarcoidosis [3], granulomatosis/granuloma [4, 5], diabetic ketoacidosis [6], and methylmethacrylate for cosmetic purposes [7] could also be causes for PTH independent hypercalcemia. However, hypercalcemia due to impaired renal calcium excretion was rarely reported. Here, we presented a case of hypocalciuria hypercalcemia with suppressed PTH levels. The mechanism could be impaired renal tubular calcium regulation.

2. Case Report

The patient was a 73-year-old man who was admitted in September 21, 2015, due to recurrent fatigue for 1 year. He was diagnosed as type 2 diabetes 18 years ago, developed chronic kidney disease 4 years ago, and began to take compound α-keto acid (2520 mg three times a day, approximately containing 600 mg calcium element). Six years ago, he was diagnosed with osteoporosis and began to take Caltrate D (600 mg calcium element) and Alphacalcidol (0.5 μg) daily. One year ago, the patient began to feel fatigue. Laboratory tests showed serum calcium elevated to 3.41 mmol/L. After stopping Caltrate D and Alphacalcidol, it fluctuated between 2.24 and 2.93 mmol/L. Two months ago, he felt fatigue again and was referred to endocrinology department. Laboratory tests showed elevated serum calcium level (3.03 mmol). No other clinical significant changes were found in thyroid function, blood gas analysis, immunologic test, protein electrophoresis, tumor markers, ACTH, and plasma total cortisol levels.

TABLE 1: The changes of the patient's serum and urine calcium levels and their related biochemical indexes in recent 7 years.

Events	2009-10-28 Calcium 600 mg/d, Alphacalcidol 50 μg/d	2011-12-16 Added compound α-keto acid (600 mg calcium/d)	2012-1 to 2013-11	2013-12-14 Initially suspected hypercalcemia during review	2014-10-25 Diagnosed as hypercalcemia; ceased calcium, Alphacalcidol	2014-11 to 2015-6	2015-09-21 This admission; ceased compound α-keto acid	2016-3-16	2016-4 to 2016-8 Compound α-keto acid (150 mg calcium/d)
Serum BUN	7.15	17.62	9.2–12.1	11.66	11.78	13.36–20.65	15.8	22.4	25.6–33.7
Serum creatinine	95.6	181.5	128.4–140.2	128.3	164.3	142.0–183.0	212.0	134.0	178.0–182.0
eGFR	N/A	34.33	46.11–51.04	50.94	35.2	31.06–34.44	29.1	44.96	31.05–31.89
PH value	N/A	N/A	N/A	N/A	N/A	N/A	7.43	N/A	N/A
Serum calcium	2.34	2.28	2.16–2.65	2.67	3.41	2.24–2.93	3.24	2.02	2.20–2.59
Serum phosphate	0.95	0.99	0.65–1.65	1.33	1.29	1.3–1.4	0.94	1.06	1.07–1.41
Urine calcium$^+$	5.01	N/A	1.63[b]	N/A	2.51	N/A	2.21	0.29	0.19–0.34
Urine volume (L)	1.50	N/A	2.4	N/A	1.50	N/A	1.00	1.6	1.4–2.0
PTH	5.48	18.05	3.58–5.19	0.76	0.82	0.79–0.82	0.79	11.44	8.12
25(OH)D	40.61	26.56	36.3–37.2	71.08	44.62	N/A	50.11	27.16	N/A
1,25(OH)$_2$D[a]	30.47	165.65	30.93	N/A	N/A	N/A	N/A	N/A	N/A
bALP	8.67	12.94	N/A	N/A	12.02	N/A	14.23	N/A	N/A
CTX	U/A	0.10	N/A	N/A	0.117	N/A	0.154	N/A	N/A

Reference value: 1,25(OH)$_2$D 39–193 pmol/L; 25(OH)D 47.7–144 pmol/L; 24-hour urine calcium 2.5–7.5 mmol/24 hours; bALP 11.4–24.6 μg/L; CTX 0.3–0.584 ng/mL; eGFR 56–122 mL/min/1.73 m^2; PTH 1.6–6.9 pmol/L; serum BUN 3.82–8.86 mmol/L; serum creatinine 53.0–140.0 μmol/L; serum calcium 2.1–2.7 mmol/L; serum phosphate 0.81–1.45 mmol/L. [a] Measurement of 1,25(OH)$_2$D was unavailable since the end of 2013. [b] 24-hour urine calcium was 1.63 mmol when serum calcium was at the level of 2.2 mmol/L.

We then comprehensively reviewed his laboratory reports in recent years (Table 1). We found his serum calcium began to raise at the end of 2013, as indicated by suppressed PTH (serum calcium 2.67 mmol/L, PTH 0.76 pmol/L), and then raised up to 3.41 mmol/L in 2014. After calcium and vitamin D restriction, his serum calcium fluctuated between 2.24 and 2.93 mmol/L, and PTH were consistently suppressed (from 0.79 to 0.82 pmol/L). Further evaluation showed that his urine calcium output decreased (1.63–2.51, reference value 2.5–7.5 mmol/24 hours) when serum calcium increased. Meanwhile, his serum 25-hydroxyvitamin D, bALP, and CTX were all in low levels. No specific signs were found by DEXA, chest and abdominal computed tomography, and bone scintigraphy.

Taken together, we suggested that this patient developed a clinical condition, featured by hypocalciuric hypercalcemia and suppressed PTH level. He was asked to cease compound α-keto acid, restrict milk intake, increase water intake, and use diuretics. His serum calcium gradually returned to normal. On March 16, 2016, he experienced recurrent cramp in both legs. Laboratory workup showed his serum calcium decreased to 2.02 mmol/L, and PTH elevated to 11.44 nmol/L. His treatment was adjusted to compound α-keto acid two tablets one day, three times one week, and he was asked to monitor serum calcium every month.

3. Discussion

Hypocalciuric hypercalcemia as familial pattern was well-known [1]. In recent two decades, acquired hypocalciuric hypercalcemia was reported and was supposed to be resulting from autoantibody against calcium-sensing receptor (CSRP) [8, 9]. A typical feature of acquired hypocalciuric hypercalcemia slightly elevated PTH level, which is due to increased set point of parathyroid cell for serum calcium. While, in this case, PTH was suppressed when serum calcium increased, and PTH elevated when serum calcium decreased, indicating normal function of CSRP in this patient's parathyroid gland. Thus, we deduced that his hypercalcemia was caused by impaired calcium excretion from urine.

In normal person, about 59% of total serum calcium is filtered into crude urine. Then, 90% of those were reabsorbed by proximal tubules, henry loop, and early distal tubules and nearly 10% reabsorbed by early collecting ducts and late distal tubular. The latter portion is relatively few but more important in calcium hemostasis because it is highly dependent on the blood calcium ion concentration. A slightly elevation of serum calcium level, under the regulation of PTH, will result in strikingly increasing calcium excretion from urine [8, 10].

In this case, the patient's serum PTH level changed corresponding to alteration of serum calcium level but failed to maintain serum calcium to the normal range. Thus, we proposed that the patient's hypocalciuric hypocalcemia resulted from impaired response of late distal tubular and early collecting ducts to the changed PTH level. We searched Medline (PubMed, update to May 2, 2016) using Mesh term "Hypocalciuric Hypercalcemia" but failed to retrieve any similar reports. We were unable to perform renal biopsy because of the patient's refusal. So, we could not, regrettably, demonstrate the exact mechanism of how the patient's renal tubular failed to respond to changed serum calcium level. The differential diagnosis of hypercalcemia without clear etiology is often very difficult; therefore, the case we presented here might provide some valuable information for future clinical practice.

4. Conclusion

PTH independent hypocalcaemia could be caused by decreased urine calcium excretion in patients with complicated clinical conditions. Calcium restriction and carefully monitoring were the key points in treatment.

Authors' Contributions

Sihao Yang and Yan Ren contributed equally to this paper.

References

[1] F. Bringhurst, M. Demay, and H. Kronenberg, "Hormones and disorders of mineral metabolism," in *Williams Textbook of Endocrinology*, S. Melmed, K. Polonsky, P. Larsen, and H. Kronenberg, Eds., pp. 1260–1277, Elsevier Sauders, Philadelphia, Pa, USA, 12th edition, 2011.

[2] T. P. Jacobs and J. P. Bilezikian, "Clinical review: rare causes of hypercalcemia," *Journal of Clinical Endocrinology and Metabolism*, vol. 90, no. 11, pp. 6316–6322, 2005.

[3] R. Lupica, M. Buemi, A. Campenni et al., "Unexpected hypercalcemia in a diabetic patient with kidney disease," *World Journal of Nephrology*, vol. 4, no. 3, pp. 438–443, 2015.

[4] P. Hardy, P. H. Morinière, B. Tribout et al., "Liver granulomatosis is not an exceptional cause of hypercalcemia with hypoparathyroidism in dialysis patients," *Journal of Nephrology*, vol. 12, no. 6, pp. 398–403, 1999.

[5] S. M. Hindi, Y. Wang, K. D. Jones et al., "A case of hypercalcemia and overexpression of CYP27B1 in skeletal muscle lesions in a patient with HIV infection after cosmetic injections with polymethylmethacrylate (PMMA) for wasting," *Calcified Tissue International*, vol. 97, no. 6, pp. 634–639, 2015.

[6] T. Makaya, S. Chatterjee, P. Arundel, C. Bevan, and N. P. Wright, "Severe hypercalcemia in diabetic ketoacidosis: a case report," *Diabetes Care*, vol. 36, no. 4, article no. e44, 2013.

[7] D. V. Rados and T. W. Furlanetto, "An unexpected cause of severe and refractory PTH-independent hypercalcemia: case report and literature review," *Archives of endocrinology and metabolism*, vol. 59, no. 3, pp. 277–280, 2015.

[8] J. C. Pallais, O. Kifor, Y.-B. Chen, D. Slovik, and E. M. Brown, "Acquired hypocalciuric hypercalcemia due to autoantibodies against the calcium-sensing receptor," *New England Journal of Medicine*, vol. 351, no. 4, pp. 362–369, 2004.

[9] N. Makita, J. Sato, K. Manaka et al., "An acquired hypocalciuric hypercalcemia autoantibody induces allosteric transition among active human Ca-sensing receptor conformations," *Proceedings of the National Academy of Sciences of the United States of America*, vol. 104, no. 13, pp. 5443–5448, 2007.

20

An Ectopic ACTH Secreting Metastatic Parotid Tumour

Thomas Dacruz,[1] Atul Kalhan,[2] Majid Rashid,[3] and Kofi Obuobie[3]

[1]*University Hospital of Wales, Cardiff, UK*
[2]*Department of Diabetes & Endocrinology, Royal Glamorgan Hospital, Mid Glamorgan CF72 8XR, UK*
[3]*Royal Gwent Hospital, Newport, UK*

Correspondence should be addressed to Atul Kalhan; atulkal31@hotmail.com

Academic Editor: Hidetoshi Ikeda

A 60-year old woman presented with features of Cushing's syndrome (CS) secondary to an ectopic adrenocorticotropic hormone (ACTH) secreting metastatic parotid tumour 3 years after excision of the original tumour. She subsequently developed fatal intestinal perforation and unfortunately died despite best possible medical measures. Ectopic ACTH secretion accounts for 5–10% of all patients presenting with ACTH dependent hypercortisolism; small cell carcinoma of lung (SCLC) and neuroendocrine tumours (NET) account for the majority of such cases. Although there are 4 previous case reports of ectopic ACTH secreting salivary tumours in literature, to our knowledge this is the first published case report in which the CS developed after 3 years of what was deemed as a successful surgical excision of primary salivary tumour. Our patient initially had nonspecific symptoms which may have contributed to a delay in diagnosis. Perforation of sigmoid colon is a recognised though underdiagnosed complication associated with steroid therapy and hypercortisolism. This case demonstrates the challenges faced in diagnosis as well as management of patients with CS apart from the practical difficulties faced while trying to identify source of ectopic ACTH.

1. Background

Cushing's syndrome (CS) is associated with a constellation of signs and symptoms related to hypercortisolism. Common conditions such as obesity, chronic alcoholism, and depression share clinical and phenotypic features which overlap with those seen in patients with CS; often it results in delayed investigations and management for the patients.

True CS can either be ACTH dependent or ACTH independent [1]. ACTH dependent CS is uncommon with 1-2 cases/million of population/per year reported in the literature, with pituitary adenoma being source of ACTH in two-thirds of such patients [1]. SCLC and pancreatic/thymic/bronchial NETs remain the commonest tumours associated with ectopic ACTH secretion [2–4]. There are rare reports linking medullary carcinoma of thyroid, phaeochromocytoma, and ovarian and salivary tumours with ectopic ACTH secretion [5, 6]. To our knowledge, there are only 4 previous case reports of ectopic ACTH secretion from a salivary gland carcinoma leading to CS [7–10]. This is also the first report of an ectopic ACTH-secreting metastatic salivary tumour in which the CS developed after 3 years of complete and what was deemed as a successful surgical excision of primary salivary tumour.

2. Case Presentation

Mrs. XX, a 60-year-old woman was hospitalised with 5-month history of worsening fatigue, leg swelling, and difficulty in walking. Her past medical history included primary hypothyroidism and hypertension. She had been diagnosed with an acinic cell carcinoma of the left parotid gland, which was resected 3 years prior to current admission. She was under follow-up of the surgical team with no obvious evidence of disease recurrence or relapse at the time of presentation.

On examination in medical assessment unit, she had florid features of CS including central obesity, plethoric face, skin thinning, purplish abdominal striae, and proximal muscle weakness. Her blood pressure was elevated with rest of the general physical and systemic examination being unremarkable.

TABLE 1: Initial routine blood test results.

Investigations	Results	Reference range
Haemoglobin	125 g/L	115–155
White blood cell count	11.5×10^9/L	4–10.5
Neutrophils	7.5×10^9/L	1.5–7.5
Platelets	318×10^9/L	150–450
Serum sodium	141 mmol/L	135–145
Serum potassium	2.6 mmol/L	3.5–5.5
Serum urea	3.6 mmol/L	2.5–7.8
Serum creatinine	51 μmol/L	50–100
Fasting blood glucose	7 mmol/L	

TABLE 2: Further investigations.

Investigations	Results	Reference range
Prolactin	429 mU/L	<560
Insulin-like growth factor 1	11 nmol/L	12.0–54.0
24-hour urinary cortisol level	4481 nmol	<146
ACTH	106 ng/L	7–63

3. Investigations

Her initial investigations results were as shown in Table 1.

On the basis of clinical suspicion of hypercortisolism, she underwent further tests as shown in Tables 2 and 3.

Magnetic Resonance Image of the Pituitary. It showed normal pituitary gland.

Abdomen/Pelvis/Thorax CT. It shows a lytic lesion on the left ischium bone suggestive of a metastatic carcinoma. A collection of gas around the sigmoid colon was noticed which was suggestive of perforated sigmoid diverticulitis.

Histopathology. Biopsy of ischial lesion showed features consistent with a metastatic poorly differentiated acinic cell carcinoma with negative staining for ACTH (Figure 2). However, the previously resected primary parotid tumour of acinic cell carcinoma were stained positively for ACTH.

4. Treatment

Our patient was commenced on metyrapone therapy on day 6 of admission with a gradual uptitration of the dose. The course of her disease was aggressive with subsequent development of intestinal perforation. Interestingly, she had minimal symptoms and signs on clinical examination suggestive of intestinal perforation with this diagnosis being only established based on the radiological investigations.

She later developed sepsis and was managed in intensive care unit. Unfortunately, despite the best possible care her condition continued to deteriorate and she died due to complications related to her ectopic ACTH related CS secondary to a metastatic salivary gland tumour.

5. Discussion

Ectopic ACTH secreting tumours are rare with a reported prevalence of 8–18% of all the patients with CS [11, 12]. The SCLC along with NETs (bronchial, thymic, and pancreatic) remains the commonest ACTH secreting tumours [2–4]. Our patient presented with CS secondary to an ectopic ACTH producing metastatic parotid tumour. In our literature search, we could only identify 4 previously reported cases of metastatic salivary tumour associated with ectopic ACTH production [5–8]. In most of the previous case reports, CS was diagnosed either at the time of diagnosis of primary salivary tumour or within months of commencement of treatment (median duration of CS diagnosis 6 months after initial salivary tumour was detected). Our patient is the first case report of an ectopic ACTH secreting salivary tumour presenting with a distant metastasis after over 3 years of being deemed cured of primary tumour (postsurgical excision).

Our patient presented with 5-month history of nonspecific features including weight gain, malaise, and leg swelling. There was a possible delay in her investigations and management due to nonspecific nature of her symptoms. An overlap of such symptoms is not uncommonly seen in obesity, depression, and chronic alcoholism which have a much higher prevalence in clinical practice.

On admission, our patient had florid signs of CS including proximal myopathy and purple striae which are considered relatively specific for CS [13]. The initial screening (24 hour UFC and ODST) tests were suggestive of hypercortisolism. An unsuppressed cortisol level on LDDST further established the biochemical evidence for CS. Elevated ACTH levels pointed towards possibility of a pituitary or ectopic source of ACTH/CRH. The MRI of pituitary gland was reported as normal in our patient. In clinical practice, it is often challenging to distinguish an ectopic ACTH secreting tumour from a pituitary source especially considering that in 40% of CD patients a MRI pituitary may be normal [14]. Inferior petrosal sinus sampling (IPSS) was considered as the next step in investigation although it could not be carried out as our patient was deemed medically unfit to undergo this invasive procedure. Previously, a HDDST was considered to be a useful additional test to distinguish pituitary from an ectopic source of ACTH. In CD, a cortisol suppression of > 50% from the basal level is noticed in only 80% of the patients undergoing HDDST, limiting the diagnostic usefulness of this test [15]. IPSS remains the gold standard to distinguish pituitary from an ectopic source of ACTH [16].

The ectopic ACTH source may not be obvious initially in patients with well-differentiated neuroendocrine tumours as these are generally slow growing and may not be visualised on routine radiological imaging. In 12% of patients, despite extensive investigations, the source of ectopic ACTH may not be identified [17]. Various modalities have been suggested to investigate and identify source of ectopic ACTH secretion including use of Somatostatin scintigraphy [18]. Proopiomelanocortin (POMC) serves as precursor molecule to ACTH and undergoes posttranslational proteolytic processing in corticotrophs. This proteolysis processing is mediated by serine proteinases such as PC1, PC2, and PC3 which are expressed only in the pituitary gland and play a role in POMC cleavage. Ectopic ACTH tumours are characterised by an abnormal circulating ACTH precursor to ACTH ratio as

TABLE 3: Dynamic tests to assess hypercortisolism.

Investigation	Procedure	Timing of the test	Results
Overnight dexamethasone test (ODST)	1 mg dexamethasone given at midnight	Measurement of 9 am cortisol	785 nmol/L
Low dose dexamethasone test (LDDST)	0.5 mg dexamethasone given every six hours for 48 hours	Cortisol measured after last dose of dexamethasone	577 nmol/L

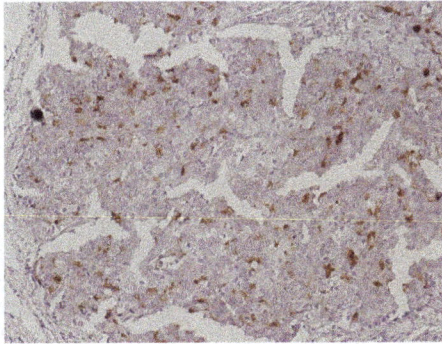

FIGURE 1: Immunohistochemical stain (×400) for ACTH showing tumour cells being positive (brown).

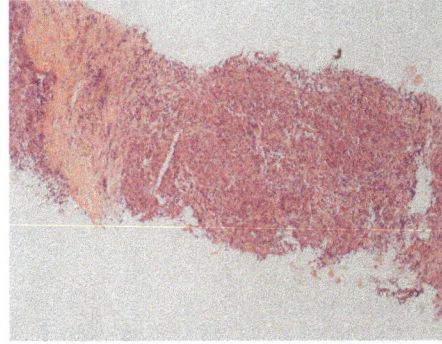

FIGURE 2: Haematoxylin and Eosin stain (×200) bony metastasis with poorly differentiated malignant epithelial cells seen.

compared to ACTH secreting pituitary adenoma due to a possible aberrant POMC processing [19, 20]. As no single imaging technique is believed to have optimal accuracy for localisation of ectopic ACTH secreting tumour, it is recommended to combine more than one imaging modality such as conventional CT along with somatostatin scintigraphy scan [18].

A whole body CT scan in our patient revealed a lytic lesion on the left ischial bone and patient went on to develop bowel perforation, with minimal features. Exogenous steroid use and CS have been associated with increased risk of intestinal perforation and sepsis [21, 22]. It is not uncommon for the cortisol excess to mask signs associated with intestinal perforation delaying the diagnosis which can potentially prove fatal as in our patient.

The ischial lytic bone lesion on histopathological analysis was confirmed to be a metastasis from the parotid gland tumour although it was stained negatively for ACTH. The immunostaining of preserved original tumour tissue was stained positively with ACTH confirming the diagnosis (Figure 1). Negative ACTH staining in ectopic tumour tissue is believed to be associated with a more aggressive disease course and a worse prognosis [23]. It is postulated that the tumour which has a high secretory rate gets depleted of all intracellular ACTH which results in negative immunostaining on histopathological analysis as may have been the case in our patient.

The further investigations and treatment were limited in our patient because of her rapid clinical deterioration. In retrospective analysis, we acknowledge the fact that there was a relative delay in initiation of metyrapone therapy in her case. Bilateral adrenalectomy should be considered as a life-preserving treatment option in patients presenting with severe ACTH dependent CS uncontrolled with medical therapy or in patients with metastatic ectopic ACTH secreting

tumours [24] although our patient was deemed an unsuitable candidate for any surgical intervention.

In summary, our patient presented with a highly aggressive ectopic ACTH secreting metastatic parotid tumour. Earlier suspicion and management of hypercortisolism could have potentially improved her prognosis although it may or may not have altered the eventual outcome.

Learning Points

(i) The signs and symptoms associated with Cushing's syndrome may be nonspecific which can potentially lead to a delay in diagnosis and management.

(ii) The presence of proximal myopathy, easy bruisability, and purple striae should prompt investigations for CS as untreated disease carries high morbidity and mortality.

(iii) Distinguishing pituitary from ectopic source of ACTH is challenging especially if there is no obvious adenoma identified on magnetic resonance imaging (MRI) of the pituitary. This is a recognised clinical scenario in up to 40% of the patients with Cushing's disease (CD).

(iv) SCLC and NETs remain the commonest tumours associated with ectopic ACTH secretion although it has been reported in association with salivary gland, medullary carcinoma of thyroid, phaeochromocytoma, and ovarian tumours.

(v) Bilateral adrenalectomy should be considered as a life-preserving treatment option in patients presenting with severe ACTH dependent CS uncontrolled with medical therapy or in patients with metastatic ectopic ACTH secreting tumours.

References

[1] H. E. Turner and J. A. H. Wass, *Oxford Handbook of Endocrinology and Diabetes*, Oxford University Press, Oxford, UK, 2nd edition, 2009.

[2] T. A. Howlett, P. L. Drury, L. Perry, I. Doniach, L. H. Rees, and G. M. Besser, "Diagnosis and management of ACTH-dependent Cushing's syndrome: comparison of the features in ectopic and pituitary ACTH production," *Clinical Endocrinology*, vol. 24, no. 6, pp. 699–713, 1986.

[3] F. A. Shepherd, J. Laskey, W. K. Evans, P. E. Goss, E. Johonsen, and F. Khamsi, "Cushing's syndrome associated with ectopic corticotropin production and small-cell lung cancer," *Journal of Clinical Oncology*, vol. 10, no. 1, pp. 21–27, 1992.

[4] L. R. Salgado, M. C. B. Villares Fragoso, M. Knoepfelmacher et al., "Ectopic ACTH syndrome: our experience with 25 cases," *European Journal of Endocrinology*, vol. 155, no. 5, pp. 725–733, 2006.

[5] R. C. Smallridge, K. Bourne, B. W. Pearson, J. A. Van Heerden, P. C. Carpenter, and W. F. Young, "Cushing's syndrome due to medullary thyroid carcinoma: diagnosis by proopiomelanocortin messenger ribonucleic acid in situ hybridization," *Journal of Clinical Endocrinology and Metabolism*, vol. 88, no. 10, pp. 4565–4568, 2003.

[6] E. H. Al Ojaimi, "Cushing's syndrome due to an ACTH-producing primary ovarian carcinoma," *Hormones*, vol. 13, no. 1, pp. 140–145, 2014.

[7] M. Sugawara and G. A. Hagen, "Ectopic ACTH syndrome due to salivary gland adenoid cystic carcinoma," *Archives of Internal Medicine*, vol. 137, no. 1, pp. 102–105, 1977.

[8] V. V. Shenoy, Z. Lwin, A. Morton, and J. Hardy, "Ectopic adrenocorticotrophic hormone syndrome associated with poor prognosis in metastatic parotid acinic cell carcinoma," *Otolaryngology—Head and Neck Surgery*, vol. 145, no. 5, pp. 878–879, 2011.

[9] L. Jamieson, S. M. Taylor, A. Smith, M. J. Bullock, and M. Davis, "Metastatic acinic cell carcinoma of the parotid gland with ectopic ACTH syndrome," *Otolaryngology—Head and Neck Surgery*, vol. 136, no. 1, pp. 149–150, 2007.

[10] V. Alcantara, E. Urgell, J. F. Sancho, and A. Chico, "Severe ectopic cushing syndrome caused by adenoid cystic carcinoma of a salivary gland," *Endocrine Practice*, vol. 19, no. 5, pp. e118–e121, 2013.

[11] B. L. Wajchenberg, B. B. Mendonca, B. Liberman et al., "Ectopic adrenocorticotropic hormone syndrome," *Endocrine Reviews*, vol. 15, no. 6, pp. 752–787, 1994.

[12] J. P. Aniszewski, W. F. Young Jr., G. B. Thompson, C. S. Grant, and J. A. Van Heerden, "Cushing syndrome due to ectopic adrenocorticotropic hormone secretion," *World Journal of Surgery*, vol. 25, no. 7, pp. 934–940, 2001.

[13] J. Newell-Price, P. Trainer, M. Besser, and A. Grossman, "The diagnosis and differential diagnosis of Cushing's syndrome and pseudo-Cushing's states," *Endocrine Reviews*, vol. 19, no. 5, pp. 647–672, 1998.

[14] C. Invitti, F. P. Giraldi, M. de Martin, and F. Cavagnini, "Diagnosis and management of Cushing's syndrome: results of an Italian multicentre study. Study Group of the Italian Society of Endocrinology on the pathophysiology of the Hypothalamic-Pituitary-Adrenal axis," *The Journal of Clinical Endocrinology & Metabolism*, vol. 84, no. 2, pp. 440–448, 1999.

[15] D. C. Aron, H. Raff, and J. W. Findling, "Effectiveness versus efficacy: the limited value in clinical practice of high dose dexamethasone suppression testing in differential diagnosis of adrenocorticotropin-dependent Cushing's syndrome," *Journal of Clinical Endocrinology and Metabolism*, vol. 82, no. 6, pp. 1780–1785, 1997.

[16] G. Reimondo, P. Paccotti, M. Minetto et al., "The corticotrophin-releasing hormone test is the most reliable non-invasive method to differentiate pituitary from ectopic ACTH secretion in Cushing's syndrome," *Clinical Endocrinology*, vol. 58, no. 6, pp. 718–724, 2003.

[17] B. L. Wajchenberg, B. B. Mendonça, B. Liberman, M. A. A. Pereira, and M. A. Kirschner, "Ectopic ACTH syndrome," *The Journal of Steroid Biochemistry and Molecular Biology*, vol. 53, no. 1–6, pp. 139–151, 1995.

[18] W. W. de Herder and S. W. J. Lamberts, "Tumor localization—the ectopic ACTH syndrome," *Journal of Clinical Endocrinology and Metabolism*, vol. 84, no. 4, pp. 1184–1185, 1999.

[19] P. M. Stewart, S. Gibson, S. R. Crosby et al., "ACTH precursors characterize the ectopic ACTH syndrome," *Clinical Endocrinology*, vol. 40, no. 2, pp. 199–204, 1994.

[20] A. C. Hale, G. M. Besser, and L. H. Rees, "Characterization of pro-opiomelanocortin-derived peptides in pituitary and ectopic adrenocorticotrophin-secreting tumours," *Journal of Endocrinology*, vol. 108, no. 1, pp. 49–56, 1986.

[21] T. Hara, H. Akutsu, T. Yamamoto, E. Ishikawa, M. Matsuda, and A. Matsumura, "Cushing's disease presenting with gastrointestinal perforation: a case report," *Endocrinology, Diabetes & Metabolism Case Reports*, vol. 11, Article ID EDM130064, 2013.

[22] K. Piekarek and L. A. Israelsson, "Perforated colonic diverticular disease: the importance of NSAIDs, opioids, corticosteroids, and calcium channel blockers," *International Journal of Colorectal Disease*, vol. 23, no. 12, pp. 1193–1197, 2008.

[23] P. J. Coates, I. Doniach, T. A. Howlett, L. H. Rees, and G. M. Besser, "Immunocytochemical study of 18 tumours causing ectopic Cushing's syndrome," *Journal of Clinical Pathology*, vol. 39, no. 9, pp. 955–960, 1986.

[24] L. K. Nieman, B. M. Biller, J. W. Findling et al., "Treatment of Cushing's syndrome: an endocrine society clinical practice guideline," *The Journal of Clinical Endocrinology & Metabolism*, vol. 100, no. 8, pp. 2807–2831, 2015.

21

Nonfunctioning Pituitary Adenoma That Changed to a Functional Gonadotropinoma

Gerson Geovany Andino-Ríos ⓘ,[1] **Lesly Portocarrero-Ortiz,**[1] **Carlos Rojas-Guerrero,**[1] **Alejandro Terrones-Lozano** ⓘ,[1] **Alma Ortiz-Plata,**[2] and **Alfredo Adolfo Reza-Albarrán** ⓘ[3]

[1]Neuroendocrinology Department, Instituto Nacional de Neurología y Neurocirugía Manuel Velasco Suárez,
  Ciudad de México, Mexico
[2]Experimental Neuropathology Laboratory, Instituto Nacional de Neurología y Neurocirugía Manuel Velasco Suárez,
  Ciudad de México, Mexico
[3]Endocrinology and Metabolism Department, Instituto Nacional de Ciencias Médicas y Nutrición Salvador Zubirán,
  Ciudad de México, Mexico

Correspondence should be addressed to Gerson Geovany Andino-Ríos; gersongandino@yahoo.com

Academic Editor: Takeshi Usui

Objective. Pituitary adenomas can be classified as clinically functional or silent. Depending on the reviewed literature, these are the first or second place in frequency of the total pituitary adenomas. Even rarer is the presence of a functional gonadotropinoma since only very few case reports exist to date. The conversion of a clinically silent to functional pituitary adenoma is extraordinarily rare; the mechanisms that explain these phenomena are unknown or not fully understood. *Methods*. We report the case of a woman who initially had a nonfunctional gonadotropinoma and in the course of her medical condition showed biochemical changes in her hormonal pituitary profile compatible with a functional gonadotropinoma. *Results*. We considered that the patient had a functional gonadotropinoma due to the hyperestrogenemia in the context of secondary amenorrhea, resolving the hyperestrogenemia after almost complete resection of the tumor. *Conclusion*. It is necessary to point out from a clinical and/or biochemical point of view the change in functionality that a nonfunctional pituitary adenoma may have. In the case of our patient, the suspicion of this change in functionality became evident when we found an increase in the FSH/LH ratio and a progressive increase in serum estradiol concentrations when the patient had amenorrhea.

1. Introduction

Nonfunctioning gonadotropinomas are the second most common type of pituitary adenoma. Its clinical diagnosis is based on the presence of symptoms associated with compression by mass effect; the true prevalence of functioning gonadotropinomas is unknown since the vast majority of reports mentioning this pituitary entity are case reports. To date, there are very few cases reported in the medical literature discussing the conversion of a nonfunctional to functional pituitary adenoma. We describe the case of a patient who initially was diagnosed with a nonfunctional gonadotropinoma that, at a later clinical follow-up, diagnosis was changed to a functional gonadotropinoma, where the main diagnostic key was the elevation of estradiol in the context of amenorrhea.

2. Case Report

A 41-year-old woman came in for consultation in July 2013. Her menarche was at age of 13, no pregnancies occurred, and her menstrual cycles were regular, every 28–30 days. At age of 36 she had noticed oligomenorrhea and subsequently amenorrhea. She also mentioned headache and blurred vision, so she was submitted to magnetic resonance imaging (MRI), which showed a pituitary adenoma of 43 × 40 × 29 mm. Her visual field test showed bilateral temporal hemianopia and she was then sent to a reference center. The first hormonal pituitary profile showed the following results: TSH: 1.9 μIU/mL (0.34–5.60), FT$_4$: 7.2 pmol/L (8.11–17.25), TT$_3$: 1.3 nmol/L (0.98–2.78), LH: 2.6 mIU/mL (2.4–12.6), FSH: 7.3 mIU/mL (3.5–12.5), estradiol 14.4 pg/mL

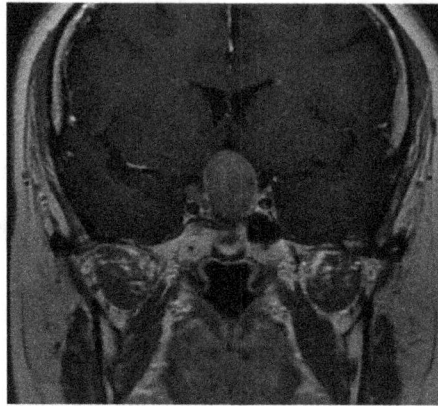

FIGURE 1: Coronal MRI T1 sequence with gadolinium. Intra- and suprasellar tumor with extension to the floor of third ventricle, after first surgery.

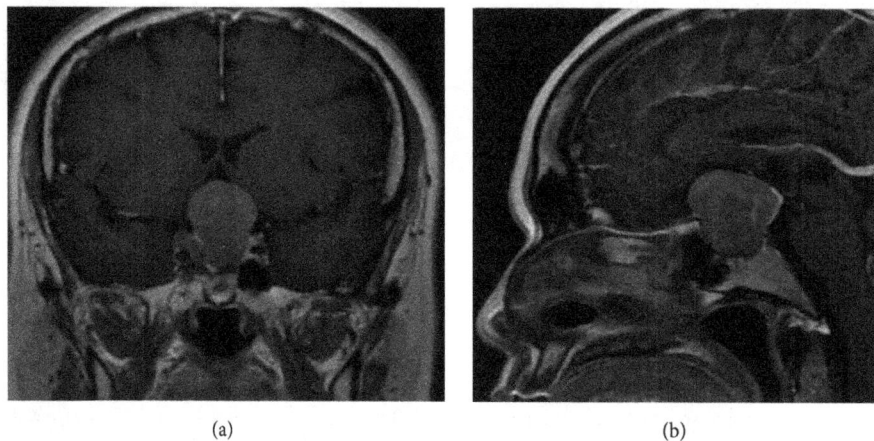

(a)   (b)

FIGURE 2: Coronal and sagittal MRI T1 sequence with gadolinium. Intra- and suprasellar tumor with tumor growth related to previous study.

(25.0–195.0), prolactin: 20.0 ng/mL (3.3–26.7), ACTH: 15.0 pg/mL (4.7–48.8), cortisol: 12.4 µg/dL (8.7–22.4), and IGF-1: 53.8 ng/mL (56–194). The patient was considered to have hypopituitarism; however, only 50 mcg oral levothyroxine treatment was started every day due to central hypothyroidism. Dynamic test was not performed to rule out secondary adrenal insufficiency due to the risk of causing pituitary apoplexy. The patient underwent transsphenoidal resection in August 2013 (Figure 1). Despite the important tumor remnant, it was not specified whether the macroscopic appearance of the tumor had any special feature that made resection difficult during surgery. Immunostaining was positive for FSH and LH. During clinical follow-up, she presented some improvement in her visual fields but amenorrhea persisted. In 2015 there was deterioration in the visual fields; new hormonal determinations showed FSH of 6.31 mIU/mL and LH of 2.20 mIU/mL, as well as increase in estradiol levels at 135 pg/mL; it was considered to perform a new tumor resection to protect the vision but a short-term surgical date could not be obtained. In March 2016, a new MRI with a focus on the sellar region was performed, finding tumor remnant growth (Figures 2(a) and 2(b)). No visual worsening was reported. A new gonadal profile was requested

which showed estradiol of 394.5 pg/mL and dissociation between FSH and LH (6.19 mIU/mL and 1.98 mIU/mL, resp.); amenorrhea persisted. After the annual biochemical monitoring of the gonadal hormones, it was concluded that the gonadotropinoma became functional, so it was decided to surgically intervene by transcranial approach that resulted in a significant reduction of the tumor lesion (Figures 3(a) and 3(b)). The decision to perform a transcranial approach was taken by the neurosurgery team due to their experience with this type of approach and the objective of resecting as much tumor tissue as possible. Ten days after the second surgery, a new gonadal profile measurement was performed: FSH 2.81 mIU/mL, LH 0.57 mIU/mL, and estradiol 20.3 pg/mL. Immunostaining index (percentage of immune-positive cells) was slightly higher for FSH (38.9%; range 31–48%) than LH (35.1%; range 29–39%). MIB-1 (Ki-67) labeling index was 1.7%. Histologically tumors cells arranged in papillary pattern were found (Figures 4(a) and 4(b)). It is noteworthy highlighting that hormonal therapy with estrogen and/or progestagens was never initiated during the entire management of the patient. Unfortunately, pelvic ultrasound could not be performed before the second surgery when the possibility of a functional gonadotropinoma was considered.

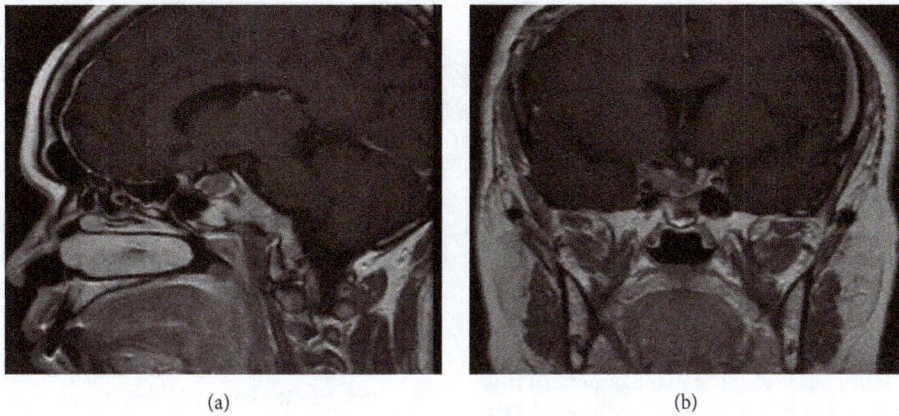

(a)   (b)

FIGURE 3: Sagittal and coronal MRI T1 sequences with gadolinium. Residual tumoral tissue only located intrasellar and right parasellar after second surgery.

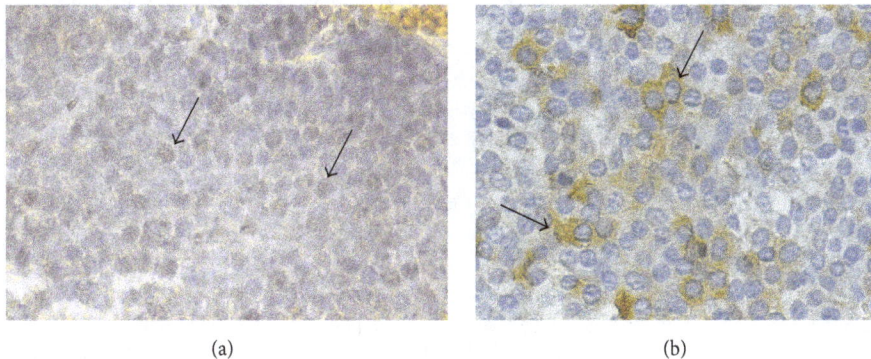

(a)   (b)

FIGURE 4: Micrography of immunohistochemistry staining with Streptavidina-Biotine technique revealed with diaminobenzidine. (a) Nuclear expression of SF-1 in the first surgery ((a), arrows). (b) Intense positivity for the FSH hormone in the second surgery ((b), arrows) (×400).

The patient is currently waiting to receive treatment with radiosurgery.

3. Discussion

Pituitary adenomas are considered the third most frequent intracranial neoplastic lesion (15%), after meningiomas and gliomas. Until recently, pituitary adenomas were considered relatively rare diseases; however, improvement in various imaging techniques has increased its detection [1]. The nonfunctioning pituitary adenomas represent 15–30% of these [2]. Nonfunctioning pituitary adenomas are considered the second most common pituitary adenoma, exceeded only by prolactinoma [3], although the silent clinical course of a large percentage of them could explain a large proportion that are not diagnosed. Usually, these tumors are manifested by the effect of mass compression, such as headache, blurred vision, and seizures. After the fourth decade of life, the nonfunctioning pituitary adenoma is the most frequent type of pituitary adenoma diagnosed. Histopathologically, most nonfunctioning pituitary adenomas have positive immunohistochemistry staining for FSH/LH [4]. The pathogenesis of functioning gonadotropinomas is unknown; several theories have been postulated, among which some that stand out are greater production of intact and biologically active FSH, hypersecretion of an abnormal form of FSH that inhibits GnRH secretion at the level of the hypothalamus, further inhibiting secretion of FSH and LH, inhibition of the union of the abnormal form of FSH to FSH receptors at the pituitary level, or loss of negative counter-regulation by estrogens towards gonadotrophins [5, 6]. Within the differential diagnoses, ovarian hyperstimulation syndrome could be the consequence of continuous hyperstimulation of biologically active forms of FSH on ovarian follicles which may lead to complications such as rupture of cysts and peritonitis, hypovolemic shock, acute renal failure, distress respiratory syndrome of the adult, and pulmonary thromboembolism [7–9]. Diagnosis of functioning gonadotropinoma may be suspected of having a profile of relative gonadal level of FSH/LH > 2, hyperestrogenemia in the context of amenorrhea, and MRI (magnetic resonance imaging) showing the presence of variable size multiseptated cysts in both ovaries. Until now, it is biochemically difficult to diagnose postmenopausal women with a functioning gonadotropinoma due to them showing constant elevated FSH levels and lack of ovarian follicles to stimulate with FSH [6, 7]. Different reviews and case reports conclude that the size of functioning gonadotropinomas is always greater than 1 cm [10]. In the case of men, FSH hypersecretion can cause testicular growth; however, this clinical data might not be recognized by the physician due to the slow evolution of testicular growth. It is controversial whether this "testicular hyperstimulation" is related to testosterone concentration or not, being that some authors report that high levels of testosterone produce greater trophic effects on seminiferous tubules, while others argue that these trophic effects are directly exerted by FSH [10–12]. In a similar way to women, all reports of functioning gonadotropinoma cases in men reveal the presence of tumors larger than 1 cm. Differential diagnoses in women include ovarian hyperstimulation syndrome, hyperandrogenic chronic anovulation syndrome, and ovarian neoplasia. In men, the differential diagnosis includes McCune-Albright syndrome, congenital testicular cysts, and malignant testicular lesions [13, 14]. The management of this sellar tumor is primarily surgical. To date, there is limited data on the experience obtained with pharmacological treatment (dopaminergic agonists or somatostatin receptor agonists), with very few and even no beneficial effects. Pharmacological treatment has been displaced by radiotherapy in its various modalities, being this the second-choice therapeutic modality [6].

The patient initially presented clinically with a nonfunctioning gonadotropinoma; subsequently, the elevated levels of gonadotrophins and estradiol were evident which led to a change in the diagnosis to a functional gonadotropinoma; such change in tumor functionality is very rare. It is known that pituitary adenomas can change their gene expression and hormonal secretion; however, the exact mechanisms that explain this phenomenon are not completely clear [15]. To date, the most classic and frequent change recognized by endocrinologists is the transformation in functionality from silent corticotropinoma to Cushing's disease. Literature case reports are not clear in establishing if there has been a change in the functional pattern of the tumors previously. In other words, published clinical findings do not show a change from a nonfunctional tumor to a pattern of gonadotrophin hypersecretion due to researchers only highlighting clinical or biochemical data on hypersecretion. In our case, biochemical finding led us to diagnose a functional tumor. We consider that the progressive increase of gonadotrophins and estradiol in a patient with a pituitary adenoma and amenorrhea may suggest the presence of a functional gonadotropinoma.

Disclosure

This research did not receive any specific grant from any funding agency in the public, commercial, or not-for-profit sector.

References

[1] E. D. Aflorei and M. Korbonits, "Epidemiology and etiopathogenesis of pituitary adenomas," *Journal of Neuro-Oncology*, vol. 117, no. 3, pp. 379–394, 2014.

[2] P. Chanson, G. Raverot, F. Castinetti, C. Cortet-Rudelli, F. Galland, and S. Salenave, "Management of clinically non-functioning pituitary adenoma," *Annales d'Endocrinologie*, vol. 76, no. 3, pp. 239–247, 2015.

[3] M. E. Molitch, "Diagnosis and treatment of pituitary adenomas: a review," *Journal of the American Medical Association*, vol. 317, no. 5, pp. 516–524, 2017.

[4] F. Castinetti, H. Dufour, S. Gaillard et al., "Non-functioning pituitary adenoma: When and how to operate? What pathologic criteria for typing?" *Annales d'Endocrinologie*, vol. 76, no. 3, pp. 220–227, 2015.

[5] J. Halupczok, B. Bidzińska-Speichert, A. Lenarcik-Kabza, G. Zieliński, A. Filus, and M. Maksymowicz, "Gonadotroph adenoma causing ovarian hyperstimulation syndrome in a premenopausal woman," *Gynecological Endocrinology*, vol. 30, no. 11, pp. 774–777, 2014.

[6] G. Ntali, C. Capatina, A. Grossman, and N. Karavitaki, "Functioning gonadotroph adenomas," *The Journal of Clinical Endocrinology & Metabolism*, vol. 99, no. 12, pp. 4423–4433, 2014.

[7] J. Halupczok, A. Kluba-Szyszka, B. Bidzińska-Speichert, and B. Knychalski, "Ovarian hyperstimulation caused by gonadotroph pituitary adenoma—review," *Advances in Clinical and Experimental Medicine*, vol. 24, no. 4, pp. 695–703, 2015.

[8] M. T. Memarzadeh, "A fatal case of ovarian hyperstimulation syndrome with perforated duodenal ulcer," *Human Reproduction*, vol. 25, no. 3, pp. 808-809, 2010.

[9] C. O. Nastri, R. A. Ferriani, I. A. Rocha, and W. P. Martins, "Ovarian hyperstimulation syndrome: Pathophysiology and prevention," *Journal of Assisted Reproduction and Genetics*, vol. 27, no. 2-3, pp. 121–128, 2010.

[10] D. L. Mana, M. S. Belingeri, M. Manavela et al., "FSH-Producing Pituitary Macroadenoma: Report of 2 Cases with Clinical Manifestations of Hormone Excess," *AACE Clinical Case Reports*, vol. 2, no. 1, pp. e7–e11, 2016.

[11] P. Dahlqvist, L.-O. D. Koskinen, T. Brännström, and E. Hägg, "Testicular enlargement in a patient with a FSH-secreting pituitary adenoma," *Endocrine Journal*, vol. 37, no. 2, pp. 289–293, 2010.

[12] R. Chamoun, L. Layfield, and W. T. Couldwell, "Gonadotroph adenoma with secondary hypersecretion of testosterone," *World Neurosurgery*, vol. 80, no. 6, pp. 900–e11, 2013.

[13] A. K. Dey, A. Dubey, K. Mittal, and S. Kale, "Spontaneous ovarian hyperstimulation syndrome - Understanding the dilemma," *Gynecological Endocrinology*, vol. 31, no. 8, pp. 587–589, 2015.

[14] G. Khanna, K. Kantawala, M. Shinawi, S. Sarwate, and L. P. Dehner, "McCune-Albright syndrome presenting with unilateral macroorchidism and bilateral testicular masses," *Pediatric Radiology*, vol. 40, no. 1, pp. S16–S20, 2010.

[15] T. Daems, J. Verhelst, A. Michotte, P. Abrams, D. Ridder, and R. Abs, "Modification of hormonal secretion in clinically silent pituitary adenomas," *The Pituitary Society*, vol. 12, no. 1, pp. 80–86, 2009.

22

A Normotensive Patient with Primary Aldosteronism

Xiao Lin, Xiaoyu Miao, Pengli Zhu, and Fan Lin

Department of VIP, Fujian Provincial Hospital, Fujian Medical University, 134 East Street, Fuzhou 350001, China

Correspondence should be addressed to Fan Lin; linfandoc@gmail.com

Academic Editor: John Broom

This study was to report a case of normotensive patient with primary aldosteronism who was admitted to our department recently. The patient was a 33-year-old male with right adrenal incidentaloma, but without any symptom. He has no history of hypertension, and blood pressure was normal when measured at multiple time points during hospitalization stay. The 24-hour ambulatory blood pressure prompted a normal blood pressure with the existence of circadian rhythm. The patient was diagnosed with primary aldosteronism by screening and confirmatory test. Due to the absence of symptom, surgery was not preferred. Blood pressure was found to be normal with the 2-month follow-up from discharge until now.

1. Introduction

Primary aldosteronism is a disease caused by increased aldosterone secreted in the zona glomerulosa of the adrenal cortex, with the symptoms of hypertension and hypokalemia as its main clinical manifestations. Although some patients with primary aldosteronism may not occur hypokalemia [1], but the vast majority of patients suffer from hypertension. Normotensive patients with primary aldosteronism are extremely rare. So far, only a total of 30 cases were reported in China and abroad [2, 3], and most of them were combined with hypokalemia. Recently, our department admitted a patient who was found with right adrenal incidentaloma by chest computed tomography (CT). Moreover, the patient was diagnosed with primary aldosteronism by screening and confirmatory test. He showed no symptom and sign, and no history and family history of hypertension, while the blood pressure and serum potassium were normal when measured at multiple time points during hospitalization stay. The case reported is shown as follows.

The patient was a 33-year-old male admitted to the hospital due to the right adrenal incidentaloma found by chest CT on August 23, 2016. The patient had no symptoms, such as dizziness, headache, chest tightness, palpitations, fatigue, and periodic paralysis, as well as no history and family history of hypertension. Physical examination showed that blood pressure was 133/83 mmHg, while his height and weight were 180 cm and 65 kg, respectively, with the body mass index of $20.1 \, \text{kg/m}^2$. The patient was conscious and without palpable evidence of thyroid enlargement. Rales were not heard from the breath of the two lungs. Heart rate of the patient was 67 beats/min with regular rhythm, and no noise was heard from auscultation areas of each valve. The whole abdomen had no tenderness, without palpable evidence of liver or spleen enlargement. No edema was found in both lower extremities. Muscle force and muscular tension of all four limbs were normal symmetry, and reflexes of bilateral tendon were also normal. After admission, the three routine examinations including blood, urine, and feces were checked to be normal, while liver and kidney functions were normal as well. Blood potassium was 3.6–3.9 mmol/l (the normal range of 3.5–5.5 mmol/l) and serum sodium was 145 mmol/l (the normal range of 137–147 mmol/l). CT scanning of the mid abdomen plus enhanced scanning suggested that a low-density nodule similar to oval shape was found in the medial limb of the right adrenal gland, with the size of approximately 1.5 cm × 1.1 cm and CT value was −14 Hu. The lesion showed mildly enhancement (Figure 1). Related hormone test was performed to determine whether the right adrenal incidentaloma had function. 24-hour urinary vanilloid myristic acid was 37.00 umol, as well as serum adrenocorticotrophic hormone (08:00) of 55.52 pg/ml, serum cortisol (08:00) of 384.90 nmol/l, and serum cortisol (16:00) of 201.80 nmol/l, which were all in normal range. 24-hour urinary cortisol was

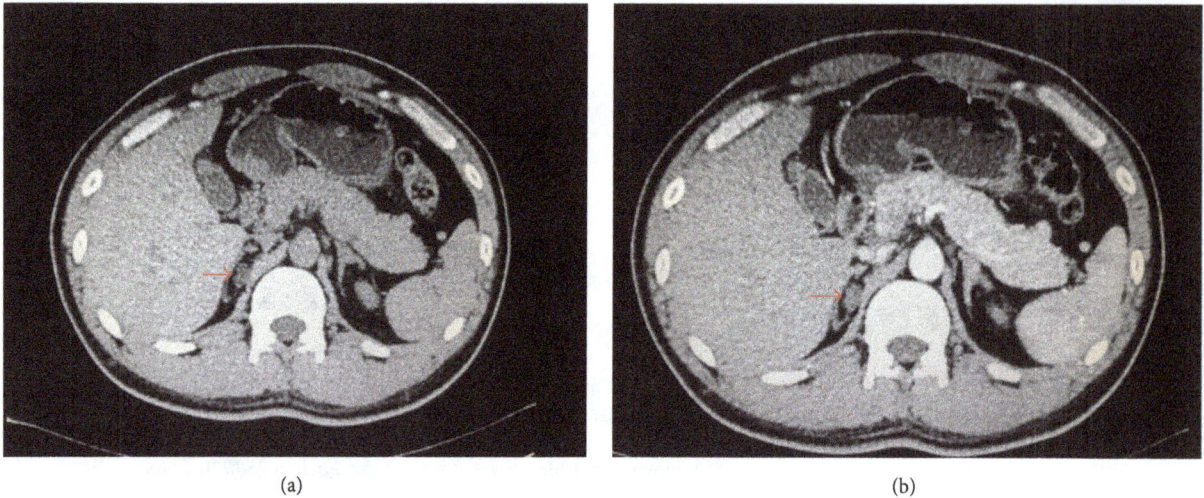

(a)   (b)

FIGURE 1: (a) Adrenal computed tomography scanning suggested right adrenal adenoma (pointed by red arrow). (b) Adrenal computed tomography enhancement indicated that the right adrenal adenoma was mildly intensified (pointed by red arrow).

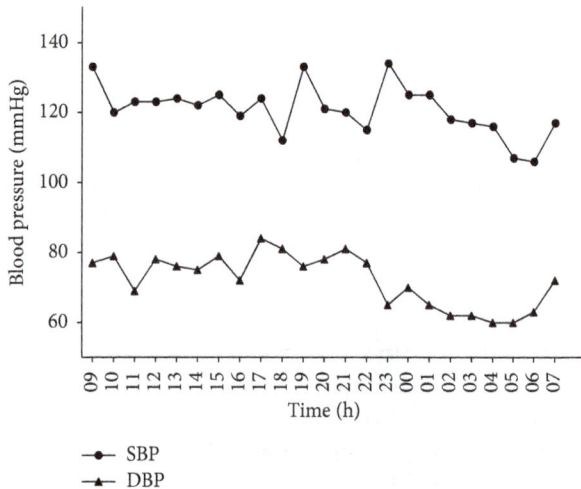

FIGURE 2: The trend of 24-hour ambulatory blood pressure of the patient.

TABLE 1: Comparison of the parameters before and after saline infusion test.

Parameters	Before	After
Serum potassium (mmol/L)	3.2	3.6
Serum sodium (mmol/L)	142	143
Serum cortisol (nmol/L)	451.70	295.10
Plasma aldosterone (ng/L)	179.93	144.68
Plasma renin activity (Ug/l·h)	0.22	0.01
Angiotensin (ng/L)	61.37	64.15

35.86 nmol (the normal range of 58.00–395.00 umol), which was a little bit low. The examinations of thyroid function, sex hormone, and growth hormone were all normal. Blood pressure of the right upper arm was measured at multiple time points during hospitalization stay, ranging between 116/60 mmHg and 133/88 mmHg. Blood pressures of the whole day by 24-hour ambulatory blood pressure monitoring were all less than 140/90 mmHg, averaged at 120/73 mmHg. The mean blood pressure at daytime was 120/75 mmHg, while it was 116/63 mmHg at night. The trend of blood pressure was dipper with double peaks and double troughs (Figure 2).

The ratio of plasma aldosterone (PAC) to plasma renin activity (PRA) was used as an indicator of screening for primary aldosteronism. The results indicated that PAC (in the supine position) was 246.21 ng/L (normal range was 59.50–173.90 ng/L) and PRA (in the supine position) was 0.10 Ug/lh (normal range was 0.05–0.79 Ug/lh), while the calculated ARR (in the supine position) was 246.21. PAC (in the erect position) was 228.33 ng/L (normal range was 65.20–295.70 ng/L), and PRA (in the erect position) was 0.35 Ug/lh (normal range was 0.93–6.56 Ug/lh), while the calculated ARR (in the erect position) was 65.24. ARRs of the patient in both supine position and erect position were greater than 50, suggesting that the possibility of primary aldosteronism was extremely great. The patient did not take any drug affecting the results of ARR and had a balanced sodium diet before screening test, as well as with normal serum potassium. According to the guidelines of the Endocrine Society of America [4], the saline infusion test was used to perform the confirmatory test of primary aldosteronism (Table 1). The results showed that PAC was 144.68 ng/L after saline infusion, which was greater than 100 ng/L, so it can be diagnosed as primary aldosteronism.

The patient had no symptom, and blood pressures were all normal when measured at multiple time points. During hospitalization stay, low serum potassium occurred once before saline infusion test. Subsequently, multiple times of the review of electrolyte demonstrated normal serum potassium. Therefore, drug therapy or surgical treatment was not performed. The patient conducted outpatient follow-up for 2 months from discharge until now without any symptoms found. Blood pressure of the right upper arm from family monitoring was 110–135/65–80 mmHg.

2. Discussion

The main clinical manifestation of primary aldosteronism is the combination with hypertension and hypokalemia. Although recent studies have found that the incidence of hypokalemia is only about 50% [5, 6] in patients with primary aldosteronism, the vast majority of patients suffer from hypertension. Based on this characteristic, the guidelines of the American Association of Endocrine [4] pointed out that indications of screening test of primary aldosteronism should include hypertension. However, there are few reports of normotensive patients with primary aldosteronism both in China and abroad. In 1972, Brooks et al. [7] first reported a normotensive patient with primary aldosteronism. To date, only a total of 30 such cases were reported in China and other countries. Rossi [8] analyzed the 26 normotensive patients with primary aldosteronism in the literature, showing that 85% of cases were from Europe and Asia, especially and mainly from Japan. Most of the patients were middle-aged and females. In addition, there were sporadic cases of familial hyperaldosteronism type I (FH-I) with normal blood pressure [2].

The patient in the current study is a young man, who was found to have right adrenal incidentaloma by chest CT. He had no history and family history of hypertension, as well as no symptoms of hypokalemia. During hospitalization stay, hypokalemia was found only once, and the remaining multiple time examinations showed normal plasma potassium. The patient was diagnosed by screening test of primary aldosteronism and confirmatory test. This finding posed a challenge to the current guidelines [4, 9] that only hypertension is used as the indicator of screening primary aldosteronism. For patient with adrenal incidentaloma who has normal blood pressure and without hypokalemia, primary aldosteronism cannot be easily excluded, which needs further screening of primary aldosteronism. From the literature, the sensitivity and specificity of saline infusion test are high. Rossi et al. performed saline infusion test for the 317 cases with ARR > 40, and, through analyzing sensitivity and specificity, 6.8 ng/dl (190 pmol/l) was selected to be the best critical value of aldosterone, with the sensitivity and specificity of 83% and 75% [10], respectively. Therefore, the case in the present study was diagnosed by this test.

For normotensive patient with primary aldosteronism, the mechanism of normal blood pressure is still unclear, which is considered to be associated with the following causes. ① Patients are still in the early stage of the disease. For example, the case reported in our study was without previous history of hypertension, while the multiple time blood pressures measured during hospitalization stay were all normal. Hypokalemia in this patient occurred only once. Markou et al. [11] reported that after 5 years of follow-up, normotensive patients with primary aldosteronism were more likely to develop hypertension than nonprimary aldosteronism patients. Therefore, as time goes by, hypertension and hypokalemia of this patient might gradually appear. ② Previous basal blood pressure of patients is low; even for the patients who have suffered from primary aldosteronism, it is still in normal range after increasing blood pressure [12].

③ Vasodilator materials are in the body of patients, such as the increased secretion or sensitivity of prostaglandin E, kallikrein, and nitric oxide, while the sensitivity of vasoconstrictor substances is reduced [8]. ④ The aldosterone escape phenomenon occurs in the patients, and its mechanism could be the inhibition of endogenous renin-angiotensin-aldosterone system due to the role of genetic and environmental factors, thereby promoting sodium excretion and vasodilatation [2, 8]. ⑤ A long-term low-sodium diet may help the patient to maintain his blood pressure normal. ⑥ A minority of FH-I patients have normal or slightly increased blood pressure, but the mechanism is unclear.

Our case report has the following limitations. ① Because the absence of symptom was found, the patient did not have the will of surgery. Therefore, it lacked pathological evidence. Now, the follow-up is conducting for the patient in the study. ② FH-I is mainly unequal genetic recombination between 11β-hydroxylase CYP11B1 and aldosterone synthase CYP11B2 to form CYP11B chimeric gene. Therefore, it results that the aldosterone secretion of the patient is regulated by ACTH, and a minority of patients with FH-I will show a normal blood pressure. The patient in our study did not receive genetic examination. If necessary, genetic screening or the fludrocortisone suppression test should be considered for this patient, in spite of the modest specificity of the latter.

In summary, it is extremely rare that the patient suffered from primary aldosteronism is with normal blood pressure and without symptoms. We realize through this case that, for adrenal incidentaloma with normal blood pressure and serum potassium, it is necessary to conduct screening test to exclude the possibility of primary aldosteronism.

Acknowledgments

This study was supported by Excellent Young Doctor Training Program in Fujian Provincial Health System (no. 2013-ZQN-ZD-4).

References

[1] J. S. Williams, G. H. Williams, A. Raji et al., "Prevalence of primary hyperaldosteronism in mild to moderate hypertension without hypokalaemia," *Journal of Human Hypertension*, vol. 20, no. 2, pp. 129–136, 2006.

[2] V. Médeau, F. Moreau, L. Trinquart et al., "Clinical and biochemical characteristics of normotensive patients with primary aldosteronism: a comparison with hypertensive cases," *Clinical Endocrinology*, vol. 69, no. 1, pp. 20–28, 2008.

[3] Y. Ito, R. Takeda, S. Karashima, Y. Yamamoto, T. Yoneda, and Y. Takeda, "Prevalence of primary aldosteronism among prehypertensive and stage 1 hypertensive subjects," *Hypertension Research*, vol. 34, no. 1, pp. 98–102, 2011.

[4] J. W. Funder, R. M. Carey, F. Mantero et al., "The management of primary aldosteronism: case detection, diagnosis, and treatment: an endocrine society clinical practice guideline," *Journal*

of Clinical Endocrinology and Metabolism, vol. 101, no. 5, pp. 1889–1916, 2016.

[5] E. Born-Frontsberg, M. Reincke, L. C. Rump et al., "Cardiovascular and cerebrovascular comorbidities of hypokalemic and normokalemic primary aldosteronism: results of the German conn's registry," *Journal of Clinical Endocrinology and Metabolism*, vol. 94, no. 4, pp. 1125–1130, 2009.

[6] S. A. Potthoff, F. Beuschlein, and O. Vonend, "Primay hyperaldosteronism—diagnostic and treatment," *Deutsche Medizinische Wochenschrift*, vol. 137, no. 48, pp. 2480–2484, 2012.

[7] R. V. Brooks, D. Felix-Davies, M. R. Lee, and P. W. Robertson, "Hyperaldosteronism from Adrenal Carcinoma," *British Medical Journal*, vol. 1, no. 5794, pp. 220–221, 1972.

[8] G. P. Rossi, "Does primary aldosteronism exist in normotensive and mildly hypertensive patients, and should we look for it," *Hypertension Research*, vol. 34, no. 1, pp. 43–46, 2011.

[9] M. Fassnacht, W. Arlt, I. Bancos et al., "Management of adrenal incidentalomas: European Society of Endocrinology Clinical Practice Guideline in collaboration with the European Network for the Study of Adrenal Tumors," *European Journal of Endocrinology*, vol. 175, no. 2, pp. G1–G34, 2016.

[10] G. P. Rossi, A. Belfiore, G. Bernini et al., "Prospective evaluation of the saline infusion test for excluding primary aldosteronism due to aldosterone-producing adenoma," *Journal of Hypertension*, vol. 25, no. 7, pp. 1433–1442, 2007.

[11] A. Markou, T. Pappa, G. Kaltsas et al., "Evidence of primary aldosteronism in a predominantly female cohort of normotensive individuals: a very high odds ratio for progression into arterial hypertension," *Journal of Clinical Endocrinology and Metabolism*, vol. 98, no. 4, pp. 1409–1416, 2013.

[12] S. Moradi, M. Shafiepour, and A. Amirbaigloo, "A woman with normotensive primary hyperaldosteronism," *Acta Medica Iranica*, vol. 54, no. 2, pp. 156–158, 2016.

23

Adrenocorticotropic Hormone Secreting Pheochromocytoma Underlying Glucocorticoid Induced Pheochromocytoma Crisis

Gil A. Geva ⓘD,[1] David J. Gross,[2] Haggi Mazeh ⓘD,[3] Karine Atlan,[4] Iddo Z. Ben-Dov,[5] and Matan Fischer ⓘD[6]

[1] The Hebrew University Hadassah Medical School, Hadassah-Hebrew University Medical Center, Jerusalem, Israel
[2] Endocrinology & Metabolism Service, Hadassah-Hebrew University Medical Center, Jerusalem, Israel
[3] Department of General Surgery, Hadassah-Hebrew University Medical Center, Jerusalem, Israel
[4] Department of Pathology, Hadassah-Hebrew University Medical Center, Jerusalem, Israel
[5] Nephrology and Hypertension Services, Hadassah-Hebrew University Medical Center, Jerusalem, Israel
[6] Department of Internal Medicine, Hadassah-Hebrew University Medical Center, Jerusalem, Israel

Correspondence should be addressed to Haggi Mazeh; hmazeh@hadassah.org.il

Academic Editor: Toshihiro Kita

Context. Pheochromocytomas are hormone secreting tumors of the medulla of the adrenal glands found in 0.1–0.5% of patients with hypertension. The vast majority of pheochromocytomas secrete catecholamines, but they have been occasionally shown to also secrete interleukins, calcitonin, testosterone, and in rare cases adrenocorticotropic hormone. Pheochromocytoma crisis is a life threatening event in which high levels of catecholamines cause a systemic reaction leading to organ failure. *Case Description.* A 70-year-old man was admitted with acute myocardial ischemia following glucocorticoid administration as part of an endocrine workup for an adrenal mass. Cardiac catheterization disclosed patent coronary arteries and he was discharged. A year later he returned with similar angina-like chest pain. During hospitalization, he suffered additional events of chest pain, shortness of breath, and palpitations following administration of glucocorticoids as preparation for intravenous contrast administration. Throughout his admission, the patient demonstrated both signs of Cushing's syndrome and high catecholamine levels. Following stabilization of vital parameters and serum electrolytes, the adrenal mass was resected surgically and was found to harbor an adrenocorticotropic hormone secreting pheochromocytoma. This is the first documented case of adrenocorticotropic hormone secreting pheochromocytoma complicated by glucocorticoid induced pheochromocytoma crisis. *Conclusion.* Care should be taken when administering high doses of glucocorticoids to patients with suspected pheochromocytoma, even in a patient with concomitant Cushing's syndrome.

1. Introduction

Pheochromocytomas are a group of hormone secreting tumors that arise from chromaffin cells in the medulla of the adrenal glands. Pheochromocytoma manifests with an array of clinical symptoms including headaches, sweating, palpitations, and hypertension. The prevalence of pheochromocytoma in patients diagnosed with hypertension is 0.1–0.5% [1]. Pheochromocytomas are usually functional and secrete catecholamines. In rare cases they have been shown to also secrete interleukins, calcitonin, and testosterone [2].

Adrenocorticotrophic hormone (ACTH) is a 39-amino acid pituitary hormone which promotes adrenal hyperplasia and glucocorticoid synthesis in response to physiological stress. Ectopic ACTH secretion accounts for 10–20% of ACTH-dependent Cushing syndrome and mostly originates from bronchial or thymic neuroendocrine tumors or small cell lung carcinomas.

We report a case of a 70-year-old man, who presented with recurrent episodes of chest pain and hypertension refractory to treatment, following glucocorticoid administration. He was found to have an ACTH secreting pheochromocytoma.

2. Case Report

A 70-year-old man presented to the emergency department at our institution, with angina-like chest pain, palpitations, and sweating.

One year prior to his current admission, he underwent endocrine evaluation following an incidental adrenal finding on imaging measuring $25 \times 34 \, \text{mm}^2$. A 24-hour urine collection for catecholamines revealed a urine epinephrine level of 150 μg (normal limit: <27 μg/day). A 1-mg overnight dexamethasone suppression test was abnormal, with serum cortisol level of 188 nmol/l (normal limit < 50 nmol/l). He then underwent an ambulatory high dose dexamethasone suppression test. That day he was referred to the emergency department due to angina-like chest pain, palpitations, and sweating. He underwent cardiac catheterization, which demonstrated no significant pathology in the coronary arteries, and was discharged the next day. Past medical history was significant for hypertension, type II diabetes mellitus, and dyslipidemia.

A year later, on current admission, the patient's electrocardiogram showed sinus rhythm, new T wave inversion in lateral and posterior leads, with no conduction abnormalities. Bedside echocardiography demonstrated hypokinesis in the distribution of the left anterior descending coronary artery. The patient underwent urgent catheterization which once again demonstrated no pathology in the coronary arteries. A subsequent echocardiogram demonstrated normal ventricular function with moderate mitral and tricuspid regurgitation.

During his stay in the coronary care unit, the patient experienced several episodes of hypertension and tachycardia, refractory to treatment with calcium channel blockers, beta and alpha adrenergic blockade, angiotensin receptor blockers, and furosemide. As part of resistant hypertension evaluation, abdominal computed tomography was performed and a $36 \times 34 \times 22 \, \text{mm}^3$ right adrenal mass was identified. The adrenal mass had a density of 39 Hounsfield units (HU) prior to intravenous contrast injection, increasing to 74 HU following contrast injection. Notably, the patient experienced a severe event of hypertension, palpitations, and chest pain following administration of 100 mg hydrocortisone as preparation for contrast agent infusion as he had received a diagnosis of sensitivity to intravenous contrast material. Plasma metanephrine was found to be 1200 pg/ml (normal < 90 pg/ml) with a normal normetanephrine level of 163 pg/ml (normal < 196 pg/ml). Plasma cortisol level at 8 am, after overnight 1-mg dexamethasone suppression, was 2770 nmol/l, while level at 8 am without dexamethasone suppression was 3292 nmol/l (normal range 100–690 nmol/l). ACTH level was 174 pmol/l (normal range 1.9–10.2 pmol/l). Renin and aldosterone levels were within normal limits.

The patient's case was presented at a multidisciplinary team meeting and surgery was advised. Following 2 weeks of alpha blockade, uneventful laparoscopic right adrenalectomy was performed, with stable blood pressure throughout the procedure. The postoperative course was uncomplicated and the patient was discharged on day two.

Pathology revealed a 36 mm pheochromocytoma of the adrenal gland with a scaled score (PASS) of 7 (vascular

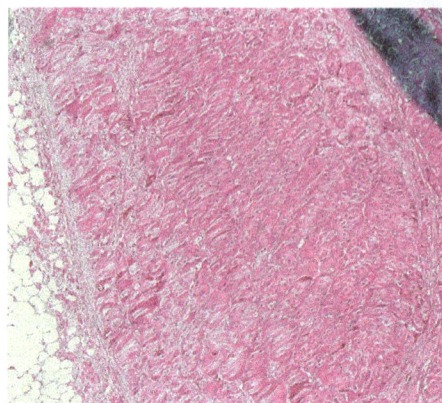

FIGURE 1: Hyperplastic adrenal cortex.

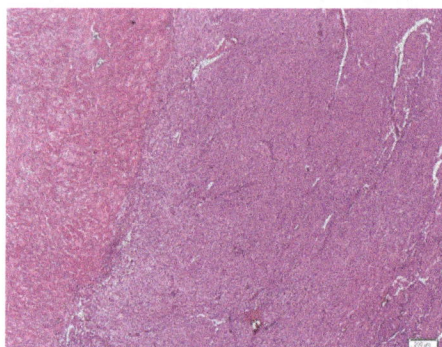

FIGURE 2: Adrenal gland, pheochromocytoma, and diffuse growth pattern with high cellularity. H&E ×40.

invasion, predominantly diffuse growth, high cellularity, and spindling of cells). Diffuse adrenal cortical hyperplasia was noted (Figure 1). Immunostaining was positive for ACTH and synaptophysin and negative for chromogranin, inhibin, calretinin, and S-100 protein. Figure 2 shows the pathology of adrenal tumor, pheochromocytoma, and diffuse growth pattern. Figure 3 depicts positive immunostraining for ACTH. Figure 4 depicts the tumor's vascular invasion, and the adrenal gland's hyperplastic cortex.

During 23 months of follow-up the patient had no cardiac events, his blood pressure decreased to 126/79, and he was able to decrease his antihypertensive medications. A CT scan performed 7 months following surgery revealed normal postoperative changes with no evidence of recurrence.

3. Discussion

Cushing's syndrome was first described in 1912 by Cushing [3]. The syndrome, which is caused by chronic exposure to abnormally high levels of the stress hormone cortisol, may present with a variety of clinical symptoms, none of which is sensitive or specific. The common manifestations include hypertension, diabetes mellitus, central obesity, proximal muscle wasting and weakness, hirsutism, red-purple striae, and oligomenorrhea in women [4].

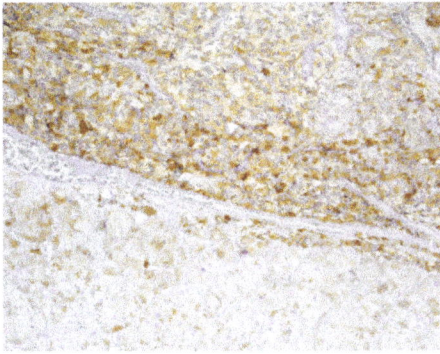

FIGURE 3: Positive Immunostaining for ACTH compatible with ectopic ACTH secretion by the tumor.

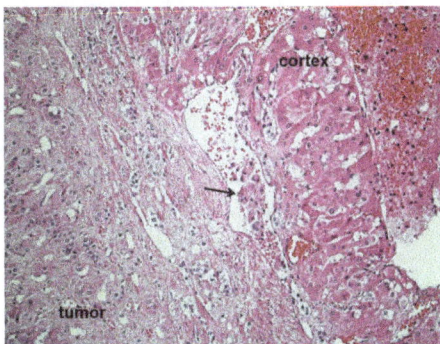

FIGURE 4: Tumor, vascular invasion at tumor edge, and hyperplastic cortex. The arrow represents vascular invasion of the tumor.

Excess ACTH accounts for 80% of cases, while the remaining 20% are ACTH-independent. Of the ACTH-dependent Cushing syndrome cases, 80%–90% are due to Cushing's disease, pituitary corticotroph adenoma [5], and 10%–20% are due to ectopic ACTH secreting tumors. Although ectopic ACTH secreting tumors are most commonly bronchial carcinoid, thymic carcinoid, or small cell lung cancer [6], more than 2 dozen cases of ACTH secreting pheochromocytomas have been described in the literature [2, 6–10].

Pheochromocytoma crisis (PC) is a potentially life threatening event caused by high levels of catecholamines secreted by the neoplastic chromaffin cells leading to organ failure [11, 12]. While many drugs have been shown to cause PC, reports of glucocorticoid induced PC are rare and mostly limited to single case reports [9, 13–17].

Our patient experienced his first event of refractory hypertension and angina-like chest pain severe enough to warrant cardiac catheterization following administration of high dose dexamethasone. The second substantial event occurred several hours after glucocorticoid administration as preparation for contrast agent infusion due to intravenous contrast sensitivity. Glucocorticoids play a fundamental part in catecholamine metabolism, production, and release both in the healthy adrenal medulla and in pheochromocytoma cells. Glucocorticoids were shown to induce, in a dose dependent manner, enzymes required for catecholamine synthesis,

including phenylethanolamine-N-methyltransferase, which converts norepinephrine to epinephrine, tyrosine hydroxylase, a rate-limiting enzyme in catecholamine metabolism, and proopiomelanocortin, an ACTH precursor [9, 13].

While a normal adrenal medulla would not be greatly affected by exogenous glucocorticoids, the loss of anatomical and cellular barriers in pheochromocytoma may increase the susceptibility of the chromaffin cells to glucocorticoids.

To the best of our knowledge this is the only published report of an ACTH secreting pheochromocytoma underlying a glucocorticoid induced PC. It is possible that Cushing's syndrome background of our patient increased his susceptibility to PC as he was constantly exposed to high levels of glucocorticoids. None of the reports regarding ACTH secreting pheochromocytoma mention a clinical state of PC, but as both these conditions are extremely rare further data are required to establish whether a pheochromocytoma with Cushing's syndrome is more likely to be complicated with pheochromocytoma crisis.

In a review of the literature, Rosas et al. [13] present 11 cases of glucocorticoid induced PC. Of those cases at least two experienced a pheochromocytoma crisis following high dose dexamethasone suppression. Given the significant risk for morbidity and mortality of pheochromocytoma crisis and the unpredictability of PC following glucocorticoid treatment, we suggest caution when administering glucocorticoids to patients with suspected pheochromocytoma.

References

[1] M. K. Pacak, D. W. M. Linehan, G. Eisenhofer, and M. M. Walther, in *Proceedings of the NIH Conference Recent Advances in Genetics, Diagnosis, Localization*, vol. 134, pp. 315–329, 2017.

[2] J. K. Laurent, L. Brunaud, M. Mathonet et al., "Ectopic hormone-secreting pheochromocytoma: A francophone observational study," *World Journal of Surgery*, vol. 36, no. 2, pp. 1382–1388, 2012.

[3] H. Cushing, "The pituitary body and its disorders: clinical states produced by disorders of the hypophysis cerebri," *Lippincott*, 1912.

[4] J. Yang, J. Shen, and P. J. Fuller, "Practical approach to diagnosing endocrine hypertension," *Nephrology*, vol. 22, no. 9, pp. 663–677, 2017.

[5] A. Lacroix, R. A. Feelders, C. A. Stratakis, and L. K. Nieman, "Cushing's syndrome," *Lancet*, vol. 386, no. 9996, pp. 913–927, 2015.

[6] E. Flynn, S. Baqar, D. Liu et al., "Bowel perforation complicating an ACTH-secreting phaeochromocytoma," *Endocrinology, Diabetes & Metabolism Case Reports*, 2016.

[7] H. Falhammar, J. Calissendorff, and C. Höybye, "Frequency of Cushing's syndrome due to ACTH-secreting adrenal medullary lesions: a retrospective study over 10 years from a single center," *Endocrine Journal*, vol. 55, no. 1, pp. 296–302, 2017.

[8] M. Fukasawa, N. Sawada, T. Miyamoto, and S. Kira, "Laparoscopic unilateral total and contralateral," *Journal of Endourology Case Reports*, vol. 2, pp. 232–234, 2016.

[9] I. Sakuma, S. Higuchi, M. Fujimoto et al., "Cushing syndrome due to ACTH-secreting pheochromocytoma, aggravated by glucocorticoid-driven positive-feedback loop," *The Journal of Clinical Endocrinology & Metabolism*, vol. 101, no. 3, pp. 841–846, 2016.

[10] L. Folkestad, M. S. Andersen, A. L. Nielsen, and D. Glintborg, "Case Report—A rare cause of Cushing's syndrome: an ACTH-secreting phaeochromocytoma," *BMJ Case Report*, vol. 14, pp. 1–4, 2014.

[11] F. M. Browers and J. W. M. Lenders, "Pheochromocytoma as an endocrine emergency," *Endocrine and Metabolic Disorders*, pp. 121–128, 2003.

[12] M. R. Sauvage and P. A. Tulasne, "Hypertensive accident in a surgical patient with unsuspected pheochromocytoma," *Anesthesia & Analgesia*, pp. 155–158, 1979.

[13] A. L. Rosas, A. A. Kasperlik-Zaluska, L. Papierska et al., "Pheochromocytoma crisis induced by glucocorticoids: a report of four cases and review of the literature," *European Journal of Endocrinology*, vol. 178, no. 2, pp. 423–429, 2008.

[14] M. F. Dupont and M. C. Battista, "Corticosteroid-induced case of a lightning pheochromocytoma crisis?: Insight into glucocorticoid receptor expression," *Integrative Cancer Science and Therapeutics*, vol. 3, pp. 345–348, 2016.

[15] E. Ogino-Nishimura, T. Nakagawa, I. Tateya, H. Hiraumi, and J. Ito, "Systemic steroid application caused sudden death of a patient with sudden deafness," *Case Reports in Otolaryngology*, vol. 2013, Article ID 734131, 4 pages, 2013.

[16] N. Takahashi, T. Shimada, K. Tanabe, and H. Yoshitomi, "Steroid-induced crisis and rhabdomyolysis in a patient with pheochromocytoma?: A case report and review," *International Journal of Cardiology*, vol. 146, pp. e41–e45, 2011.

[17] D. Won, Y. Sun, Y. Kim, and D. Hoon, "Pheochromocytoma crisis after a dexamethasone suppression test for adrenal incidentaloma," *Endocr*, pp. 213–219, 2010.

24

Pituitary Adenoma and Hyperprolactinemia Accompanied by Idiopathic Granulomatous Mastitis

Sebahattin Destek,[1] Vahit Onur Gul,[2] Serkan Ahioglu,[3] and Kursat Rahmi Serin[4]

[1]*Department of General Surgery, Bezmialem Vakıf University School of Medicine, Istanbul, Turkey*
[2]*General Surgery Department, Edremit Government Hospital, Edremit, 10300 Balikesir, Turkey*
[3]*Biochemistry Department, Edremit State Hospital, Edremit, 10300 Balikesir, Turkey*
[4]*General Surgery Department, Liv Hospital, Ulus, Istanbul, Turkey*

Correspondence should be addressed to Vahit Onur Gul; vonurgul@hotmail.com

Academic Editor: John Broom

Idiopathic granulomatous mastitis (IGM) is a rare chronic inflammatory disease of the breast, and its etiology remains not fully elucidated. IGM is observed more often in patients with autoimmune disease. Hyperprolactinemia is observed during pregnancy, lactation, and a history of oral contraceptive use. A 39-year-old patient with no history of oral contraceptive use presented with complaints such as redness, pain, and swelling in her left breast. Ultrasound and magnetic resonance imaging (MRI) revealed a suspicious inflamed mass lesion. Core biopsy was performed to exclude breast cancer and to further diagnose. The breast abscess was drained and steroids were given for treatment. In order to monitor any progression during the three months of treatment, hormone levels were routinely examined. Prolactin level was above the reference range, and pituitary MRI revealed a pituitary prolactinoma. After treatment with prolactin inhibitors, IGM also improved with hyperprolactinemia. This report emphasizes attention to hyperprolactinemia in cases of IGM diagnosis and treatment.

1. Introduction

IGM is a recurrent chronic inflammatory disease characterized by noncaseating granuloma, lobule inflammation, and rare breast abscess formation. Clinical and radiological features may be indistinguishable from breast cancer [1]. The etiology is not fully elucidated [2]. IGM is observed more often in patients with autoimmune diseases, hyperprolactinemia conditions such as pituitary adenomas, during pregnancy and/or lactation, and a history of oral contraceptive use [2, 3]. In the absence of pregnancy and/or lactation, with no history of oral contraceptive use, and/or any additional illness, it is necessary to evaluate prolactin levels during the process of analyzing IGM etiology. If positive, high prolactin levels should be treated primarily.

2. Case Report

A thirty-nine-year-old single patient with no children and no history of oral contraceptive use was admitted to our clinic with complaints of redness, pain, and swelling in her left breast (Figure 1). She had no additional illness or complaints (BMI: 33.3). She was a tobacco user (5–10 units/day), within the normal weight category, and had three gravidity. Breast ultrasound revealed irregular limited solid heterogeneous hypoechoic mass lesions suspicious for malignancy; the largest one was 16 mm in diameter. There were no lymph nodes in the left axilla. The mass was categorized BIRADS-4 in breast ultrasonography. Breast MRI revealed heterogeneous enhancement with 3.5 × 5 cm of inflammatory area at the left breast upper outer quadrant. Biopsy was recommended for differential diagnosis of inflammatory breast cancer (Figure 2). Serum C reactive protein (CRP) was high (12.4 mg/l), sedimentation rate was high (37 mm/h), and CA 125 and CA 15-3 levels were normal. Gram (+) cocci were observed in the breast abscess stain; however, abscess culture results were negative. IGM was diagnosed with core biopsy examination (Figure 3). The breast abscess was drained and steroids were given for two months (Prednol

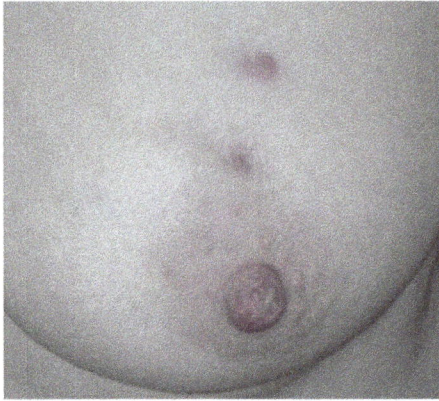

FIGURE 1: Left breast IGM 1.

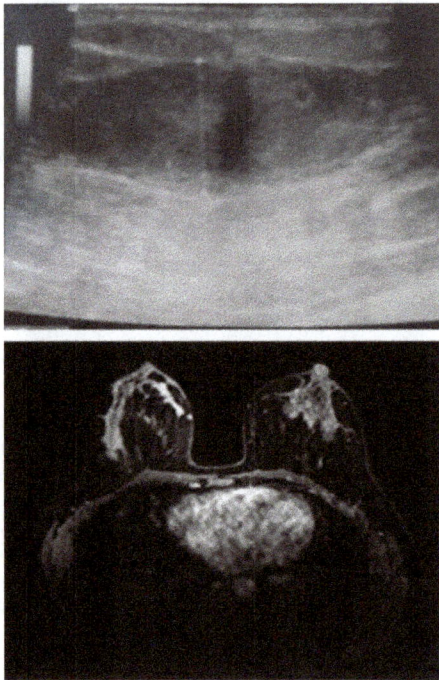

FIGURE 2: IGM breast USG and MRI.

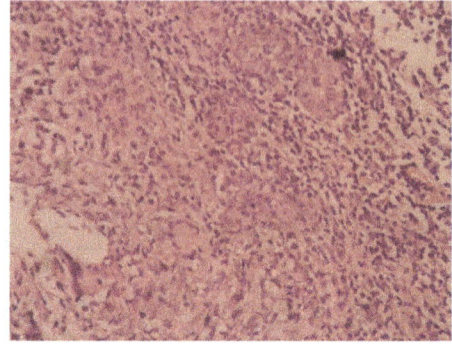

FIGURE 3: IGM histopathology H-E ×40.

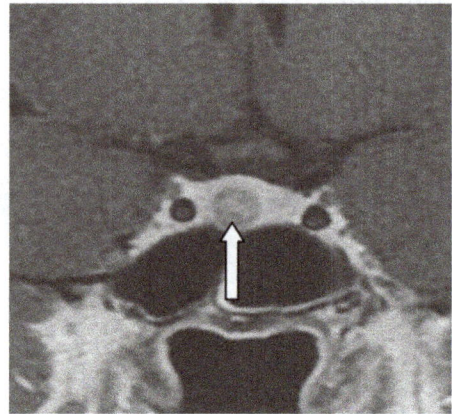

FIGURE 4: MRI of the pituitary microadenoma.

Prolactin levels returned to normal and there was resolution of IGM after 4 months. Follow-up included monitoring of CRP levels. No recurrences were observed during a four-year follow-up period.

3. Discussion

In 1972, Kessler and Wolloch first defined granulomatous mastitis (GM) [1, 2]. GM can be idiopathic (primary) and specific (secondary) [2, 3]. Secondary GM involves caseation necrosis and emerges with a variety of infectious conditions such as vasculitis, sarcoidosis, tuberculosis, actinomycosis, and blastomycosis filariasis [2, 3]. IGM is detected in less than 1% of breast biopsies performed in women [1, 3]. It is also called idiopathic granulomatous lobulitis or idiopathic granulomatous lobular mastitis. It is often seen in women between the second and fourth decade of life. It is rarely detected in men [1]. This case report involved a 39-year-old woman.

The etiology of IGM is not fully understood, but autoimmune and hormonal disorders are often discussed as causes [2, 3]. IGM etiology, on the basis of inflammation and autoimmune effect, is reported to be in various pathological gene disorders [4]. IGM may appear together with autoimmune disorders such as Sjögren's syndrome, erythema nodosum, and arthritis [2, 4]. It is suggested that IGM can develop

4 mg/day/oral and 0.1% betamethasone pomade) and empiric antibiotics (cefuroxime axetil 500 mg tablets 2 × 1) were given during treatment for ten days. After two months of treatment, there was no improvement. Therefore, body serum hormone profiles were examined. Growth hormone, insulin-like growth factor, thyroid stimulating hormone, estradiol, luteinizing hormone, and follicle-stimulating hormone were normal. However, serum prolactin was elevated (351 ng/ml). Pituitary MRI revealed a 7 × 4 mm sized microadenoma causing pituitary prolactinoma (Figure 4). In order to treat hyperprolactinemia, prolactin inhibitor (Cabergoline) was given to the patient. Cabergoline was started at 1 mg per week; then it increased for six weeks. After prolactin levels returned to normal, it was reduced. Cabergoline treatment was continued for two years.

when T-lymphocytes mediated autoimmune reaction occurs against lobular epithelial cells and gastric secretions [2, 3]. Also, a close relationship between IGM and hormonal conditions such as pregnancy, lactation, use of oral contraceptives, and hyperprolactinemia has been demonstrated. In addition IGM is associated with α1-antitrypsin deficiency, diabetes, breast trauma, obesity, race, smoking, and infectious agents. IGM is more prevalent in the Mediterranean Region and in Asia [2]. This case report involved a tobacco user with normal weight and no history of oral contraceptive use.

A close association between IGM and hyperprolactinemia has been reported [2, 5]. Also, according to multiple reports, prolactin levels are important in recurrent cases [2, 4]. Hyperprolactinemia is mostly seen due to intense physiological conditions drugs such as phenothiazine, metoclopramide, risperidone, and pituitary adenomas [2, 5]. Researchers have demonstrated a relationship between IGM and pituitary adenoma that causes hyperprolactinemia [6, 7]. Prolactin plays a role in the inflammatory pathogenesis of the breast [7, 8]. Prolactin has a very important place in the proliferation and differentiation of normal breast epithelial tissue and in stimulating lactation after pregnancy [8]. Prolactin levels and/or increased expression of prolactin is thought to play a role in breast fibrocystic changes, ductal ectasia, benign breast lesions, and IGM and even in the development of breast carcinoma [8]. It has been reported that prolactin antagonist therapies cure IGM successfully when used in the treatment of hyperprolactinemia [5, 7]. In the case presented here, a pituitary adenoma causing hyperprolactinemia was found.

IGM presents with complaints such as painful breast mass, redness, abscess, and fistula and sometimes mimics cancer because of withdrawal of the nipple and peau d'orange appearance. It is rarely accompanied with axillary lymphadenopathy [3]. Usually, there is unilateral breast involvement; patients with bilateral breast involvement quarter are seen in [3, 4]. Hypoechoic tubular structures and nodules are seen in breast ultrasound; nodular opacities and focal asymmetry are seen in mammography. MRI findings are often nonspecific. Radiological results also mimic inflammatory breast cancer [1, 3].

Generally, in the absence of secondary infection, there is no growth in abscess culture [2, 3].

Gram stain and cultures should be performed in addition to PAS (periodic acid shift) staining for fungi and Ziehl-Neelsen stain for tuberculosis [3, 9]. IGM is diagnosed by the exclusion of other specific diseases that cause GM. A definite diagnosis is made by cytologic examination of fine needle and histopathological examination of core or excisional biopsies. Noncaseating granuloma in the lobular areas, giant cells, chronic inflammation, and microabscesses are seen in biopsy [9]. We applied Tru-cut biopsy in our patient and found similar clinical and radiological features to breast carcinoma.

Corticosteroids are the most common drugs administered for the treatment of IGM [3]. Other drugs used include anti-inflammatory drugs and immunosuppressive agents such as colchicine, methotrexate, or azathioprine [9]. Wide local excision or mastectomy can be applied in cases of medical treatment resistance, recurrent abscess, or fistula [10].

Recurrence rates can rise up to 50%. Follow-up recommendations include 3–6-month intervals for the first 2 years [9, 10]. In this case report, the breast abscess was drained and steroids, antibiotics, and prolactin inhibitor therapy was given to the patient. No recurrence was observed at four-year follow-up.

4. Conclusion

IGM is a disease associated with autoimmunity and hormonal disorders. When investigating the etiology of IGM, prolactin levels should always be checked. Prolactin elevation should be monitored particularly closely and continuously and for a prolonged period of time in severe cases. Prolactin elevation is known to increase immunity and inflammation. While investigating the causes of hyperprolactinemia, the primary focus should be the presence of a pituitary adenoma. Prolactin inhibitors will improve treatment success of IGM with reducing recurrence in cases with prolactin elevation.

Disclosure

This paper is not based on a previous communication to a society or meeting.

References

[1] R. T. Fazzio, S. S. Shah, N. P. Sandhu, and K. N. Glazebrook, "Idiopathic granulomatous mastitis: imaging update and review," *Insights into Imaging*, vol. 7, no. 4, pp. 531–539, 2016.

[2] F. Altintoprak, T. Kivilcim, and O. V. Ozkan, "Aetiology of idiopathic granulomatous mastitis," *World Journal of Clinical Cases*, vol. 2, no. 12, pp. 852–854, 2014.

[3] D. Diesing, R. Axt-Fliedner, D. Hornung, J. M. Weiss, K. Diedrich, and M. Friedrich, "Granulomatous mastitis," *Archives of Gynecology and Obstetrics*, vol. 269, no. 4, pp. 233–236, 2004.

[4] S. Destek, V. O. Gul, and S. Ahioglu, "A variety of gene polymorphisms associated with idiopathic granulomatous mastitis," *Journal of Surgical Case Reports*, vol. 2016, no. 9, Article ID rjw156, 2016.

[5] C. Lin, C. Hsu, T. Tsao, and J. Chou, "Idiopathic granulomatous mastitis associated with risperidone-induced hyperprolactinemia," *Diagnostic Pathology*, vol. 7, article no. 2, 2012.

[6] P. H. Rowe, "Granulomatous mastitis associated with a pituitary prolactinoma," *The British Journal of Clinical Practice*, vol. 38, no. 1, pp. 32–34, 1984.

[7] A. Nikolaev, C. N. Blake, and D. L. Carlson, "Association between hyperprolactinemia and granulomatous mastitis," *The Breast Journal*, vol. 22, no. 2, pp. 224–231, 2016.

[8] E. F. Need, V. Atashgaran, W. V. Ingman, and P. Dasari, "Hormonal regulation of the immune microenvironment in the mammary gland," *Journal of Mammary Gland Biology and Neoplasia*, vol. 19, no. 2, pp. 229–239, 2014.

[9] J. R. Benson and D. Dumitru, "Idiopathic granulomatous mastitis: presentation, investigation and management," *Future Oncology*, vol. 12, no. 11, pp. 1381–1394, 2016.

25

Severe Hyperthyroidism Complicated by Agranulocytosis Treated with Therapeutic Plasma Exchange: Case Report and Review of the Literature

Vishnu Garla ⓘ, Karthik Kovvuru, Shradha Ahuja, Venkatataman Palabindala, Bharat Malhotra ⓘ, and Sohail Abdul Salim

Department of Internal Medicine, University of Mississippi Medical Center, Jackson, MS, USA

Correspondence should be addressed to Vishnu Garla; vishnu.garla@gmail.com

Academic Editor: Osamu Isozaki

Aim. To present a case of Graves' disease complicated by methimazole induced agranulocytosis treated with therapeutic plasma exchange (TPE) and review of the literature. *Case Presentation.* A 21-year-old patient with a history of Graves' disease presented to the endocrine clinic. His history was significant for heat intolerance, weight loss, and tremors. Upon examination he had tachycardia, smooth goiter, thyroid bruit, and hyperactive reflexes. He was started on methimazole and metoprolol and thyroidectomy was to be done once his thyroid function tests normalized. On follow-up, the patient symptoms persisted. Complete blood count done showed a white blood cell count of 2100 (4000–11,000 cells/cu mm) with a neutrophil count of 400 cells/cu mm, consistent with neutropenia. He was admitted to the hospital and underwent 3 cycles of TPE and was also given filgrastim. He improved clinically and his thyroxine (T4) levels also came down. Thyroidectomy was done. He was discharged on levothyroxine for postsurgical hypothyroidism. *Conclusion.* Plasmapheresis may be useful in the treatment of hyperthyroidism. It works by removing protein bound hormones and also possibly inflammatory cytokines. Further studies are needed to clarify the role of various modalities of TPE in the treatment of hyperthyroidism.

1. Introduction

Hyperthyroidism is an overproduction and persistent release of thyroid hormones, while thyrotoxicosis refers to the set of clinical manifestations secondary to excessive thyroid hormone action on the tissues [1]. Conventionally thyrotoxicosis is treated medically using agents which inhibit the synthesis and release of thyroid hormones [2]. TPE was first used as a modality in the treatment of hyperthyroidism in the 1970s; however, till this date the role of TPE in the treatment of hyperthyroidism is unclear [3, 4].

We present a case of Graves' disease complicated by agranulocytosis treated with TPE along with a pertinent review of the literature.

2. Case Description

A 21-year-old male patient presented to the emergency department with neck pain and dysphagia. He had been diagnosed with Graves' disease about 4 years ago; however, he was not taking any medication for the last 2 years. Upon further enquiry, the patient admitted to a history of weight loss, palpitations, tremors, and lack of sleep. Vital signs showed a heart rate of 130/minute, blood pressure of 132/67 mm Hg, respiratory rate of 18/minute, and temperature of 97.8. Examination revealed an anxious patient with bilateral lid lag, large smooth goiter with a thyroid bruit, and tremors of upper extremities. Laboratory assessment revealed a suppressed TSH, high free t4, free t3, positive antithyrotropin receptor antibodies (TRab), and thyroid stimulating immunoglobulin (TSI) confirming the diagnosis of Graves' disease (Table 1). Ultrasound of the neck showed an enlarged hypervascular thyroid gland consistent with Graves' disease. Methimazole and atenolol were started. Thyroidectomy was planned to be done once the thyroid function tests normalized. The patient was discharged from the hospital and was to follow up in the endocrine clinic in 1 month. Upon follow-up in the endocrine clinic, the patient admitted that he had been noncompliant with his medications for a week. He also complained of heat

TABLE 1: Laboratory assessment on admission.

TSH (0.27–4.2 mcIu/ml)	<0.01
Free t4 (0.9–1.7 ng/dl)	>7.77
Free t3 (0.8–2.0 ng/ml)	>6.51
WBC (4000–11,000 cells/cu mm)	2.1
Absolute neutrophil count	0.4
TRab (0–1.75 IU/L)	26
TSI (0–1.3)	5.5

intolerance, weight loss, insomnia, palpitations, and a sore throat. Again noted on exam were tachycardia, a smooth goiter with bruit, tremors, and hyperactive reflexes in all extremities. TSH was suppressed, free t4 and total t3 were high, and complete blood count showed a low white blood cell count (WBC) and low absolute neutrophil count. A diagnosis of methimazole induced agranulocytosis was made and the patient was admitted to the hospital.

Hematology was consulted for TPE to control hyperthyroidism and also administration of filgrastim for neutropenia. Three treatments of plasma exchanges were done 2 days apart. The replacement fluid used was half albumin and half plasma. Filgrastim was administered daily. WBC and neutrophil counts improved significantly and normalized. Patient continued to improve clinically and his free t4, previously in the unmeasurable range, did come down. Thyroidectomy was done and pathology revealed an enlarged thyroid with diffuse hyperplasia. Postoperatively, he developed hypocalcemia and was treated with calcium carbonate. Levothyroxine was started for the treatment of postsurgical hypothyroidism. Upon follow-up, a month later in the endocrine clinic, the patient was doing well on levothyroxine.

3. Methods and Results

We searched PubMed using the following key words: hyperthyroidism and plasmapheresis. We restricted our search to publications in "English" and involving "human subjects." Abstract of meetings and unpublished results were not included in our study. The last search was done on 6/27/2017.

The initial search resulted in 91 articles; 64 articles were excluded based on the title and abstract. Eligibility criteria were those articles which used TPE to treat hyperthyroidism. 27 articles met the inclusion criteria and were included (Table 2) [4–30].

4. Discussion

Thyroxine (T4) has the highest concentration among iodothyronines in the plasma and is produced exclusively by the thyroid; triiodothyronine (T3) is primarily derived (about 80%) from the peripheral tissues by deiodination of T4. T4 is about 68% bound to thyroxine binding globulin (TBG), 11% to transthyretin, and 20% to albumin. T3 is 80% bound to TBG, 9% to transthyretin, and 11% to albumin [1]. This extensive protein binding aids in the clearance

of thyroid hormones during therapeutic plasma exchange (TPE) [31].

TPE is an extracorporeal blood purification technique used to for eliminating large molecular substances from the plasma [30]. In contrast to dialysis which cannot clear protein bound substances, TPE can clear protein bound substances [13]. The process involves passing the patient's blood through a medical device and separating the plasma out; it is then replaced with a colloid (albumin or plasma) or a combination of crystalloid and colloid. TPE clears thyroid hormones which are protein bound; the colloid used to replace the plasma provides new binding sites for thyroid hormone which are cleared during the next TPE session [6]. Besides thyroid hormones, TPE may help in the clearance of cytokines, deiodinase enzyme, and Graves' antibodies which help not only in the resolution of thyrotoxicosis but also of Graves' ophthalmopathy and pretibial myxedema [31].

There are a number of replacement fluids available, plasma as a replacement fluid offers the advantage of not depleting coagulation factors and also replenishing thyroxine binding globulin [20]. Human albumin offers the advantage of having a larger pool of low affinity binding sites for thyroid hormone [9]. We recommend plasma as the replacement fluid in patients with coagulation disorders or those who are going for surgery.

TPE was first used for the treatment of hyperthyroidism in 1970 by Ashkar et al. on 3 cases of thyroid storm [4]. Our literature review showed that TPE was used in 16 cases not responding to standard treatment, 13 cases of agranulocytosis or other side effects of thionamides, 8 cases of amiodarone induced thyrotoxicosis, and 5 cases for preparation of thyroidectomy. Petry et al. used TPE for the treatment of thyroid storm in postsleeve pneumonectomy patient who did not respond to the conventional treatment and thyroidectomy was considered high risk [22]. Jha et al. reported a case of thyroid storm secondary to excessive consumption thyroid supplements successfully treated with TPE. TPE was particularly useful as the patient had been taking excessive supplements for six days making the use of gastric decontamination and cholestyramine less useful [30].

Lew et al. used double filtration plasmapheresis (DFPP) in a patient with Graves' disease who needed surgical debridement. DFPP is a process where the plasma is first separated from the blood and then large molecules like immunoglobulins and lipoproteins are removed. The advantage would be lesser removal of coagulation factors making it useful in a patient who has to undergo surgery; however, small molecules may not be removed effectively by this procedure [11]. Koball et al. used a single pass albumin dialysis (SPAD) in a patient who had no clinical improvement after two sessions of plasmapheresis. Albumin dialysis has been used to eliminate toxins which accumulate in liver failure. The authors hypothesized that since this was a continuous procedure it would be effective in removing a greater quantity of hormone from the blood. It was also noted that if the plasmapheresis was followed by SPAD it decreased the chance of rebound increase of thyroid hormones [13].

The American society of apheresis categorizes the use of TPE in the treatment of hyperthyroidism as category III

TABLE 2: Literature review.

Authors	Cases	Indication	Indication for plasmapheresis	Outcome
Kaderli et al.	3	Amiodarone induced thyrotoxicosis	Amiodarone induced thyrotoxicosis	Underwent thyroidectomy
Min et al.	1	Graves' disease	Elevated liver function tests	Biochemical improvement with about 40% decrease in total T3
Aydemir et al.	1	Graves' disease	Jaundice	Biochemical improvement with greater than 60% decrease in FT4 and FT3
Bilir et al.	1	Graves' disease	Drug induced angioneurotic edema	Underwent thyroidectomy
Carhill et al.	2	Graves' disease	(1) Increase in transaminases (2) Unresponsive to standard treatment	Clinical and biochemical improvement
Vyas et al.	1	Exogenous intoxication	Exogenous etiology	Clinical and biochemical improvement
Lew et al.	1	Graves' disease	Agranulocytosis and hemophagocytosis	Clinical and biochemical improvement with greater than 80% decrease in FT4 and FT3
Enghofer et al.	1	Graves' disease	Fulminant hepatitis	Underwent thyroidectomy
Koball et al.	1	Unknown	Preparation for urgent thyroidectomy	Clinical and biochemical improvement
Ezer et al.	11	(7) Graves' disease (3) Toxic multinodular goiter (1) Iodine induced thyrotoxicosis	(7) Unresponsive to standard treatment (3) Agranulocytosis (1) Emergent preparation for thyroidectomy	Clinical improvement noted
Adali et al.	1	Gestational hyperthyroidism sec to molar pregnancy	Emergent preparation for thyroidectomy	Biochemical improvement with >80% decrease in FT3 and >75% decrease in FT4
Pasimeni et al.	1	Contrast induced hyperthyroidism	Unresponsive to methimazole	Clinical and biochemical improvement
Azezli et al.	1	Gestational hyperthyroidism sec to molar pregnancy	Preparation for emergent thyroidectomy	Clinical and biochemical improvement with 75.1% decrease in free t3 and 63.1% decrease in free t4
Erbil et al.	1	Gestational hyperthyroidism sec to molar pregnancy	Unresponsive to propylthiouracil	Biochemical improvement
Guvenc et al.	1	Toxic multinodular goiter	Agranulocytosis	Clinical and biochemical improvement
Ozbey et al.	4	Graves' disease	(1) Agranulocytosis (1) PTU induced vasculitis (1) Drug induced urticarial (1) Hepatotoxicity	Decrease in TT3 by about 40–78% and FT4 by >69%

TABLE 2: Continued.

Authors	Cases	Indication	Indication for plasmapheresis	Outcome
Diamond et al.	3	Amiodarone induced thyrotoxicosis	Unresponsive to standard treatment	Clinical improvement in 2 patients Mild decrease in the FT4
Petry et al.	1	Graves' disease	Status after sleeve pneumonectomy	Clinical and biochemical improvement
Ozdemir et al.	1	Hyperthyroidism	Unresponsive to standard treatment	Clinical and biochemical improvement with 60% decrease in FT4 and 75% decrease in FT3
Segers et al.	5	Thyrotoxicosis	Thyrotoxicosis	Clinical improvement. Decrease in FT3 of 63.5% and FT4 by 57.8%
Ligtenberg et al.		Preparation for surgery	Preparation for surgery	Decrease in FT3 of 7% and 18% Decrease in FT4 of 0% and 33%
Samaras et al.	1	Amiodarone induced thyrotoxicosis	Unresponsive to standard treatment	Failure of treatment resulting in death of the patient Decrease in TT3 and TT4 noted after TPE with rebound increase in levels later
Aghini-Lombardi et al.	2	Amiodarone induced thyrotoxicosis	Adjunct to methimazole	Decrease in FT4 and FT3 Normalization of TT4 and TT3
De Rosa et al.	1	Hyperthyroidism	Agranulocytosis	Biochemical improvement with 51% decrease in FT3, 47% decrease in FT4, 60% decrease in TT3, and 53% decrease in TT4
Binimelis et al.	6	Levothyroxine intoxication	Cardiac and neurological symptoms	Clinical and biochemical improvement in 15 days
Jha et al.	1	Medicinal thyroid overdose	Medicinal thyroid overdose	Clinical and biochemical improvement with 43% decrease in TT4 and 68% decrease in TT3
Ashkar et al.	3	Hyperthyroidism	Severe hyperthyroidism	Clinical improvement in 2-3 days

Ft4: free thyroxine, Ft3: free triiodothyronine, TT4: total thyroxine, TT3: total triiodothyronine, and TPE: therapeutic plasma exchange.

which states that the role of TPE has not been established in the treatment of thyroid storm. The recommended frequency of treatment is daily to once in three days till clinical improvement is noted [3].

TPE in the treatment of hyperthyroidism can be used when conventional treatment is not working or contraindicated. As noted in our literature review, it can be used in a variety of scenarios with clinical and biochemical improvement. Limitations of TPE include lack of wide spread availability, potential for hemodynamic instability, and the risk of infections.

5. Conclusions

In summary, TPE is a useful adjunct in the treatment of hyperthyroidism; its use is suggested in cases with severe thyrotoxicosis with cardiac or neurological complications, or when standard antithyroid treatments are either unresponsive or contraindicated. It is also a useful adjunct in treating cases with levothyroxine overdose. TPE should be done daily till clinical improvement is noted. Thyroid hormone status is monitored by checking free t4 and free t3 before and after every TPE session; however, clinical and biochemical dissociation may exist. More research is needed into the usefulness of DFPP and SPAD in the treatment of hyperthyroidism.

References

[1] S. Melmed, K. P. onsky, P. Larsen, and H. Kronenberg, *Williams Textbook of Endocrinology*, S. Mandel and P. Larsen, Eds., Elsevier, 12 edition, 2011.

[2] H. J. Baskin, R. H. Cobin, D. S. Duick et al., "American association of clinical endocrinologists medical guidelines for clinical practice for the evaluation and treatment of hyperthyroidism and hypothyroidism," *Endocrine Practice*, vol. 8, no. 6, pp. 457–469, 2002.

[3] J. Schwartz, A. Padmanabhan, N. Aqui et al., "Guidelines on the use of therapeutic apheresis in clinical practice-evidence-based approach from the writing committee of the american society for apheresis: the seventh special issue," *Journal of Clinical Apheresis*, vol. 31, no. 3, pp. 149–162, 2016.

[4] F. S. Ashkar, R. B. Katims, W. M. Smoak, and A. J. Gilson, "Thyroid storm treatment with blood exchange and plasmapheresis," *Journal of the American Medical Association*, vol. 214, no. 7, pp. 1275–1279, 1970.

[5] R. M. Kaderli, R. Fahrner, E. R. Christ et al., "Total thyroidectomy for amiodarone-induced thyrotoxicosis in the hyperthyroid state," *Experimental and Clinical Endocrinology & Diabetes*, vol. 124, no. 1, pp. 45–48, 2016.

[6] S. H. Min, A. Phung, T. J. Oh et al., "Therapeutic plasmapheresis enabling radioactive iodine treatment in a patient with thyrotoxicosis," *Journal of Korean Medical Science*, vol. 30, no. 10, pp. 1531–1534, 2015.

[7] S. Aydemir, Y. Ustundag, T. Bayraktaroglu, I. O. Tekin, I. Peksoy, and A. U. Unal, "Fulminant hepatic failure associated with propylthiouracil: a case report with treatment emphasis on the use of plasmapheresis," *Journal of Clinical Apheresis*, vol. 20, no. 4, pp. 235–238, 2005.

[8] B. Ekiz Bilir, N. Soysal Atile, O. Kirkizlar et al., "Effectiveness of preoperative plasmapheresis in a pregnancy complicated by hyperthyroidism and anti-thyroid drug-associated angioedema," *Gynecological Endocrinology*, vol. 29, no. 5, pp. 508–510, 2013.

[9] A. Carhill, A. Gutierrez, R. Lakhia, and R. Nalini, "Surviving the storm: two cases of thyroid storm successfully treated with plasmapheresis," *BMJ Case Reports*, vol. 2012, 2012.

[10] A. A. Vyas, P. Vyas, N. L. Fillipon, R. Vijayakrishnan, and N. Trivedi, "Successful treatment of thyroid storm with plasmapheresis in a patient with methimazole-induced agranulocytosis." *Endocrine practice : official journal of the American College of Endocrinology and the American Association of Clinical Endocrinologists*, vol. 16, no. 4, pp. 673–676, 2010.

[11] W. H. Lew, C.-J. Chang, J.-D. Lin, C.-Y. Cheng, Y.-K. Chen, and T.-I. Lee, "Successful preoperative treatment of a Graves' disease patient with agranulocytosis and hemophagocytosis using double filtration plasmapheresis," *Journal of Clinical Apheresis*, vol. 26, no. 3, pp. 159–161, 2011.

[12] M. Enghofer, K. Badenhoop, S. Zeuzem et al., "Fulminant hepatitis A in a patient with severe hyperthyroidism: rapid recovery from hepatic coma after plasmapheresis and total thyroidectomy," *The Journal of Clinical Endocrinology & Metabolism*, vol. 85, no. 5, pp. 1765–1769, 2000.

[13] S. Koball, H. Hickstein, M. Gloger et al., "Treatment of thyrotoxic crisis with plasmapheresis and single pass albumin dialysis: a case report: Thoughts and progress," *Artificial Organs*, vol. 34, no. 2, pp. E55–E58, 2010.

[14] A. Ezer, K. Caliskan, A. Parlakgumus, S. Belli, I. Kozanoglu, and S. Yildirim, "Preoperative therapeutic plasma exchange in patients with thyrotoxicosis," *Journal of Clinical Apheresis*, vol. 24, no. 3, pp. 111–114, 2009.

[15] E. Adali, R. Yildizhan, A. Kolusari, M. Kurdoglu, and N. Turan, "The use of plasmapheresis for rapid hormonal control in severe hyperthyroidism caused by a partial molar pregnancy," *Archives of Gynecology and Obstetrics*, vol. 279, no. 4, pp. 569–571, 2009.

[16] G. Pasimeni, F. Caroli, G. Spriano, M. Antonini, R. Baldelli, and M. Appetecchia, "Refractory thyrotoxicosis induced by iodinated contrast agents treated with therapeutic plasma exchange. A case report," *Journal of Clinical Apheresis*, vol. 23, no. 2, pp. 92–95, 2008.

[17] A. Azezli, T. Bayraktaroglu, S. Topuz, and S. Kalayoglu-Besisik, "Hyperthyroidism in molar pregnancy: rapid preoperative preparation by plasmapheresis and complete improvement after evacuation," *Transfusion and Apheresis Science*, vol. 36, no. 1, pp. 87–89, 2007.

[18] Y. Erbil, D. Tihan, A. Azezli et al., "Severe hyperthyroidism requiring therapeutic plasmapheresis in a patient with hydatidiform mole," *Gynecological Endocrinology*, vol. 22, no. 7, pp. 402–404, 2006.

[19] B. Guvenc, C. Unsal, E. Gurkan, and S. Dincer, "Plasmapheresis in the treatment of hyperthyroidism associated with agranulocytosis: a case report," *Journal of Clinical Apheresis*, vol. 19, no. 3, pp. 148–150, 2004.

[20] N. Ozbey, S. Kalayoglu-Besisik, N. Gul, A. Bozbora, E. Sencer, and S. Molvalilar, "Therapeutic plasmapheresis in patients with severe hyperthyroidism in whom antithyroid drugs are contraindicated," *International Journal of Clinical Practice*, vol. 58, no. 6, pp. 554–558, 2004.

[21] T. H. Diamond, R. Rajagopal, K. Ganda et al., "Plasmapheresis as a potential treatment option for amiodarone-induced thyrotoxicosis [4] (multiple letters)," *Internal Medicine Journal*, vol. 34, no. 6, pp. 369–371, 2004.

[22] J. Petry, P. E. Y. Van Schil, P. Abrams, and P. G. Jorens, "Plasmapheresis as effective treatment for thyrotoxic storm after sleeve pneumonectomy," *The Annals of Thoracic Surgery*, vol. 77, no. 5, pp. 1839–1841, 2004.

[23] S. Ozdemir, M. A. Buyukbese, P. Kadioglu, T. Soyasal, H. Senturk, and P. Akin, "Plasmapheresis: an effective therapy for refractory hyperthyroidism in the elderly," *Indian Journal of Medical Sciences*, vol. 56, no. 2, pp. 65–68, 2002.

[24] O. Segers, H. Spapen, L. Steenssens, R. Cytryn, M. H. Jonckheer, and L. Vanhaelst, "Treatment of severe iodine-induced hyperthyroidism with plasmapheresis." *Acta clinica Belgica*, vol. 43, no. 5, pp. 335–343, 1988.

[25] J. Ligtenberg, J. Tulleken, and J. Zijlstra, "Plasmapheresis in thyrotoxicosis [4]," *Annals of Internal Medicine*, vol. 131, no. 1, pp. 71-72, 1999.

[26] K. Samaras and G. M. Marel, "Failure of plasmapheresis, corticosteroids and thionamides to ameliorate a case of protracted amiodarone-induced thyroiditis," *Clinical Endocrinology*, vol. 45, no. 3, pp. 365–368, 1996.

[27] F. Aghini-Lombardi, S. Mariotti, P. V. Fosella et al., "Treatment of amiodarone iodine-induced thyrotoxicosis with plasmapheresis and methimazole," *Journal of Endocrinological Investigation*, vol. 16, no. 10, pp. 823–826, 1993.

Severe Hyperthyroidism Complicated by Agranulocytosis Treated with Therapeutic Plasma Exchange...

109

[28] G. De Rosa, A. Testa, G. Menichella et al., "Plasmapheresis in the therapy of hyperthyroidism associated with leukopenia," *Haematologica*, vol. 76, no. 1, pp. 72–74, 1991.

[29] J. Binimelis, L. Bassas, L. Marruecos et al., "Massive thyroxine intoxication: evaluation of plasma extraction," *Intensive Care Medicine*, vol. 13, no. 1, pp. 33–38, 1987.

[30] S. Jha, S. Waghdhare, R. Reddi, and P. Bhattacharya, "Thyroid storm due to inappropriate administration of a compounded thyroid hormone preparation successfully treated with plasmapheresis," *Thyroid*, vol. 22, no. 12, pp. 1283–1286, 2012.

[31] C. Muller, P. Perrin, B. Faller, S. Richter, and F. Chantrel, "Role of plasma exchange in the thyroid storm," *Therapeutic Apheresis and Dialysis*, vol. 15, no. 6, pp. 522–531, 2011.

Anaplastic Spindle Cell Squamous Carcinoma Arising from Tall Cell Variant Papillary Carcinoma of the Thyroid Gland: A Case Report and Review of the Literature

Darren K. Patten,[1,2] Alia Ahmed,[3] Owain Greaves,[4] Roberto Dina,[5] Rashpal Flora,[5] and Neil Tolley[1]

[1]*Department of Surgery, Hammersmith Hospital, Imperial College Healthcare NHS Trust, London, UK*
[2]*Department of Surgery and Cancer, The Imperial Centre for Translational and Experimental Medicine, Imperial College London, Hammersmith Campus, London, UK*
[3]*Department of General Medicine, Wexham Park Hospital, NHS Frimley Health Foundation Trust, London, UK*
[4]*Department of Life Sciences, Imperial College London, London, UK*
[5]*Department of Histopathology, Hammersmith Hospital, Imperial College Healthcare NHS Trust, London, UK*

Correspondence should be addressed to Darren K. Patten; darren.patten@gmail.com

Academic Editor: Najmul Islam

Tall cell variant (TCV) of papillary thyroid carcinoma (PTC), an aggressive form of thyroid cancer, is characterised by 50% of cells with height that is three times greater than the width. Very rarely, some of these cancers can progress to spindle cell squamous carcinoma (SCSC) resulting in cancers with elements of both SCSC and TCV PTC. Here we report a case of SCSC arising from TCV PTC. In addition to this case, we have performed a literature review and compiled all published reports of SCSC arising from TCV PTC, including the nature of treatment and the prognosis for each of the 20 patients recorded. This is intended for use as a guide for clinicians in what the most appropriate treatment options may be for a newly diagnosed patient. Due to the rarity coupled with diagnosis occurring at a very advanced stage of disease progression, performing clinical trials is difficult and therefore drawing conclusions on optimal treatment methods remains a challenge.

1. Introduction

First described by Hawk and Hazard in 1976, tall cell variant (TCV) of papillary thyroid carcinoma (PTC) is defined as an aggressive thyroid tumour, with 50 per cent of cells having height at least two or three times greater than width and bearing nuclear characteristics of PTC [1, 2]. Interestingly, some cases of TCV PTC progress to spindle cell squamous carcinoma (SCSC) which is a rare form of anaplastic carcinoma, consisting of both spindle cell elements and squamous islands with focal keratinization [3, 4]. TCV PTC associated with SCSC can be divided into three types as described by Gopal et al. [5]. We present a rare case of type 1 anaplastic SCSC arising from TCV PTC, highlighting the diagnostic

challenges, as well as a review of the literature of all reported type 1 cases.

2. Case

In April 2011, a 51-year-old man presented to his primary care physician with symptoms of a mild sore throat and haemoptysis. Antibiotics were commenced for a presumed bacterial infection. He presented again two months later with shortness of breath and stridor and was referred to an Otolaryngologist for further care. Clinically, the patient was euthyroid and examination of the neck revealed a right-sided thyroid swelling with no lymphadenopathy. Blood tests were performed, including full blood count, thyroid function,

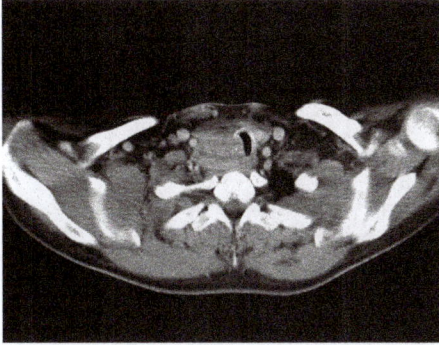

FIGURE 1: Neck CT scan showing the invasion of the trachea.

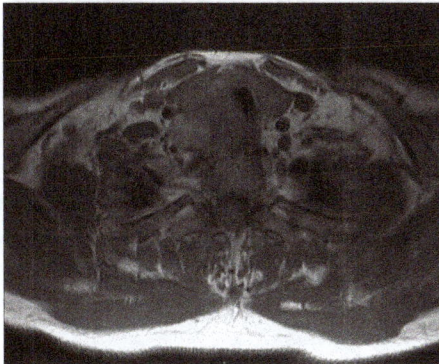

FIGURE 2: T1 MRI of neck showing invasion of trachea.

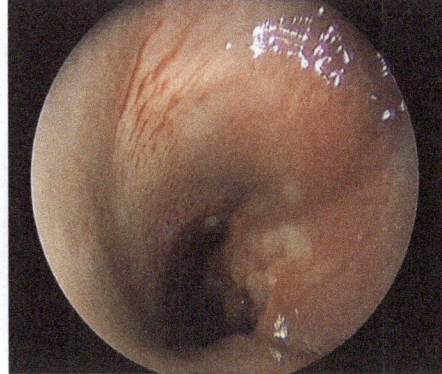

FIGURE 3: Tracheoscopy showing invasion of trachea from thyroid tumour.

calcium, phosphate, and vitamin D levels, and were all normal. The patient subsequently underwent an ultrasound scan (USS) and fine needle aspiration of the thyroid gland and was prescribed a short course of oral prednisolone. The results of the fine needle aspiration cytology (FNAC) suggested papillary carcinoma of the thyroid. Following steroid treatment, the patient was experiencing worsening haemoptysis, shortness of breath, and stridor associated with dizziness. The initial computer tomography (CT) scan of his neck revealed a mass extending from the posterior aspect of the right thyroid lobe, and further CT and magnetic resonance imaging (MRI) scan of the neck demonstrated that the thyroid mass had eroded into the trachea (Figures 1 and 2). Oral dexamethasone was commenced and the patient was referred to Hammersmith Hospital. A tracheoscopy was performed and vertical intraluminal tumour involvement was measured at 5 cm (Figure 3). The patient had no known drug allergies and his past medical history included hypercholesterolaemia which was controlled with medication.

The patient underwent a total thyroidectomy in September 2011, manubrial split (with levels 6 and 7 node dissection), and tracheal resection. End-to-end tracheal anastomosis was achieved with insertion of a tracheal stent and formation of a tracheostomy. The right recurrent laryngeal nerve was sacrificed owing to extensive tumour infiltration. Intraoperatively, the resected trachea was sent for frozen section histological analysis. The superior and inferior margins of the tracheal resection were clear of tumour and the specimen was

reported as a moderately to poorly differentiated squamous cell carcinoma of the thyroid invading and ulcerating the tracheal mucosa.

Although the patient was found to be hypocalcaemic postoperatively, he made an uncomplicated recovery and the tracheostomy was removed 14 days following surgery. He was discharged with calcium supplementation. The case was discussed at the Thyroid Cancer Multidisciplinary Team Meeting where a decision was made to offer the patient a course of chemoradiotherapy.

Unfortunately, the patient died 4 weeks following hospital discharge.

3. Materials and Methods

The literature review was performed using the PubMed database from 1961 to 2012. The terms "thyroid" and "thyroid gland" were used in conjunction with "tall cell variant papillary carcinoma" and/or "squamous cell carcinoma" or "spindle cell squamous cell carcinoma." A total of 162 articles were generated from the search of which only articles with cases documenting SCSC arising from TCV were included. Of the 162 articles, 3 were identified and a total number of 19 cases of documented SCSC arising from TCV PTC were included (Supplementary Table 1 in Supplementary Material available online at https://doi.org/10.1155/2017/4581626).

4. Histology

The thyroid contained a 5 cm tumour which showed two distinct morphologies. Part of the tumour (which was predominantly centred in the thyroid) showed features of papillary carcinoma including papillary architecture (with tall, well-formed papillae) and tumour cells that were columnar in shape, with nuclei showing overlapping, clearing, and pseudoinclusions (Figure 4(a)). As the length of the tumour cells was more than twice the width, the appearances were interpreted as those of the tall cell variant (of papillary carcinoma).

In addition, approximately 60–70% of the tumour showed features of moderately to poorly differentiated squamous cell

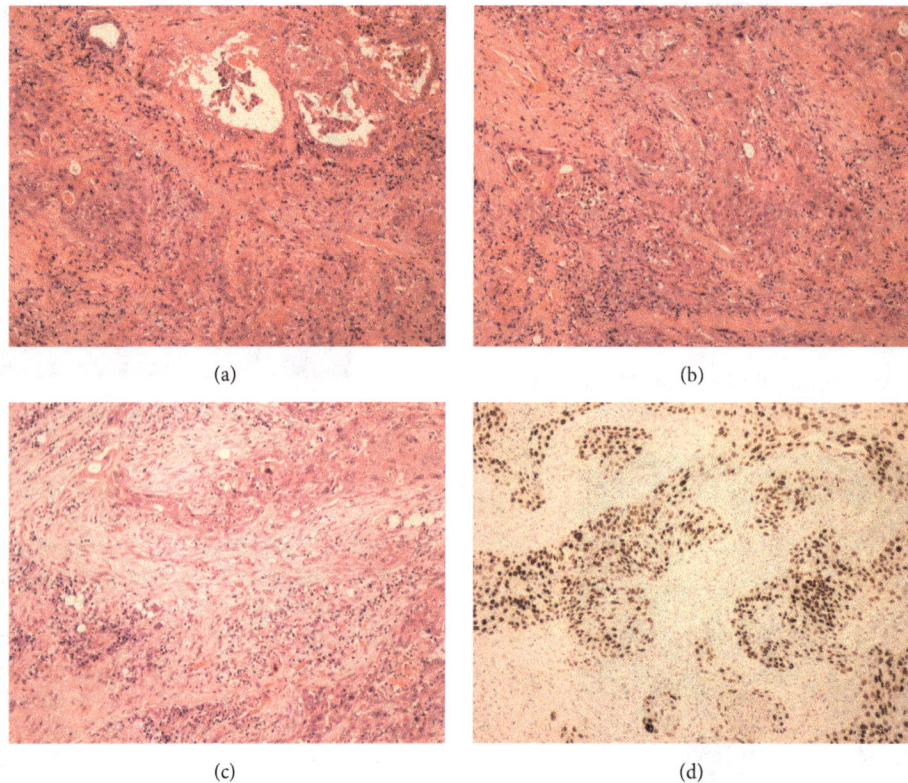

FIGURE 4: Histology of the tumour. (a) Features of papillary carcinoma including papillary architecture (with tall, well-formed papillae) and tumour cells that were columnar in shape, with nuclei showing overlapping, clearing, and pseudoinclusions. (b) Moderately to poorly differentiated squamous cell carcinoma. (c) Moderately to poorly differentiated squamous cell carcinoma with spindle cell elements. (d) Positive for (nuclear) thyroid transcription factor-1 (TTF-1) and Galectin-3 (cytoplasmic) in both components.

carcinoma (Figure 4(b)) with spindle cell elements (Figure 4(c)).

The two components were intimately admixed and there were areas of transition from the papillary component to the squamous component.

Immunohistochemical analysis showed positivity for (nuclear) thyroid transcription factor-1 (TTF-1) and Galectin-3 (cytoplasmic) in both components (Figure 4(d)). Thyroglobulin was expressed in the papillary component, but not the squamous/spindle cell component. P63 was positive in the squamous component. The Ki67 proliferation index varied between 5% in the papillary component and 40% in the squamous component.

Extensive extrathyroidal extension was noted with invasion of the trachea and skeletal muscle. There was also widespread lymphovascular invasion and metastatic tumour was present in three lymph nodes.

5. Discussion

Thyroid carcinoma, being the most common endocrine malignancy, has an overall estimated incidence of 7.7 per 100,000.

TCV PTC is an aggressive tumour characterised by its tall columnar shape, with a height : width ratio of 2-3 : 1 and abundant eosinophilic or oxyphilic cytoplasm [1, 2,

6, 7]. Although a rare occurrence, TCV PTC may transform into anaplastic SCSC. TCV PTC is associated with adverse prognostic features including large tumour size, extrathyroidal extension, and vascular invasion, with a high incidence of locoregional recurrence, distant metastasis, and shorter disease-free survival [6, 8–14]. In addition, TCV possesses a more aggressive phenotype than conventional PTC, independent of age, gender, and tumour size [15]. On close examination of the cell cycle regulatory proteins such as p27, Ki67 cyclin D1, and P53 and eukaryotic translation initiation factors 4E and 2 alpha expression, TCV exhibits a molecular profile which is comparable to thyroid tumours with an unfavourable prognosis [4, 16–19].

Three main types of anaplastic SCSC arising from TCV PTC have been described by Gopal et al. based on histological examination: type 1 is defined by the presence of both TCV and SCSC within the initial resection; type 2 occurs when the SCSC component arises as a recurrence or metastasis in patients with a known history of TCV; type 3 is defined as SCSC presenting as a primary laryngeal squamous cell carcinoma in patients with or without a known history of TCV [5].

This case presented some diagnostic difficulties. Ultrasound guided FNAC is a useful tool in the investigation workup of thyromegaly but has proven to be misleading in many studies [20–22]. The initial FNAC result, in this

TABLE 1: The table shows demographics, clinicopathologic features, treatment, outcome, and follow-up of patients with anaplastic SCSC arising from TCV PTC. (Data based on the 20 reported cases including present case.)

Patient demographics & clinicopathologic features	
Number of patients	20
Median age (years)	71
Male : female ratio	1 : 1.5
Thyroid swelling	80% (16/20)
Thyroid nodule(s)	20% (4/20)
Thyroid profile	
Euthyroid	5% (1/20)
Not reported	95% (19/20)
Treatment	
Surgery	5% (1/20)
Surgery + chemotherapy/radiotherapy	5% (1/20)
Not reported	90% (18/20)
Outcome & follow-up	
Alive	5% (1/20)
Death from tumour	5% (1/20)
Disease-free follow-up	6 months
Follow-up not reported	90% (18/20)

case, suggested PTC, which was misleading. When assessing the time course and severity of the patient's progressive symptoms coupled with the results of the CT and MRI scans, a working diagnosis of PTC becomes less likely. Secondly, the tracheal resection sent frozen section histological analysis revealed a diagnosis of moderately to poorly differentiated squamous cell carcinoma (SCC). This scenario implied that there was a greater possibility that the patient possessed two primary tumours (PTC and laryngeal SCC) as opposed to both tumour components arising from the thyroid gland.

The patient presented in this case was eventually defined as having the type 1 variant of anaplastic SCSC arising from TCV PTC owing to the histological assessment of the resected specimen which revealed both SCSC and TCV. Although TTF-1 reactivity has also been shown to be present in primary squamous tumours of the lung [23, 24], its positivity along with Galectin-3 within the SCSC component implies that the latter originated from the thyroid gland.

On careful review on the current literature documenting anaplastic SCSC arising from TCV PTC, only the case series presented by Gopal et al. [5] (14 cases), Saunders and Nayar [25] (1 case), and Johnson et al. [6] (4 cases) have cases that demonstrate type 1 variant of this rare disease. Although Gopal et al. present 18 cases of type 1 anaplastic SCSC arising from TCV PTC only 14 of these are documented to have an SCSC component along with the TCV component of tumour [5]. Of the 5 cases presented by Bronner and LiVolsi, only 4 fall within the type 1 scenario [3] (Supplementary Table 1).

The median age at presentation is 71 years with females being more affected than males (1.5 : 1, resp.) (Table 1). Of the 20 cases reviewed, 16 (80%) presented with a rapidly enlarging thyroid mass whereas 4 (20%) presented with a

thyroid nodule. Thyroid profile status was difficult to ascertain owing to a lack of reporting. With regard to treatment, the patient in this case underwent a total thyroidectomy and another patient underwent completion thyroidectomy and adjuvant chemoradiotherapy; 90% (18/20) of cases did not have documented treatment regimes. Regarding outcome and follow-up, 1 patient of 20 was reported to be alive after 6 months and the patient in this case deceased 4 weeks following surgery; 18 of 20 cases (90%) did not have documented prognosis and follow-up. The lack of outcome reporting is due to the rarity as well as aggressiveness (with survival rates of 20% at one year) of this unusual type of thyroid tumour and therefore makes development of an optimal treatment strategy a definite challenge [26].

The difficulties highlighted by this case are, firstly, the diagnosis of type 1 SCSC arising from TCV PTV. This is essentially a histological diagnosis, and as shown in this case, the FNAC results can be unreliable. Secondly, the rarity of this type of thyroid carcinoma coupled with late presentation has not allowed for a treatment regime to be established. When considering other types of aggressive thyroid tumours (e.g., anaplastic thyroid carcinoma) and their treatment, it is possible to suggest the use of chemoradiation coupled following surgical resection [27]. Another problem in the identification of new treatments for the type of thyroid carcinoma reported in this case is the rarity and aggressiveness of the tumour, rendering difficulty in recruiting patients who are clinically suited to participate in clinical trials.

6. Conclusion

We present the 20th documented case of type 1 anaplastic SCSC arising from TCV PTC highlighting the challenges in the diagnostic workup and a thorough review of all cases in the medical literature. This extremely rare neoplastic phenomenon forms a very small percentage of thyroid carcinomas and with its rarity and highly advanced stage of disease progression at presentation, recruiting patients to participate in clinical trials will inevitably lead to poor response rates from conventional and even newly emerging treatment regimens.

References

[1] W. A. Hawk and J. B. Hazard, "The many appearances of papillary carcinoma of the thyroid," *Cleveland Clinic Quarterly*, vol. 43, no. 4, pp. 207–216, 1976.

[2] R. Ghossein and V. A. Livolsi, "Papillary thyroid carcinoma tall cell variant," *Thyroid*, vol. 18, no. 11, pp. 1179–1181, 2008.

[3] M. P. Bronner and V. A. LiVolsi, "Spindle cell squamous carcinoma of the thyroid: an unusual anaplastic tumor associated with tall cell papillary cancer," *Modern Pathology*, vol. 4, no. 5, pp. 637–643, 1991.

[4] C. G. Kleer, T. J. Giordano, and M. J. Merino, "Squamous cell carcinoma of the thyroid: an aggressive tumor associated with tall cell variant of papillary thyroid carcinoma," *Modern Pathology*, vol. 13, no. 7, pp. 742–746, 2000.

[5] P. P. Gopal, K. T. Montone, Z. Baloch, M. Tuluc, and V. Livolsi, "The variable presentations of anaplastic spindle cell squamous carcinoma associated with tall cell variant of papillary thyroid carcinoma," *Thyroid*, vol. 21, no. 5, pp. 493–499, 2011.

[6] T. L. Johnson, R. V. Lloyd, N. W. Thompson, W. H. Beierwaltes, and J. C. Sisson, "Prognostic implications of the tall cell variant of papillary thyroid carcinoma," *American Journal of Surgical Pathology*, vol. 12, no. 1, pp. 22–27, 1988.

[7] S. Prendiville, K. D. Burman, M. D. Ringel et al., "Tall cell variant: an aggressive form of papillary thyroid carcinoma," *Otolaryngology—Head and Neck Surgery*, vol. 122, no. 3, pp. 352–357, 2000.

[8] A. Flint, R. D. Davenport, and R. V. Lloyd, "The tall cell variant of papillary carcinoma of the thyroid gland: comparison with the common form of papillary carcinoma by DNA and morphometric analysis," *Archives of Pathology and Laboratory Medicine*, vol. 115, no. 2, pp. 169–171, 1991.

[9] Y. Ito, M. Hirokawa, M. Fukushima et al., "Prevalence and prognostic significance of poor differentiation and tall cell variant in papillary carcinoma in Japan," *World Journal of Surgery*, vol. 32, no. 7, pp. 1535–1545, 2008.

[10] R. Jobran, Z. W. Baloch, V. Aviles, E. F. Rosato, S. Schwartz, and V. A. LiVolsi, "Tall cell papillary carcinoma of the thyroid: metastatic to the pancreas," *Thyroid*, vol. 10, no. 2, pp. 185–187, 2000.

[11] E. Lawrence, S. T. Lord, Y. Leon et al., "Tall cell papillary thyroid carcinoma metastatic to femur: evidence for thyroid hormone synthesis within the femur," *American Journal of the Medical Sciences*, vol. 322, no. 2, pp. 103–108, 2001.

[12] A. K.-C. Leung, S.-M. Chow, and S. C. K. Law, "Clinical features and outcome of the tall cell variant of papillary thyroid carcinoma," *Laryngoscope*, vol. 118, no. 1, pp. 32–38, 2008.

[13] J. J. Michels, M. Jacques, M. Henry-Amar, and S. Bardet, "Prevalence and prognostic significance of tall cell variant of papillary thyroid carcinoma," *Human Pathology*, vol. 38, no. 2, pp. 212–219, 2007.

[14] M. L. Ostrowski and M. J. Merino, "Tall cell variant of papillary thyroid carcinoma: a reassessment and immunohistochemical study with comparison to the usual type of papillary carcinoma of the thyroid," *American Journal of Surgical Pathology*, vol. 20, no. 8, pp. 964–974, 1996.

[15] R. A. Ghossein, R. Leboeuf, K. N. Patel et al., "Tall cell variant of papillary thyroid carcinoma without extrathyroid extension: biologic behavior and clinical implications," *Thyroid*, vol. 17, no. 7, pp. 655–661, 2007.

[16] T. C. Putti and T. A. Bhuiya, "Mixed columnar cell and tall cell variant of papillary carcinoma of thyroid: a case report and review of the literature," *Pathology*, vol. 32, no. 4, pp. 286–289, 2000.

[17] G. Tallini, G. Garcia-Rostan, A. Herrero et al., "Downregulation of p27KIP1 and Ki67/Mib1 labelling index support the classification of thyroid carcinoma into prognostically relevant categories," *The American Journal of Surgical Pathology*, vol. 23, no. 6, pp. 678–685, 1999.

[18] S. Wang, R. V. Lloyd, M. J. Hutzler et al., "Expression of eukaryotic translation initiation factors 4E and 2α correlates with the progression of thyroid carcinoma," *Thyroid*, vol. 11, no. 12, pp. 1101–1107, 2001.

[19] S. Wang, R. V. Lloyd, M. J. Hutzler, M. S. Safran, N. A. Patwardhan, and A. Khan, "The role of cell cycle regulatory protein, cyclin D1, in the progression of thyroid cancer," *Modern Pathology*, vol. 13, no. 8, pp. 882–887, 2000.

[20] D. K. Patten, R. Flora, N. Tolley, and F. Palazzo, "Sporadic medullary thyroid carcinoma with a pedunculated intraluminal internal jugular vein recurrence: a case report and literature review," *International Journal of Surgery Case Reports*, vol. 3, no. 2, pp. 92–96, 2012.

[21] D. K. Patten, Z. Wani, and N. Tolley, "Solitary Langerhan's histiocytosis of the thyroid gland: a case report and literature review," *Head and Neck Pathology*, vol. 6, no. 2, pp. 279–289, 2012.

[22] D. K. Patten, M. Fazel, R. Dina, and N. Tolley, "Solitary extramedullary plasmacytoma of the thyroid involved by papillary carcinoma: a case report and review of the literature," *Endocrine Pathology*, vol. 22, no. 3, pp. 155–158, 2011.

[23] P. A. Bejarano, R. P. Baughman, P. W. Biddinger et al., "Surfactant proteins and thyroid transcription factor-1 in pulmonary and breast carcinomas," *Modern Pathology*, vol. 9, no. 4, pp. 445–452, 1996.

[24] H. A. Harlamert, J. Mira, P. A. Bejarano et al., "Thyroid transcription factor-1 and cytokeratins 7 and 20 in pulmonary and breast carcinoma," *Acta Cytologica*, vol. 42, no. 6, pp. 1382–1388, 1998.

[25] C. A. Saunders and R. Nayar, "Anaplastic spindle-cell squamous carcinoma arising in association with tall-cell papillary cancer of the thyroid: a potential pitfall," *Diagnostic Cytopathology*, vol. 21, no. 6, pp. 413–418, 1999.

[26] S. Walsh, R. Prichard, and A. D. K. Hill, "Emerging therapies for thyroid carcinoma," *Surgeon*, vol. 10, no. 1, pp. 53–58, 2012.

[27] A. T. Swaak-Kragten, J. H. W. de Wilt, P. I. M. Schmitz, M. Bontenbal, and P. C. Levendag, "Multimodality treatment for anaplastic thyroid carcinoma—treatment outcome in 75 patients," *Radiotherapy and Oncology*, vol. 92, no. 1, pp. 100–104, 2009.

27

Recurrent Episodes of Thyrotoxicosis in a Man following Pregnancies of his Spouse with Hashimoto's Thyroiditis

Regina Belokovskaya[1] and Alice C. Levine[2]

[1]Internal Medicine Department, Mount Sinai St. Luke's and Roosevelt Hospitals, Icahn School of Medicine at Mount Sinai,
1111 Amsterdam Avenue, New York, NY 10025, USA
[2]Division of Endocrinology, Metabolism and Bone Diseases, Icahn School of Medicine at Mount Sinai, 1 Gustave L. Levy Place,
P.O. Box 1055, New York, NY 10029, USA

Correspondence should be addressed to Regina Belokovskaya; rbelokovskaya@chpnet.org

Academic Editor: Thomas Grüning

Over an 8-year period, a male patient presented three times to an endocrinologist with strikingly similar presentations, including palpitations, anxiety, and tremors. Each of his presentations occurred following either the birth of one of his two children or his wife's late termination of pregnancy. This patient's illness followed the typical time course of silent thyroiditis: hyperthyroidism, followed by euthyroidism, a late hypothyroid phase, and then a complete resolution of symptoms and normalization of thyroid function tests over a period of several months. We discuss the curious clinical presentation, diagnostic evaluation, and a literature review of alternate explanations for this patient's condition, including a discussion of the impact of seasonal shift, spousal's autoimmune disease, stress, and evolutionary changes in males postpartum. Although the differential diagnosis is broad in this case and the thyrotoxicosis could have coincidentally followed pregnancies of the patient's wife, documented hormonal changes in men during postpartum period in conjunction with the timeline of the patient's condition are suggestive of recurrent "sympathetic" postpartum thyroiditis. To our knowledge, this is the first case report of recurrent painless thyroiditis in a man following pregnancies of his wife with Hashimoto's thyroiditis.

1. Introduction

Silent thyroiditis, also known as painless or subacute lymphocytic thyroiditis, is one of several autoimmune thyroid disorders [1]. The clinical presentation of postpartum thyroiditis is virtually identical to that of silent thyroiditis, except that postpartum thyroiditis occurs in women within 1 year after delivery and rarely develops one month postpartum. It is typically associated with the development of either transient hyperthyroidism or hypothyroidism or both up to 1 year postpartum with eventual return to a euthyroid state [2, 3]. Usually, patients have a brief phase of thyrotoxicosis lasting 2–4 weeks, followed by hypothyroidism for 4–12 weeks and then resolution and a return to euthyroidism [4]. In the United States, postpartum thyroiditis occurs in approximately 5–10% of women. The incidence can be greater in certain high-risk populations, including those with a history of

autoimmune disorders, with previous thyroid dysfunction including previous postpartum thyroiditis (70% chance of recurrence with subsequent pregnancies), and/or having a family history of thyroid dysfunction [5, 6]. We present a curious case of a man who developed painless thyroiditis three times coinciding with the postpartum period of his wife with Hashimoto's thyroiditis.

2. Case Report

A 33-year-old male, with a past medical history of hyperlipidemia, seasonal allergies, and occasional sleep problems, originally presented feeling anxious, hot, and jittery, with recent weight loss and increased frequency of his bowel movements. He appeared slightly anxious, but the rest of exam was unremarkable, including thyroid examination which did not reveal any enlargement, tenderness,

TABLE 1: Profile of thyroid function tests and timeline of patient's wife postpartum period.

Date	TSH (0.34– 5.60 μIU/Ml)	T4, total (5.0– 12.2 MCG/DL)	T4, free (0.60– 1.10 NG/DL)	T3, free (2.50– 3.90 Pg/mL)	Thyroglobulin AB (0.0–4.1 U/mL)	TPO (microsomal) AB (0.0–5.6 IU/mL)
June 2007 (1 year after miscarriage)	4.09	7.2				
September 2007 (1 year and 3 months after miscarriage)	2.78	7.9				
June 2011 (4 months postpartum)	0.07		3.30	9.80	448.3	>1000.0
July 2011 (5 months postpartum)	0.11		2.50	6.60		
August 2011 (6 months postpartum)	1.57		0.40	2.60		
September 2011 (7 months postpartum)	5.73		0.80	3.30	521.1	>1000.0
June 2012 (1 year and 4 months postpartum)	2.83		0.90	2.98	139.2	237.2
September 2014 (1 month postpartum, 2nd baby)	0.08		2.04	6.00	333.1	>1000.0
January 2015 (5 months postpartum, 2nd baby)	4.90		0.89	3.04		

or nodules. These symptoms were first reported in 2006 following his wife's late termination of pregnancy performed because of congenital abnormalities noted on prenatal evaluation. He was diagnosed with subacute thyroiditis at that time (no laboratory values are available from his initial presentation) with subsequent normalization of his TSH to the high normal range (4.09, reference range of 0.34–5.60 μIU/Ml) in 2007 and resolution of symptoms. In 2011, several months after his wife's delivery of a healthy baby boy, the patient, who was 38 years old at the time, again presented with symptoms of hyperthyroidism including palpitations, anxiety, and tremors. The TSH was suppressed at 0.07 μIU/Ml (0.34–5.60 μIU/Ml), an elevated free T4 of 3.30 ng/dL (0.60–1.10 ng/dL), free T3 of 9.80 ng/dL (2.50–3.90 ng/dL), thyroglobulin Ab of 448.3 U/Ml (0.0–4.1 U/Ml), and TPO (microsomal Ab) >1000.0 IU/Ml (0.0–5.6 IU/Ml). A markedly decreased thyroid uptake of 0.2% (normal range 10 to 30%) on a nuclear medicine scan was suggestive of the diagnosis of silent thyroiditis. The patient was started on a beta-blocker, propranolol, for symptom control. Several months later, his labs revealed a mildly elevated TSH of 5.73, free T4 of 0.80, free T3 of 3.30, thyroglobulin Ab of 521.1, and TPO of >1000.0 consistent with the hypothyroid phase of thyroiditis. He reported feeling tired, although he no longer experienced heat intolerance or tremors. His weight was stable and his anxiety had significantly subsided. In September 2014, following the birth of his daughter, the patient presented with a similar clinical presentation and a suppressed TSH (0.08 μIU/Ml), elevated free T4 (2.04 ng/dL), elevated free T3 (6.0 ng/dL), thyroglobulin Ab (333.1 U/Ml), and TPO of >1000 IU/Ml. During a follow-up visit, in January 2015, the patient presented in late slightly hypothyroid phase of thyroiditis with TSH of 4.9 μIU/Ml, free T3 of 3.4 Pg/mL,

and free T4 of 0.89 NG/DL. TSH from May 2015 is still elevated at 5.0 μIU/Ml and he is now feeling tired and complaining of weight gain. These TFTs were consistent with recurrent painless thyroiditis that coincided with his wife's posttermination and postpartum periods. Table 1 summarizes these findings.

Of note, the patient's wife did not experience any similar symptoms during or following the three pregnancies. She has a history of Hashimoto's thyroiditis, diagnosed in 2011, when she initially presented with TSH of 96 μIU/Ml, and is maintained on levothyroxine with dose adjustments during gestation.

3. Discussion

The case presented here describes recurrent episodes of thyrotoxicosis in a man following pregnancies of his spouse who has treated Hashimoto's thyroiditis. The differential diagnosis for his presentation is broad, and multiple factors might have contributed to this patient's condition. For instance, the thyroid supplementation of the patient's wife suggests that surreptitious ingestion of thyroid hormones is possible. However, the cyclical course of this patient's disease is not consistent with exogenous thyroid hormone use. Given that the recurrent abnormal TFT levels occurred in the summer months, seasonal variations in thyroid levels must be considered, though these are unlikely to be solely responsible for the thyroid hormone variations. The time course of the disease is on the other hand consistent with silent thyroiditis. Patient transitioned from a state of hyperthyroidism to a state of mild hypothyroidism, followed by a resolution of thyroid function tests over a 3-4-month period. Documented hormonal changes in men, during postpartum period, whether stress related or evolutionary in nature, are suggestive of the diagnosis of "sympathetic" postpartum thyroiditis.

Research shows that the environmental impact of living with a spouse suffering from an autoimmune disease should not be ignored. Hemminki et al. looked at epidemiology of Grave's disease and the evidence of familial risks between family members. The study found a high disease concordance of 2.75 between spouses in Swedish population over the course of 20 years, which suggests the operation of some form of environmental sharing. The study mentions similar correlation between spouses and rheumatoid arthritis and amyotrophic lateral sclerosis. Shared smoking habits, psychosocial risk factors, stress, and infections are believed to be the mechanism behind the spouse correlation, all of which may precipitate many autoimmune conditions [7]. Emilsson et al. argued that first-degree relatives and spouses of individuals with celiac disease are at increased risk of nonceliac autoimmune disease. He also suggested that possible sharing of microbiome and the environment with their spouse might impact the risk of developing and diagnosing other autoimmune diseases [8].

Cyclical thyroid hormone changes found in this patient could have been caused by seasonal shifts. In a study about physiological variations in thyroid hormones Fisher states that the levels of T4 are statistically higher in winter as opposed to summer, although the variation is minimal. He attributes this variation to an effect of cold, which accelerates the peripheral metabolism of thyroid hormone during the winter months [9]. A study by Smals et al. found a seasonal variation in circulating serum T4 and T3 levels, inversely correlating with the seasonally altering environmental temperature. Lowest serum T4 and T3 levels were found in the summer [10].

Given that the cycles of thyroid hormone shifts in this patient coincided with his wife's pregnancies, it is important to consider the likelihood of men experiencing similar hormonal changes to women during the postpartum period. In a study by Storey et al. hormone concentrations and responses to infant stimuli in expectant and new fathers living with their partners were measured in order to determine whether men can experience changes that parallel the dramatic shifts seen in pregnant women. The result was that men and women had similar stage-specific differences in hormone levels, including higher concentrations of prolactin and cortisol in the period just before the births and lower postnatal concentrations of testosterone and estradiol. Men reporting pregnancy symptoms and men reporting strong emotional responses to the stimuli had significantly higher prolactin concentrations and experienced a larger testosterone decrease between the two blood samples than men without these responses. The pattern of hormonal change in men demonstrated in this study and its absence in nonpaternal species suggests that hormones may play a role in priming males to provide care for their offspring. From an evolutionary standpoint, it appears that the testosterone decrease in the postnatal period may reduce male's tendencies to engage in nonnurturing behaviors and thus promote greater paternal responsiveness [11].

Considering the similarities in the presentation of autoimmune thyroid diseases, one must often rely on the most common manifestation to determine the diagnosis. For a patient suffering from silent thyroiditis, a presence of ophthalmopathy and/or a thyroid bruit during the thyrotoxic stage would be a strong indication of Grave's disease. Neither presentation was found in this patient. Grave's disease was definitively ruled out by a markedly decreased thyroid uptake on a nuclear medicine scan. Most patients with silent thyroiditis have normal thyroid function at one year. In patients suffering from postpartum thyroiditis, 30 to 50% of patients develop permanent hypothyroidism within nine years [12, 13]. Such appears to be the case with this patient as his TSH levels were found to be elevated during the last two visits. Though the timing of this patient's symptoms is strongly suggestive of postpartum thyroiditis, a causal relationship between episodes of recurrent painless thyroiditis (silent thyroiditis) and spousal postpartum periods has not yet been established.

4. Conclusion

The case presented here poses a question whether hormonal changes seen during a postpartum period in a female can manifest themselves in the male spouse. To our knowledge, this is the first case report of a recurrent and possibly "sympathetic" postpartum thyroiditis in a male. Although differential diagnosis is broad, a plausible link between the postpartum period and the coinciding thyrotoxicosis in the male spouse has been presented. A number of documented cases showed that levels of several hormones in men change significantly during their spouse's postpartum period. Such changes, as described, may actually serve an evolutionary purpose. An alternative explanation for our patient's symptoms was established by the inclusion of studies showing a link between living with a spouse suffering from an autoimmune disease and the likelihood of the male partner developing a similar condition. Though more research is required to establish causality, postpartum thyroiditis should be considered as a possible diagnosis for a male patient presenting with anxiety, palpitations, weight loss, and tremors coinciding with postpartum period of his partner.

References

[1] D. S. Ross, "Syndromes of thyrotoxicosis with low radioactive iodine uptake," *Endocrinology and Metabolism Clinics of North America*, vol. 27, no. 1, pp. 169–185, 1998.

[2] J. H. Lazarus, "Thyroid disorders associated with pregnancy: etiology, diagnosis, management," *Treatments in Endocrinology*, vol. 4, no. 1, pp. 31–41, 2005.

[3] M. H. Samuels, "Subacute, silent, and postpartum thyroiditis," *Medical Clinics of North America*, vol. 96, no. 2, pp. 223–233, 2012.

[4] A. Stagnaro-Green, "Approach to the patient with postpartum thyroiditis," *Journal of Clinical Endocrinology and Metabolism*, vol. 97, no. 2, pp. 334–342, 2012.

[5] American Thyroid Association, 2014, http://www.thyroid.org/wp-content/uploads/patients/brochures/Postpartum_Thyroiditis_brochure.pdf.

[6] J. H. Lazarus, F. Ammari, R. Oretti, A. B. Parkes, C. J. Richards, and B. Harris, "Clinical aspects of recurrent postpartum thyroiditis," *British Journal of General Practice*, vol. 47, no. 418, pp. 305–308, 1997.

[7] K. Hemminki, X. Li, J. Sundquist, and K. Sundquist, "The epidemiology of Graves' disease: evidence of a genetic and an environmental contribution," *Journal of Autoimmunity*, vol. 34, no. 3, pp. J307–J313, 2010.

[8] L. Emilsson, C. Wijmenga, J. A. Murray, and J. F. Ludvigsson, "Autoimmune disease in first-degree relatives and spouses of individuals with celiac disease," *Clinical Gastroenterology and Hepatology*, vol. 13, no. 7, pp. 1271–1277.e2, 2015.

[9] D. A. Fisher, "Physiological variations in thyroid hormones: physiological and pathophysiological considerations," *Clinical Chemistry*, vol. 42, no. 1, pp. 135–139, 1996.

[10] A. G. H. Smals, H. A. Ross, and P. W. C. Kloppenborg, "Seasonal variation in serum T3 and T4 levels in man," *Journal of Clinical Endocrinology and Metabolism*, vol. 44, no. 5, pp. 998–1001, 1977.

[11] A. E. Storey, C. J. Walsh, R. L. Quinton, and K. E. Wynne-Edwards, "Hormonal correlates of paternal responsiveness in new and expectant fathers," *Evolution and Human Behavior*, vol. 21, no. 2, pp. 79–95, 2000.

[12] A. Stagnaro-Green, "Clinical review 152: postpartum thyroiditis," *Journal of Clinical Endocrinology and Metabolism*, vol. 87, no. 9, pp. 4042–4047, 2002.

[13] L. D. K. E. Premawardhana, A. B. Parkes, F. Ammari et al., "Postpartum thyroiditis and long-term thyroid status: prognostic influence of thyroid peroxidase antibodies and ultrasound echogenicity," *The Journal of Clinical Endocrinology & Metabolism*, vol. 85, no. 1, pp. 71–75, 2000.

28

Primary Mucosa-Associated Lymphoid Tissue Lymphoma of Thyroid with the Serial Ultrasound Findings

Eon Ju Jeon, Ho Sang Shon, and Eui Dal Jung

Department of Internal Medicine, Catholic University of Daegu, School of Medicine, Daegu 42472, Republic of Korea

Correspondence should be addressed to Eui Dal Jung; jed15@cu.ac.kr

Academic Editor: John Broom

Extranodal marginal zone lymphoma of mucosa-associated lymphoid tissue (MALT) of the thyroid gland is uncommon. Even though its natural history is not well defined, it is known to be indolent course. We present a case of primary MALT thyroid lymphoma with the serial sonographic findings in the patient presenting as the focal nodule. A 45-year-old woman visited our hospital for neck examination. Initially, fine-needle aspiration cytology in the focal hypoechoic lesion in the left thyroid lobe on ultrasound sonography was performed and consistent with Hashimoto's thyroiditis. However, the results of serial ultrasounds and core-needle biopsy revealed an extranodal marginal zone lymphoma of MALT on 4-year follow-up. Patients with a focal hypoechoic nodule with linear echogenic strands and segmental pattern in the background of Hashimoto's thyroiditis on ultrasonography should undergo careful surveillance for malignancy. Serial sonographic features in this case are meaningful in the understanding of the natural history of the extranodal marginal zone lymphoma of MALT of the thyroid.

1. Introduction

Primary thyroid lymphoma is a rare thyroid tumor, accounting for approximately 2–8% of thyroid malignancies and for 1-2% of extrathyroid lymphomas [1–3]. The most of thyroid lymphomas are non-Hodgkin's lymphomas of B cell origin. The most common subtype is diffuse large B cell lymphoma (DLBL) and the other subtype is an extranodal marginal zone lymphoma of MALT comprising 6% to 27% of thyroid lymphomas [1]. Extranodal marginal zone lymphoma of MALT is rare and it can occur in a variety of organs, including the orbit, conjunctiva, salivary glands, skin, thyroid glands, and lung even though the most common sites are stomach and intestine [2]. These tumors are often localized and of indolent clinical behavior.

Because thyroid gland has no native lymphoid tissue, thyroid lymphoma is thought to develop from chronic autoimmune thyroiditis such as Hashimoto's thyroiditis [1, 4, 5]. In addition, because thyroid gland is not a mucosal organ, extranodal marginal zone lymphoma of MALT of the thyroid is thought to be common occurring in chronic autoimmune thyroiditis. However, the mechanism of underlying malignant transformation has yet to be clearly elucidated.

For the evaluation of the thyroid nodule, fine-needle aspiration cytology (FNAC) is relatively accurate test and can be easily performed. Nevertheless, the diagnosis of thyroid lymphoma using FNAC or core-needle biopsy (CNB) is difficult. Therefore, there are often cases that are diagnosed with immunohistochemical stating after surgery.

Although there are several studies about extranodal marginal zone lymphoma of MALT accompanied with Hashimoto's thyroiditis, we herein report the experience with the serial ultrasound findings and FNAC results of the course of primary MALT thyroid lymphoma in the patient with focal nodule and Hashimoto's thyroiditis.

2. Case Report

A 45-year-old woman visited our hospital for neck examination in March 2010. The mild goiter had been present over several years. However, she does not have further evaluation about it. In the meantime, there is no significant change of the goiter. There were no symptoms such as dyspnea, hoarseness, pain, and the difficulty of swallowing. There was no change of weight, fever, or night sweats. She had no history of thyroid disease or radiation exposure. She did not smoke and

(a)

(b)

(c)

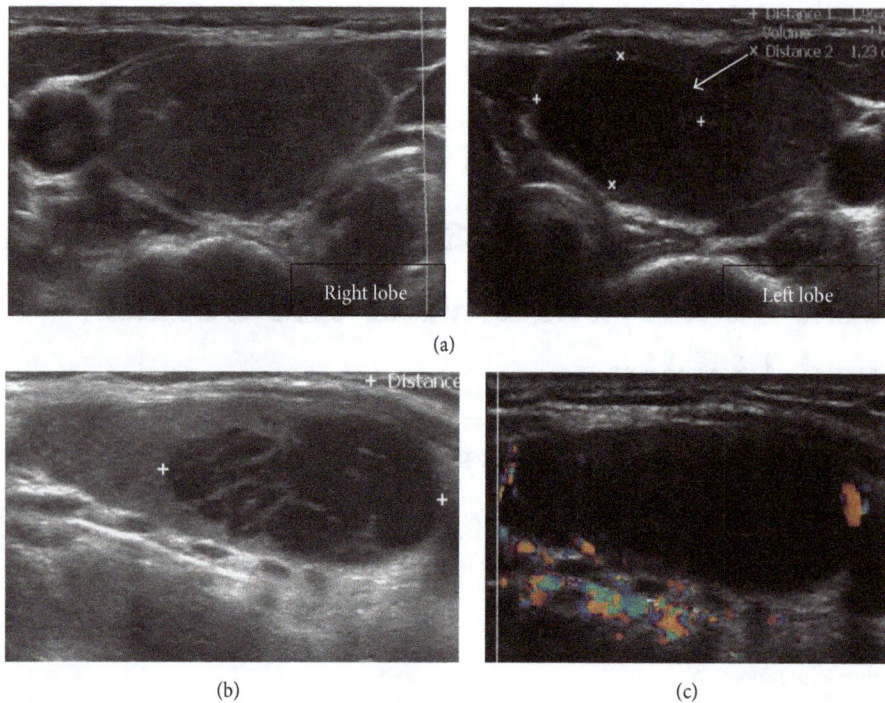

FIGURE 1: (a) Thyroid ultrasound shows a markedly hypoechoic area (arrow), with interspersed linear echogenic strands pattern in transverse view and (b) longitudinal view. (c) Color Doppler image shows a left thyroid nodule with peripheral increased blood flows in longitudinal view during a first visit.

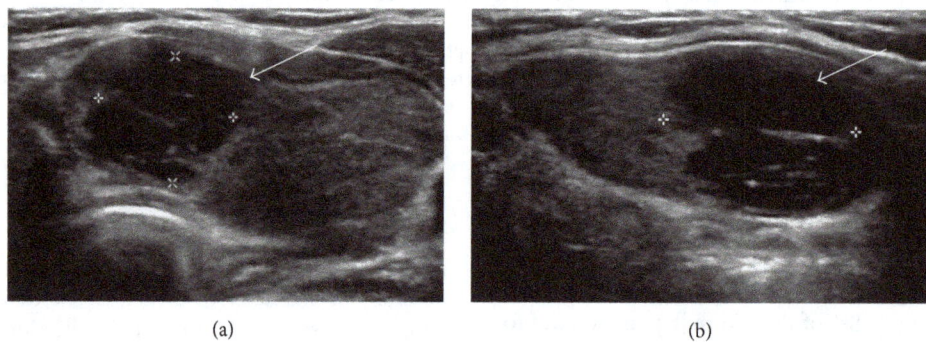

(a)

(b)

FIGURE 2: Four years later, image of the left thyroid nodule (a) in transverse view and (b) longitudinal view.

had no familial history of endocrine disorders. On physical examination, the thyroid was diffusely enlarged and there is no palpable nodule and focal tenderness on neck. There is no hepatomegaly and splenomegaly on abdomen. Her physical examination was otherwise unremarkable. Her blood pressure was 120/70 mmHg and body temperature was 36.8°C.

The laboratory findings were as follows: thyroid function tests: free T4, 0.864 ng/dL (normal range, 0.8 to 1.9 ng/dL); T3, 1.08 ng/dL (normal range, 0.6 to 1.7 ng/mL); thyroid stimulating hormone (TSH), 7.89 μIU/mL (normal range, 0.4 to 4.7 μIU/mL); antithyroglobulin antibody level increase, 1 : 25; antimicrosomal antibodies, negative. Subclinical hypothyroidism was suspected.

Initial ultrasonography (US) revealed diffuse enlargement of both thyroid glands, with heterogeneous background parenchyma and a focal hypoechoic nodule measuring 1.9 × 1.2 × 2.4 cm in upper portion of the left thyroid gland (Figure 1). US-guided fine-needle aspiration cytology (FNAC) showed the presence of lymphocyte. There were no malignant findings. Therefore, the nodule was suspicious of the lymphocytic thyroiditis lesion. Six months and one year later, US-guided FNAC was followed. There were no significant changes of the size and finding on US. The results of FNAC showed lymphocytes repeatedly. However, on follow-up four years later, the results of FNAC showed atypical lymphoid proliferation in February 2014 (Figure 2). US-guided CNB was performed, which showed thyroid follicular atrophy and lymphocyte infiltration in the interstitial tissue. In the immunohistochemistry stain, CD20 was positive and CD5 was negative. The histological findings were suggestive of B

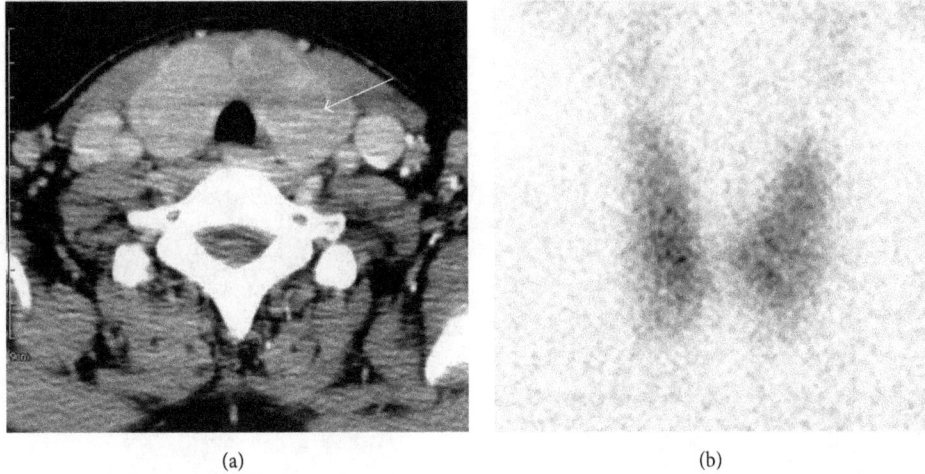

(a)   (b)

Figure 3: (a) Neck computed tomography shows 1.9×1.2 cm sized hypodense mass involving thyroid isthmus in the left thyroid. (b) Thyroid scan with Tc-^{99}m pertechnetate shows diffuse and even uptake in both thyroid glands.

cell lineage. Cervical contrast-enhanced computer tomography (CT) showed a low-density nodule in the same area and benign or intermediate nature lymph nodes in levels of lb and lla both of the lateral neck (Figure 3(a)). Thyroid scan showed diffuse and even uptake (Figure 3(b)). All the hematological and biochemical investigations were within the normal range. She underwent total thyroidectomy and lateral neck node dissection. The specimen included the $6.5 \times 4.5 \times 3.5$ cm left thyroid lobe and $7.2 \times 3.3 \times 3.0$ cm right thyroid lobe. The tumor size was 1.5×1.0 cm.

On microscopic examination of the tumor margin, the findings showed diffuse lymphocytic infiltration in the normal thyroid parenchyma, thyroid follicular atrophy, and the formation of the lymphoid follicles (Figure 4(a)). This was compatible with Hashimoto's thyroiditis. The tumor was diffusely replaced by an atypical lymphocyte with small and centrocyte-like cell. These cells gave rise to numerous lymphoepithelial lesions (Figure 4(b)). The metastasis of central neck node was not evident. Immunohistochemistry showed CD20 positivity, CD5 negativity, and cytokeratin positivity. She was diagnosed with the MALT lymphoma (Figures 4(c) and 4(d)). Postoperative ^{18}F-fluorodeoxyglucose positron emission tomography of the neck performed and revealed the uptake in the cervical, axillary, and iliac lymph nodes. Using the Ann Arbor staging system, she was at stage IIIE, and R-CHOP chemotherapy was considered.

3. Discussion

Primary thyroid lymphoma is a rare thyroid tumor, and most of them are DLBL of B cell origin. Extranodal marginal zone lymphoma of MALT of the thyroid has been reported to vary between 6 and 27% according to the literature [1]. Primary thyroid lymphoma is usually occurring in patients with Hashimoto's thyroiditis. Extranodal marginal zone lymphoma of MALT has an indolent course, while DLBL has the aggressive progress. The diagnosis of the extranodal marginal

zone lymphoma of MALT is often delayed because systemic symptoms do not appear well.

Thus, although lymphoma of the thyroid gland is relatively rare, there are a few studies. However, the development of an extranodal marginal zone lymphoma of MALT has been linked to chronic autoimmune disease such as Hashimoto's thyroiditis and it is interesting. In the normal condition, thyroid gland is an organ that lacks the lymph nodes; however, if the autoimmune disease is accompanied, it acquired the infiltration of lymphocytes into lymphoid tissue [5–7]. B cells are present and the differentiation of plasma cells appeared in this tissue. That is very similar to MALT. DLBP is present in the transition between the DLBL and the extranodal marginal zone lymphoma of MALT, and DLBL is thought to be rapidly converted from an extranodal marginal zone lymphoma of MALT. In Korea, since Lee et al. reported an extranodal marginal zone lymphoma of MALT at first [8], it has gradually been known about the clinicopathologic characteristics [9, 10]. Most had a history of long-term Hashimoto's thyroiditis. Some did not accompany Hashimoto's thyroiditis. It was reported that de novo extranodal marginal zone lymphoma of MALT may occur without the preceding thyroiditis. Most of cases have an abrupt change in size and compressive symptoms were developed by mass effects.

In the diagnosis of the thyroid lymphoma, it is important that clinicians suspect it. Most patients with thyroid lymphoma showed rapidly increased goiter between 1 and 3 months at about 70%, and in approximately 30% the patients complained of obstructive symptoms such as hoarseness [1, 3, 11, 12]. It was involved with unilateral lobe or both lobes of thyroid. It was hard and there was no pain. Therefore, in patients with Hashimoto's thyroiditis, extranodal marginal zone lymphoma of MALT should be suspected if thyroid grows rapidly and they had compressive symptoms between the weeks or months. The most common cause of sudden increases for differential diagnosis is bleeding of benign tumor of the thyroid gland. However, in this case, the patient mainly complained of pain and it usually disappears in a

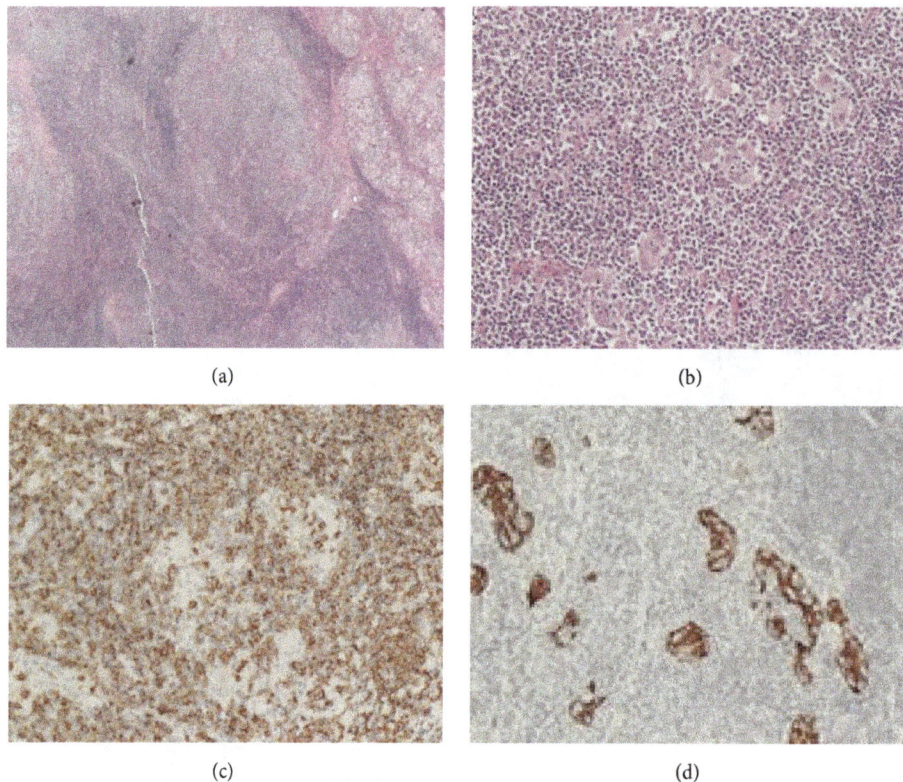

FIGURE 4: (a) Microscopic finding shows the extranodal marginal zone lymphoma of MALT in a background of Hashimoto's thyroiditis (H&E stain, ×20). (b) Microscopic finding of the thyroid mass shows marked lymphocytic infiltration and a few degenerated follicles (H&E stain, ×200). (c) Immunohistochemical findings disclose diffuse positive staining for CD20 (immunohistochemistry, ×200). (d) Immunostaining for cytokeratin highlights lymphoepithelial lesions (immunohistochemistry, ×200).

few days. If the goiter becomes large rapidly causing pressure symptoms, it should consider the possibility of anaplastic cancer or thyroid lymphoma. Typical symptoms of lymphoma such as fever, night sweat, and weight loss are rare [3]. Extranodal marginal zone lymphoma of MALT is slowly proceeding and tends to remain localized for long time.

Even though this patient had no symptoms except stable bulging neck, she had a medical checkup by chance and was diagnosed with subclinical hypothyroidism due to Hashimoto's thyroiditis and focal nodule. Initially, FNAC in the focal hypoechoic lesion in the left thyroid lobe on US was performed and consistent with Hashimoto's thyroiditis. However, the results of serial USs and CNB revealed an extranodal marginal zone lymphoma of MALT on 4-year follow-up. Recently, thyroid nodules even if they are not palpable are detected easily with the spreads of US and US-guided FNAC is available. Therefore, the diagnostic accuracy of the first-line US and FNAC of an extranodal marginal zone lymphoma of MALT of the thyroid compared with these of differentiated thyroid cancer is low and varies widely. Considering that there was no change in thyroid lesions on sequential US follow-up, this case is a possibility that the diagnosis had been delayed due to the limits of FNAC compared to the insidious onset of it. In general, the US findings that suggest thyroid malignancy are well known as follows: marked hypoechogenicity, irregular margins, and a taller-than-wide shape. However, the characteristic US features of the extranodal marginal zone lymphoma of MALT are not known well. At present, Orita et al. reported characteristic US features of MALT lymphoma of the salivary and thyroid gland [13]. Mainly, two US patterns were observed for the extranodal marginal zone lymphoma of MALT: the interspersed linear echogenic strands pattern and the segmental pattern. In this patient, US feature was similar to linear echogenic strands pattern that are considered to be fibrous bands (Figures 1 and 2).

In the case of an extranodal marginal zone lymphoma of MALT accompanied with Hashimoto's thyroiditis, the pathological and immunohistochemical examination of the tissue is required to confirm it because of coexisting neoplastic lesions and reactive lesions [6]. Even though there are no specific markers, extranodal marginal zone lymphoma of MALT can be diagnosed immunohistologically, by the presence of immunoglobulin light chain, CD20, and Bcl-2 and the absence of CD5, CD10, and CD23.

The prognosis of the extranodal marginal zone lymphoma of MALT localized to the thyroid is excellent and the 5-year disease-specific survival rates for it are more than 95%; however, it is known to poor prognosis in the advanced stage involving extrathyroid invasion and transforming to a higher grade. The current optimal guidelines for treatment and follow-up are not conclusive.

In conclusion, the extranodal marginal zone lymphoma of MALT of the thyroid gland is rare and not fully understood.

In this case, despite short-term follow-up of 4 years, serial sonographic features may be meaning in the understanding of an indolent course and the knowledge of serial changes of an extranodal marginal zone lymphoma of MALT of the thyroid. Because even the clinical prognosis is worse in the advanced stage of it, patients with a focal thyroid nodule that characterized the linear echogenic strands and segmental pattern in the background of Hashimoto's thyroiditis on ultrasonography should undergo further evaluation and careful surveillance for the possibility of an extranodal marginal zone lymphoma of MALT.

References

[1] S. Widder and J. L. Pasieka, "Primary thyroid lymphomas," *Current Treatment Options in Oncology*, vol. 5, no. 4, pp. 307–313, 2004.

[2] S. N. Malek, A. J. Hatfield, and I. W. Flinn, "MALT Lymphomas," *Current Treatment Options in Oncology*, vol. 4, no. 4, pp. 269–279, 2003.

[3] S. M. Ansell, C. S. Grant, and T. M. Habermann, "Primary thyroid lymphoma," *Seminars in Oncology*, vol. 26, no. 3, pp. 316–323, 1999.

[4] F. Matsuzuka, A. Miyauchi, S. Katayama et al., "Clinical aspects of primary thyroid lymphoma: diagnosis and treatment based on our experience of 119 cases," *Thyroid*, vol. 3, no. 2, pp. 93–99, 1993.

[5] L. E. Holm, H. Blomgren, and T. Lowhagen, "Cancer risks in patients with chronic lymphocytic thyroiditis," *The New England Journal of Medicine*, vol. 312, no. 10, pp. 601–604, 1985.

[6] A. Graff-Baker, J. A. Sosa, and S. A. Roman, "Primary thyroid lymphoma: a review of recent developments in diagnosis and histology-driven treatment," *Current Opinion in Oncology*, vol. 22, no. 1, pp. 17–22, 2010.

[7] E. Hyjek and P. G. Isaacson, "Primary B cell lymphoma of the thyroid and its relationship to Hashimoto's Thyroiditis," *Human Pathology*, vol. 19, no. 11, pp. 1315–1326, 1988.

[8] T. Y. Lee, E. S. Ryoo, I. S. Nam, G. Y. Hong et al., "A case of MALT lymphoma of the thyroid accompany in Hashimoto's thyroiditis," *The Korean Journal of Medicine*, vol. 61, pp. 281–285, 2001.

[9] O. N. Kong, S. H. Joo, S. H. Shin et al., "A case of thyroid MALT lymphoma without autoimmune thyroiditis," *Journal of Korean Society of Endocrinology*, vol. 20, no. 3, pp. 268–272, 2005.

[10] J. H. Cho, Y. H. Park, W. S. Kim et al., "High incidence of mucosa-associated lymphoid tissue in primary thyroid lymphoma: a clinicopathologic study of 18 cases in the Korean population," *Leukemia and Lymphoma*, vol. 47, no. 10, pp. 2128–2131, 2006.

[11] L. D. Green, L. Mack, and J. L. Pasieka, "Anaplastic thyroid cancer and primary thyroid lymphoma: a review of these rare thyroid malignancies," *Journal of Surgical Oncology*, vol. 94, no. 8, pp. 725–736, 2006.

[12] N. Latheef, V. Shenoy, M. P. Kamath, M. C. Hegde, and A. R. Rao, "Maltoma of thyroid: a rare thyroid tumour," *Case Reports in Otolaryngology*, vol. 2013, Article ID 740241, 3 pages, 2013.

[13] Y. Orita, Y. Sato, N. Kimura et al., "Characteristic ultrasound features of mucosa-associated lymphoid tissue lymphoma of the salivary and thyroid gland," *Acta Oto-Laryngologica*, vol. 134, no. 1, pp. 93–99, 2014.

29

Adrenal Ganglioneuroblastoma in Adults: A Case Report and Review of the Literature

Stefano Benedini,[1,2] **Giorgia Grassi,**[1,2] **Carmen Aresta,**[1,2] **Antonietta Tufano,**[2] **Luca Fabio Carmignani,**[3] **Barbara Rubino,**[4] **Livio Luzi,**[1,2] **and Sabrina Corbetta**[5]

[1]*Department of Biomedical Sciences for Health, Università degli Studi di Milano, Milan, Italy*
[2]*Endocrinology Unit, IRCCS Policlinico San Donato, San Donato Milanese, Italy*
[3]*Urology Department, IRCCS Policlinico San Donato, San Donato Milanese, Italy*
[4]*Pathology Department, IRCCS Policlinico San Donato, San Donato Milanese, Italy*
[5]*Endocrinology Service, Department of Biomedical Sciences for Health, University of Milan,*
IRCCS Istituto Ortopedico Galeazzi, Milan, Italy

Correspondence should be addressed to Stefano Benedini; stefano.benedini@unimi.it

Academic Editor: Carlo Capella

Incidentally discovered adrenal masses are very common given the increased number of imaging studies performed in recent years. We here report a clinical case of a 20-year-old woman who presented with left flank pain. Ultrasound examination revealed a contralateral adrenal mass, which was confirmed at computed tomography (CT) scan. Hormonal hypersecretion was excluded. Given the size ($11 \times 10 \times 7$ cm) and the uncertain nature of the mass, it was surgically removed and sent for pathological analyses. Conclusive diagnosis was ganglioneuroblastoma. Ganglioneuroblastoma is an uncommon malignant tumor, extremely rare in adults, particularly in females. This neoplasm is frequently localized in adrenal gland.

1. Introduction

One of the most common unexpected findings revealed by imaging studies is an adrenal mass, called incidentaloma, which occurs in about 2–4% of the radiological studies performed for other reasons [1]. The preliminary evaluation of the mass is aimed to distinguish benign from malign lesions and to exclude hormonal hypersecretion. Most adrenal masses are small nonfunctioning adrenocortical adenomas, which do not require treatment or follow-up. Nevertheless, if the mass shows hormonal hypersecretion or malignancy is suspected, surgery is recommended [2].

Ganglioneuroblastoma (GNB) represents a rare cause of adrenal tumor in adults. Preoperative suspicion is challenging and the final diagnosis is often made by the pathologist after surgical removal.

2. Case Presentation

A 20-year-old Caucasian woman was admitted through the Emergency Department for right flank pain. Abdominal ultrasound examination was performed and a contralateral adrenal mass was incidentally found. Subsequently, the patient underwent computed tomography (CT) to confirm the finding. The mass in left adrenal lodge was solid and measured $11 \times 10 \times 7$ cm, showing heterogeneous density (varying 17–40 HU) and calcifications (Figure 1). Dynamic analysis revealed a progressive and modest contrast enhancement in venous phase.

The patient was addressed to the Endocrine Unit for biochemical evaluation of the adrenal mass.

She was in good clinical conditions and the complete physical examination was negative; in particular, no Cushing stigmata or hirsutism was present. Her height was 153 cm,

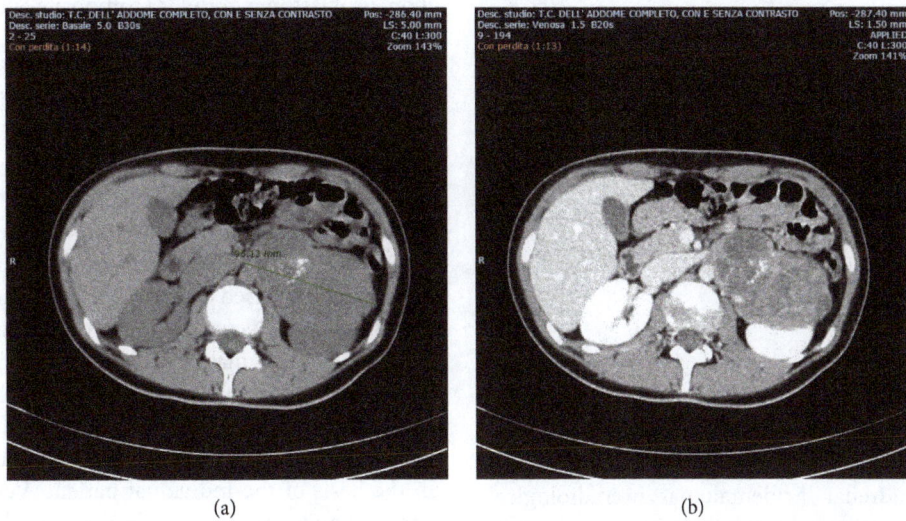

(a)   (b)

FIGURE 1: Abdominal CT scan with and without contrast enhancement: presence of a big and heterogeneous mass with calcification in left adrenal lodge (b). Dynamic analysis revealed a progressive and modest contrast enhancement in venous phase (a).

weight 48.5 kg (BMI 20.7 Kg/m^2), blood pressure was 110/70 mmHg, pulse rate 64 beats/min, and SpO$_2$ 99% (room air). There was no family history of relevant morbidities. She was active smoker and suffered from patent foramen ovale of the heart and focal nodular hyperplasia of the liver.

Results of the complete blood count, plasma levels of electrolytes, tests of coagulation, kidney, liver, and thyroid function were normal. Adrenal function evaluation revealed that urinary metanephrines and normetanephrines in the normal range, DHEA-S 1500 ng/ml (350–4300), aldosterone 457.2 pg/ml (37–150), renin 1.5 ng/ml/h (1.0–2.4), aldosterone-renin ratio 30.48, basal cortisol, and 17-OH-progesterone were normal both in basal condition and after stimulation with ACTH 250 mcg. Regrettably the patient was on contraceptive estroprogestinic therapy at the time of hormonal evaluation.

Considering the size and the undetermined radiological features, the adrenal mass met the criteria for surgical removal according the most recent international guidelines [2].

The patient was admitted to the Department of Urology where she underwent transabdominal adrenalectomy. The adrenal mass incorporated the renal hilum, aorta, and superior mesenteric arteria; therefore intraoperative decision to perform additional left nephrectomy was taken. There were no complications after surgery.

The surgical sample sent for pathological examination included left kidney, left adrenal gland, and two lymph nodes (celiac and paraaortic). The tumor grossly was grey and multilobulated, replaced the entire adrenal gland, measured 11 × 10 × 7 cm, weighed 195 g, and incorporated arterial and venous vessels of renal hilum and sparing renal parenchyma.

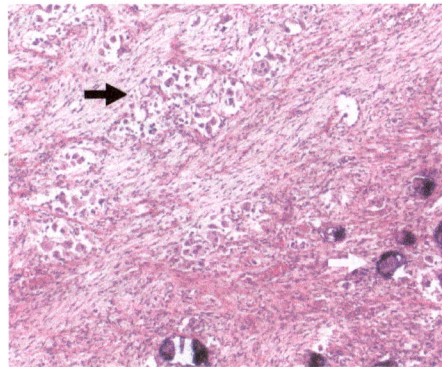

FIGURE 2: Histological examination (hematoxylin and eosin stain, 10x): high proportion of ganglion cells (black arrow) in spindle stroma and dystrophic calcification (white arrow).

The histological report described a spindle cell stroma in a fibrillary matrix interspersed with scattered nests of primitive neuroblasts and high proportion of differentiating elements (ganglion cells) (Figure 2), placing the tumor in a favorable subgroup (ganglioneuroblastoma intermixed). Localization was found in both lymph nodes. These findings were consistent with intermixed stroma-rich ganglioneuroblastoma (GNB) according to Shimada et al., arising from the adrenal and with metastatic extension to ipsilateral lymph nodes [3]. The mitosis-karyorrhexis index (MKI) was <2%. In this case, any N-MYC amplification was detected and any deletion of the short arm of the chromosome 1. Chemotherapy was not proposed based on the favorable histology. Any disease recurrence occurred in the 21-month follow-up from surgery.

TABLE 1: Causes of adrenal masses.

(i) *Cystic masses*: endothelial cyst, pseudocyst, and hydatid cyst

(ii) *Solid masses*: adenoma, nodular hyperplasia, carcinoma, metastases, pheochromocytoma, neuroblastic tumors, neurofibroma, schwannoma, leiomyoma, angiosarcoma, hamartoma, tuberculoma, and amyloidosis

(iii) *Fat-containing masses*: lipoma and myelolipoma

Modified from Arnaldi and Boscaro [1].

3. Discussion

Incidentally discovered adrenal masses are becoming more common with the imaging technological advances and the increased number of imaging studies performed. Nowadays the prevalence of adrenal incidentalomas in radiological studies has come close to the autoptic data: approximately 2–4% in adult age, increasing up to 10% in elderly population. Their differential diagnosis must consider a wide range of pathologies (Table 1). The prevalence of different etiologies varies among the studies; however, it is likely that the majority consists in nonfunctioning adenomas. Other frequently reported lesions are cortisol secreting adenomas, pheochromocytomas, primitive carcinomas, and distant metastatic lesions. In a study including 1111 adult patients with adrenal incidentalomas, GNB was diagnosed in only one case [4]. It is important to point out that the majority of adrenal lesions do not come to surgery; therefore pathological diagnoses of most adrenal incidentalomas remain unknown [1].

Peripheral neuroblastic tumors (PNTs) are a group of tumors arising from sympathetic ganglion cells. In two-thirds of the cases, PNTs arise in the adrenal gland or the retroperitoneal paravertebral ganglia. PNTs represent one of the most frequent solid tumors in children, while the occurrence in adults is very rare. Overall survival in infants is very high (91%) and progressively declines parallel to the increased age at diagnosis. In a study performed on RARECAREnet and involving very few cases, 5-year survival was reported to be 48% in adolescents (15–24 years) and 40% in adults (25–64 years) [5]. The vast majority of PNTs are sporadic and family history is reported only in a small percentage of cases [6]. Conditions such as Hirschsprung's disease and central hypoventilation, Turner syndrome, and Neurofibromatosis 1 seem to confer an increased risk of developing neuroblastic tumors, according to the literature [7–9]. No association with patent foramen ovale or focal nodular hyperplasia has been reported. PNTs are made up of two components: neuroblastic cells, with different degrees of differentiation, and Schwannian cells. The International Neuroblastoma Pathology Classification (INPC) distinguishes four pathological groups according to the different proportion of ganglion and Schwann cells: neuroblastoma (Schwannian stroma-poor, undifferentiated/poorly, differentiated/differentiating), ganglioneuroblastoma intermixed (Schwannian stroma-rich), ganglioneuroma (Schwannian stroma-dominant), and ganglioneuroblastoma nodular (composite Schwannian stroma-rich/stroma-dominant/stroma-poor) [3]. Clinic presentation is variable and the most common symptoms include pain or compression of the abdominal viscera. Metastatic dissemination occurs in about 40% of patients and involves more frequently bone and bone marrow. Catecholamines secretion is documented in more than 70% of cases [10]. The International Neuroblastoma Risk Group Consensus Pretreatment Classification Scheme defines prognosis and design treatment programs based on the stage of the tumor (according to the International Neuroblastoma Risk Group Staging System, INRGSS), age at diagnosis, pathology (INPC), and gene expression abnormalities (MYCN gene amplification, 11q aberration, and ploidy) (Table 2) [11]. Therapeutic modalities include surgery, radiotherapy, and chemotherapy combined on the basis of the individual patient. Very low risk group is treated only with surgery, followed by observation. Radiotherapy and chemotherapy are reserved for the higher risk groups, combined in different protocols [5].

Revision of the published literature in PubMed retrieved 15 cases of adult-onset adrenal GNB (Table 3) [12, 13]. The majority of patients were male and mean age at diagnosis was 38.9 years (21–67 years). Clinic was not specific and often represented by pain or other symptoms due to compression. Catecholamines secretion was documented only in 4 cases. Left adrenal gland was more frequently involved, and in one case bilateral tumors were reported. Imaging features of GNB varied from oval and homogeneous masses to heterogeneous, infiltrating, and calcified lesions. Because most of the lesions grew silently, at time of diagnosis big masses were found (mean size 10.44 cm). In locally advanced PNTs with potentially associated surgery-related complications, presurgical chemotherapy should be administered in order to shrink the tumor and enable safe resection saving other abdominal viscera involved [14]. Neuroblastic origin of the tumor was suspected preoperatively in just few cases, suggesting that though the radiological appearances of adrenal GNB have been described in detail [15], the preoperative diagnosis remains challenging and may be misleading. Consequently patients were addressed straight to surgery and the definitive etiology was histologically defined. Metastases were found at diagnosis in half of the patient and occurred in lymph nodes, liver, or bone marrow. The presence of metastases does not seem to correlate with the size or the histopathological subtype of the tumor. Most of the patients were treated only with surgery, showing no recurrence during follow-up (mean follow-up duration 20.9 months). Metastases were detected after 2.5 years in a patient who refused radio- and chemotherapy after surgical removal. One patient died 3 months after diagnosis due to heart failure.

No long-term data in adults have been reported due to the small series of patients.

There is no evidence about the most appropriate follow-up for adrenal GNB in adults.

TABLE 2: International Neuroblastoma Risk Group Consensus Pretreatment Classification Scheme.

INRG Stage	Age (months)	INPC group	Grade of differentiation	MYCN gene	11q aberration	Ploidy	Pretreatment risk group
L1/L2		GN maturing; GNB intermixed					Very low
L1 Localized tumor confined to one body compartment and with absence of image-defined risk factors		Any, except GN maturing or GNB intermixed		NA			Very low
				Amplified			High
	<18	Any, except GN maturing or GNB intermixed		NA	No		Low
					Yes		Intermediate
L2 Locoregional tumor with presence of one or more image-defined risk factor			Differentiating	NA	No		Low
					Yes		Intermediate
	≥18	GNB nodular; NB	Poorly differentiated or undifferentiated	NA			Intermediate
				Amplified			High
M Distant metastatic disease (except MS)	<18			NA		Hyperploid	Low
	<12			NA		Diploid	Intermediate
	12–18			NA		Diploid	Intermediate
	<18			Amplified			High
	≥18						High
MS Metastatic disease confined to skin, liver, and/or bone marrow in children <18 months				NA	no		Very low
					yes		High
				Amplified			High

INRG: International Neuroblastoma Risk Group; INCP: International Neuroblastoma Pathology Classification; GN = ganglioneuroma; GNB = ganglioneuroblastoma; NB = neuroblastoma; NA: not amplified; modified from Cohn et al. [11].

TABLE 3: Reported cases of adult-onset adrenal GNB in literature.

First Author (year)	Age (years)	Gender	Symptoms	Size (cm)	Side	Imaging	Hormonal activity	Metastases	Preliminary diagnosis	Histopathology	Treatment	Follow-up
Butz (1940)	25	M						Liver				
Cameron (1967)	58	F	Diarrhea		Right		↑ urinary catecholamines, vanilmandelic acid and homovanilmandelic acid	Absent	Pheochromocytoma	Pheochromocytoma	Surgery	3.5 years, no recurrence
Takahashi (1988)	21	M	Asymptomatic	8.8	Left		↑ urinary vanilmandelic acid	Lymph nodes	Neuroblastoma		Surgery + RT + CT	8 months, no recurrence
Koizumi (1992)	47	F	Fatigue, low back pain	9	Right	Heterogeneous	↑ urinary catecholamines, vanilmandelic acid and homovanilmandelic acid	Bone marrow	None		None	3 months, dead
Higuchi (1993)	29	M		11			↑ urinary catecholamines	Bone marrow			Surgery	10 months, no recurrence
Hiroshige (1995)	35	M	Asymptomatic	10	Left	Heterogeneous and calcifications	None	Absent	Carcinoma, neuroblastoma		Surgery	2 years, no recurrence
Mehta (1997)	22	M		9	Bilateral						Surgery	
Rousseau (1998)		F			Left			Liver			Surgery + RT + CT	
Fujiwara (2000)	25	M	Headache, palpitations, hypertension, weight loss	9	Left	Ovalar, heterogeneous, calcifications	None	Absent	Pheochromocytoma	GNB intermixed + pheochromocytoma	Surgery	5 years, no recurrence
Slapa (2002)	20	F	Asymptomatic	18			None	Absent			Surgery	1 year, no recurrence
Koike (2003)	50	M	Asymptomatic	4,5	Right	Ovalar, necrotic central area	None		Pheochromocytoma, adrenal malignancy, neuroblastic tumor		Surgery	2.5 years, no recurrence
Gunlusoy (2004)	59	M	Right flank and epigastric pain, malaise, anemia, weight loss, microscopic hematuria	12	Right	Lobulated, necrotic areas	None	Lymph nodes	None		Surgery	
Mizuno (2010)	53	M	Increased frequency of urination	11	Right	Smooth margins, homogeneous	None	Lumbar spine	None	GNB nodular	Surgery	Recurrence after 2.5 years

TABLE 3: Continued.

First Author (year)	Age (years)	Gender	Symptoms	Size (cm)	Side	Imaging	Hormonal activity	Metastases	Preliminary diagnosis	Histopathology	Treatment	Follow-up
Bolzacchini (2015)	63	M	Asymptomatic	5	Left	Irregular margins, heterogeneous	None	Absent	None	GNB nodular	Surgery	6 months, no recurrence
Qiu (2015)	27	F	Pain	11	Left	Ovalar, cystic-solid	None	Absent	Pheochromocytoma	GNB intermixed	Surgery	5 months, no recurrence
Present case (2015)	21	F	Asymptomatic	11	Left	Lobulated, heterogeneous, calcifications	None	Lymph nodes	Adrenal carcinoma, leiomyosarcoma	GNB intermixed	Surgery	21 months, no recurrence

Modified from Bolzacchini et al. [12, 13].

References

[1] G. Arnaldi and M. Boscaro, "Adrenal incidentaloma," *Best Practice & Research: Clinical Endocrinology & Metabolism*, vol. 26, no. 4, pp. 405–419, 2012.

[2] M. Fassnacht, W. Arlt, I. Bancos et al., "Management of adrenal incidentalomas: European society of endocrinology clinical practice guideline in collaboration with the european network for the study of adrenal tumors," *European Journal of Endocrinology*, vol. 175, no. 2, pp. G1–G34, 2016.

[3] H. Shimada, I. M. Ambros, L. P. Dehner et al., "The International Neuroblastoma Pathology Classification (the Shimada system)," *Cancer*, vol. 86, no. 2, pp. 364–372, 1999.

[4] A. A. Kasperlik-Zaluska, E. Roslonowska, J. Slowinska-Srzednicka et al., "1,111 Patients with adrenal incidentalomas observed at a single endocrinological center: incidence of chromaffin tumors," *Annals of the New York Academy of Sciences*, vol. 1073, pp. 38–46, 2006.

[5] R. Luksch, M. R. Castellani, P. Collini et al., "Neuroblastoma (Peripheral neuroblastic tumours)," *Critical Reviews in Oncology/Hematology*, vol. 107, pp. 163–181, 2016.

[6] A. Claviez, M. Lakomek, J. Ritter et al., "Low occurrence of familial neuroblastomas and ganglioneuromas in five consecutive GPOH neuroblastoma treatment studies," *European Journal of Cancer*, vol. 40, no. 18, pp. 2760–2765, 2004.

[7] D. E. Weese-Mayer, C. M. Rand, A. Zhou, M. S. Carroll, and C. E. Hunt, "Congenital central hypoventilation syndrome: a bedside-to-bench success story for advancing early diagnosis and treatment and improved survival and quality of life," *Pediatric Research*, vol. 81, no. 1-2, pp. 192–201, 2016.

[8] J. Blatt, A. F. Olshan, P. A. Lee, and J. L. Ross, "Neuroblastoma and related tumors in Turner's syndrome," *The Journal of Pediatrics*, vol. 131, no. 5, pp. 666–670, 1997.

[9] P. Origone, R. Defferrari, K. Mazzocco, C. Lo Cunsolo, B. De Bernardi, and G. P. Tonini, "Homozygous inactivation of NF1 gene in a patient with familial NF1 and disseminated neuroblastoma," *American Journal of Medical Genetics*, vol. 118, no. 4, pp. 309–313, 2003.

[10] E. H. LaBrosse, C. Com-Nougué, J. M. Zucker et al., "Urinary excretion of 3-methoxy-4-hydroxymandelic acid and 3-methoxy-4-hydroxyphenylacetic acid by 288 patients with neuroblastoma and related neural crest tumors," *Cancer Res*, vol. 40, no. 6, pp. 1995–2001, 1980.

[11] S. L. Cohn, A. D. J. Pearson, W. B. London et al., "The International Neuroblastoma Risk Group (INRG) classification system: an INRG task force report," *Journal of Clinical Oncology*, vol. 27, no. 2, pp. 289–297, 2009.

[12] E. Bolzacchini, B. Martinelli, and G. Pinotti, *Adult onset of ganglioneuroblastoma of the adrenal gland: case report and review of the literature. Surg Case Rep*, 1, 79, 2015.

[13] W. Qiu, T. Li, X. D. Sun, and G. Y. Lv, "Onset of adrenal ganglioneuroblastoma in an adult after delivery," *Annals of Surgical Treatment and Research*, vol. 89, no. 4, pp. 220–223, 2015.

[14] G. Cecchetto, V. Mosseri, B. De Bernardi et al., "Surgical risk factors in primary surgery for localized neuroblastoma: the LNESG1 study of the European international society of pediatric oncology neuroblastoma group," *Journal of Clinical Oncology*, vol. 23, no. 33, pp. 8483–8489, 2005.

[15] Y.-K. Guo, Z.-G. Yang, Y. Li et al., "Uncommon adrenal masses: CT and MRI features with histopathologic correlation," *European Journal of Radiology*, vol. 62, no. 3, pp. 359–370, 2007.

30

Spontaneous Regression of Metastatic Papillary Thyroid Cancer in a Lymph Node

Jien Shim,[1] **Jianyu Rao,**[2] **and Run Yu** (iD)[1]

[1]*Division of Endocrinology, Diabetes, and Metabolism, Department of Medicine, University of California, Los Angeles, David Geffen School of Medicine, Los Angeles, CA 90095, USA*
[2]*Department of Pathology and Laboratory Medicine, University of California, Los Angeles, David Geffen School of Medicine, Los Angeles, CA 90095, USA*

Correspondence should be addressed to Run Yu; runyu@mednet.ucla.edu

Academic Editor: Carlo Capella

Spontaneous regression of cancer is defined as disappearance of cancer in the absence of specific therapy. In thyroid cancer patients with biochemically incomplete response to initial treatments, spontaneous decline in thyroglobulin levels without any cancer treatment is a well-known phenomenon; however, spontaneous regression of persistent or recurrent structural disease has not been reported. We here present a case of papillary thyroid cancer in a 58-year-old female who underwent total thyroidectomy and two radioiodine ablations. She had persistently elevated thyroglobulin levels. Six years after her initial treatments, she had biopsy-proven cervical lymph node metastasis. The patient opted not to undergo any further treatment. Over the course of the next 10 years, without any additional treatment, the lymph node disappeared and her thyroglobulin levels decreased to almost undetectable ranges, implying near-complete regression. Our case illustrates that metastatic papillary thyroid cancer in lymph nodes can regress spontaneously.

1. Introduction

Spontaneous regression of cancer is an extremely rare event where a malignant tumor disappears in the absence of anti-cancer treatment [1–3]. It has been reported in various types of cancer, but complete regression has not been reported in structurally evident papillary thyroid cancer. Here, we report a case of metastatic papillary thyroid cancer in a lymph node that regressed spontaneously.

2. Case Presentation

A 58-year-old female with papillary thyroid cancer presented to the endocrinology clinic for follow-up. Patient had been first diagnosed with papillary thyroid cancer 6 years before at an outside clinic. She had undergone total thyroidectomy shortly after diagnosis, followed by radioiodine therapy with 150 mCi of I-131. She had postsurgical hypothyroidism, treated with levothyroxine 200 mcg orally daily, which suppressed her thyroid-stimulating hormone (TSH)

to 0.02 mcIU/mL (reference range: 0.3–4.7). Levothyroxine dose was periodically titrated to keep TSH suppressed while keeping the patient clinically euthyroid. One year after total thyroidectomy and radioiodine therapy, she had persistently elevated thyroglobulin (Tg) level of 11.4 ng/dL (3–40) with undetectable thyroglobulin antibodies (TgAb) (Figure 1). She underwent a whole body scan with 4 mCi of I-131, which did not show any residual tumors in the thyroid bed or metastatic disease. Ultrasound of the neck did not detect suspicious lesions. Fluorodeoxyglucose positron emission tomography (FDG-PET) showed abnormal foci in the left lower anterior neck, right lower neck, and right upper neck, suspicious for metastatic lymph nodes. Magnetic resonance imaging (MRI) and computed tomography (CT) of the neck at the same time did not identify any abnormalities. The lymph nodes were characterized as benign appearing, the largest one measuring 16.7 mm on the left at level IB. Two years after radioactive iodine ablation, PET/CT again identified abnormal foci in the left lower neck and right upper neck, consistent with malignant lymph nodes. Three years after the

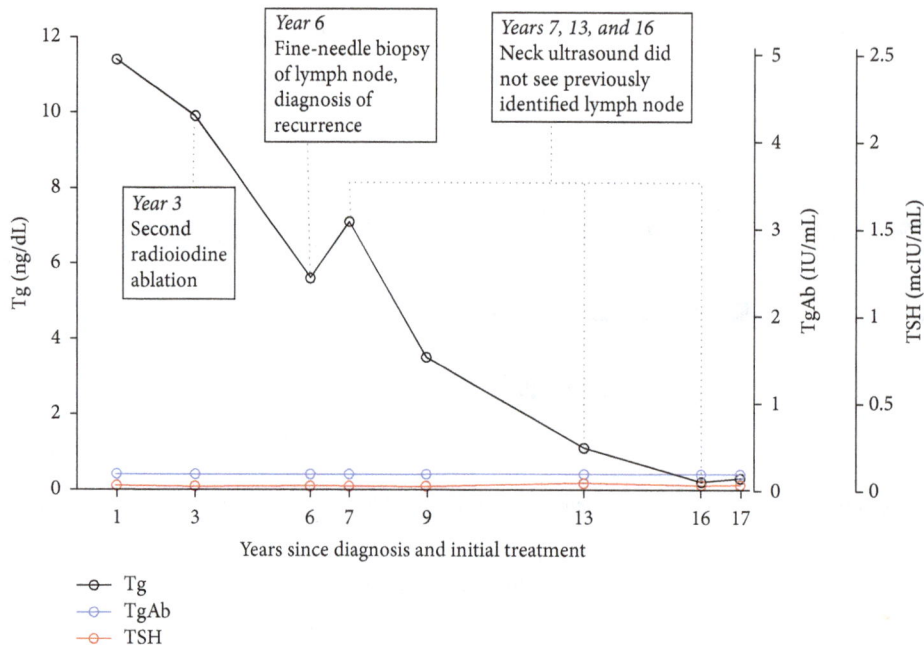

FIGURE 1: Time course of thyroglobulin (Tg), thyroglobulin antibody (TgAb), and TSH after initial treatment of papillary thyroid cancer.

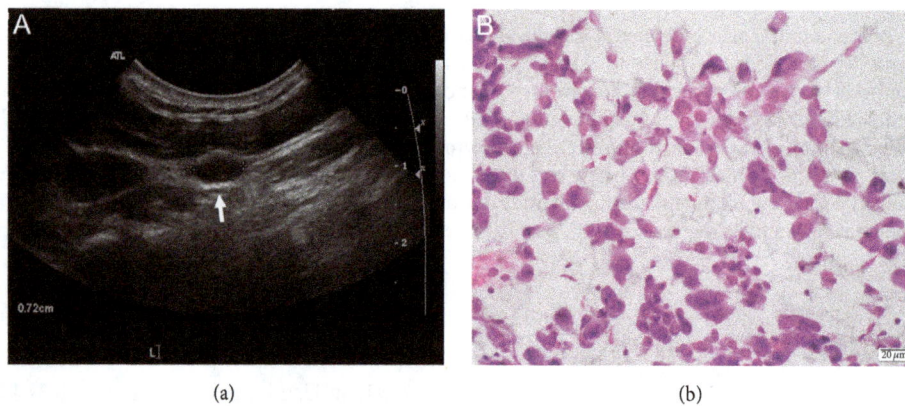

(a)

(b)

FIGURE 2: Metastatic papillary thyroid cancer in a lymph node. (a) Ultrasound image of the lymph node (arrow). (b) Cytological features of cells (Giemsa stain) obtained from the lymph node by fine-needle aspiration. Note the cytological features typical of papillary thyroid cancer cells. See text for detail.

first radioactive iodine ablation, patient's Tg was still elevated at 9.9 ng/dL with undetectable TgAb. Patient underwent second radioiodine ablation with 150 mCi of I-131. A whole body scan after I-131 radioiodine ablation did not show any abnormal activity.

At the endocrine clinic, 6 years after her total thyroidectomy and first radioactive iodine ablation and 3 years after the second radioactive iodine ablation, the patient felt well without dysphagia, dysphonia, or dyspnea. Her past medical history included type 2 diabetes. She had no family history of thyroid cancer. Her medications included aspirin 81 mg daily, sitagliptin-metformin 50–500 mg daily, and levothyroxine 137 mcg daily. Physical examination findings were unremarkable. Her serum Tg measured at 5.6 ng/mL with undetectable TgAb. TSH was <0.02 mcIU/mL and free T4

was 2.5 ng/dL (reference range 0.8–1.6 ng/dL). Neck ultrasound showed several lymph nodes on the left lateral neck and left submandibular region, measuring 0.5 cm to 0.8 cm (Figure 2). No abnormal masses were identified in the region of the thyroid bed. One of the enlarged lymph nodes measuring 0.8 cm in largest dimension was biopsied by fine-needle aspiration (FNA). Cytology showed moderately cellular, scattered clusters and sheets of moderately atypical epithelial cells with irregular nuclear contours, nuclear grooving, and numerous intranuclear pseudoinclusions, diagnostic of metastatic papillary thyroid carcinoma (Figure 2). Patient opted not to undergo surgery but rather to be monitored.

One year after the FNA, neck ultrasound no longer detects the previously identified abnormal appearing lymph nodes. Her Tg still measured 7.1 ng/mL with undetectable

TgAb and suppressed TSH. The patient had sporadic follow-up with our clinic, but subsequent Tg levels over the next 10 years gradually declined (Figure 1) with undetectable TgAb and suppressed TSH. Neck ultrasound at 6 and 9 years after metastatic lymph node diagnosis (and 12 and 15 years after initial treatments with total thyroidectomy and first radioiodine ablation) did not identify any abnormalities, including lymphadenopathy.

3. Discussion

This case illustrates unprecedented spontaneous regression of papillary thyroid cancer metastasis in a lymph node. Spontaneous cancer regression is a rare phenomenon that has been reported in various types of cancers, including neuroblastoma, choriocarcinoma, malignant melanoma, lymphoma, renal cell carcinoma, and breast and colon cancer [1–3]. The mechanism of spontaneous regression is poorly understood, but a few of the proposed mechanisms include immune mediation, growth factor and cytokine-mediated mechanism, and hormonal mediation [4].

This is the first report of biopsy-proven metastatic differentiated thyroid cancer in a lymph node that regressed without any treatment. Differentiated thyroid cancer prognosis depends on the stage and the initial response to therapy during follow-up [5]. This is reflected in American Thyroid Association Dynamic Risk Stratification where individual cases are categorized as excellent response, biochemically incomplete response, structurally incomplete response, or indeterminate response [5]. Spontaneous remission of thyroid cancer in patients with biochemically incomplete response (but without structural disease) to initial therapy is an established phenomenon [6, 7]. Elevated Tg levels may spontaneously decline over time in patients without structural disease. Structural disease is defined as having imaging evidence of recurrence. In one study, after total thyroidectomy for differentiated thyroid cancer, 33.7% of patients with biochemically incomplete response had no evidence of disease after 10 years of follow-up, only managed with levothyroxine therapy with adequate suppression of TSH [6]. Spontaneous *partial* remission of metastatic papillary thyroid cancer has also been reported. High dose of I-131 therapy achieved long-term remission in 20 children exposed to Chernobyl disaster [7]. Children diagnosed with differentiated thyroid cancer with pulmonary metastasis underwent treatment with multiple I-131 ablation (total average dose 24.2 GBq, which is more than 600 mCi) in the initial 5 years after diagnosis; median Tg level was 5.6 ng/dL after the last I-131 treatment, but, 12 years later, more than 10 patients had Tg levels <1 ng/dL without any additional treatment. With regard to lung metastases, all patients showed stable partial remission. This illustrates that metastatic disease of differentiated thyroid cancer may not progress and even regress over years without additional therapy. Spontaneous regression of structurally incomplete response to initial papillary thyroid cancer treatment is exceedingly rare. In the only study that we can find addressing the question, a single patient of the 153 (0.7%) with structurally incomplete response had no evidence of disease at final follow-up without any additional therapy, but

no details of the patient were given [6]. Our patient had biopsy-proven papillary thyroid cancer grossly involving a lymph node that regressed within a year without any cancer treatment other than suppressive doses of levothyroxine. She had both biochemically and structurally incomplete response to initial total thyroidectomy and radioiodine ablation as shown by elevated nonstimulated Tg levels for many years and suspicious lymph node on ultrasound that was confirmed by cytology. To our knowledge, our patient represents the first described case in the literature on spontaneous, nearly complete regression of metastatic papillary thyroid cancer in lymph node or in any other organs. In particular, her structural disease had completely regressed on imaging at follow-up, unlike the children who had stable partial remission of lung metastases [7]. Surgical resection is typically the mainstay of treatment for recurrent structural thyroid cancer. In retrospect, aggressive management of our patient's isolated lymph node with surgery could have posed greater risks (e.g., perioperative risks and surgical complications) than observation alone. As seen in our case, active surveillance is a reasonable approach to small volume disease recurrence. Further studies are necessary to determine if observation alone has greater benefit in survival and quality of life than active treatment to eradicate the metastatic lesions, especially for stable, small volume recurrences.

Our case is one of a kind in the thyroid cancer literature, illustrating both a more rapid structural regression after lymph node biopsy and a slower biochemical regression of metastatic papillary cancer. Spontaneous regression of cancer after lymph node biopsy has been reported in other types of cancers. A metastatic non-small-cell lung cancer with primary tumor measuring 6 cm and mediastinal lymph node metastases regressed after paratracheal lymph node biopsy [8]. One theory to explain this phenomenon is that lymph node biopsy causes architectural destruction causing antigen release and triggering an immunological response [9]. The time course of cancer regression is usually within months of lymph node biopsy, similar to the course of spontaneous regression in our patient which happened within a year after fine-needle biopsy, making immunological mechanism in our case plausible. The spontaneous regression of papillary thyroid cancer in a lymph node in our case is different from partial primary tumor regression in papillary thyroid cancer [9]. First, the spontaneous regression in our case is virtually complete. Second, histologically, the lymph nodes in our case did not exhibit extensive fibrosis or lymphocytic infiltrate as shown in two cases of papillary thyroid microcarcinoma that regressed to less than 1.5 mm with metastasis to lymph nodes [10]. The slower biochemical regression of metastatic papillary cancer in our patient can be seen in 1/3 of patients with biochemical incomplete response to initial therapy, the mechanism for which remains unclear [6].

Spontaneous regression of metastatic papillary thyroid cancer in lymph nodes may not be very rare as currently believed. Patients with small recurrences may not have masses large enough to be detected on routine surveillance imaging, thus classifying them as biochemically incomplete rather than structurally incomplete. Perhaps spontaneous regression of differentiated thyroid cancer with structural metastases may be more common than we currently think. Our case further suggests that active surveillance is a reasonable approach to the management of small volume of recurrent metastatic papillary thyroid cancer.

References

[1] T. C. Everson, "Spontaneous regression of cancer," *Annals of the New York Academy of Sciences*, vol. 114, no. 2, pp. 721–735, 1964.

[2] J. Sasaki, H. Kurihara, Y. Nakano, K. Kotani, E. Tame, and A. Sasaki, "Apparent spontaneous regression of malignant neoplasms after radiography: Report of four cases," *International Journal of Surgery Case Reports*, vol. 25, pp. 40–43, 2016.

[3] K. Chida, K. Nakanishi, H. Shomura et al., "Spontaneous regression of transverse colon cancer: a case report," *Surgical Case Reports*, vol. 3, no. 1, 2017.

[4] R. J. Papac, "Spontaneous regression of cancer: possible mechanisms," *In Vivo*, vol. 12, no. 6, pp. 571–578, 1998.

[5] R. M. Tuttle, H. Tala, J. Shah et al., "Estimating risk of recurrence in differentiated thyroid cancer after total thyroidectomy and radioactive iodine remnant ablation: using response to therapy variables to modify the initial risk estimates predicted by the new American thyroid association staging system," *Thyroid*, vol. 20, no. 12, pp. 1341–1349, 2010.

[6] F. Vaisman, D. Momesso, D. A. Bulzico et al., "Spontaneous remission in thyroid cancer patients after biochemical incomplete response to initial therapy," *Clinical Endocrinology*, vol. 77, no. 1, pp. 132–138, 2012.

[7] J. Biko, C. Reiners, M. C. Kreissl, F. A. Verburg, Y. Demidchik, and V. Drozd, "Favourable course of disease after incomplete remission on 131I therapy in children with pulmonary metastases of papillary thyroid carcinoma: 10 years follow-up," *European Journal of Nuclear Medicine and Molecular Imaging*, vol. 38, no. 4, pp. 651–655, 2011.

[8] A. Lopez-Pastorini, T. Plönes, M. Brockmann, C. Ludwig, F. Beckers, and E. Stoelben, "Spontaneous regression of non-small cell lung cancer after biopsy of a mediastinal lymph node metastasis: A case report," *Journal of Medical Case Reports*, vol. 9, no. 1, article no. 217, 2015.

[9] G. B. Challis and H. J. Stam, "The spontaneous regression of cancer. A review of cases from 1900 to 1987," *Acta Oncologica*, vol. 29, no. 5, pp. 545–550, 1990.

[10] K. W. Simpson and J. Albores-Saavedra, "Unusual findings in papillary thyroid microcarcinoma suggesting partial regression: a study of two cases," *Annals of Diagnostic Pathology*, vol. 11, no. 2, pp. 97–102, 2007.

31

Hashimoto's Thyroiditis and Graves' Disease in One Patient: The Extremes of Thyroid Dysfunction Associated with Interferon Treatment

R. H. Bishay[1,2] and R. C. Y. Chen[1,2]

[1]*Department of Endocrinology and Metabolism, Concord Repatriation General Hospital, Concord, NSW 2139, Australia*
[2]*Concord Clinical School, Sydney Medical School, University of Sydney, Sydney, NSW 2005, Australia*

Correspondence should be addressed to R. H. Bishay; ramy.bishay@sswahs.nsw.gov.au

Academic Editor: Osamu Isozaki

Autoimmune thyroid disease associated with interferon therapy can manifest as destructive thyroiditis, Graves' Hyperthyroidism, and autoimmune (often subclinical) hypothyroidism, the latter persisting in many patients. There are scare reports of a single patient developing extremes of autoimmune thyroid disease activated by the immunomodulatory effects of interferon. A 60-year-old man received 48 weeks of pegylated interferon and ribavirin therapy for chronic HCV. Six months into treatment, he reported fatigue, weight gain, and slowed cognition. Serum thyroid stimulating hormone (TSH) was 58.8 mIU/L [0.27–4.2], fT4 11.1 pmol/L [12–25], and fT3 4.2 pmol/L [2.5–6.0] with elevated anti-TPO (983 IU/mL [<35]) and anti-TG (733 U/mL [<80]) antibodies. He commenced thyroxine with initial clinical and biochemical resolution but developed symptoms of hyperthyroidism with weight loss and tremor 14 months later. Serum TSH was <0.02 mIU/L, fT4 54.3 pmol/L, and fT3 20.2 pmol/L, with an elevated TSH receptor (TRAb, 4.0 U/L [<1.0]), anti-TPO (1,163 IU/mL) and anti-TG (114 U/mL) antibodies. Technetium scan confirmed Graves' Disease with bilateral diffuse increased tracer uptake (5.9% [0.5–3.5%]). The patient commenced carbimazole therapy for 6 months. Treatment was ceased following spontaneous clinical and biochemical remission (TSH 3.84 mIU/L, fT4 17pmol/L, fT3 4.5 pmol/L, and TRAb <1 U/L). This raises the need to monitor thyroid function closely in patients both during and following completion of interferon treatment.

1. Background

Approximately 3% of the world population, or 180 million people, are infected with hepatitis C virus (HCV) and 38–76% will have at least one extrahepatic manifestation [1]. In a large cohort of US adults with HCV, a small but appreciable proportion will develop clinically significant autoimmune thyroid disease (AITD) (adjusted HR 1.13), making AITD the commonest endocrinopathy in HCV patients [2].

Exogenous exposure to interferon- (IFN-) based therapies has long been known to have a predilection for causing AITD. The IFNs are a family of cytokine proteins produced by white blood cells, fibroblasts, and cells of the adaptive immune system. Congruent with their name, they interfere with viral replication among other functions. There are three main groups of IFN, namely, alpha (α), beta (β), and gamma (γ). Interferon-α is commonly used for its clinical ability to alter the immune response in a variety of conditions such as HCV and multiple sclerosis. Prior to the advent of directly acting antiviral drugs (DAAs), combination of pegylated IFN-α and ribavirin therapy remained the gold standard for treatment of patients with chronic HCV infection; however in many parts of the world (including Australia) IFN-α based therapies are still being used [3]. Numerous reports of AITD have been reported in HCV patients in the setting of current or following IFN-based treatment [4–6]. Data from three studies on 421 patients who were antibody negative prior to IFN-α therapy showed anti-TPO positivity in 9.5%, and over half (58%) of those patients developed overt AITD. Overall, pooling the incident rates from six studies, AITD seems to affect 2.7 to 10%, or an average of 6%, of IFN-α treated patients [6].

Hypothyroidism is the dominant form of thyroid dysfunction but studies vary on its incidence, from 66 to 97% of cases [6]. Furthermore, over 87% of hypothyroid patients are also positive for anti-TPO antibodies, reflecting its basis as an autoimmune process. Importantly, autoimmune hypothyroidism may persist in 56 to 59% of patients. Incidence of hyperthyroidism varies among studies as well, with approximately 25% to 60% suffering from transient thyrotoxicosis and the remainder having scintigraphic and/or biochemical evidence of Graves' Hyperthyroidism, many of which required treatment [6]. In contrast, a large study of 869 HCV patients receiving IFN-α reported biphasic thyroiditis responsible for the majority of AITD cases (58%) [7].

With some exceptions, there are very few case reports reporting extremes of AITD in a single patient in association with IFN-α treatment [8, 9]. The "swinging thyroid" concept was illustrated in two recent cases, where the characteristic biphasic pattern of thyroiditis, initial TRAb-negative thyrotoxicosis with subsequent development of clinical and biochemical hypothyroidism, was then followed by biochemical and scintigraphic evidence of Graves' Hyperthyroidism [8]. To date, there are scarce reports documenting the development of initial clinical and biochemical hypothyroidism associated with high titres of anti-TPO with subsequent development of Graves' Disease in a single patient, illustrating a novel clinical pattern of AITD. This case also highlights the importance of understanding the pathophysiological mechanism underpinning the unpredictable course of autoimmune disease associated with IFN-α, as discussed below.

2. Case Presentation

A 60-year-old man originally from China with no prior history of thyroid or autoimmune disease received a standard course of 48-week pegylated IFN-α and ribavirin therapy for chronic HCV (genotype 1b) with achievement of sustained virological response. He had compensated chronic liver disease with cirrhosis (Child-Pugh A) without other complications and no other reported medical problems. He denied previous use of amiodarone, lithium, medications, or supplements containing iodine or exposure to contrast. He was a nonsmoker and did not drink alcohol. Six months after commencing treatment, he reported fatigue, weight gain of 3 kg, and slowed cognition at a routine clinical visit. He denied changes to his skin, hair, or bowel habits. On examination, his vital signs were normal. His weight was 78 kg with a body mass index (BMI) of 26.8 kg/m^2. There was no goitre and there were no signs of oedema, dermopathy, ophthalmopathy, or lymphadenopathy. Cardiac, respiratory, and gastrointestinal examinations were normal and in particular no stigmata of chronic liver disease was present. A peripheral neurological examination including reflexes was normal.

Serum biochemistry including electrolytes, renal function, and full blood count were within normal limits, with no biochemical or serological evidence of decompensated liver disease. Alpha-fetoprotein (AFP) was normal at 3.5 kIU/L [normal, 0.0–6.0]. Pretreatment HCV quantitative RNA was >3,000,000 IU/mL and was undetectable 6 months after

commencing treatment. A recent abdominal ultrasound revealed a radiologically normal liver with no signs of portal hypertension or hepatic lesions. His serum thyroid stimulating hormone (TSH) prior to therapy was 1.65 mIU/L [normal, 0.27–4.2] with a normal free T4 (fT4) of 14.5 pmol/L [normal, 12–25]. The TSH at the time of review (i.e., 6 months later) was 58.8 mIU/L, free T4 was 11.1 pmol/L, and free T3 was 4.2 pmol/L [normal, 2.5–6.0] (Figure 1(a)). Anti-TPO (983 IU/mL, normal <35) and anti-TG (733 U/mL, normal <80) antibodies were elevated (Figure 1(b)).

Given his symptoms and biochemical evidence of autoimmune hypothyroidism, the patient was commenced on standard adult thyroxine replacement therapy at 100 mcg daily. His symptoms improved and there was full clinical and biochemical resolution of his hypothyroid state. Fourteen months later, he returned for follow-up reporting symptoms of hyperthyroidism with weight loss, tremor, and palpitations. He had lost 5 kg of weight. At the time of review, serum TSH was suppressed at <0.02 mIU/L with elevated fT4 of 54.3 pmol/L, fT3 of 20.2 pmol/L, and an elevated TRAb of 4.0 U/L (normal <1.0), with anti-TPO (1,163 IU/mL) and anti-TG (114 U/mL) antibodies. Technetium scan revealed bilateral diffuse increased tracer uptake (5.9%, normal 0.5–3.5%), consistent with Graves' Disease (Figure 2).

The patient's thyroxine was ceased and he was placed on antithyroid treatment with carbimazole 5 mg TDS. He self-ceased therapy 6 months later, with serendipitous clinical and biochemical remission. His serum TSH was 3.84 mIU/L, fT4 17 pmol/L, and fT3 4.5 pmol/L, but with persistently elevated anti-TPO at 383 IU/mL. Anti-TG 23 U/mL and TRAb < 1 U/L were normal. At the time of writing, the patient remained clinically and biochemically euthyroid.

3. Discussion

Development of hypothyroidism with subsequent Graves' Disease represents a rare and novel clinical pattern of AITD following IFN-α therapy. Although IFN-α associated AITD has been described for more than 30 years, the immunological mechanisms have only been recently elucidated [8, 10]. This is clinically relevant in many parts of the world, including Australia, where IFN-α based therapies are still being used to treat chronic HCV infection. For example, although DAAs are becoming standard of care globally, treatment for HCV genotype 1 (54% of diagnosed cases in the Australian population) involves weekly pegylated IFN injections, with twice-a-day ribavirin tablets and a once-a-day tablet of simeprevir (Olysio). For genotype 3 (37% of the population), the mainstay of therapy is a combination of weekly pegylated IFN injections and daily ribavirin tablets over a period of 26 weeks [3]. Thus, IFN-α is still being used countrywide and in many parts of the world, making the adverse effects of IFN-α therapy relevant to hepatologists, endocrinologists, and primary care physicians.

Patients with chronic HCV without prior treatment with IFN-α already have modulation of the immune system. In particular, the cytotoxic response of CD4 T-cells is primed by high levels of circulating interferon-γ (IFN-γ) and interleukin-2 (IL-2). When exogenous IFN-α is administered,

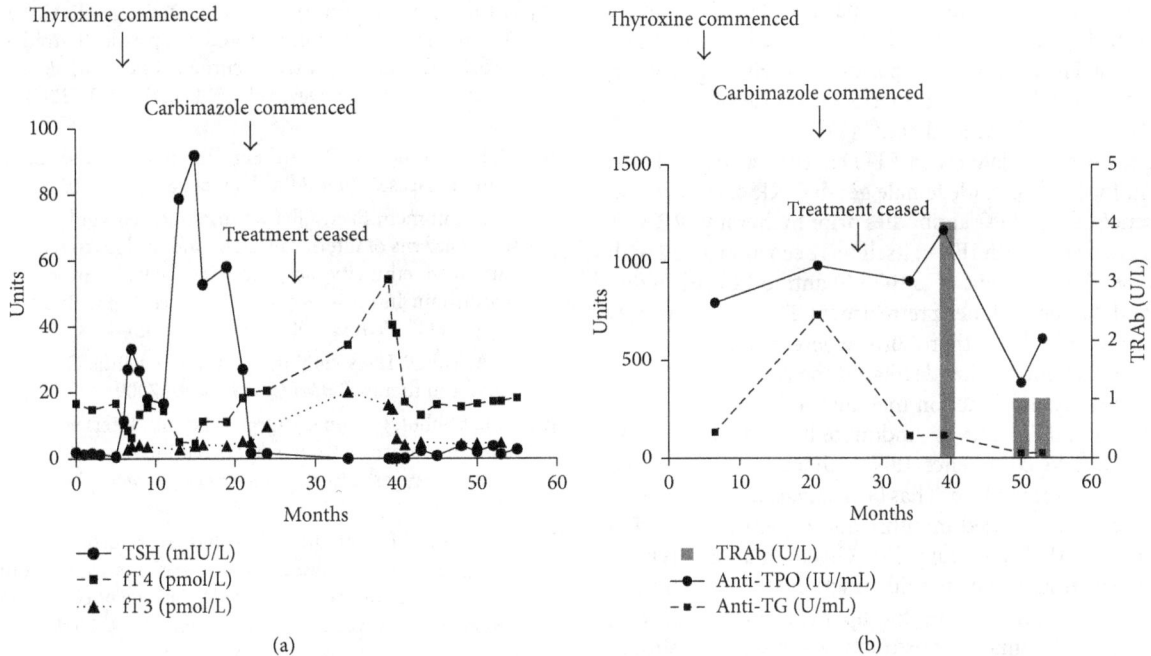

FIGURE 1: (a) Temporal pattern of thyroid function tests showing both hypothyroidism and subsequent T3-toxicosis, consistent with Graves' Disease. (b) Thyroid antibodies showing persistently elevated anti-TPO and later development of thyrotoxicosis with positive TRAb titres. TSH, *thyroid stimulating hormone*; fT4, *free thyroxine*; fT3, *free triiodothyronine*; anti-TPO, *anti-thyroperoxidase antibody*; anti-TG, *anti-thyroglobulin antibody*; TRAb, *TSH receptor antibody.*

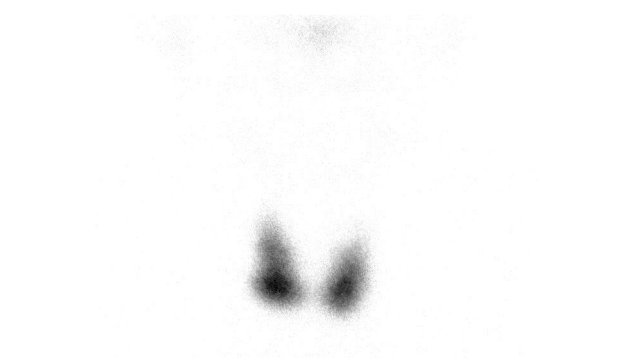

FIGURE 2: Technetium scan revealing bilateral diffuse increased tracer uptake at 5.9% [normal 0.5–3.5%], consistent with Graves' Disease.

the cytotoxic activation of CD4 T-cells is amplified further, primarily via a Th1 mediated pathway, and interacts with abnormally expressed major histocompatibility complex class I antigen surface expression on thyrocytes. The end result is apoptosis and destruction of thyrocytes and thyroid follicles [8]. Exogenous IFN-α may also influence switching to a Th2 pathway, which can result in the development of autoantibodies (e.g., anti-TPO, anti-TG) resulting in thyrotoxicosis, due to thyroid follicular rupture and release of stored thyroid hormones into the circulation. Thyroiditis is confirmed by low pertechnetate uptake scan and positive thyroid autoantibody titres. Thionamides are contraindicated in this scenario given the likelihood of exacerbating thyroid dysfunction,

and corticosteroids are ineffective. Following depletion of thyroid hormone reserve, hypothyroidism may ensue and subsequently recover, though many patients will remain hypothyroid [6]. Interestingly, our index patient developed autoimmune hyperthyroidism consistent with Graves' Disease, with positive TRAb-antibody titres, T3-toxicosis, and confirmatory scintigraphy, following initial hypothyroidism. The fact that Graves' Disease, which is thought to be due to a Th2 mediated production of stimulating TRAb, is much less common in IFN-α treated patients suggests that IFN-α preferentially activates Th1 immunity which in turn leads to the higher rate of destructive thyroiditis seen in these patients. This is consistent with previous reports that IFN-α may have suppressive effects on Th2 immunity [11] and supports the results from several studies which illustrate that the predominant form of AITD in IFN-α treated patients is indeed autoimmune hypothyroidism [6].

As to why Graves' Disease develops later, even after cessation of IFN-α, is unknown. It has been proposed that there is further modulation of the immune system in a genetically susceptible individual via a Th2 mechanism, resulting in the production of TSH stimulating immunoglobulin (TSI) [8]. In contrast to hypothyroidism or biphasic thyroiditis, the Graves' Disease may develop much later after treatment, as in the index patient, who became thyrotoxic 9 months after completing IFN-α treatment. Overall, IFN-α induced AITD can occur from as early as 4 weeks to as late as 23 months, with a median onset of 17 weeks after commencing IFN-α [12]. However, one study failed to reveal a difference with respect to the type of AITD that developed and onset of disease.

Furthermore, a small study of 94 patients failed to find a relationship between AITD in IFN-α treated patients and pretreatment HCV virological parameters, HCV genotype, total dose of pegylated IFN-α or ribavirin, use of nonpegylated IFN-α, or virological outcome [10].

Risk factors associated with AITD in the setting of IFN-α treatment for HCV include female gender (RR 4.4) as well as the presence of anti-TPO antibodies prior to therapy (RR 3.9); however treatment with IFN-α itself has been associated with the *de novo* development of anti-TPO antibodies [6]. Being female and having a higher pretreatment TSH were strongly associated with biphasic thyroiditis, whereas Asian ethnicity and being a current smoker decreased the risk [7]. Arguably, pretreatment thyroid function may be used to predict those who develop AITD but is undoubtedly indicated in all patients about to commence IFN-α therapy. Although no clear guidelines are in place, it has been suggested that thyroid function tests be assessed monthly and 6 months following completion of IFN-α therapy [8]. Given this case report, it may be suggested that thyroid function tests be assessed for a longer period of time, for up to 2 years, following IFN-α therapy. Ultimately, posttherapy surveillance should be individualised based on patient symptoms, personal or family history of thyroid disease, and presence of anti-thyroid antibodies.

Authors' Contribution

R. H. Bishay was involved in the care of the patient, prepared the paper, and collected the patient data and consent. R. C. Y. Chen was involved in the care of the patient in a supervisory role and assisted with the editing of the paper.

References

[1] A. Galossi, R. Guarisco, L. Bellis, and C. Puoti, "Extrahepatic manifestations of chronic HCV infection," *Journal of Gastrointestinal and Liver Diseases*, vol. 16, no. 1, pp. 65–73, 2007.

[2] T. P. Giordano, L. Henderson, O. Landgren et al., "Risk of non-Hodgkin lymphoma and lymphoproliferative precursor diseases in US veterans with hepatitis C virus," *The Journal of the American Medical Association*, vol. 297, no. 18, pp. 2010–2017, 2007.

[3] Hepatitis Australia, *Need-To-Know News on Hepatitis C Treatment—May 2015*, Hepatitis Australia, Sydney, Australia, 2015, http://www.hepatitisaustralia.com.

[4] A. Antonelli, C. Ferri, and P. Fallahi, "Hepatitis C: thyroid dysfunction in patients with hepatitis C on IFN-α therapy," *Nature Reviews Gastroenterology and Hepatology*, vol. 6, no. 11, pp. 633–635, 2009.

[5] P. Fallahi, S. M. Ferrari, U. Politti, D. Giuggioli, C. Ferri, and A. Antonelli, "Autoimmune and neoplastic thyroid diseases associated with hepatitis C chronic infection," *International Journal of Endocrinology*, vol. 2014, Article ID 935131, 9 pages, 2014.

[6] M. F. Prummel and P. Laurberg, "Interferon-α and autoimmune thyroid disease," *Thyroid*, vol. 13, no. 6, pp. 547–551, 2003.

[7] J. S. Mammen, S. R. Ghazarian, A. Rosen, and P. W. Ladenson, "Patterns of interferon-alpha-induced thyroid dysfunction vary with ethnicity, sex, smoking status, and pretreatment thyrotropin in an international cohort of patients treated for hepatitis C," *Thyroid*, vol. 23, no. 9, pp. 1151–1158, 2013.

[8] H. A. Tran, "The swinging thyroid in hepatitis C infection and interferon therapy," *BMJ Case Reports*, 2009.

[9] N. L. Bohbot, J. Young, J. Orgiazzi et al., "Interferon-α-induced hyperthyroidism: a three-stage evolution from silent thyroiditis towards Graves' disease," *European Journal of Endocrinology*, vol. 154, no. 3, pp. 367–372, 2006.

[10] E. Vezali, I. Elefsiniotis, C. Mihas, E. Konstantinou, and G. Saroglou, "Thyroid dysfunction in patients with chronic hepatitis C: virus- or therapy-related?" *Journal of Gastroenterology and Hepatology*, vol. 24, no. 6, pp. 1024–1029, 2009.

[11] C. Carella, G. Mazziotti, G. Amato, L. E. Braverman, and E. Roti, "Interferon-α-related thyroid disease: pathophysiological, epidemiological, and clinical aspects," *The Journal of Clinical Endocrinology & Metabolism*, vol. 89, no. 8, pp. 3656–3661, 2004.

[12] T. Okanoue, S. Sakamoto, Y. Itoh et al., "Side effects of high-dose interferon therapy for chronic hepatitis C," *Journal of Hepatology*, vol. 25, no. 3, pp. 283–291, 1996.

32

Recurrent Thyrotoxicosis due to Both Graves' Disease and Hashimoto's Thyroiditis in the Same Three Patients

Ashley Schaffer, Vidya Puthenpura, and Ian Marshall

Department of Pediatrics, Rutgers-Robert Wood Johnson Medical School, 89 French Street, New Brunswick, NJ 08901, USA

Correspondence should be addressed to Ian Marshall; marshaia@rwjms.rutgers.edu

Academic Editor: Mihail A. Boyanov

Hashimoto's thyroiditis (HT) and Graves' disease (GD) are the 2 most common autoimmune disease processes affecting the thyroid gland. The relationship between the two is complex and not clearly understood. It has been theorized that HT and GD are 2 separate disease processes due to unique genetic differences demonstrated by genome studies. On the other hand, based on occurrence of both HT and GD in monozygotic twins and within the same family, they have been regarded to represent 2 ends of the same spectrum. This case report describes 3 patients who presented with thyrotoxicosis due to both GD and HT. The initial presentation was thyrotoxicosis due to GD treated with antithyroid medication followed by temporary resolution. They all subsequently experienced recurrence of thyrotoxicosis in the form of Hashitoxicosis due to HT, and then eventually all developed thyrotoxicosis due to GD, requiring radioablation therapy.

1. Introduction

Hashimoto's thyroiditis (HT) and Graves' disease (GD) are 2 autoimmune thyroid diseases that account for the majority of acquired thyroid dysfunction in the pediatric population [1, 2]. It has been suggested that they are 2 entirely separate disease processes due to unique genetic differences demonstrated by genome studies [3]. On the other hand, based on occurrence of both HT and GD in monozygotic twins [4, 5] and in the same family [6, 7], they have been regarded to represent 2 ends of the same spectrum. A common mechanism proposed for their development is loss of tolerance to multiple thyroid antigens, including TSH receptor (TSHR), thyroglobulin, and thyroid peroxidase [8]. This leads to T lymphocyte infiltration of the thyroid gland [9] that can then follow 2 separate pathways, depending on the balance between T-helper 1 (Th1) and T-helper 2 (Th2) cells. Th1-cell-mediated autoimmunity leads to thyroid cell apoptosis and hypothyroidism in HT while a hyperreactive Th2-mediated humoral response against TSHR with stimulatory antibodies results in GD thyrotoxicosis [10, 11].

Although the exact incidence of HT in the pediatric population is unknown, it is much more frequent than GD [12]. As the presentation is usually asymptomatic, the diagnosis is commonly made incidentally by routine biochemical testing [13]. Clinically, HT can present with a firm, nontender goiter and occasionally with clinical evidence of hypothyroidism [13]. Rarely, HT can present with Hashitoxicosis, which is a transient form of thyrotoxicosis that results from release of preformed thyroid hormone due to inflammatory destruction of thyroid cells [14]. As inflammation resolves and because thyroid hormone release is not due to ongoing stimulation of TSHR, resolution typically occurs within a few months. It is usually asymptomatic, with typically only mild clinical symptoms of thyrotoxicosis if present [15].

Although GD is much less frequent than HT, with an incidence of about 1 : 10,000, it is the most common cause of thyrotoxicosis in the pediatric population [16]. Clinically, GD can present with a firm, nontender goiter, ophthalmopathy, a peripheral tremor, tongue fasciculations, tachycardia, and/or hypertension [1].

Diagnosis of HT is confirmed by presence of anti-thyroid peroxidase antibodies (anti-TPO Ab) and anti-thyroglobulin antibodies (anti-TG Ab) [17]. Diagnostic testing for GD relies on identification of TSHR autoantibodies that are measured by 2 different assays. The first is a radioreceptor assay that measures the ability of TSHR autoantibodies to compete with radiolabeled thyroid stimulating hormone (TSH) to bind to TSHR. These are commonly referred to as TSH binding inhibitor immunoglobulins (TBII) [18]. The second diagnostic test is a bioassay that measures the ability of TSHR autoantibodies to stimulate TSHR activity via cyclic adenosine monophosphate (cAMP) production [18]. These antibodies, which are known as thyroid stimulating immunoglobulins (TSIG), are the direct cause of thyrotoxicosis in GD.

Interestingly, anti-TPO Ab and anti-TG Ab can be detected in up to 70% of patients with GD, in addition to TBII and TSIG antibodies at the time of diagnosis [19]. However, the converse is not true in HT, where only TPO and/or TG antibodies are typically elevated [19].

We report 3 patients who presented with biochemical and clinical thyrotoxicosis due to GD and then after presumed spontaneous resolution of initial thyrotoxicosis experienced recurrence of biochemical thyrotoxicosis due to Hashitoxicosis, followed by a third period of biochemical and clinical thyrotoxicosis due to GD.

2. Case Presentation

Case 1. A 15-year-old female was diagnosed with thyrotoxicosis based on elevated free T4 (FT4) of 2.4 ng/dL (0.9–1.4) and suppressed TSH of 0.02 mIU/L (0.5–4.3) identified in work-up for irregular menses. Additional testing demonstrated elevated anti-TPO Ab at 180 IU/mL (0–35) and anti-TG Ab at 136 IU/mL (0–20); TBII were elevated at 22% (≤16), with TSIG within the normal range at 119% (≤125). Physical examination revealed a firm, nontender goiter only. I[123] thyroid uptake and scan revealed increased 4-hour uptake at 34% (5–15%) and 24-hour uptake at 62% (15–35%).

Thyrotoxicosis due to GD was diagnosed but not treated due to absence of significant symptoms. After 6 months, worsening biochemical thyrotoxicosis associated with palpitations, insomnia, loss of weight, tongue fasciculations, peripheral tremor, tachycardia, and hypertension developed. Testing showed peak FT4 of 10.4 ng/dL and suppressed TSH of 0.01 mIU/L. TBII antibodies had increased to 49% with TSIG positive at 158%. Methimazole (MMI) therapy was started, with biochemical and clinical resolution of thyrotoxicosis within 2 months. After 18 months on therapy, with GD antibodies negative, MMI was discontinued to assess spontaneous resolution. She remained biochemically and clinically euthyroid for 4 months off MMI. Biochemical thyrotoxicosis without clinical symptoms developed after 4 months (peak FT4 of 2.4 ng/dL and TSH of 0.01 mIU/mL) with repeat anti-TPO and TG antibody levels at >1000 IU/mL and 147 IU/mL, respectively, and TBII and TSIG remaining negative. Repeat I[123] thyroid uptake and scan revealed low 4-hour uptake of 2.5% and low 24-hour I[123] uptake of 2.3%. This presentation was consistent with Hashitoxicosis, and because of mild nature and anticipation of its transient course antithyroid therapy was not initiated.

After 6 weeks, primary hypothyroidism actually developed (FT4 of 0.6 ng/dL and TSH of 25.66 mIU/mL) for which thyroxine replacement therapy was started. However, within 3 months, clinical and biochemical thyrotoxicosis was diagnosed which, despite discontinuation of therapy, deteriorated (peak FT4 of 3.9 ng/dL and TSH of 0.01 mIU/mL). Repeat I[123] thyroid uptake and scan revealed elevated 4-hour and 24-hour uptake at 34% and 62%, respectively. [131]I radioiodine ablation (RAI) was successfully performed with development of primary hypothyroidism within 2 months when thyroxine replacement therapy was restarted.

Case 2. A 14-year-old male presented with a 2-month history of palpations, jitteriness, insomnia, heat intolerance, and 10 lb weight loss. Initial examination revealed a nontender, firm goiter, tongue fasciculations, peripheral tremor, increased deep tendon reflexes, tachycardia, and hypertension. He was diagnosed with thyrotoxicosis due to GD based on wFT4 of 5.6 ng/dL and TSH of <0.01 mIU/mL and positive TBII at 34% (≤16) and TSIG at 130% (≤125); anti-TPO Ab and anti-TG Ab were positive at 107 IU/mL (<35) and 90 IU/mL (<20), respectively. He was treated with MMI therapy, which was then discontinued after 24 months, after which he remained clinically and biochemically euthyroid for a 12-month period.

Although asymptomatic, follow-up testing revealed biochemical thyrotoxicosis (peak FT4 of 3.9 ng/dL and TSH of 0.01 mIU/mL), with anti-TPO and anti-TG Ab levels at 308 IU/mL and 147 IU/mL, respectively, and negative TBII and TSIG antibody levels. I[123] thyroid uptake and scan demonstrated low 4-hour uptake of 3% and 24-hour uptake of 5%. Hashitoxicosis was then diagnosed but did not require treatment. However, subsequent clinical and biochemical monitoring revealed increasing FT4 levels with associated development of clinical thyrotoxicosis. Repeat I[123] thyroid uptake and scan demonstrated elevated 4-hour and 24-hour uptakes at 70% and 82%, respectively. He underwent RAI with development of hypothyroidism within 1 month for which he has been on thyroxine replacement therapy.

Case 3. The fraternal twin sister of Case 1 presented at 17 years of age to our emergency room with jitteriness, anxiety, tongue fasciculations, peripheral tremor, and hypertension and tachycardia. Testing showed extremely elevated FT4 at >7.77 ng/dL (0.9–1.8) with TSH suppressed at 0.01 mIU/mL (0.35–5.5); TSIG was positive at 432% (<140) and TBII at 83.2% (≤16), with positive anti-TPO Ab at 606 IU/mL (<35); anti-TG Ab was negative. She was diagnosed with thyrotoxicosis due to GD for which she was started on MMI therapy. After therapy for 18 months and with negative TSIG and TBII antibodies, a trial off MMI was initiated. She remained clinically and biochemically euthyroid off MMI for a period of 12 months at which time biochemical thyrotoxicosis developed. FT4 peaked at 3.0 ng/dL with TSH suppressed at 0.002 mIU/mL. Anti-TPO Ab remained positive at 612 IU/mL with TSIG and TBII levels still negative. She remained asymptomatic. I[123] thyroid uptake and scan revealed low 4-hour uptake of 2.9% (5–15) and low 24-hour uptake of 4.7% (10–35), suggestive of Hashitoxicosis. Subsequently, she developed clinical signs of thyrotoxicosis with peak FT4 of 7.4 ng/dL and suppressed TSH at 0.001 mIU/mL. TSIG and TBII were now positive at 506% and 78.3%, respectively, with anti-TPO Ab positive at >900 IU/mL. MMI was restarted for recurrence of thyrotoxicosis due to GD followed by RAI after her repeat I^{123} thyroid uptake and scan revealed elevated 4-hour and 24-hour uptakes of 66 and 68%, respectively. Subsequent to RAI, she developed primary hypothyroidism that was treated with thyroxine replacement therapy.

3. Discussion

These are three very interesting patients who presented with 3 phases of thyrotoxicosis, initially with both biochemical and clinical thyrotoxicosis due to GD, followed by off MMI therapy by recurrence of biochemical thyrotoxicosis only due to Hashitoxicosis, and then again with both biochemical and clinical thyrotoxicosis due to GD.

The exact relationship between HT and GD continues to be debated. They have been suggested to be 2 separate disease processes partly based on whole-genome scanning studies in humans that revealed unique differences between loci associated with HT and GD [3]. Alternatively, they have been regarded as 2 ends of the same spectrum. This is based on reports that describe the occurrence of HT in one and GD in the second of monozygotic twins [4, 5, 20], the occurrence of HT and GD in the same family [6], and HT following GD in the same patient [21].

It cannot be argued that Hashitoxicosis and not GD was the cause of the initial thyrotoxicosis in all 3 patients. Based on the severity of thyrotoxicosis, presence of clinical symptoms and signs, need for pharmacological therapy, duration of thyrotoxicosis, and presence of positive TSIG and TBII antibodies, it is reasonable to conclude that the etiology of the initial thyrotoxicosis was GD.

The recurrence of thyrotoxicosis, associated with presence of HT antibodies when GD antibodies remained negative, and mild course associated with absence of clinical symptoms and signs were all suggestive of Hashitoxicosis and not GD. Furthermore, repeat I^{123} uptake and scans revealed uptake indicative of an inflammatory thyroiditis associated with HT and not increased uptake diagnostic for GD.

Another possible but unlikely explanation, at least for the transition from thyrotoxicosis to eventual hypothyroidism in the patients, could have been occurrence of TSHR autoantibodies in GD that inhibit TSH binding to TSHR (TSHR blocking antibodies or TSH stimulation blocking immunoglobulins) with subsequent hypothyroidism [18]. However, not only is presence of these antibodies an extremely rare biochemical phenomenon, but also negative TBII testing at that time suggested absence of these and other TSHR autoantibodies.

We believe this report is important as not only is it the first to report thyrotoxicosis due to GD, then due to Hashitoxicosis, and then due to GD in the same individuals, but also the cooccurrence of these 2 autoimmune processes highlights the concept that these are not separate processes but parts of the same autoimmune spectrum.

References

[1] I. Hunter, S. A. Greene, T. M. MacDonald, and A. D. Morris, "Prevalence and aetiology of hypothyroidism in the young," *Archives of Disease in Childhood*, vol. 83, no. 3, pp. 207–210, 2000.

[2] M. Segni, E. Leonardi, B. Mazzoncini, I. Pucarelli, and A. M. Pasquino, "Special features of Graves' disease in early childhood," *Thyroid*, vol. 9, no. 9, pp. 871–877, 1999.

[3] S. M. McLachlan, Y. Nagayama, P. N. Pichurin et al., "The link between Graves' disease and Hashimoto's thyroiditis: a role for regulatory T cells," *Endocrinology*, vol. 148, no. 12, pp. 5724–5733, 2007.

[4] G. Aust, K. Krohn, N. G. Morgenthaler et al., "Graves' disease and Hashimoto's thyroiditis in monozygotic twins: case study as well as transcriptomic and immunohistological analysis of thyroid tissues," *European Journal of Endocrinology*, vol. 154, no. 1, pp. 13–20, 2006.

[5] J.-I. Tani, K. Yoshida, H. Fukazawa et al., "Hyperthyroid Graves' disease and primary hypothyroidism caused by TSH receptor antibodies in monozygotic twins: case reports," *Endocrine Journal*, vol. 45, no. 1, pp. 117–121, 1998.

[6] M. P. Desai and S. Karandikar, "Autoimmune thyroid disease in childhood: a study of children and their families," *Indian Pediatrics*, vol. 36, no. 7, pp. 659–668, 1999.

[7] H. Tamai, H. Uno, Y. Hirota et al., "Immunogenetics of Hashimoto's and Grave's diseases," *Journal of Clinical Endocrinology and Metabolism*, vol. 60, no. 1, pp. 62–66, 1985.

[8] S. M. McLachlan and B. Rapoport, "Breaking tolerance to thyroid antigens: changing concepts in thyroid autoimmunity," *Endocrine Reviews*, vol. 35, no. 1, pp. 59–105, 2014.

[9] S. Fountoulakis and A. Tsatsoulis, "On the pathogenesis of autoimmune thyroid disease: a unifying hypothesis," *Clinical Endocrinology*, vol. 60, no. 4, pp. 397–409, 2004.

[10] M. O. Canning, C. Ruwhof, and H. A. Drexhage, "Aberrancies in antigen-presenting cells and T cells in autoimmune thyroid disease. A role in faulty tolerance induction," *Autoimmunity*, vol. 36, no. 6-7, pp. 429–442, 2003.

[11] C. Phenekos, A. Vryonidou, A. D. Gritzapis, C. N. Baxevanis, M. Goula, and M. Papamichail, "Th1 and Th2 serum cytokine profiles characterize patients with Hashimoto's thyroiditis (Th1) and Graves' disease (Th2)," *NeuroimmunoModulation*, vol. 11, no. 4, pp. 209–213, 2004.

[12] K. Zaletel and S. Gaberšček, "Hashimoto's thyroiditis: from genes to the disease," *Current Genomics*, vol. 12, no. 8, pp. 576–588, 2011.

[13] A. Fava, R. Oliverio, S. Giuliano et al., "Clinical evolution of autoimmune thyroiditis in children and adolescents," *Thyroid*, vol. 19, no. 4, pp. 361–367, 2009.

[14] Z. M. Nabhan, N. C. Kreher, and E. A. Eugster, "Hashitoxicosis in children: clinical features and natural history," *The Journal of Pediatrics*, vol. 146, no. 4, pp. 533–536, 2005.

[15] M. Wasniewska, A. Corrias, M. Salerno et al., "Outcomes of children with hashitoxicosis," *Hormone Research in Paediatrics*, vol. 77, no. 1, pp. 36–40, 2012.

[16] S. Rivkees and D. Mattison, "Propylthiouracil (PTU) hepatoxicity in children and recommendations for discontinuation of use," *International Journal of Pediatric Endocrinology*, vol. 2009, p. 132041, 2009.

[17] M. Cappa, C. Bizzarri, and F. Crea, "Autoimmune thyroid diseases in children," *Journal of Thyroid Research*, vol. 2011, Article ID 675703, 13 pages, 2011.

[18] S. M. McLachlan and B. Rapoport, "Thyrotropin-blocking auto-antibodies and thyroid-stimulating autoantibodies: potential mechanisms involved in the pendulum swinging from hypothyroidism to hyperthyroidism or vice versa," *Thyroid*, vol. 23, no. 1, pp. 14–24, 2013.

[19] A. Lahoti and G. R. Frank, "Laboratory thyroid function testing: do abnormalities always mean pathology?" *Clinical Pediatrics*, vol. 52, no. 4, pp. 287–296, 2013.

[20] A. Iicki, C. Marcus, and F. A. Karlsson, "Hyperthyroidism and hypothyroidism in monozygotic twins: detection of stimulating and blocking THS receptor antibodies using the FRTL5-cell line," *Journal of Endocrinological Investigation*, vol. 13, no. 4, pp. 327–331, 1990.

[21] H. Umar, N. Muallima, J. M. F. Adam, and H. Sanusi, "Hashimoto's thyroiditis following Graves' disease," *Acta Medica Indonesiana*, vol. 42, no. 1, pp. 31–35, 2010.

33

Diabetes Mellitus with Poor Glycemic Control as a Consequence of Inappropriate Injection Technique

Ramesh Sharma Poudel ⓘ,[1] Shakti Shrestha ⓘ,[2] Sushma Bhandari,[1] Rano Mal Piryani,[3] and Shital Adhikari ⓘ[3]

[1]Hospital Pharmacy, Chitwan Medical College Teaching Hospital, Chitwan, Nepal
[2]Department of Pharmacy, Shree Medical and Technical College, Chitwan, Nepal
[3]Department of Internal Medicine, Chitwan Medical College Teaching Hospital, Chitwan, Nepal

Correspondence should be addressed to Ramesh Sharma Poudel; poudel.ramesh@cmc.edu.np

Academic Editor: John Broom

Majority of patients with diabetes mellitus (DM), who are on insulin therapy, use insulin pen for convenience, accuracy, and comfort. Some patients may require two different types of insulin preparations for better glycemic control. We have reported a case of poor glycemic control as a consequence of inappropriate insulin injection technique. A 57-year-old man with type 2 DM had been using premix insulin 30 : 70 for his glycemic control for the last 12 years. On follow-up visit, his blood sugar level (BSL) had increased; therefore the treating physician increased the dose of premix insulin and added basal insulin with the aim of controlling his blood sugar level. Despite these changes, his BSL was significantly higher than his previous level. On investigation, the cause of his poor glycemic control was found to be due to inadequate delivery of insulin (primarily premix) as a consequence of lack of priming and incompatibility of single insulin pen for two cartridges. His basal insulin was discontinued and the patient along with his grandson was instructed to administer insulin correctly. After correction of the errors, the patient had a better glycemic control.

1. Introduction

Insulin therapy is an effective treatment for controlling blood sugar level (BSL) in type 1 diabetes, gestational diabetes, and certain type 2 diabetes incidences including failure of oral hypoglycemic agents. Sometimes more than one type of insulin is prescribed for better glycemic control. Nowadays insulin pens are preferred for convenience over traditional insulin syringe and vial to inject insulin. Use of pen improves adherence to treatment [1], offers lesser pain during administration [2], and enhances patient confidence in selecting the correct dose of insulin [3, 4]. Correct insulin delivery is critical for better diabetes control [5]. Faulty injection technique not only results in inadequate glycemic control [6] but also results in hypoglycemia [7] and insulin allergy [8, 9]. In this study, we report a case of poor glycemic control as a consequence of inappropriate insulin injection technique.

2. Case Report

A 57-year-old man with a 15-year history of type 2 diabetes mellitus visited the outpatient clinic of a hospital for regular check-up. He had been using premix insulin 30 : 70 (Huminsulin 30/70, Lilly Frances S.A.S., 67640 Fegersheim, France) through HumaPen Ergo II (Eli Lilly and Company, Pharmaceutical Delivery System, Lilly Corporate Centre, Indianapolis, IN 46285, USA), 20 units before lunch and 6 units before dinner, to control his BSL for the last 12 years. The patient was also receiving treatment for dilated cardiomyopathy with left ventricle ejection fraction of 20%, hypertension, and chronic kidney disease. On follow-up examination, his fasting (before breakfast) and postprandial (after 2 hours of main meal) BSL were 192 mg/dl and 499 mg/dl, respectively. To control his increased BSL, the treating physician increased the dose of premix insulin 30 : 70 to 28 units in the morning and 14 units in the evening. Additionally, he was advised to

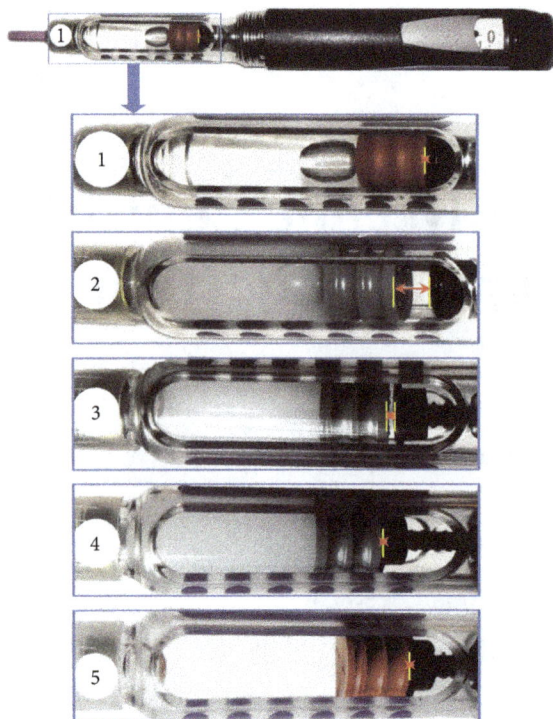

FIGURE 1: Illustration of insulin delivery during faulty injection technique. Numbers 1–5 demonstrate each of the highlighted steps of the delivery. The cartridge plungers in red and grey are basal and premix (30/70) insulin, respectively. In steps 2 and 3, two yellow lines represent the gap between screw (black) and cartridge plunger (grey) during delivery while a single yellow line represents no gap (steps 1 and 4-5). Details of the figure have been mentioned in the Discussion.

use 10 units of basal insulin glargine (Glaritus, Wockhardt Limited, H-14/2 MIDC, Waluj, Aurangabad 431 136), which was from different pharmaceutical company, once daily at 8 pm. Then, physician requested the patient to visit hospital after 2 weeks. On subsequent follow-up visit, BSL of the patient was found to be dramatically high (fasting: 342 mg/dl and postprandial: 554 mg/dl) despite regular use of insulin. The physician requested the patient to get admitted to the hospital in order to control his BSL. However, the patient did not comply with the request, and the physician referred the patient to medication counseling centre of the hospital pharmacy for assessment of insulin injection technique.

Assessment of his insulin injection technique by a registered pharmacist revealed that the patient was using a single insulin pen (HumaPen Ergo II) for two different insulin preparations (Huminsulin 30/70 and Glaritus) without considering priming and compatibility of the insulin pen for two different cartridges. This resulted in either no release of insulin (steps 2 to 3 in Figure 1) or inadequate delivery of premix insulin 30 : 70 (steps 3 to 4 in Figure 1). Also, the premix insulin was not resuspended by patient or his grandson prior to use and the needle was removed immediately after completely inserting the thumb bottom causing insufficient delivery. There was also lack of knowledge on priming of

insulin pen. It was found that the insulin pen was stored in a clay pot. The patient and his grandson were educated about the gap between the screw of insulin pen and cartridge plunger, caused by the use of two different cartridges with different dosages in the same insulin pen without considering priming and compatibility of insulin pen for two cartridges. The counseling pharmacist demonstrated the occasions of no insulin delivery (steps 2 to 3 in Figure 1) and inadequate delivery (steps 3 to 4 in Figure 1) in this case, and his grandson was oriented to appropriate injection technique. Furthermore, the pharmacist also reported the recommending physician about inappropriate insulin injection technique of patient and requested adjusting the dose of insulin. The physician discontinued the basal insulin but advised to continue the premix insulin (28 units in the morning and 14 units in the evening). Four days later, the fasting (before breakfast) and postprandial (after 2 hours of main meal) BSL were found to be 138 mg/dl and 216 mg/dl, respectively. We reinforced the proper injection technique to the patient and his grandson and requested them to visit the hospital after one week for reassessment of the injection technique and determination of fasting and postprandial BSL. Then a plan to adjust the treatment was explained to the patient and his accompanying grandson. Unfortunately, the patient did not visit the hospital for further follow-up. Therefore, we were unable to calculate the mean and standard deviation of fasting and postprandial sugar levels, which require multiple values over a period of time. Hence, the evaluation of the differences over time in terms of statistical significance is not reported. The patient's grandson, on behalf of the patient, has provided written informed consent for the publication of the case report.

3. Discussion

Correct insulin injection technique is critical to ensure optimal glycemic control while faulty injection technique can result in inadequate glycemic control, hypoglycemia, and insulin allergy [6–10]. Of all parts an insulin pen consists of a cartridge holder that holds the insulin cartridge, a dose knob to measure the dose, a screw to push the dialed dose of insulin out of the cartridge, a pen needle to inject insulin, and a pen cap to cover the needle and cartrige holder. Some patients may require two different insulin preparations for better glycemic control. Patients who are using two types of insulin preparations need to consider using two insulin pens for injecting the required doses of insulin. While using single pen for two different cartridges, patients need to consider priming before each injection and compatibility of insulin pen for different cartridges. But, in our case, the patient was using a single insulin pen for two different cartridges that were not completely compatible. Moreover, the patient did not consider priming before each injection probably due to lack of proper education on insulin injection technique causing poor glycemic control. The dose knob was initially set at the required units of insulin. On pressing the thumb button the screw inside the insulin pen moved downward to push the cartridge plunger of the cartridge and the dialed dose of insulin was injected through the needle. However, the screw did not retract back to its original position but remained at the position it was initially dialed to. Therefore, subsequent insulin injection from the same cartridge was affected. For this reason, patients need to use two insulin pens for two different cartridges or consider to prime before each injection confirming that single insulin pen is compatible for two different cartridges to inject appropriate dose of insulin. Hence, in our case, due to the variation in the dose of two insulin reparations without priming, the position of the screw was not at the same level corresponding to the level of cartridge plunger in the cartridge (steps 2 and 3 in Figure 1). Subsequently, insulin would not have been injected from the cartridge till the screw would have reached to the level of cartridge plunger in the cartridge. Figure 1 illustrates the insulin delivery through the use of single insulin pen for two different cartridges without considering priming where the patient had used the cartridges of both insulin preparations for 14 days. It can be observed in the figure that the screw was initially tightly attached to cartilage plunger in case of basal insulin with the red cartridge plunger at approximately 140 units (step 1); therefore, the dialed dose of insulin was delivered from the pen. When the cartilage of basal insulin was replaced with premixed insulin in the morning which had cartridge plunger (grey) at approximately 172 units (had used for last 14 days), a gap could be observed between screw and cartridge plunger (approximately 32 units as in step 2). On dialing and pressing 28 units (morning dose) the screw moved 28 units below. However, approximately 4-unit gap still prevailed between the cartridge plunger and screw (step 3), causing no delivery of premix insulin at this time. In the evening 14 units was dialed and pressed. But due to 4-unit gap in step 3, only about 10-unit premix insulin could be delivered (step 4), resulting in insufficient insulin delivery at this time. The cartridge plunger would be moving to approximately 182 units after the evening dose of premix insulin. Similarly, at about 8 pm the premix insulin cartridge was removed and replaced by basal insulin cartridge (plunger with red color). As a result, the screw which had remained at 182 units at the end of evening dose of premix insulin would now move upward and be set at level of approximately 140 units (corresponding to cartilage plunger of basal insulin) and the screw would be tightly attached to cartridge plunger (step 5). On dialing and pressing the 10-unit dose of basal insulin, the screw would move down 10 units to deliver the set dose (insufficient delivery may occur in case of no priming of the pen) and be set at approximately 150 units. Next day premix insulin cartridge (grey) would be replaced by the basal insulin cartridge (red) in the same pen and gaps as shown in step 2 and step 3 would continue to repeat without considering priming.

Although many manufacturers now provide free insulin pens, majority of the patients in our setting need to purchase it due to insufficient distribution and unawareness of patients about the free supply of pens. This encourages patients to use single pen for compatible insulin cartridges to save money. In the present case, the patient was also found to be using the premix insulin without resuspension. A large multicentered study suggests a link between higher consumption of insulin and insufficient mixing of cloudy (premix) insulin prior to use [6]. Patient and his accompanying grandson were trained on the correct insulin technique according to the

reference of Forum for Injection Technique and Therapy: Expert Recommendations [11]. Such incidences of errors might be due to lower doctor-to-population ratio in the present healthcare setting of Nepal [12]. Therefore, patient-doctor interaction is restricted due to time limitation [13]. Moreover, the role of pharmacist is usually undermined [14, 15] and majority of community pharmacy professionals have inadequate knowledge and practice on injection technique [16, 17]. Such problem in low-resource setting can be overcome by educating patients through trained comprehensive diabetes educator [18] and subsequent reinforcement and reassessment of insulin injection technique of patients [6].

Our case report highlights the need for continued assessment and education regarding insulin injection technique by trained healthcare professionals, even though the patients are often properly instructed on its correct administration before the initiation of a therapy.

4. Conclusion

Use of single insulin pen for two different cartridges without considering priming and their compatibility results in no or inadequate insulin delivery, causing poor glycemic control. Therefore, the healthcare professionals should consider reassessment and reinforcement of insulin injection technique during follow-up visits by patients.

Acknowledgments

The authors acknowledged the patient and their relative for their participation in this study. The authors are also grateful to Mr. Santosh Sigdel, a Senior Lecturer, Boston International College, Chitwan, Nepal, and Mr. Praves Lamichhane, Faculty of Science, The University of Sydney, Sydney, Australia, for English editing.

References

[1] W. C. Lee, S. Balu, D. Cobden, A. V. Joshi, and C. L. Pashos, "Medication adherence and the associated health-economic impact among patients with type 2 diabetes mellitus converting to insulin pen therapy: An analysis of third-party managed care claims data," *Clinical Therapeutics*, vol. 28, no. 10, pp. 1712–1725, 2006.

[2] A. Ahmann, S. L. Szeinbach, J. Gill, L. Traylor, and S. K. Garg, "Comparing patient preferences and healthcare provider recommendations with the pen versus vial-and-syringe insulin delivery in patients with type 2 diabetes," *Diabetes Technology & Therapeutics*, vol. 16, no. 2, pp. 76–83, 2014.

[3] S. Brunton, "Initiating insulin therapy in type 2 diabetes: Benefits of insulin analogs and insulin pens," *Diabetes Technology & Therapeutics*, vol. 10, no. 4, pp. 247–256, 2008.

[4] J. E. Thurman, "Insulin pen injection devices for management of patients with type 2 diabetes: Considerations based on an endocrinologist's practical experience in the United States," *Endocrine Practice*, vol. 13, no. 6, pp. 672–678, 2007.

[5] G. Grassi, P. Scuntero, R. Trepiccioni, F. Marubbi, and K. Strauss, "Optimizing insulin injection technique and its effect on blood glucose control," *Journal of Clinical & Translational Endocrinology*, vol. 1, no. 4, pp. 145–150, 2014.

[6] A. H. Frid, L. J. Hirsch, A. R. Menchior, D. R. Morel, and K. W. Strauss, "Worldwide injection technique questionnaire study: population parameters and injection practices," *Mayo Clinic Proceedings*, vol. 91, no. 9, pp. 1212–1223, 2016.

[7] B. Karges, B. O. Boehm, and W. Karges, "Early hypoglycaemia after accidental intramuscular injection of insulin glargine," *Diabetic Medicine*, vol. 22, no. 10, pp. 1444-1445, 2005.

[8] P. P. Chakraborty, S. N. Biswas, and S. Patra, "Faulty injection technique: a preventable but often overlooked factor in insulin allergy," *Diabetes Therapy*, vol. 7, no. 1, pp. 163–167, 2016.

[9] T. Sanyal, S. Ghosh, S. Chowdhury, and S. Mukherjee, "Can a faulty injection technique lead to a localized insulin allergy?" *Indian Journal of Endocrinology and Metabolism*, vol. 17, no. 1, pp. S358–S359, 2013.

[10] A. Frid, L. Hirsch, R. Gaspar et al., "The third injection technique workshop in athens (TITAN)," *Diabetes & Metabolism*, vol. 36, no. 2, pp. S19–S29, 2010.

[11] A. H. Frid, G. Kreugel, G. Grassi et al., "New insulin delivery recommendations," *Mayo Clinic Proceedings*, vol. 91, no. 9, pp. 1231-1255, 2016.

[12] C. Shrestha and R. Bhandari, "Insight into human resources for health status," *Health Prospect*, vol. 11, pp. 40–44, 2013.

[13] J. Moshang, "Getting the job done: The diabetes nurse specialist," *International Journal of Clinical Practice*, vol. 61, no. 9, pp. 1429-1431, 2007.

[14] B. K. Poudel and I. Ishii, "Hospital pharmacy service in developing nations: the case of Nepal," *Research in Social & Administrative Pharmacy*, vol. 12, no. 6, pp. 1038-1039, 2016.

[15] R. S. Poudel and A. Prajapati, "Hospital pharmacy profession in Nepal through the eye of a pharmacist," *Journal of Chitwan Medical College*, vol. 6, no. 16, pp. 56-57, 2017.

[16] S. Gyawali, D. S. Rathore, K. Adhikari, P. R. Shankar, V. K. Kc, and S. Basnet, "Pharmacy practice and injection use in community pharmacies in Pokhara city, Western Nepal," *BMC Health Services Research*, vol. 14, p. 190, 2015.

[17] M. Shrestha, R. Maharjan, A. Prajapati, S. Ghimire, N. Shrestha, and A. Banstola, "Assessment of knowledge and practice of community pharmacy personnel on diabetes mellitus management in Kathmandu district: A cross sectional descriptive study," *Journal of Diabetes and Metabolic Disorders*, vol. 14, no. 1, article no. 71, 2015.

[18] M. D. Bhattarai, "Comprehensive diabetes and non-communicable disease educator in the low-resource settings," *Journal of Nepal Medical Association*, vol. 54, no. 202, pp. 94–103, 2016.

34

Remarkable Presentation: Anaplastic Thyroid Carcinoma Arising from Chronic Hyperthyroidism

Habib G. Zalzal ⓘ,[1] Jeffson Chung ⓘ,[1] and Jessica A. Perini[2]

[1]*Department of Otolaryngology-Head and Neck Surgery, West Virginia University School of Medicine, Morgantown, WV, USA*
[2]*Section of Endocrinology, Department of Internal Medicine, West Virginia University School of Medicine, Morgantown, WV, USA*

Correspondence should be addressed to Jeffson Chung; jeffson.chung@hsc.wvu.edu

Academic Editor: Carlo Capella

Background. Undifferentiated anaplastic carcinoma rarely develops from chronic hyperthyroidism. Although acute hyperthyroidism can develop prior to anaplastic transformation, chronic hyperthyroidism was thought to be a protective measure against thyroid malignancy. *Methods.* A 79-year-old female presented acutely to the hospital with dyspnea. She had been taking methimazole for chronic hyperthyroidism due to toxic thyroid nodules, previously biopsied as benign. Upon admission, imaging showed tracheal compression, requiring a total thyroidectomy with tracheostomy for airway management. *Results.* Pathology demonstrated undifferentiated anaplastic thyroid carcinoma. The patient passed away shortly after hospital discharge. Despite treatment with methimazole for many years, abrupt enlargement of her toxic multinodular goiter was consistent with malignant transformation. Chronic hyperthyroidism and toxic nodules are rarely associated with thyroid malignancy, with only one previous report documenting association with anaplastic thyroid carcinoma. *Conclusion.* Progressive thyroid enlargement and acute worsening of previously controlled hyperthyroidism should promote concern for disease regardless of baseline thyroid function.

1. Introduction

Historically, chronic hyperthyroidism had been considered protective against thyroid carcinoma. Some data suggest a lower incidence of papillary thyroid cancer in those with lower TSH levels [1]. This presumably arises from a decreased stimulatory effect on thyroid tissue presented by the low serum thyroid stimulatory hormone (TSH) found in hyperthyroidism. However, with the increasing incidence of thyroid cancer seen over the past years, there appears to be an improved understanding that thyroid carcinomas can also arise in glands that are thyrotoxic due to Graves' disease, toxic multinodular goiter, and autonomously functioning thyroid adenomas [2]. Recent review of the literature has shown the risk of malignancy associated with toxic hot nodules ranges from 1 to 10.3% [2] or even up to 15% in those with Graves' disease [3]. Most of these documented malignancies are differentiated thyroid carcinomas and very rarely medullary thyroid cancer [4].

Anaplastic thyroid carcinoma (ATC) represents one of the most aggressive endocrine tumors and constitutes approximately between 1.6 and 5% of all thyroid malignancies [5]. ATC comes with a dismal prognosis limited to a 10–20% mean survival at 12 months [6]. Patients with ATC experience significant local compressive symptoms due to a rapidly evolving central neck mass (77%) along with dysphagia (40%), hoarseness (40%), and stridor (24%) [7]. Metastases are noted in 50% of patients at the time of diagnosis, most commonly in the lungs (80%), bone (6–16%), and brain (5–13%) [7]. Not uncommonly patients also develop thyrotoxicosis. Although thyrotoxicosis can develop in a gland with ATC, it is rare to find ATC develop from underlying longstanding hyperthyroidism. We found only one other case in the literature of ATC arising from a patient with chronic hyperthyroidism [8]. In this report, we present our experience with a patient who developed ATC after many years of hyperthyroidism and toxic multinodular goiter.

2. Patient

A 79-year-old Caucasian female presented to our institution with chest pain, dyspnea, and a rapidly enlarging thyroid

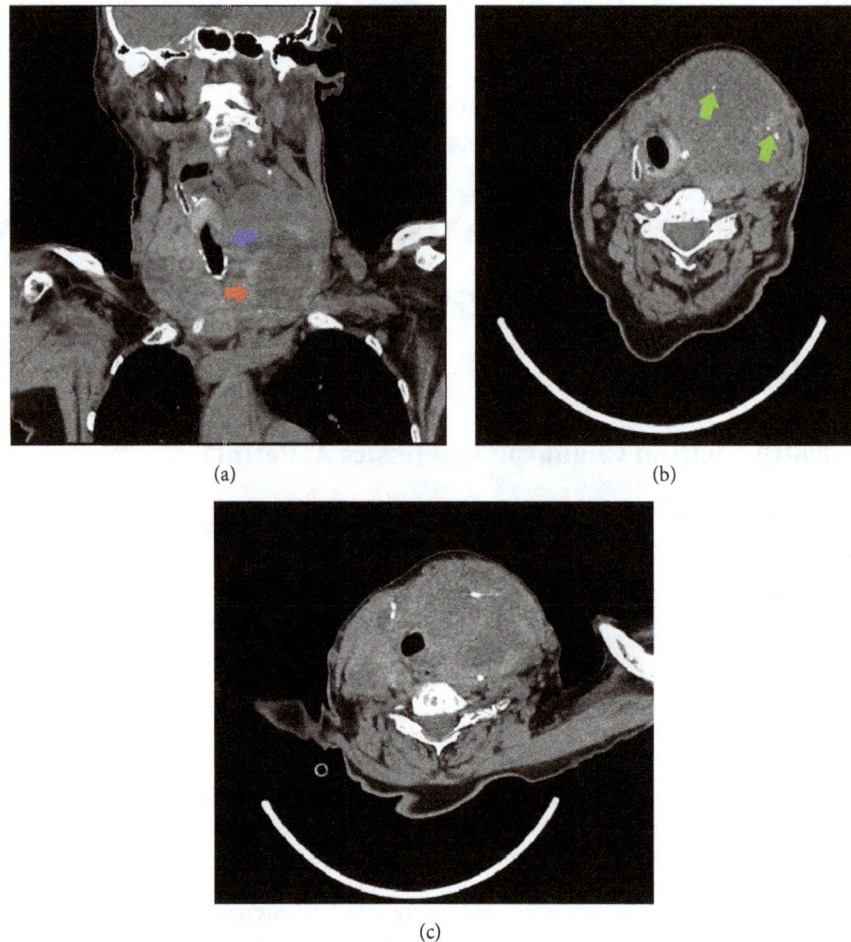

(a)

(b)

(c)

FIGURE 1: Significantly enlarged thyroid mass causing tracheal deviation to the right (blue arrow) with hypoattenuation within the left thyroid lobe (red arrow) (a). Scattered calcifications (green arrows) apparent within the lesion (b) with extension into the anterior mediastinum and continued deviation of the trachea (c).

goiter. The patient endorsed that she was previously quite healthy aside from stable hyperthyroidism and a nonenlarging thyroid goiter. Her thyroid had been overactive for years, treated with stable dose of 7.5 mg daily of methimazole for at least the past four years. In 2002, 2003, and 2010, she had had thyroid uptake scans indicating heterogeneous elevated uptake consistent with toxic multinodular goiter and a cold area was identified in the lower right lobe. In 2000 and 2010, she had biopsies of the nodules of the right and left lobes with benign results. Since treatment with methimazole, she had been asymptomatic up until three months prior to presentation, living a mostly independent and having active lifestyle that included cooking, gardening, and daily errands.

The patient's family became concerned approximately three months before presentation to our facility because the patient lost a significant amount of weight while her goiter rapidly enlarged. Soon after, she had sudden "terrible pain" in the left side of her neck, diagnosed as an internal jugular vein thrombus. At the time of this diagnosis, her thyroid measured 8.4 × 12 cm. She saw her endocrinologist who noted that her thyroid was hyperfunctioning again and no longer controlled with her daily dose of methimazole,

which was subsequently increased. A month later, her labs showed that her thyroid was even more overactive. Her dose of methimazole was subsequently increased to 30 mg per day. She was evaluated for surgery the following month, but surgery was deferred due to uncontrolled hyperthyroidism. The day prior to presentation at our institution she developed chest pressure and tightness when lying down. A computed tomography (CT) scan of her chest and neck showed that her thyroid had grown to 9.8 × 13.2 cm.

Upon admission, her TSH measured <0.003 μIU/L (reference range 0.5–4.70 μIU/mL), free serum thyroxine (T$_4$) measured 1.56 ng/dL (reference range 0.7–1.25 ng/dL), and free serum triiodothyronine (T$_3$) measured 2.4 pg/mL (reference range 1.7–3.7 pg/mL). Ultrasound of her thyroid showed gross enlargement of both thyroid lobes with the largest nodules measuring 9.7 cm in the left lobe and 5.1 cm in the right lobe. Subsequent CT scan of her chest showed the mass extending into the anterior mediastinum with scattered calcifications within the mass (Figure 1). There was narrowing of the trachea in addition to multiple pulmonary masses throughout the visualized lung fields. She was continued on methimazole (20 mg twice a day) while hospitalized

(a)

(b)

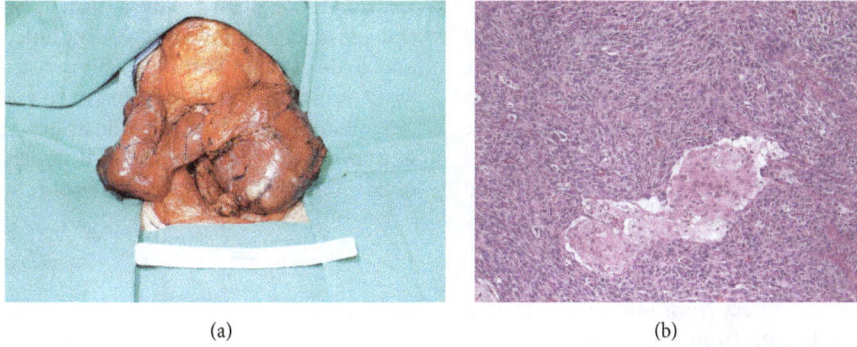

FIGURE 2: (a) Intraoperative photograph of total thyroid specimen, greatest dimension 8.7 cm in size. (b) Microscopic pathology of squamoid and undifferentiated thyroid cells.

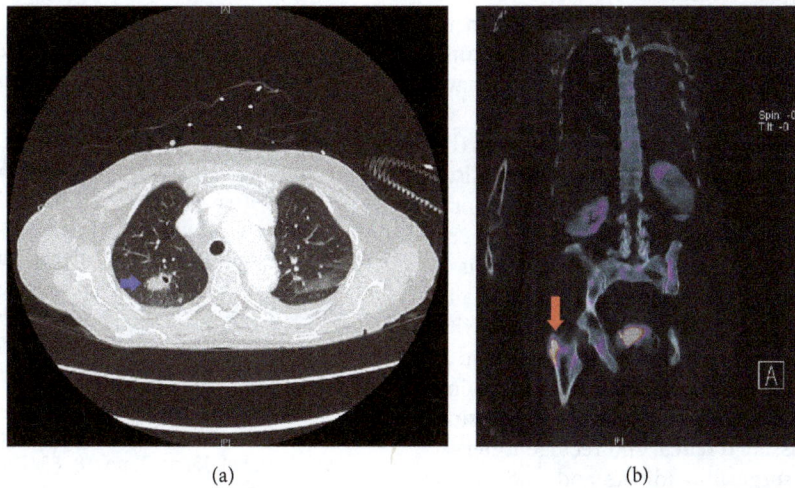

(a)

(b)

FIGURE 3: Metastatic work-up demonstrates a pulmonary nodule within the right upper lobe (1.1×2.1 cm) with central cavitation (blue arrow) (a) and increased 99 mTc HDP uptake within the right intratrochanteric femur positive for a destructive lytic lesion (red arrow) (b).

and started on propranolol and prednisone for symptomatic control. Her free T_4 improved and free T_3 remained within normal limits on this regimen.

Due to dyspnea and malignancy concerns, she underwent a total thyroidectomy two weeks after admission to obtain a pathologic diagnosis. Intraoperative findings included involvement of the left recurrent laryngeal nerve and tracheal invasion. Intraoperative biopsies sent for frozen section analysis were reported as poorly differentiated carcinoma, suggestive of anaplastic thyroid carcinoma (Figure 2). As a result, a prophylactic tracheostomy was placed. The final pathology report confirmed undifferentiated anaplastic carcinoma (8.7 cm) involving the left thyroid, positive for lymphatic involvement (2/5 central nodes) and extrathyroidal extension to the pretracheal cartilage. Surgical margins were positive along the left middle and inferior pole. The right thyroid lobe had multiple benign nodes. Subsequent whole-body CT and nuclear medicine scan found multiple bilateral pulmonary nodules with central cavitation and a destructive right intertrochanteric lytic lesion with pathological fracture (Figure 3). The final staging was pT4b N1b M1 anaplastic thyroid carcinoma (American Joint Committee on Cancer 7th Edition). Chemotherapy was recommended for her ATC,

as she was deemed not a candidate for radiation therapy. The patient's family chose to pursue chemotherapy closer to home. The patient quickly deteriorated towards the end of her hospitalization and missed several follow-up appointments with her medical oncologist upon discharge. She passed away at home within a month after leaving the hospital.

3. Discussion

Chronic hyperthyroidism had long been thought to be protective against the development of malignancy within the thyroid gland [2]. Thus, development of thyroid cancer within a hyperthyroid gland was thought to be uncommon. However, meta-analyses have shown that thyroid cancer can in fact develop in hyperthyroid glands, although it is not common, and most of the malignancies identified in hyperfunctioning thyroid glands have been differentiated thyroid cancers. Conversely, acute thyroiditis can develop in association with thyroid malignancies. For example, rare cases of "malignant pseudothyroiditis" have been described wherein local parathyroid malignancies or metastatic lesions to the thyroid prompted thyroid inflammation and thyrotoxicosis [9]. ATC is also associated with acute thyrotoxicosis that develops around the time of acute malignant transformation [2, 10]. A 2007 review of the association between ATC and thyrotoxicosis outlines eight cases in the literature [10]. The authors discuss the development of acute thyrotoxicosis with anaplastic thyroid cancer as a consequence of rapid leakage of thyroid hormone into the bloodstream from destroyed thyrocytes. Phillips et al. argue that the acute hyperthyroid state in ATC is caused by a hyperfunctioning metastatic tumor [10]. Thyrotoxicosis associated with ATC has been termed "anaplastic pseudothyroiditis" [11].

This situation, however, differs from our patient in that thyrotoxicosis did not originate from the anaplastic tumor but predated the malignant transformation by several years. Our case shows the unique condition in which anaplastic thyroid cancer developed from a hyperthyroid patient despite several years of methimazole treatment. ATC is associated with a previous history of thyroid goiter and is known to be more common in geographic regions of endemic iodine deficiency [7] but not associated with glands that have previously been hyperfunctioning.

To our knowledge, a 2014 report by Marcelino et al. is the only published case that associates chronic hyperthyroidism with subsequent development of ATC [8]. Their study reports a similar presentation in a 70-year-old male who had been diagnosed with a toxic nodule three years prior to diagnosis of ATC. He was conservatively managed with methimazole and β-adrenergic blockers. Three years later, he re-presented with dyspnea, hoarseness, and dysphagia similar to our patient. A subsequent neck CT scan showed a suspicious mass involving the left thyroid lobe and isthmus ($7 \times 6 \times 5$ cm), with invasion of the surrounding soft tissue, trachea, and recurrent nerve. Their patient was not a surgical candidate and underwent radiotherapy without much improvement in thyroid size before passing away several weeks later of airway compression [8]. Similar to Marcelino et al., previous work-up of our patient's thyroid nodules, including biopsies of bilateral nodules, was negative for malignancy. While her thyroid uptake scans previously identified a cold nodule in the lower right thyroid lobe, her surgical pathologic specimen of the left thyroid lobe identified the anaplastic carcinomic tissue while her right thyroid nodule was negative for anaplastic disease. In addition, previous thyroid scans had elevated and patchy uptake in the left lobe despite the pathologic finding. The development of ATC from differentiated thyroid carcinoma is well established [7], although our patient did not have this diagnosis, based on the negative FNA years prior. Whether our patient developed "de novo" ATC similar to what was theorized by Marcelino et al. is debatable, but plausible considering the fact that the previously toxic left thyroid nodule was the one which developed ATC in our patient. This was despite the presence of a cold nodule in the right thyroid lobe which remained negative for malignancy after removal.

Undifferentiated anaplastic thyroid carcinoma is a rare and underreported condition in the setting of chronic hyperthyroidism. There exists only one other reported case of this association in the literature, also involving a septuagenarian who developed rapid thyroid enlargement with tracheal compression years after diagnosis and control of hyperthyroidism with methimazole. While current recommendations for treatment of hyperthyroidism involve medical therapy, the presence of any nontoxic nodule in the thyroid, and any toxic nodule with suspicious features, should warrant work-up with ultrasound, fine needle aspirate, and ongoing surveillance. Our case demonstrates that even those with negative biopsy and longstanding hyperthyroidism are at risk of development of anaplastic thyroid carcinoma.

References

[1] E. Fiore, T. Rago, M. A. Provenzale et al., "Lower levels of TSH are associated with a lower risk of papillary thyroid cancer in patients with thyroid nodular disease: thyroid autonomy may play a protective role," *Endocrine-Related Cancer*, vol. 16, no. 4, pp. 1251–1260, 2009.

[2] K. Pazaitou-Panayiotou, K. Michalakis, and R. Paschke, "Thyroid cancer in patients with hyperthyroidism," *Hormone and Metabolic Research*, vol. 44, no. 4, pp. 255–262, 2012.

[3] J. L. Kraimps, M. H. Bouin-Pineau, M. Mathonnet et al., "Multicentre study of thyroid nodules in patients with Graves' disease," *British Journal of Surgery*, vol. 87, no. 8, pp. 1111–1113, 2000.

[4] K. Pazaitou-Panayiotou, P. Perros, M. Boudina et al., "Mortality from thyroid cancer in patients with hyperthyroidism: The Theagenion Cancer Hospital experience," *European Journal of Endocrinology*, vol. 159, no. 6, pp. 799–803, 2008.

[5] V. Kumar, B. Blanchon, X. Gu et al., "Anaplastic thyroid cancer and hyperthyroidism," *Endocrine Pathology*, vol. 16, no. 3, pp. 245–250, 2005.

[6] J. L. Pasieka, "Anaplastic thyroid cancer," *Current Opinion in Oncology*, vol. 15, no. 1, pp. 78–83, 2003.

[7] G. Nagaiah, A. Hossain, C. J. Mooney, J. Parmentier, and S. C. Remick, "Anaplastic thyroid cancer: a review of epidemiology, pathogenesis, and treatment," *Journal of Oncology*, vol. 2011, Article ID 542358, pp. 1–13, 2011.

[8] M. Marcelino, P. Marques, L. Lopes, V. Leite, and J. J. de Castro, "Anaplastic carcinoma and toxic multinodular goiter: an unusual presentation," *European Thyroid Journal*, 2014.

[9] I. B. Rosen, H. G. Strawbridge, P. G. Walfish, and J. Bain, "Malignant pseudothyroiditis: A new clinical entity," *The American Journal of Surgery*, vol. 136, no. 4, pp. 445–449, 1978.

[10] J. S. Phillips, D. R. Pledger, and A. W. Hilger, "Rapid thyrotoxicosis in anaplastic thyroid carcinoma," *The Journal of Laryngology & Otology*, vol. 121, no. 7, pp. 695–697, 2007.

[11] S. Basaria, R. Udelsman, J. Tejedor-Sojo, W. H. Westra, and A. S. Krasner, "Anaplastic pseudothyroiditis," *Clinical Endocrinology*, vol. 56, no. 4, pp. 553–555, 2002.

35

DKA with Severe Hypertriglyceridemia and Cerebral Edema in an Adolescent Boy: A Case Study and Review of the Literature

Tansit Saengkaew, Taninee Sahakitrungruang,
Suttipong Wacharasindhu, and Vichit Supornsilchai

Division of Endocrinology, Department of Pediatrics, Faculty of Medicine, Chulalongkorn University, Bangkok 10330, Thailand

Correspondence should be addressed to Tansit Saengkaew; tansitpedpsu@gmail.com

Academic Editor: Wayne V. Moore

A 13-year-old adolescent boy with type 1 diabetes mellitus (1b) presented with diabetic ketoacidosis (DKA) and cerebral edema. Grossly lipemic serum and lipemia retinals due to extremely high triglyceride (TG) level were observed without evidence of xanthoma or xanthelasma. Cerebral edema was treated by appropriate ventilation and mannitol administration. Normal saline was carefully given and regular insulin was titrated according to blood sugar levels. Triglyceride levels were reduced from 9,800 mg/dL to normal range within 9 days after conventional treatment was commenced without antilipid medication. Based on our review of the literature, this is the first reported case of confirmed pediatric DKA with severe hypertriglyceridemia and cerebral edema. In patients with DKA and hypertriglyceridemia, clinicians should be mindful of the possibility of associated acute pancreatitis and cerebral edema.

1. Introduction

Diabetic ketoacidosis (DKA) is a common presentation of type 1 diabetes mellitus that requires urgent treatment. Diagnostic criteria for DKA include hyperglycemia (BS > 200 mg/dL), ketosis, and metabolic acidosis. The most serious complication in delayed diagnosis of DKA is cerebral edema, a complication that increases patient morbidity and mortality. Acute pancreatitis (AP), peripheral venous thrombosis, pulmonary edema, and rhabdomyolysis are only rarely found in patients with DKA [1].

Severe hypertriglyceridemia (TG > 1,000 mg/dL) is another rare complication found in DKA patients. Severe hypertriglyceridemia can increase risk of acute pancreatitis, especially in patients with TG levels higher than 1,000–1,772 mg/dL [2, 3]. Prevalence of severe hypertriglyceridemia was found in about 8% of adults with DKA [4], but few data have been reported in children with severity ranging from asymptomatic to severe acute pancreatitis. The mechanism of hypertriglyceridemia in DKA that has been proposed involves increased free fatty acid (FFA) secretion from adipocytes by counterregulatory hormone stimulation, which results in decreased clearance of VLDL-TG [5]. Recommended treatment includes intravenous fluid and insulin administration appropriated to DKA treatment guidelines. Plasmapheresis or heparinization was used in some reported cases to decrease triglyceride level in adults [6–13]. The objective of this report is to present and describe the clinical features, laboratory investigations, case management, and natural course of hypertriglyceridemia in a 13-year-old adolescent boy with DKA. A review of the literature relating to hypertriglyceridemia and its manifestations in children with DKA was performed and is included in this report for purposes of comparison with our patient.

We searched all English articles that were published and shown in PubMed, MEDLINE, and Web of Science up to August 2015. The keywords were DKA, hypertriglyceridemia, cerebral edema, and acute pancreatitis. We selected only publications (retrospective cohort studies and case reports) about children, adolescents, and young adults who presented with DKA and hypertriglyceridemia. All clinical and laboratory data including age at presentation, initial TG level, diagnosis and treatment of acute pancreatitis, and duration of TG return to normal range were reviewed and summarized.

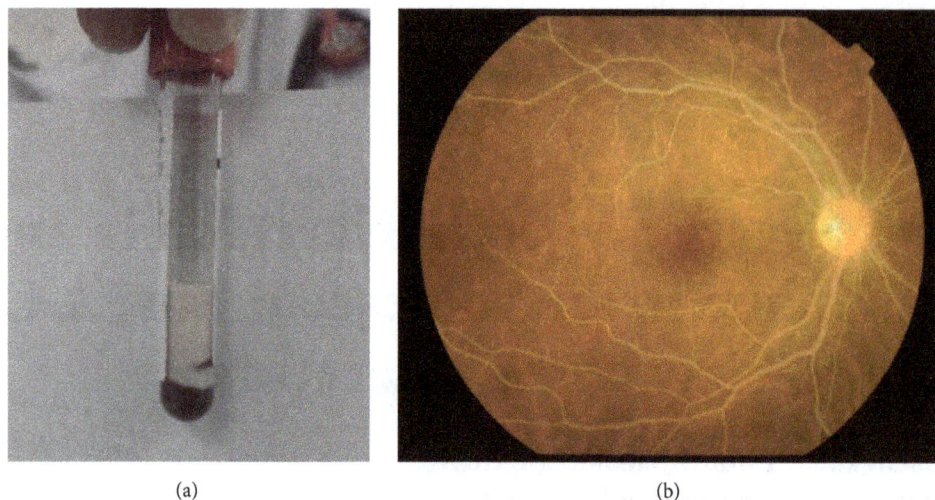

(a)   (b)

FIGURE 1: Images describing lipemic serum (a) and lipemia retinals, whitish, creamy vessels of retina (b).

2. Case Presentation

A 13-year-old boy with type 1 diabetes mellitus (T1DM) presented at the Emergency Department of King Chulalongkorn Memorial Hospital (Bangkok, Thailand) with Kussmaul breathing and confusion, after having malaise and polyuria for one month and epigastric pain for 2 days. He was diagnosed with T1DM at another hospital one year earlier and was being treated with insulin, metformin, and glipizide. Our patient reported having discontinued all medications for 6 months prior to this admission. His maternal grandmother was diagnosed with type 2 diabetes mellitus at the age of 40 and her condition was reported as being effectively controlled with oral hypoglycemic drugs. No family history of dyslipidemia was reported. On admission, our patient was confused, agitated, and disoriented regarding time, place, and persons. Vital signs revealed body temperature of 38.5°C, pulse rate 128, respiratory rate 26/min with Kussmaul pattern, and blood pressure 156/102 mmHg. Anthropometric measurements showed weight of 43 kg, height 152 cm, and body mass index (BMI) 18.61 kg/m^2. There was no eruptive or tuberous xanthoma or xanthelasma at the skin. Ophthalmologic examination revealed presence of whitish, creamy vessels of retinas, called lipemia retinals (Figure 1(a)). No focal neurologic deficit was noted.

At presentation, our patient was found to have DKA, with initial BS of 513 mg/dL, venous blood gas with pH 7.062, pCO$_2$ 22.4 mmHg, HCO$_3$ 6.4, and BE −21.7 mEq/L, and serum ketone 3.2 mmol/L. His blood demonstrated a grossly lipemic appearance (Figure 1(b)) and his lipemic condition disturbed the results of other biochemical blood investigations. Cerebral edema was diagnosed according to 1 major criterion (alteration and fluctuation of consciousness) and 2 minor criteria (lethargy and diastolic blood pressure >90 mmHg). CT of the brain was not performed due to the unstable clinical condition of our patient. He was intubated due to deterioration of consciousness and cerebral edema. Mannitol (0.5 mg/kg) was subsequently administered and 3%

NaCl was given intravenously to maintain a hypernatremic state for purposes of decreasing intracranial pressure. Normal saline was carefully given and regular insulin was then started and titrated to 0.2 units/kg/hr according to patient blood sugar levels. He was out of DKA as defined by pH > 7.3, bicarbonate > 15 mmol/L, and serum ketone negative, within 24 hours. Lipid profiles were analyzed on the second day of admission, with results revealing triglyceride of 9,810 mg/dL, cholesterol 705 mg/dL, LDL 254 mg/dL, and HDL 6 mg/dL. Patient had no abdominal pain and serum amylase was 57 IU/L. Therefore, acute pancreatitis was excluded. Triglyceride level was reduced to 377 mg/dL within 9 days of admission (Figure 2) without the use of antilipid medication. Our patient was extubated within 2 days of admission after recovery from DKA and cerebral edema. His father's lipid profiles showed cholesterol of 215 mg/dL, triglyceride 111 mg/dL, LDL 144 mg/dL, and HDL 50 mg/dL. His mother's lipid profiles showed cholesterol of 167 mg/dL, triglyceride 75 mg/dL, LDL 101 mg/dL, and HDL 47 mg/dL.

After discharge from the hospital, T1DM treatment with basal-bolus insulin regimen was commenced. Our patient continued to have HbA1c-related complications (10–15%) due to poor self-treatment compliance. Although he developed DKA twice as a result, his TG levels remained within normal range.

3. Discussion

Two large series reported data in adult DKA with severe hypertriglyceridemia [4, 19]. Fulop and Eder found that 15 of 136 (11%) DKA patients had severe hypertriglyceridemia (TG > 1,000 mg/dL), but only one patient developed acute pancreatitis [19]. Incidence of severe hypertriglyceridemia was similarly found in 8 of 100 (12.5%) adult DKA patients in the other of the two studies, with half of the patients developing acute pancreatitis [4]. In children, most cases were individually presented in patient case reports (Table 1). All reported cases had TG levels higher than 1,000 mg/dL,

TABLE 1: Literature review of pediatric DKA patients with hypertriglyceridemia.

Patients	Age (year)	Peak TG (mg/dL)	Acute pancreatitis	Cerebral edema	Treatment with antilipid medication	Time to normalized TG level (days, (TG level))
Cywinski et al., 1965 [14]	12.5	>1,000	Yes	Suspected	No	7 (232)
Blackett et al., 1986 [6]	13	14,461	No	Suspected	No	7 (122)
Slyper et al., 1994 [15]	14	3,119	Yes	Suspected	No	NA
Kadota-Shinozaki et al., 1997 [16]	19	3,386	Yes	No	No	2 (483)
Hahn et al., 2010 [10]	20	15,000	Yes	No	No	3 (506)
Williamson et al., 2012 [12]	8	10,852	No	No	No	17 (NA)
Lutfi et al., 2012 [11]	10	16,334	Yes	No	Fenofibrate, plasmapheresis	1.5 (1,100)
Kota et al., 2012 [17]	12	1,020	Yes	No	No	3 (340)
Aboulhosn and Arnason, 2013 [13]	18	1,724	Yes	No	No	NA
Wolfgram and Macdonald, 2013 [18]	10	8,300	Yes	No	No	NA
Our case	**13**	**9,810**	**No**	**Yes**	**No**	**9 (377)**

NA, not available.

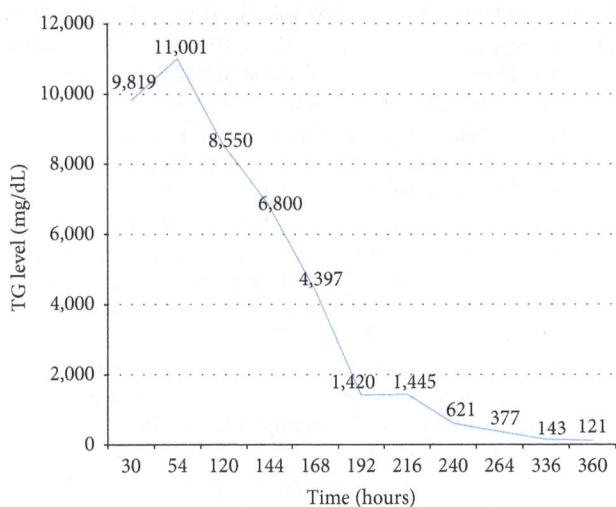

FIGURE 2: Triglyceride levels after DKA treatment.

supporting the hypothesis that elevated TG (>1,000 mg/dL) is a risk factor for acute pancreatitis [2, 3]. However, 3 out of 11 patients (2.8%) did not develop acute pancreatitis. One pediatric patient did not develop acute pancreatitis, even though he had extremely high TG level (14,461 mg/dL) [6]. As such, other risk factors for this condition need to be identified. Accordingly, clinical investigations for acute pancreatitis should be routine in all cases presenting with TG level higher than 1,000 mg/dL to ensure early and proper management.

The postulated mechanism of hypertriglyceridemia in DKA patients centers on lack of insulin action, which activates lipolysis in adipose tissue that then results in free fatty acid (FFA) formation and increases in VLDL formation by the liver [19]. In addition, insulin normally inhibits ApoC-III expression, which plays a major role in inhibiting lipoprotein lipase (LPL) and hepatic lipase (HL). This results in decreased hydrolysis and delayed VLDL-TG clearances

from plasma. As a result, ApoC-III increases in an insulin-deficient state, with a subsequent increase in plasma TG level [5]. Severe hypertriglyceridemia-induced pancreatitis develops as a result of increased FFA levels that are produced from triglyceride hydrolysis by pancreatic lipase and insulin deficiency. High FFA levels cause acute pancreatitis as a result of capillary endothelium and pancreatic acinar cell destruction [14, 20].

Appropriate management of DKA with hypertriglyceridemia includes intravenous fluid and insulin administration according to DKA guideline, because the major mechanism of hypertriglyceridemia is insulin deficiency. Plasma TG level was gradually reduced to less than 500 mg/dL within 3–17 days in most cases. However, 9 of 15 patients reviewed by Fulop and Eder had normal plasma TG concentrations for up to 6 months without any lipid-lowering agent [19]. One patient reported by Lutfi et al. who had extremely high TG level (16,334 mg/dL) with renal insufficiency and who failed with conservative treatment was successfully treated by plasmapheresis [11]. TG levels were reduced from 5,093 to 1,157 mg/dL in that study. Heparinization was also reported as an alternative treatment for hypertriglyceridemia in adult DKA patients, together with fluid and insulin administration [8]. In that study, TG levels were reduced from 8,701 mg/dL to normal range within 2 days of treatment without abnormal bleeding.

Cerebral edema was suspected in 3 pediatric cases from the literature review and one case from the present report. All 3 cases from the literature had abnormal pupillary reflex with unconsciousness, but all had spontaneous recovery without treatment by mannitol or hypertonic saline. To our knowledge and based on our review of the literature, the association between severe hypertriglyceridemia and cerebral edema is unclear. The hypothesized mechanism is that hyperviscosity due to extremely high TG level likely causes decreased cerebral blood flow, which may correlate with cerebral edema [21]. Yuen et al. found that severe dehydration and hypertriglyceridemia aggravated cerebral hypoperfusion, which had the effect of worsening cerebral edema.

The weakness of our case was that serum lipase test was not done and contrast enhanced CT of the abdomen was not performed. Even though the patient had no abdominal pain and normal amylase level, acute pancreatitis could not be absolutely excluded.

In this case report, we presented a pediatric DKA patient with cerebral edema and severe hypertriglyceridemia. In patients with DKA and hypertriglyceridemia caused by severe insulin deficiency, clinicians should be mindful of the possibility of associated acute pancreatitis and cerebral edema. Triglyceride levels were gradually decreased to normal range within 9 days after standard intravenous fluid and insulin administration was commenced.

Acknowledgments

The authors gratefully acknowledge all pediatric residents and nurses at King Chulalongkorn Memorial Hospital for providing exceptional patient care.

References

[1] J. I. Wolfsdorf, J. Allgrove, M. E. Craig et al., "Ispad clinical practice consensus guidelines 2014. Diabetic ketoacidosis and hyperglycemic hyperosmolar state," *Pediatric Diabetes*, vol. 15, supplement 20, pp. 154–179, 2014.

[2] V. G. Athyros, O. I. Giouleme, N. L. Nikolaidis et al., "Long-term follow-up of patients with acute hypertriglyceridemia-induced pancreatitis," *Journal of Clinical Gastroenterology*, vol. 34, no. 4, pp. 472–475, 2002.

[3] S. Sandhu, A. Al-Sarraf, C. Taraboanta, J. Frohlich, and G. A. Francis, "Incidence of pancreatitis, secondary causes, and treatment of patients referred to a specialty lipid clinic with severe hypertriglyceridemia: a retrospective cohort study," *Lipids in Health and Disease*, vol. 10, article 157, 2011.

[4] S. Nair, D. Yadav, and C. S. Pitchumoni, "Association of diabetic ketoacidosis and acute pancreatitis: observations in 100 consecutive episodes of DKA," *American Journal of Gastroenterology*, vol. 95, no. 10, pp. 2795–2800, 2000.

[5] S. Qu, T. Zhang, and H. H. Dong, "Effect of hepatic insulin expression on lipid metabolism in diabetic mice," *Journal of Diabetes*, 2015.

[6] P. R. Blackett, J. H. Holcombe, P. Alaupovic, and J. D. Fesmire, "Plasma lipids and apolipoproteins in a 13-year-old boy with diabetic ketoacidosis and extreme hyperlipidemia," *The American Journal of the Medical Sciences*, vol. 291, no. 5, pp. 342–346, 1986.

[7] M. J. Rumbak, T. A. Hughes, and A. E. Kitabchi, "Pseudonormoglycemia in diabetic ketoacidosis with elevated triglycerides," *American Journal of Emergency Medicine*, vol. 9, no. 1, pp. 61–63, 1991.

[8] R. P. Cole, "Heparin treatment for severe hypertriglyceridemia in diabetic ketoacidosis," *Archives of Internal Medicine*, vol. 169, no. 15, pp. 1439–1441, 2009.

[9] J. Wolfsdorf, M. E. Craig, D. Daneman et al., "Diabetic ketoacidosis in children and adolescents with diabetes," *Pediatric Diabetes*, vol. 10, supplement 12, pp. 118–133, 2009.

[10] S. J. Hahn, J.-H. Park, J. H. Lee, J. K. Lee, and K.-A. Kim, "Severe hypertriglyceridemia in diabetic ketoacidosis accompanied by acute pancreatitis: case report," *Journal of Korean Medical Science*, vol. 25, no. 9, pp. 1375–1378, 2010.

[11] R. Lutfi, J. Huang, and H. R. Wong, "Plasmapheresis to treat hypertriglyceridemia in a child with diabetic ketoacidosis and pancreatitis," *Pediatrics*, vol. 129, no. 1, pp. e195–e198, 2012.

[12] S. Williamson, V. Alexander, and S. A. Greene, "Severe hyperlipidaemia complicating diabetic ketoacidosis," *Archives of Disease in Childhood*, vol. 97, no. 8, p. 735, 2012.

[13] K. Aboulhosn and T. Arnason, "Acute pancreatitis and severe hypertriglyceridaemia masking unsuspected underlying diabetic ketoacidosis," *BMJ Case Reports*, vol. 2013, 2013.

[14] J. S. Cywinski, F. A. Walker, H. White, and H. S. Traisman, "Juvenile diabetes mellitus associated with acute pancreatitis," *Acta paediatrica Scandinavica*, vol. 54, no. 6, pp. 597–602, 1965.

[15] A. H. Slyper, D. T. Wyatt, and C. W. Brown, "Clinical and/or biochemical pancreatitis in diabetic ketoacidosis," *Journal of Pediatric Endocrinology*, vol. 7, no. 3, pp. 261–264, 1994.

[16] A. Kadota-Shinozaki, T.-A. Nakamura, H. Hidaka et al., "Diabetic lipemia with maturity-onset diabetes of the young," *Internal Medicine*, vol. 36, no. 8, pp. 571–574, 1997.

[17] S. K. Kota, S. Jammula, S. K. Kota, L. K. Meher, and K. D. Modi, "Acute pancreatitis in association with diabetic ketoacidosis in a newly diagnosed type 1 diabetes mellitus patient; case based review," *International Journal of Clinical Cases and Investigations*, vol. 4, no. 1, pp. 54–60, 2012.

[18] P. M. Wolfgram and M. J. Macdonald, "Severe hypertriglyceridemia causing acute pancreatitis in a child with new onset type i diabetes mellitus presenting in ketoacidosis," *Journal of Pediatric Intensive Care*, vol. 2, no. 2, pp. 77–80, 2013.

[19] M. Fulop and H. Eder, "Severe hypertriglyceridemia in diabetic ketosis," *The American Journal of the Medical Sciences*, vol. 300, no. 6, pp. 361–365, 1990.

[20] A. Chait and J. D. Brunzell, "Chylomicronemia syndrome," *Advances in Internal Medicine*, vol. 37, pp. 249–273, 1992.

[21] N. Yuen, S. E. Anderson, N. Glaser, D. J. Tancredi, and M. E. O'Donnell, "Cerebral blood flow and cerebral edema in rats with diabetic ketoacidosis," *Diabetes*, vol. 57, no. 10, pp. 2588–2594, 2008.

36

Internal Spreading of Papillary Thyroid Carcinoma: A Case Report and Systemic Review

Hui Jin,[1,2] **Huanhuan Yan** ⓘ**,**[1,2] **Huamei Tang,**[3] **Miao Zheng,**[1,2] **Chaojie Wu,**[1,2] **and Jun Liu** ⓘ[1,2]

[1]*Shanghai General Hospital of Nanjing Medical University, Shanghai 201620, China*
[2]*Department of Breast-Thyroid-Vascular Surgery, Shanghai General Hospital, Shanghai Jiaotong University, Shanghai 201620, China*
[3]*Pathological Center of School of Medicine, Shanghai Jiaotong University, Shanghai 201620, China*

Correspondence should be addressed to Jun Liu; liujun95039@163.com

Academic Editor: Carlo Capella

An 18-year-old female diagnosed finally as PTC with intrathyroid spread was reported, and the diagnosis and surgical treatment of internal spreading of PTC were discussed. One lump was found on the thyroid isthmus by physical examination and B ultrasound, and multiple nodular shadows were found by CT. This patient finally underwent total thyroidectomy with bilateral central node dissection due to multifocal papillary thyroid carcinoma except PTC in the isthmus found in right lobe by intraoperative frozen section. The pathological section showed a major thyroid carcinoma in thyroid isthmus with scattered micropapillary carcinoma around it in the whole thyroid gland. The small lesions are distributed around central lesion in a radial form and the number of small lesions decreases with increased distance from central lesion. PTC with internal spread should be distinguished from multifocal PTC and poorly differentiated PTC in pathology. Thyroid cancerous node had a large diameter; it was likely to have internal spread. Combined imaging before surgery should be valued to diagnose PTC with internal spread. Preoperative CT and intraoperative frozen section are helpful for surgical volume selection of PTC with internal spread.

1. Case Abstract

An 18-year-old female patient was hospitalized due to "a touchable lump on the right of thyroid isthmus" which has been found for about 2 months. The patient has congenital heart disease history and no thyroid disease history in her family. *Physical Examination.* Bilateral thyroid was slightly swollen. A hard lump about 20 × 10 mm could be touched on thyroid isthmus and could move up and down when swallowing. No vascular murmur could be heard. *Laboratory Examination.* Routine blood examination and the level of thyroid hormone were normal. *B Ultrasound.* Echo of thyroid was even, and a low echo tubercle, with size 11 × 20 mm, aspect ratio 0.55, unclear border, and irregular shapes, could be observed on the right side of thyroid isthmus. Multiple dot-like calcification and blood flow signals could be observed (Figure 1(a)). *CT Scan.* Multiple nodular

shadows of lower density could be observed in thyroid and some were calcified with a larger one located in isthmus, about 17 × 10 mm, and the rest were normal (Figure 1(b)). *FNA.* Cells were arranged closely and overlapped presenting papillary structure. Cell nucleus ditches could be observed (Figure 1(c)). We diagnosed it preoperatively as papillary thyroid carcinoma (PTC). *Echocardiography.* Congenital heart disease with ventricular septal defect, left to right shunt, and mild pulmonary hypertension.

A hard lump of size 20 × 15 mm and unclear border could be seen on the isthmus of thyroid during surgery. Nanometer carbon tracer was injected into bilateral thyroid to help us to distinguish lymph nodes from parathyroid glands. At first, the right thyroidectomy + isthmectomy with right central node dissection was performed. However, the intraoperative frozen section not only confirmed the preoperative diagnosis of PTC on the thyroid isthmus, in

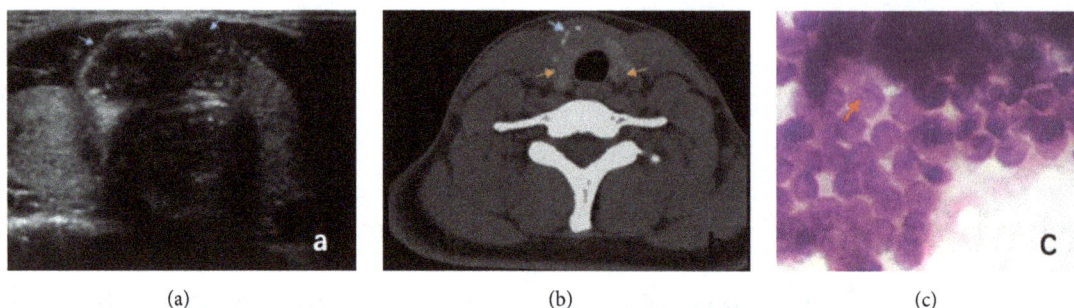

(a) (b) (c)

FIGURE 1: (a) *B Ultrasound*. Blue arrow for the low echo tubercle in the thyroid isthmus. (b) *CT Scan*. Yellow arrow for thyroid multiple lower density nodule; blue arrow for calcification. (c) *FNA*. Red arrow for cell nucleus ditch.

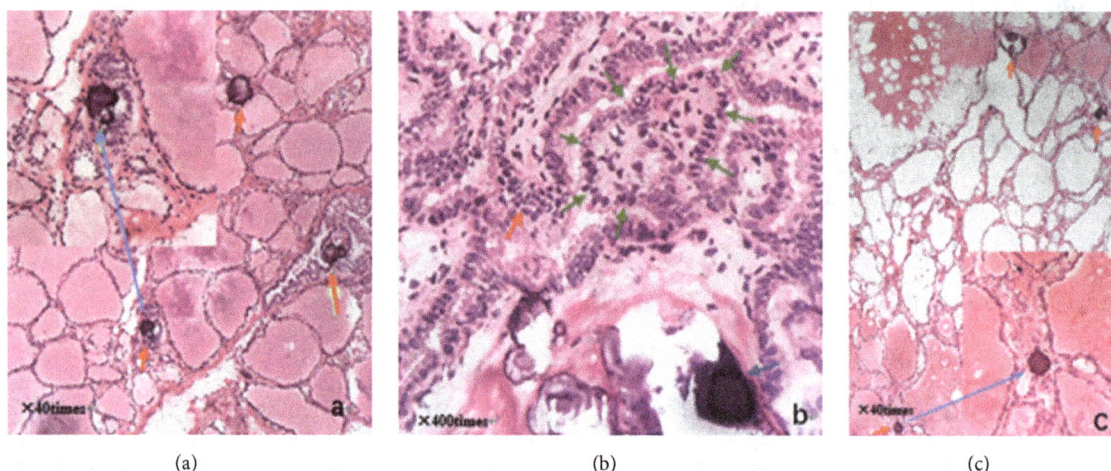

(a) (b) (c)

FIGURE 2: (a) Intraoperative frozen pathology of right thyroid lobe: red arrow for psammoma body. (b) Intraoperative frozen pathology of thyroid isthmus: red arrow for heterocyst; blue arrow for psammoma body; green arrow for papillary structure. (c) Intraoperative frozen pathology of left thyroid lobe: red arrow for psammoma body.

which disordered and branched papillary structure, scattered psammoma bodies, frosted-glass-like cell nucleus, larger nucleus, nucleus grooves, and intranuclear pseudoinclusions were found (Figure 2(b)), but also showed multifocal papillary thyroid carcinoma (MPTC) in right thyroid lobe as multiple psammoma bodies and papillary structure could be found in it (Figure 2(a)). Subsequently, left thyroidectomy and left central node dissection were added, and then the operation was finally ended. Multiple psammoma bodies and heterotypic cells were also found in left thyroid lobe on intraoperative frozen section (Figure 2(c)). The patient was discharged 3 days after operation without any symptoms of hypoparathyroidism and recurrence of laryngeal nerve injury.

Postoperative pathology showed that micropapillary carcinomas scattered around a major thyroid carcinoma ($22 \times 11 \times 20$ mm) in thyroid isthmus, and scattered micropapillary carcinoma also existed on both thyroid right lobe and left lobe (Figures 3–5). Immunohistochemistry showed CK19 (+), HBME-1 (+), TG (+), TTF-1 (+), TPO (+), CD56 (−), ki67 (about 3%), and beta-catenin (+). And 2 out of 3 central lymph nodes with metastasis were found. Interestingly, it

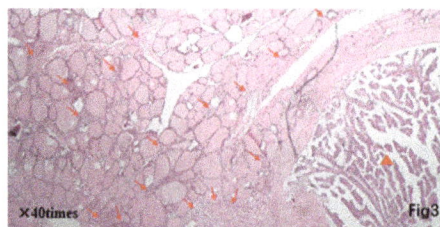

FIGURE 3: Red triangle for large carcinoma lesions at the lower right corner; red arrow for small lesions composed of dozens of heterocyst reunion on the left side.

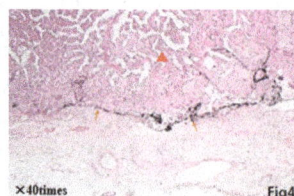

FIGURE 4: Red triangle for large carcinoma lesions; yellow arrow for tracer dye black lymphatic vessels.

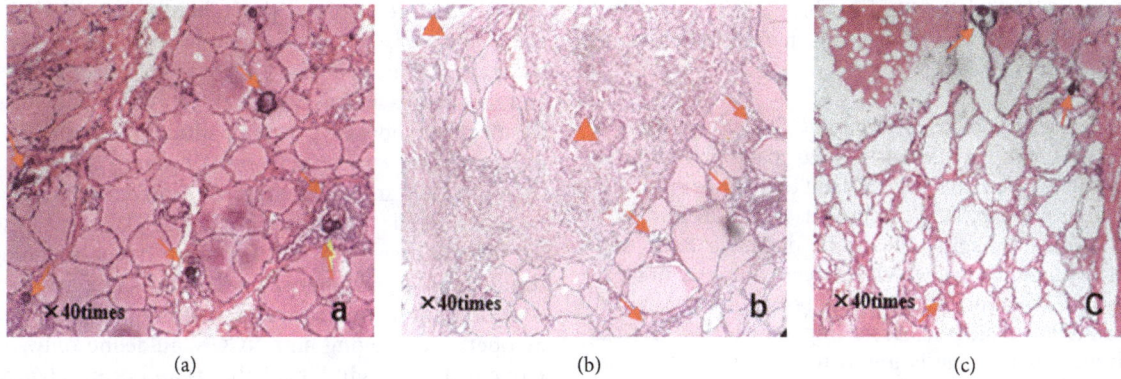

FIGURE 5: (a) Pathology section of right thyroid lobe: red arrow for psammoma body. (b) Pathology section of thyroid isthmus: red triangle for large carcinoma lesions; red arrow for small lesions composed of dozens of heterocyst. (c) Pathology section of left thyroid lobe: red arrow for psammoma body.

can be observed that some small lesions are distributed around central lesion in radial form and the number of small lesions decreases with increased distance from central lesion on postoperative pathological sections. A larger carcinoma lesion (lower and right corner) with some small lesions composed of tens of heterocysts (upper-left section) can be observed in Figure 3. A spread lesion in the lymph-vessel blackened by nanometer carbon tracer and blackened lymph-vessels in the lesion were showed in Figure 4. Intraoperative frozen sections were analyzed again and the number of satellite lesions in the left lobe and right lobe was counted under the same magnification. It can also be observed that some small lesions are distributed around central lesion in radial form and the number of satellite lesions decreases with increased distance from central lesion, and the central lesion is just the PTC in the isthmus near the right lobe. The number of satellite lesions in the right lobe is more than that in left lobe (Figure 5). Therefore, the final pathological diagnosis was considered as PTC with intrathyroid spread.

2. Discussion

2.1. Diagnosis and Identification of Internal Spread of PTC.
PTC is the most common type of thyroid cancer, taking around 70%~80% [1]. Internal spread of PTC is one of the metastasis ways of thyroid cancer. There is a connection among lesions including a major one and small lesions in the surrounding parts. It is usually spread by the abundant lymphatic networks in thyroid. In this case, it can be observed from postoperative pathological sections that some small lesions are distributed around central lesion in radial form and the number of small lesions decreases with increased distance from central lesion. Therefore, it was considered as internal spread of thyroid carcinoma. A larger carcinoma lesion has increased possibility of internal spread. When a satellite lesion is as small as the accumulation of tens of cancer cells, medical imaging does not always reflect abnormal signs; when it grows to a certain size, preoperative diagnosis is similar to MPTC.

PTC with internal spread should be distinguished from MPTC and poorly differentiated papillary carcinoma. MPTC is one of the clinical characteristics of PTC and exists as multiple independent carcinoma lesions in thyroid. Its malignancy is higher than single lesion carcinoma of thyroid. It is closely associated with lymphatic metastasis, recurrence, and prognosis. The incidence of MPTC is about 18%~87% in PTC [2, 3]. MPTC is one form of PTC and featured by invasion into lymph node and tissue around thyroid and recurrence. The lymphatic metastasis rate of MPTC is close to 60%. MPTC can be classified into three types according to the locations: (1) MPTC in unilateral thyroid: preoperative diagnosis finds no tubercle in opposite thyroid; (2) MPTC in unilateral thyroid: preoperative diagnosis finds tubercles in opposite thyroid but considers them as benign tubercles; (3) MPTC are distributed in bilateral thyroid. Hashimoto's thyroiditis (HT) and hereditary thyroid cancer are the risk factors of MPTC. Other clinical statistics also reflect PTC combined with HT has higher incidence of MPTC [4, 5]. HT affects the whole thyroid gland. It finally results as diffuse destroyed thyroid cells and higher TSH level, and the latter may stimulate the proliferation of papillary cancer cells. The malignant tubercle developed based on this type of diffuse lesion often bears multiple lesions [6, 7]. The tubercles of multilesion carcinoma are similar and not directly associated. According to the available clinical data, internal spread of PTC is a special type for PTC. Compared with MPTC, the surrounding lesions are smaller and only can be observed under a microscope. As it is not a macroscopic tubercle, it cannot be touched in surgery. Under microscope, larger cancerous tubercles surrounded by tens or hundreds of small cancerous nests in radial form can be observed. The number of small tubercles and cluster degree decrease with increased distance from large tubercles, which indicates internal spread of thyroid carcinoma.

Poorly differentiated thyroid cancer is seldom composed of single structure and often exists as the combination of island, beam, or solid structures in different proportions. Solid structure is very common. The tumor cells do not have the thyroid follicles typical nuclear features of PTC, spread along the lymphatic vessels and thyroid follicles side clearance.

2.2. Preoperative Diagnosis of Internal Spread of Thyroid Papillary Carcinoma.

While it is easy to make preoperative diagnosis of PTC, it is extremely difficult to diagnose internal spread of thyroid papillary carcinoma. B ultrasound is a preferred medical imaging means to diagnose a thyroid disease. If a tubercle of low echo, irregular form, unclear border, and calcification is found, the possibility of thyroid cancer should be considered. According to historical clinical data analysis, if a tubercle is found to have any 3 features above, over 90% of pathology literature reports the specificity of malignant tubercle. In this case, the low echo tubercle in isthmus has irregular form, unclear border, and strong echo, which highly suggests the possibility of malignant tubercle. For suspected malignant tubercle and the lymph gland with possibility of metastasis, fine needle aspiration (FNA) under guidance of B ultrasound is very significant to the identification of thyroid tubercle, malignant or not, and determination of lymph node dissection scope. As proved by multiple statistics, the coincidence rate of FNA diagnosis and postoperative pathological sections is above 90% [8]. According to the result of FNA for calcified tubercles, it was found that cells are arranged closely and overlapped presenting papillary structure. Nucleus grooves of cells could be seen. The case was diagnosed as PTC (Figure 1(c)).

It can be found from this case that CT is very significant to comprehensive diagnosis of thyroid diseases. Due to the damaged iodine-storing cells in thyroid cancer, a low-density zone can be seen in CT image. In this case, CT image showed multiple low-density tubercle shadows in addition to the tubercle in isthmus, and B ultrasound image showed even echo of thyroid. We tried to analyze that, in the early stage of internal spread of thyroid papillary carcinoma, a macroscopic tubercle was not yet formed in the surrounding but the gather of cells only. US is the common method for thyroid cancer diagnosis with high sensitivity within 1 mm. CT is a useful complement for US in judging the invasion of adjacent tissues, and the involved lymph node in some areas [9–11]. Why were the multiple low-density tubercle shadows found by CT but not by US in our case? One reason may be that US evaluation is operator dependent. The other reason may be that US is not sensitive to this kind of small foci of intrathyroid spread of PTC.

For the diagnosis of internal spread of PTC, it is essential to combine multiple diagnosis means based on medical history and correctly judge the distribution of major tubercle and surrounding lesions and metastasis of neck lymphatic. In this case, B ultrasound report hinted a tubercle is at the right side of isthmus while CT showed multiple low-density tubercle shadows. As B ultrasound was limited by human factors, diagnosis scope might be shrunken resulting in a negative result, and the CT scanning way could just make up this defect of B ultrasound.

2.3. Intraoperative Frozen Pathology Section Is Helpful to Guide the Way of Surgery in the Case of Internal Spread of PTC.

In this case, according to the result of B ultrasound and CT before surgery, the tubercle was located on the right side of isthmus. Meanwhile, considering the age of the patient, the primary plan was to resect right thyroid and its isthmus and perform central lymph node dissection. Result of intraoperative frozen pathology section showed that micropapillary carcinomas were dispersed in the isthmus of thyroid gland and right thyroid. After knowing this result, we considered the possibility of MPTC, and resect the left lobe, and sent for intraoperative frozen pathology. The result showed psammoma bodies and some heterocyst. We considered it as micropapillary carcinomas. If according to preoperative imaging and NCCN guideline only, resection scope included right lobe, isthmus and central lymph node. The result of intraoperative frozen pathology section guided us to resect all thyroid tissue and central lymph node. We thought that the satellite lesions were small in the early stage of metastasis, not large enough to be found in imaging. If internal spread of thyroid papillary carcinoma was not certain, we should pay attention to the result of intraoperative frozen pathology section.

If the case was diagnosed as internal spread of PTC, surgery scope should refer to MPTC. For internal spread of thyroid, resection scope does not vary greatly with MPTC. Most statistical results support whole resection, even though central lesion and satellite lesion are limited to one side. Related data statistics about internal metastasis of PTC are still in short supply. There are research reports about primary multifocal carcinoma. For the cases diagnosed as single-sided multifocal PTC, offside thyroid was cut within half a year and the relevance ratio of opposite neoplastic foci was as high as 69.1%. For patients with HT of B ultrasound and thyroid function, even though multiple lesions are in single side, both sides should be cut off. Multifocal carcinoma is an independent risk factor of lymphatic metastasis. It is safe to perform whole cutting and central lymph node dissection. For skipping lymphatic metastasis, functional lymph node dissection should be performed.

3. Conclusion

This is a typical case of internal spread of PTC as a major thyroid carcinoma in thyroid isthmus with scattered micropapillary carcinoma around it in the whole thyroid gland. PTC with internal spread should be distinguished from multifocal PTC and poorly differentiated PTC in pathology. Combined imaging, as B ultrasound, CT, and FNA, before surgery should be valued. Sometimes, even though B ultrasound report showed no abnormality of multiple lesions, we could not eliminate the possibility of internal metastasis of PTC. Especially when cancerous nodule had a large diameter, it was likely to have internal metastasis. Preoperative CT and intraoperative frozen section are helpful for surgical volume selection of PTC with internal spread.

References

[1] G. Pellegriti, F. Frasca, C. Regalbuto, S. Squatrito, and R. Vigneri, "Worldwide increasing incidence of thyroid cancer: update on epidemiology and risk factors," *Journal of Cancer Epidemiology*, vol. 2013, Article ID 965212, 10 pages, 2013.

[2] T. M. Shattuck, W. H. Westra, P. W. Ladenson, and A. Arnold, "Independent clonal origins of distinct tumor foci in multifocal papillary thyroid carcinoma," *The New England Journal of Medicine*, vol. 352, no. 23, pp. 2406–2412, 2005.

[3] S. Y. Park, Y. J. Park, Y. J. Lee et al., "Analysis of differential BRAF V600E mutational status in multifocal papillary thyroid carcinoma: evidence of independent clonal origin in distinct tumor foci," *Cancer*, vol. 107, no. 8, pp. 1831–1838, 2006.

[4] X. Liu, L. Zhu, D. Cui et al., "Coexistence of histologically confirmed Hashimoto's thyroiditis with different stages of papillary thyroid carcinoma in a consecutive Chinese cohort," *International Journal of Endocrinology*, vol. 2014, Article ID 769294, 7 pages, 2014.

[5] Y. Zhang, J. Dai, T. Wu, N. Yang, and Z. Yin, "The study of the coexistence of Hashimoto's thyroiditis with papillary thyroid carcinoma," *Journal of Cancer Research and Clinical Oncology*, vol. 140, no. 6, pp. 1021–1026, 2014.

[6] E. Zeindl-Eberhart, S. Liebmann, P. R. Jungblut et al., "Influence of RET/PTC1 and RET/PTC3 oncoproteins in radiation-induced papillary thyroid carcinomas on amounts of cytoskeletal protein species," *Amino Acids*, vol. 41, no. 2, pp. 415–425, 2011.

[7] V. Guarino, M. D. Castellone, E. Avilla, and R. M. Melillo, "Thyroid cancer and inflammation," *Molecular and Cellular Endocrinology*, vol. 321, no. 1, pp. 94–102, 2010.

[8] C. Asteria, A. Giovanardi, A. Pizzocaro et al., "US-elastography in the differential diagnosis of benign and malignant thyroid nodules," *Thyroid*, vol. 18, no. 5, pp. 523–531, 2008.

[9] J. M. Ní Mhuircheartaigh, B. Siewert, and M. R. Sun, "Correlation between the size of incidental thyroid nodules detected on CT, MRI or PET-CT and subsequent ultrasound," *Clinical Imaging*, vol. 40, no. 6, pp. 1162–1166, 2016.

[10] V. Summaria, V. Rufini, P. Mirk, A. M. Costantini, F. Reale, and G. Maresca, "Diagnostic imaging of differentiated thyroid carcinoma.," *Rays*, vol. 25, no. 2, pp. 177–190, 2000.

[11] C. Ogawa, M. Kammori, H. Onose et al., "Utilization of three-dimensional computed tomography for papillary thyroid carcinoma arising in the thyroglossal duct remnant: report of a case," *Surgery Today*, vol. 40, no. 7, pp. 650–653, 2010.

37

Bilateral Carotid-Cavernous Fistulas: An Uncommon Cause of Pituitary Enlargement and Hypopituitarism

Anthony Liberatore and Ronald M. Lechan

Department of Medicine, Division of Endocrinology, Diabetes and Metabolism, Tupper Research Institute, Tufts Medical Center, Boston, MA 02111, USA

Correspondence should be addressed to Anthony Liberatore; anthony.liberatore@lawrencegeneral.org

Academic Editor: Yuji Moriwaki

Carotid-cavernous fistulas (CCFs) are rare, pathologic communications of the carotid artery and the venous plexus of the cavernous sinus. They can develop spontaneously in certain at risk individuals or following traumatic head injury. Typical clinical manifestations include headache, proptosis, orbital pain, and diplopia. We report a case of bilateral carotid-cavernous fistulas associated with these symptoms and also with pituitary enlargement and hypopituitarism, which improved following surgical intervention. Arterialization of the cavernous sinus and elevated portal pressure may interfere with normal venous drainage and the conveyance of inhibiting and releasing hormones from the hypothalamus, resulting in pituitary enlargement and hypopituitarism. This condition should be considered in the differential diagnosis of hypopituitarism associated with anterior pituitary enlargement.

1. Introduction

Diffuse enlargement of the anterior pituitary gland can be associated with a number of physiological and pathologic clinical conditions. Physiologic enlargement is seen during adolescence and pregnancy and after menopause [1, 2] and can occur with long-standing primary hypothyroidism, hypogonadism, or hypoadrenalism due to thyrotroph, gonadotroph, or corticotroph hyperplasia, respectively [1, 3]. A variety of pathologic conditions also result in diffuse enlargement of the anterior pituitary and can be associated with varying degrees of hypopituitarism including infiltrative and inflammatory disorders such as hemochromatosis, amyloidosis, sarcoidosis, Langerhans cell histiocytosis, lymphocytic and granulomatous hypophysitis, Wegener's granulomatosis, necrotizing infundibular hypophysitis, and Erdheim-Chester disease; infectious disorders including bacterial, fungal, and parasitic disease; and neoplastic disorders including germinoma, metastatic carcinoma, myeloma, lymphoma, and leukemia [4–7]. Other rare causes include ectopic or excess secretion of GHRH or CRH from a ganglioneuroma or carcinoid tumor [8–10] and germline mutations of *PROP1* [11]. Transient pituitary enlargement has also been reported after bilateral cavernous sinus thrombosis [12].

An underrecognized and uncommon cause of pituitary enlargement is vascular congestion from carotid-cavernous fistulas (CCFs). CCFs are rare arteriovenous shunts that permit blood flow from the carotid artery into the cavernous sinus. The cavernous sinus contains a venous plexus that drains the confluent veins emanating from anterior and posterior pituitary. Thereby, arterialized blood in the cavernous sinus can disrupt normal venous pituitary drainage and cause pituitary enlargement [13], hypoperfusion [14], and hypopituitarism [15, 16]. To increase awareness of this disorder and the characteristics of its presentation, we report a case of 53-year-old woman found to have bilateral CCFs while being evaluated for pituitary enlargement and hypopituitarism. The fistulas were repaired surgically resulting in reduction in pituitary size and eventual recovery of her hypothalamic-pituitary-adrenal axis. However she has ongoing central hypothyroidism.

2. Case Report

A 53-year-old woman was referred to the emergency department with a left, cranial nerve VI palsy and enlarged pituitary on head MRI. For the three months prior to admission, she

(a)   (b)

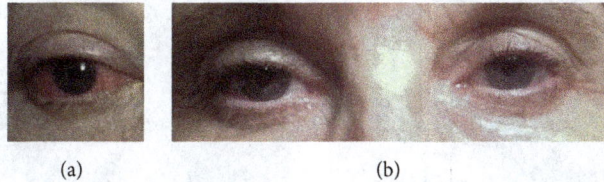

FIGURE 1: Patient's eye findings on presentation (a) and 1 month after embolization (b). Initial periorbital edema, chemosis, proptosis, and conjunctival injection dramatically improved with coiling.

had complaints of headaches, sinus pressure, and bilateral eye redness and had been evaluated by several physicians. On these occasions, she was treated for seasonal allergies with short courses of antibiotics and corticosteroids, but without significant improvement in her symptoms. Two weeks prior to admission, while driving, she developed acute-onset diplopia with lightheadedness and vertigo. Her visual symptoms improved if she covered her left eye. These new symptoms lead to referral to an otolaryngologist and then an ophthalmologist who obtained MRI which revealed pituitary enlargement. She was sent to the emergency room following the discovery of the pituitary abnormality.

In the emergency department, she had a notable, isolated, left, cranial nerve VI palsy, periorbital edema, bilateral conjunctival injection with chemosis (Figure 1(a)), and a delayed relaxation phase of her biceps reflex. Given the pituitary enlargement, she was admitted to the Neurosurgery service. Ophthalmology was consulted and their evaluation noted elevated intraocular pressure, 26 mmHg on the right and 21 mmHg on the left (normal 10–20 mmHg). Fundoscopic examination revealed sharp optic discs. Her initial blood pressure was 137/67 mmHg with pulse 65 beats per minute. There was no postural change in her vital signs. Laboratory testing revealed a serum sodium of 142 mmol/L (135–145), potassium 4 mmol/L (3.6–5.1), random cortisol undetectable, and ACTH 5.5 pmol/L. A 250-μg cosyntropin stimulation test was performed the following morning. Basal cortisol was 27.6 nmol/L, 30 minute cortisol 405 nmol/L, and 60-minute maximum 488 nmol/L. TSH was normal at 2.21 mIU/L (0.4–4.8) and free thyroxine was borderline low, 9.78 pmol/L (9–19). Prolactin was elevated at 1.7 nmol/L (0.17–1.3). Other anterior pituitary function tests were normal and age-appropriate (IGF-1 17.03 nmol/L [11–30.5]; FSH 61.4 IU/L [26.7–133.4]). Glucocorticoids and levothyroxine were started.

Noncontrast head MRI revealed an enlarged pituitary measuring 1.1 cm AP × 0.9 cm superior-inferior × 1.4 cm transverse with upward convexity into the suprasellar cistern (Figures 2(a) and 2(b)). There was no cavernous sinus invasion. Note, however, was made of bilateral, low-signal foci in the cavernous sinuses raising the question of aneurysms or venous flow. MRA confirmed intense early postcontrast enhancement within the cavernous sinuses, adjacent to the internal carotid arteries, consistent with bilateral CCFs (Figure 3). She was taken to the operating room for bilateral endovascular fistula coiling. Within 48 hours, her diplopia improved, steroids were tapered, and she was discharged on

hydrocortisone 10 mg with breakfast and 5 mg with supper and a weight-based dose of levothyroxine, 75 mcg once a day.

The patient thereafter was evaluated regularly in the outpatient endocrine clinic at follow-up appointments. At 1 month, significant improvements in eye signs were noted (Figure 1(b)). A head MRI at 4 months showed that the pituitary had decreased in size to 1.3 cm AP × 0.7 cm superior-inferior × 1.2 cm transverse (Figures 2(c) and 2(d)). An early morning cortisol checked 24 hours after the last dose of hydrocortisone was 444 nmol/L and FT4 was 19.3 pmol/dL. Prolactin had decreased to 0.65 nmol/L. As it appeared her adrenal and thyroid axes were recovering; hydrocortisone and levothyroxine were discontinued. Two weeks later, thyroid function tests off of levothyroxine showed persistent central hypothyroidism (TSH 0.87 mIU/L, FT4 7.7 pmol/L, and TT3 1.25 pmol/L [1.08–3.08]) and therefore, levothyroxine was resumed. A second 250 μg cosyntropin stimulation test was performed to further evaluate the hypothalamic-pituitary-adrenal axis. Baseline cortisol was 182 nmol/L, 30-minute cortisol was 477 nmol/L, and 60-minute cortisol was 571 nmol/L. An overnight metyrapone test was then performed to confirm recovery of the pituitary-adrenal axis. After a late night dose of metyrapone, 35 mg/kg, the patient returned for early morning blood work. Morning ACTH was 62 pmol/L with 11-deoxycortisol level >300 nmol/L, demonstrating normal adrenal function and recovery of the pituitary-adrenal axis. While the shunt was cured by embolization, the requirement for levothyroxine suggested residual anterior pituitary dysfunction.

Although the patient was noted to have joint laxity and skin features suggestive of Ehlers-Danlos syndrome, genetic testing for this condition was negative.

3. Discussion

The cavernous sinuses contain the internal carotid artery, cranial nerves III, IV, V1, V2, and VI, sympathetic fibers, and a venous plexus that drains the confluent veins emanating from anterior and posterior pituitary [13]. Carotid-cavernous fistulas are rare arteriovenous shunts that permit blood flow from the carotid artery into the cavernous sinus. Abnormal flow into the cavernous sinus due to a carotid-cavernous fistula can disrupt normal venous pituitary drainage and can be acute or subacute, depending on the rate of blood flow.

CCFs can be classified into types A, B, C, or D by angiographic criteria [17]. Type A is a direct shunt between the internal carotid artery and the cavernous sinus [17]. Type

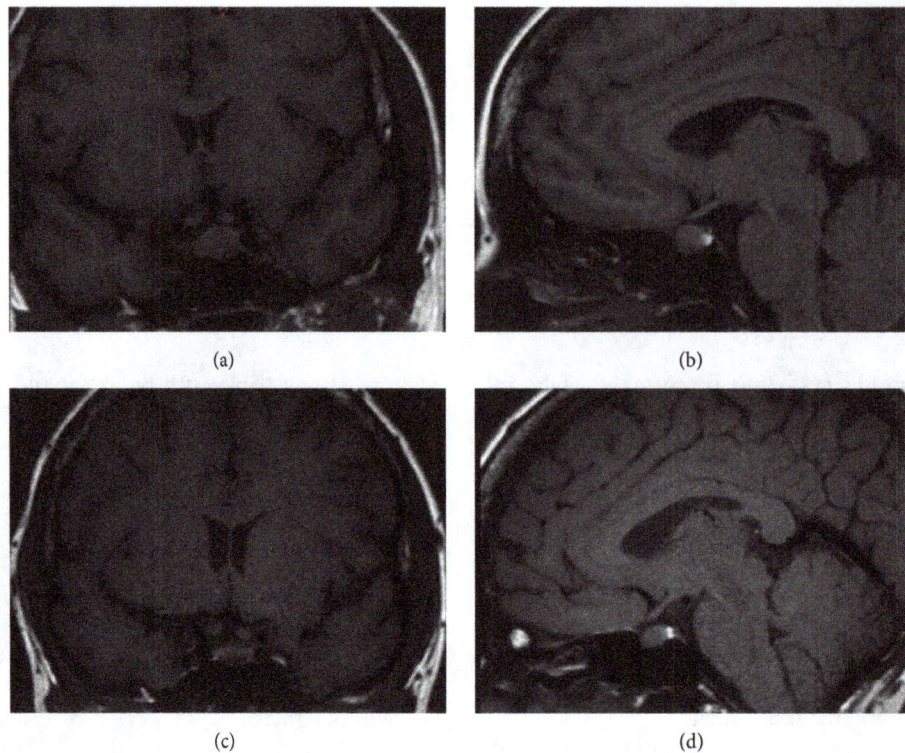

(a)

(b)

(c)

(d)

Figure 2: Sella MRI images showing pituitary enlargement at presentation (a, b) and 4 months after embolization (c, d), showing significant reduction in size.

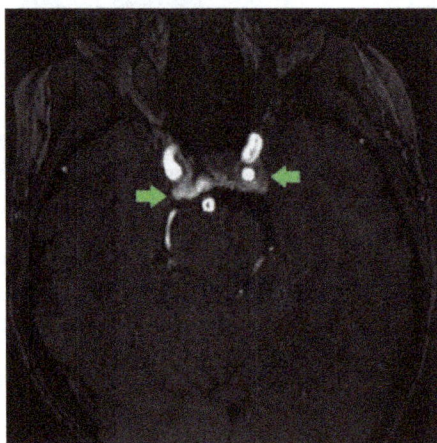

Figure 3: Axial head MRA image demonstrating flow-related contrast from the internal carotid arteries entering the cavernous sinuses (arrows), suggesting bilateral carotid-cavernous fistulas.

the spontaneous or iatrogenic rupture of a carotid aneurysm within the cavernous sinus [17–20]. Signs and symptoms of a high-flow, type A CCF include acute-onset headache, diplopia, proptosis, chemosis, orbital pain, and orbital bruit [18]. Types B, C, and D are low-flow shunts and account for approximately 25% of all CCFs. These typically have symptoms similar to direct CCFs but with a more insidious onset [18]. Patients are often treated for myriad conditions from keratoconjunctivitis to presumed thyroid ophthalmopathy to idiopathic orbital inflammatory disease before the dural shunt is diagnosed. Visual loss is more common with high-flow shunts but can occur in 20–30% of low-flow shunts due to ischemic optic neuropathy, chorioretinal dysfunction, or uncontrolled glaucoma, due to elevated venous pressure and, in turn, intraopthalmic pressure [21]. Predisposing factors in the development of spontaneous CCFs include connective tissue disorders such as Ehlers-Danlos type IV, fibromuscular dysplasia, and pseudoxanthoma elasticum, hypertension, atherosclerosis, and pregnancy [18, 21]. Between 10 and 60% of types B–D shunts can resolve spontaneously, possibly due to thrombosis of the affected area of the cavernous sinus [17]. Noninvasive imaging by CT, MR, or CT/MR angiography is often done as a first-line study in patients with symptoms suggestive of CCF [18]. Findings include cavernous sinus enlargement, proptosis, extraocular muscle enlargement, or superior ophthalmic vein dilation [18]. The gold-standard diagnostic test is catheter cerebral angiography, which carries a morbidity rate of less than 1% when done by experienced neuroradiologists [21]. First-line treatment of CCF is transarterial or transvenous coil or liquid embolization to occlude

B is a dural shunt between the meningeal branches of the internal carotid artery and the cavernous sinus [17]. Type C is a dural shunt between meningeal branches of the external carotid artery and the cavernous sinus [17]. Type D is a simultaneous shunt between the meningeal branches of both the internal and external carotid arteries and the cavernous sinus [17]. Type A CCFs account for approximately 75–80% of all CCFs [18]. They are high-flow shunts that typically result from basilar skull fracture, although they can occur from flow through the fistula while maintaining normal flow in the carotid artery [18]. The possibility of adverse events, however, is significantly higher in patients with underlying connective tissue disorders [21]. In one series of Ehlers-Danlos patients, for example, mortality following treatment of CCFs was as high as 59%, 23% of which was directly due to diagnostic or therapeutic procedures themselves [21, 22]. These patients are at increased risk due friability of vessels, propensity to develop arterial dissections, aneurysms, and rupture due to type III collagen defects in the vessel walls [22, 23].

The largest treatment series of indirect, dural CCF cases described 135 patients, followed for an average of 56 months [24]. Patients were mostly female, 73%, with a mean age of 60 years [24]. Presenting signs and symptoms, in order of declining frequency, were arterialization of conjunctival veins (93%), chemosis (87%), proptosis (81%), diplopia with ophthalmoparesis (68%), cranial bruit (49%), retroorbital headache (34%), elevated intraocular pressure (34%), and diminished visual acuity (31%) [24]. In the patients who underwent endovascular vascular surgery, there was a cure rate of 90% [24].

There are rare case reports in the literature of hypopituitarism caused by carotid artery aneurysms. A recent review by Hanak et. al. [25] identified 40 cases of cerebral aneurysms with intrasellar extension, 90% of which were of the ICA. In this series, endocrinopathy was noted in 57% of unruptured aneurysms, 40% of aneurysms that later ruptured, and 83% of aneurysms associated with concurrent pituitary adenomas. Elevated prolactin was the most common finding (90%), followed by gonadotropin deficiency (82%), ACTH deficiency (70%), and TSH deficiency (60%) [25]. Most cases appear to be due to mass effect directly on the pituitary, stalk, or hypothalamus [25–28]. A series of 4087 patients diagnosed with hypopituitarism estimated that the etiology was from an intrasellar aneurysm in 7 patients or 0.17% [26]. The two prior English-literature case reports of hypopituitarism associated with CCFs also report that direct mass effect from the fistulas on either the stalk [15] or pituitary gland itself [16] was a likely etiology for pituitary dysfunction.

Anterior pituitary dysfunction in this patient, however, would not appear to be due to a space occupying mass as seen with aneurysms. More likely, it was due to impaired venous drainage from the pituitary and/or hypothalamus due to increased venous pressure in the confluent veins and/or portal veins, the latter interfering with conveyance of hypothalamic releasing/inhibitory factors to the anterior pituitary. Venous congestion was also likely responsible for the enlargement of the anterior pituitary. Normalization of cortisol and prolactin following correction of the AV shunt in our patient supports this hypothesis, although her ongoing central hypothyroidism raises concern that this condition can result in permanent deficits. The paucity of cases reporting hypopituitarism [15, 16] in association with CCF suggests that it is either uncommon or an underrecognized complication.

Anterior pituitary enlargement and palsy of cranial nerve VI in this patient initially raised the possibility of an inflammatory disorder of the pituitary or a pituitary adenoma. Indeed, hypophysitis, particularly granulomatous hypophysitis, can present as a sellar mass associated with cranial nerve

palsies due to involvement of the adjacent cavernous sinus [29] as can occur with other inflammatory disorders of the pituitary including Sjögren's syndrome [30, 31], sarcoidosis [32], Wegener's granulomatosis [33, 34], tuberculosis [35], syphilis [36, 37], and fungal infections [38]. Langerhans histiocytosis, germinoma, and lymphoma may also be associated with similar findings but often associated with central diabetes insipidus [39–41]. A distinguishing feature that separates these disorders from individuals with CCF, however, is the presence of proptosis, conjunctival chemosis, and/or corkscrew episcleral blood vessels which occurs in the majority of cases as was present in the case presented herein [18].

In conclusion, patients suspected of having a CCF should have an assessment of anterior pituitary function, particularly of their thyroid and adrenal axes. If deficiencies are detected, these patients should be treated with hormone replacement therapy to minimize the possibility of complications. After a successful intervention, pituitary function should be reassessed because at least some recovery is possible over the ensuing months. Carotid-cavernous fistula should be considered in the differential diagnosis of pituitary enlargement on imaging studies, particularly when associated with orbital congestion.

Acknowledgments

The authors would like to thank Dr. Gregory Lee and Dr. Thomas Hedges of Tufts Medical Center Department of Ophthalmology for external eye images presented with this report.

References

[1] S. M. C. De Sousa, P. Earls, and A. I. McCormack, "Pituitary hyperplasia: case series and literature review of an underrecognised and heterogeneous condition," *Endocrinology, Diabetes & Metabolism Case Reports*, Article ID 150017, 2015.

[2] A. Tsunoda, O. Okuda, and K. Sato, "MR height of the pituitary gland as a function of age and sex: especially physiological hypertrophy in adolescence and in climacterium," *American Journal of Neuroradiology*, vol. 18, no. 3, pp. 551–554, 1997.

[3] J. Zhou, L. Ruan, H. Li, Q. Wang, F. Zheng, and F. Wu, "Addison's disease with pituitary hyperplasia: a case report and review of the literature," *Endocrine*, vol. 35, no. 3, pp. 285–289, 2009.

[4] M. T. McDermott, "Infiltrative disorders of the pituitary gland," in *Diseases of the Pituitary: Diagnosis and Treatment*, M. E. Wierman, Ed., pp. 305–322, Humana Press, Totowa, NJ, USA, 1997.

[5] K. Manaka, N. Makita, and T. Iiri, "Erdheim-Chester disease and pituitary involvement: a unique case and the literature," *Endocrine Journal*, vol. 61, no. 2, pp. 185–194, 2014.

[6] D. M. McLaughlin, W. J. Gray, F. G. C. Jones et al., "Plasmacytoma: an unusual cause of a pituitary mass lesion. A case report and a review of the literature," *Pituitary*, vol. 7, no. 3, pp. 179–181, 2004.

[7] A. Gutenberg, J. J. Bell, I. Lupi et al., "Pituitary and systemic autoimmunity in a case of intrasellar germinoma," *Pituitary*, vol. 14, no. 4, pp. 388–394, 2011.

[8] D. E. Schteingart, R. V. Lloyd, H. Akil et al., "Cushing's syndrome secondary to ectopic corticotropin-releasing hormone-adrenocorticotropin secretion," *The Journal of Clinical Endocrinology & Metabolism*, vol. 63, no. 3, pp. 770–775, 1986.

[9] S. Ezzat, S. L. Asa, L. Stefaneanu et al., "Somatotroph hyperplasia without pituitary adenoma associated with a long standing growth hormone-releasing hormone-producing bronchial carcinoid," *The Journal of Clinical Endocrinology & Metabolism*, vol. 78, no. 3, pp. 555–560, 1994.

[10] S. Melmed, "Acromegaly," *The New England Journal of Medicine*, vol. 355, no. 24, pp. 2558–2573, 2006.

[11] A. Voutetakis, M. Argyropoulou, A. Sertedaki et al., "Pituitary magnetic resonance imaging in 15 patients with prop1 gene mutations: pituitary enlargement may originate from the intermediate lobe," *Journal of Clinical Endocrinology and Metabolism*, vol. 89, no. 5, pp. 2200–2206, 2004.

[12] M. Joubert, R. Verdon, and Y. Reznik, "Transient pituitary enlargement with central hypogonadism secondary to bilateral cavernous sinus thrombosis: pituitary oedema?" *European Journal of Endocrinology*, vol. 160, no. 5, pp. 873–875, 2009.

[13] N. Sato, C. M. Putman, J. C. Chaloupka, B. J. Glenn, F. Vinuela, and G. Sze, "Pituitary gland enlargement secondary to dural arteriovenous fistula in the cavernous sinus: appearance at MR imaging," *Radiology*, vol. 203, no. 1, pp. 263–267, 1997.

[14] Y. Shigematsu, Y. Korogi, M. Kitajima et al., "Abnormal perfusion of the pituitary gland secondary to dural arteriovenous fistulas in the cavernous sinus: dynamic MR findings," *American Journal of Neuroradiology*, vol. 24, no. 5, pp. 930–936, 2003.

[15] A. Goto, Y. Takahashi, M. Kishimoto et al., "Hypopituitarism caused by bilateral internal carotid artery aneurysms with a carotid-cavernous fistula," *Internal Medicine*, vol. 47, no. 8, pp. 815–816, 2008.

[16] S. S. Yarandi, M. A. Khoshnoodi, and P. Chandra, "Hypopituitarism caused by carotid cavernous fistula," *Internal Medicine*, vol. 50, no. 10, pp. 1105–1108, 2011.

[17] D. L. Barrow, R. H. Spector, I. F. Braun, J. A. Landman, S. C. Tindall, and G. T. Tindall, "Classification and treatment of spontaneous carotid cavernous sinus fistulas," *Journal of Neurosurgery*, vol. 62, no. 2, pp. 248–256, 1985.

[18] J. A. Ellis, H. Goldstein, E. S. Connolly Jr., and P. M. Meyers, "Carotid-cavernous fistulas," *Neurosurgical Focus*, vol. 32, no. 5, p. E9, 2012.

[19] W. Mustafa, K. Kadziolka, R. Anxionnat, and L. Pierot, "Direct carotid-cavernous fistula following intracavernous carotid aneurysm treatment with a flow-diverter stent: a case report," *Interventional Neuroradiology*, vol. 16, no. 4, pp. 447–450, 2010.

[20] N. Kobayashi, S. Miyachi, M. Negoro et al., "Endovascular treatment strategy for direct carotid-cavernous fistulas resulting from rupture of intracavernous carotid aneurysms," *American Journal of Neuroradiology*, vol. 24, no. 9, pp. 1789–1796, 2003.

[21] N. R. Miller, "Diagnosis and management of dural carotid-cavernous sinus fistulas," *Neurosurgical Focus*, vol. 23, no. 5, article E13, 2007.

[22] I. Linfante, E. Lin, E. Knott, B. Katzen, and G. Dabus, "Endovascular repair of direct carotid-cavernous fistula in Ehlers-Danlos type IV," *Journal of NeuroInterventional Surgery*, vol. 7, article e3, 2015.

[23] W. I. Schievink, D. G. Piepgras, F. Earnest IV, and H. Gordon, "Spontaneous carotid-cavernous fistulae in Ehlers-Danlos syndrome Type IV. Case report," *Journal of Neurosurgery*, vol. 74, no. 6, pp. 991–998, 1991.

[24] P. M. Meyers, V. V. Halbach, C. F. Dowd et al., "Dural carotid cavernous fistula: definitive endovascular management and long-term follow-up," *American Journal of Ophthalmology*, vol. 134, no. 1, pp. 85–92, 2002.

[25] B. W. Hanak, G. Zada, V. V. Nayar et al., "Cerebral aneurysms with intrasellar extension: a systematic review of clinical, anatomical, and treatment characteristics—a review," *Journal of Neurosurgery*, vol. 116, no. 1, pp. 164–173, 2012.

[26] H. M. Heshmati, V. Fatourechi, S. A. Dagam, and D. G. Piepgras, "Hypopituitarism caused by intrasellar aneurysms," *Mayo Clinic Proceedings*, vol. 76, no. 8, pp. 789–793, 2001.

[27] D. Ding, G. U. Mehta, and K. C. Liu, "Pituitary insufficiency from large unruptured supraclinoid internal carotid artery aneurysm," *British Journal of Neurosurgery*, vol. 28, no. 2, pp. 290–292, 2014.

[28] P. M. Munarriz, I. Paredes, M. Cicuendez, and A. Lagares, "Acute confusional syndrome and hypopituitarism produced by a giant aneurysm of internal carotid artery," *The American Journal of the Medical Sciences*, vol. 346, no. 2, p. 147, 2013.

[29] B. H. M. Hunn, W. G. Martin, S. Simpson Jr., and C. A. Mclean, "Idiopathic granulomatous hypophysitis: a systematic review of 82 cases in the literature," *Pituitary*, vol. 17, no. 4, pp. 357–365, 2014.

[30] V. V. Ashraf, R. Bhasi, R. P. Kumar, and A. S. Girija, "Primary Sjögren's syndrome manifesting as multiple cranial neuropathies: MRI findings," *Annals of Indian Academy of Neurology*, vol. 12, no. 2, pp. 124–126, 2009.

[31] M. Colaci, G. Cassone, A. Manfredi, M. Sebastiani, D. Giuggioli, and C. Ferri, "Neurologic complications associated with Sjögren's disease: case reports and modern pathogenic dilemma," *Case Reports in Neurological Medicine*, vol. 2014, Article ID 590292, 11 pages, 2014.

[32] J. Anthony, G. J. Esper, and A. Ioachimescu, "Hypothalamic-pituitary sarcoidosis with vision loss and hypopituitarism: case series and literature review," *Pituitary*, vol. 19, no. 1, pp. 19–29, 2016.

[33] M. Goyal, W. Kucharczyk, and E. Keystone, "Granulomatous hypophysitis due to Wegener's granulomatosis," *American Journal of Neuroradiology*, vol. 21, no. 8, pp. 1466–1469, 2000.

[34] H. Nishino, F. A. Rubino, R. A. DeRemee, J. W. Swanson, and J. E. Parisi, "Neurological involvement in Wegener's granulomatosis: an analysis of 324 consecutive patients at the Mayo Clinic," *Annals of Neurology*, vol. 33, no. 1, pp. 4–9, 1993.

[35] M. C. Sharma, R. Arora, A. K. Mahapatra, P. Sarat-Chandra, S. B. Gaikwad, and C. Sarkar, "Intrasellar tuberculoma—an enigmatic pituitary infection: a series of 18 cases," *Clinical Neurology and Neurosurgery*, vol. 102, no. 2, pp. 72–77, 2000.

[36] S. Alqahtani, "Acute cranial neuropathies heralding neurosyphilis in a human immunodeficiency virus-infected patient," *American Journal of Case Reports*, vol. 15, pp. 411–415, 2014.

[37] L. Bricaire, C. Van Haecke, S. Laurent-Roussel et al., "The great imitator in endocrinology: a painful hypophysitis mimicking a pituitary tumor," *Journal of Clinical Endocrinology and Metabolism*, vol. 100, no. 8, pp. 2837–2840, 2015.

[38] A. E. Merkler, N. Gaines, H. Baradaran et al., "Direct Invasion of the optic nerves, chiasm, and tracts by Cryptococcus neoformans in an immunocompetent host," *The Neurohospitalist*, vol. 5, no. 4, pp. 217–222, 2015.

[39] P. Makras, C. Samara, M. Antoniou et al., "Evolving radiological features of hypothalamo-pituitary lesions in adult patients with Langerhans cell histiocytosis (LCH)," *Neuroradiology*, vol. 48, no. 1, pp. 37–44, 2006.

[40] D. Belen, A. Çolak, and O. E. Özean, "CNS involvement of Langerhans cell histiocytosis. Report of 23 surgically treated cases," *Neurosurgical Review*, vol. 19, no. 4, pp. 247–252, 1996.

[41] A. Giustina, M. Gola, M. Doga, and E. A. Rosei, "Clinical review 136: primary lymphoma of the pituitary: an emerging clinical entity," *Journal of Clinical Endocrinology and Metabolism*, vol. 86, no. 10, pp. 4567–4575, 2001.

38

A Case of Pneumothorax after Treatment with Lenvatinib for Anaplastic Thyroid Cancer with Lung Metastasis

Haruhiko Yamazaki ⓘ,[1] **Hiroyuki Iwasaki,**[1] **Toshinari Yamashita,**[1] **Tatsuya Yoshida,**[1] **Nobuyasu Suganuma,**[1] **Takashi Yamanaka,**[1] **Katsuhiko Masudo,**[2] **Hirotaka Nakayama,**[3] **Kaori Kohagura,**[3] **Yasushi Rino,**[3] **and Munetaka Masuda**[3]

[1]*Department of Breast and Endocrine Surgery, Kanagawa Cancer Center, Yokohama, Japan*
[2]*Department of Breast and Thyroid Surgery, Yokohama City University Medical Center, Yokohama, Japan*
[3]*Department of Surgery, Yokohama City University School of Medicine, Yokohama, Japan*

Correspondence should be addressed to Haruhiko Yamazaki; h.yamazaki0413@kcch.jp

Academic Editor: John Broom

A 63-year-old man was diagnosed with multiple lung metastases from anaplastic thyroid cancer and received lenvatinib. Follow-up computed tomography on day 34 of lenvatinib treatment showed pneumothorax. The pneumothorax was temporarily improved with chest drainage. However, pleurodesis was performed to treat a relapse of the pneumothorax. Pneumothorax during chemotherapy for a malignant tumor is considered a relatively rare complication. This case is the first documentation that pneumothorax may develop during lenvatinib treatment. The possible development of pneumothorax should be considered when lenvatinib is used in patients with lung metastasis.

1. Introduction

The incidence of anaplastic thyroid carcinoma (ATC) is 1 to 2% of all thyroid malignancies and is less frequent. However, the prognosis is extremely poor and the 1-year survival rate is reported as 18% [1]. Lenvatinib has a high antitumor effect on thyroid cancer including ATC [2, 3]. In general, pneumothorax during chemotherapy for a malignant tumor is considered a relatively rare complication [4]. Cases of pneumothorax after treatment with lenvatinib have not been reported. Here we report a case of pneumothorax after treatment with lenvatinib for ATC with lung metastasis.

2. Case Report

A 63-year-old man with a history of treatment for hypertension, hyperuricemia, benign prostatic hyperplasia, sleep apnea syndrome, and bronchial asthma consulted with a nearby doctor regarding hoarseness and mild swallowing difficulty. Computed tomography (CT) findings suggested thyroid cancer with lung metastases, and he visited our hospital (Figure 1). He was hospitalized on the same day as presentation, and a needle biopsy from thyroid tumor resulted in a diagnosis of anaplastic thyroid cancer (ATC). Lenvatinib (24 mg) was started the day after hospitalization. On day 6 of lenvatinib treatment, CT of the primary tumor and lung metastases showed stable disease. He was discharged with no adverse events. On day 20 of lenvatinib administration, the patient developed grade 3 hand–foot syndrome and the lenvatinib was reduced to 20 mg/day. Follow-up CT on day 34 of lenvatinib treatment showed pneumothorax, and he was urgently hospitalized. The patient's height was 174 cm, weight was 79 kg, body temperature was 36.3°C, and blood oxygen saturation was 98% on room air, and he had no breathing difficulty. His blood test results were as follows: thyroid-stimulating hormone, 9.13 μIU/mL; free triiodothyronine, 2.58 pg/mL; and free thyroxine, 1.01 ng/mL. CT showed right pneumothorax, and air was observed inside part of the lung metastases (Figure 2). We established chest drainage, and the pneumothorax improved the next day.

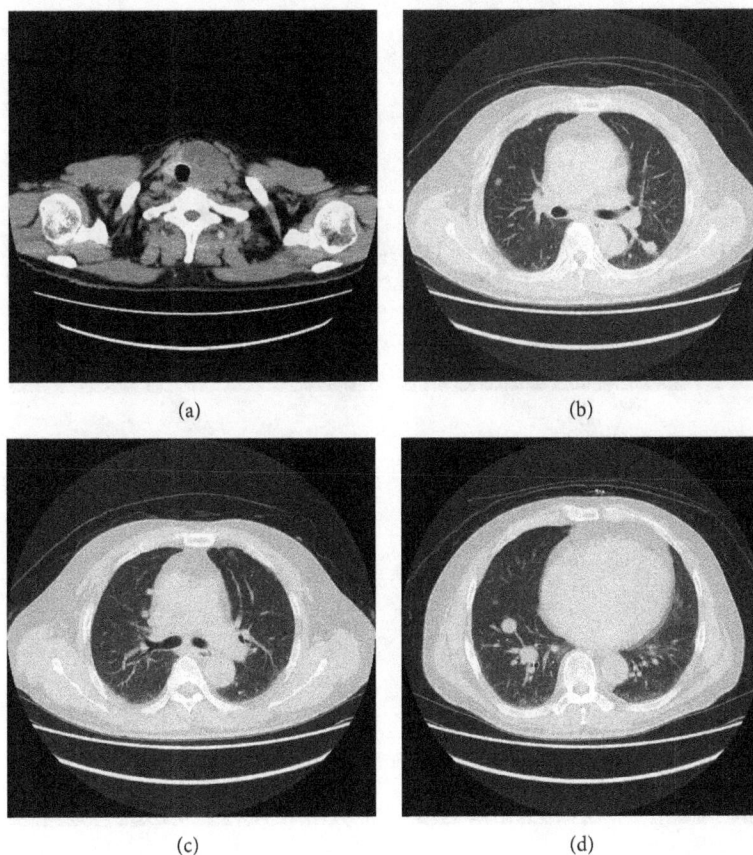

FIGURE 1: (a–d) Computed tomography showed tumor with eggshell calcification of the thyroid left lobe and multiple lung metastases. There were no bulla and bleb.

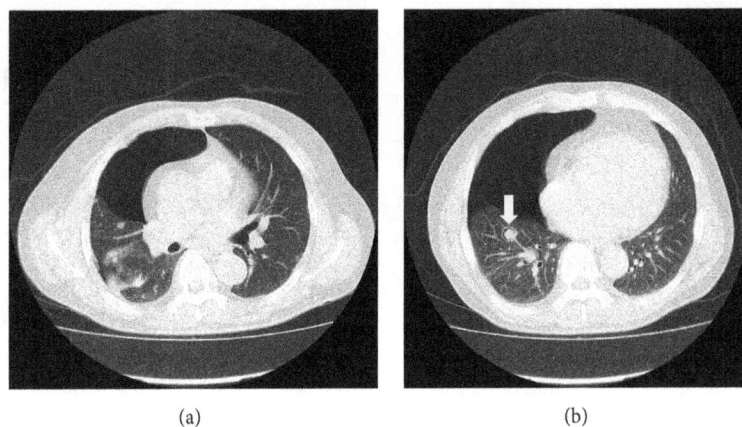

FIGURE 2: (a, b) Follow-up computed tomography on day 34 of lenvatinib start showed the right pneumothorax and the air was recognized inside a part of lung metastases (arrow).

However, his swallowing difficulty became exacerbated, and the lenvatinib was increased to 24 mg/day. The pneumothorax was resolved and he was discharged 3 days after hospitalization. At 19 days after discharge, the lenvatinib was reduced to 20 mg/day because of grade 1 pneumothorax and grade 3 proteinuria. Three days later, the pneumothorax became exacerbated and we reestablished chest drainage after emergency hospitalization. Despite the chest drainage, an air leak persisted and the lenvatinib was reduced to 14 mg/day. However, pleurodesis was performed 10 days after starting chest drainage because of continuing air leakage. We removed the chest drain because the pneumothorax had improved the next day. However, the pneumothorax recurred the same day, and we re-started the chest drainage. We removed the chest drain 5 days later, and he was discharged the next day. CT of the primary tumor on day 73 of lenvatinib treatment showed

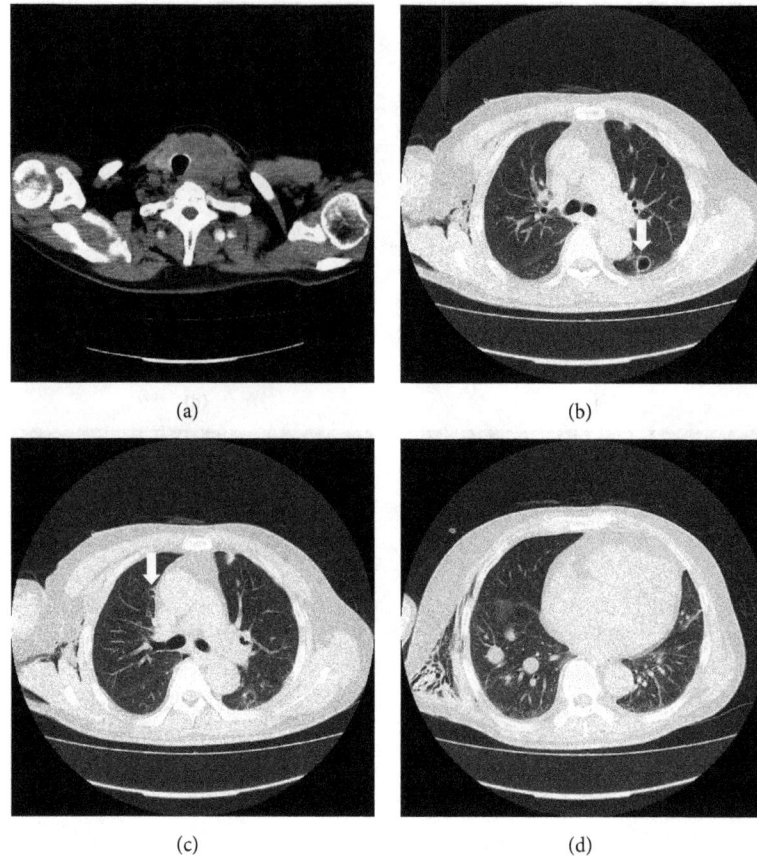

(a)   (b)

(c)   (d)

FIGURE 3: (a–d) Computed tomography on day 73 of lenvatinib start showed that primary tumor was stable disease and there is no recurrence of pneumothorax. Thin wall cavitations were observed in the metastatic lesions (arrow).

stable disease, and the thin-walled cavitations were observed in the metastatic lesions (Figure 3). The patient developed no further recurrences of pneumothorax.

3. Discussion

Lenvatinib is an oral multitargeted tyrosine kinase inhibitor of vascular endothelial growth factors 1, 2, and 3; fibroblast growth factor receptors 1 through 4; platelet-derived growth factor receptor α; and the RET and KIT signaling networks. The SELECT trial and a phase II trial conducted in Japan showed that lenvatinib was effective for unresectable thyroid cancer [2, 3]. In the SELECT trial, hypertension was the most frequent adverse event (67.8%), followed by diarrhea (59.4%) and fatigue (59.0%) [2]. However, the occurrence of pneumothorax was not reported. Primary spontaneous pneumothorax is mainly caused by the rupture of a bleb or of a bulla [5]. In this case, however, the CT before the treatment of lenvatinib did not show such lesion. We observed lesions that caused thin wall cavitation by CT after improvement of pneumothorax, which we hypothesise to be the source of the air leak. In general, pneumothorax during chemotherapy for a malignant tumor is considered a relatively rare complication [4]. The reported incidence rate is relatively high in patients with sarcoma (about 2%) [6].

Various causes of pneumothorax during chemotherapy have been surmised. Yamada et al. [7] classified them as follows: rupture of bullae or blebs directly under the pleura during chemotherapy, formation of bronchopleural fistulas secondary to tumor necrosis, development of pleural lesions secondary to damage to the lung parenchyma induced by chemotherapy or radiation therapy, formation of cavities or emphysematous lesions in the peripheral tissues with subsequent rupture by the check-valve mechanism because of obstruction or stenosis of bronchi due to tumors, and elevation of intrathoracic pressure caused by vomiting as a side effect of chemotherapy, resulting in rupture of the pleura. In this case, air was observed inside part of the lung metastases; therefore, the second mechanism (formation of bronchopleural fistulas secondary to tumor necrosis) was considered to be involved in the onset of pneumothorax. Pneumothorax has also been reported in association with other molecular-targeted drugs, including sunitinib for renal cell cancer [8], pazopanib for soft tissue sarcoma [9], and bevacizumab for colon cancer or breast cancer [10, 11]. These patients also had lung metastasis, and the mechanism of onset was similar to our case. In our case, the pneumothorax temporarily improved with chest drainage, but it subsequently recurred and pleurodesis was performed. The pneumothorax recurred again immediately after pleurodesis and finally improved with chest drainage. The series of treatments took 1 month to complete. In some reported cases, however, the treatment lasted several months [7, 11]. Pleurodesis is an indication for patients who cannot or refuse to undergo surgery [12]. Bleeding tendency and delayed wound healing are adverse effects of lenvatinib, so withdrawal of the medication is necessary before surgery. Our patient had a risk of sudden death due to the increase in size of the primary lesion, and long-term withdrawal of lenvatinib was difficult. Therefore, surgery was not considered a treatment option. In some cases, it is necessary to reduce, withdraw, or change the patient's anticancer drugs to allow for treatment of pneumothorax; during that time, however, the primary lesion may progress. The possible onset of pneumothorax must be considered when lenvatinib is used for thyroid cancer in patients with lung metastasis.

Acknowledgments

The authors thank Angela Morben, DVM, ELS, from Edanz Group (https://www.edanzediting.com/ac) for editing a draft of this manuscript.

References

[1] I. Sugitani, A. Miyauchi, K. Sugino, T. Okamoto, A. Yoshida, and S. Suzuki, "Prognostic factors and treatment outcomes for anaplastic thyroid carcinoma: ATC research consortium of Japan cohort study of 677 patients," *World Journal of Surgery*, vol. 36, no. 6, pp. 1247–1254, 2012.

[2] M. Schlumberger, M. Tahara, L. J. Wirth et al., "Lenvatinib versus placebo in radioiodine-refractory thyroid cancer," *The New England Journal of Medicine*, vol. 372, no. 7, pp. 621–630, 2015.

[3] S. Takahashi, M. Tahara, N. Kiyota et al., "Phase II study of lenvatinib (LEN), a multi-targeted tyrosine kinase inhibitor, in patients (PTS) with all histologic subtypes of advanced thyroid cancer (differentiated, medullary and anaplastic)," *Annals of Oncology*, vol. 25, no. suppl_4, pp. iv340–iv356, 2014.

[4] R. S. Lai, R. P. Perng, and S. C. Chang, "Primary lung cancer complicated with pneumothorax," *Japanese Journal of Clinical Oncology*, vol. 22, no. 3, pp. 194–197, 1992.

[5] R. d. Lyra, "Etiology of primary spontaneous pneumothorax," *Jornal Brasileiro de Pneumologia*, vol. 42, no. 3, pp. 222–226, 2016.

[6] J. B. Hoag, M. Sherman, Q. Fasihuddin, and M. E. Lund, "A comprehensive review of spontaneous pneumothorax complicating sarcoma," *Chest*, vol. 138, no. 3, pp. 510–518, 2010.

[7] N. Yamada, N. Abe, K. Usui et al., "Clinical analysis of 12 cases of pneumothorax during intensive chemotherapy for malignant neoplasms," *Gan To Kagaku Ryoho*, vol. 37, pp. 1519–1523, 2010.

[8] A. Katta, M. J. Fesler, A. Tan, G. Vuong, and J. M. Richart, "Spontaneous bilateral pneumothorax in metastatic renal cell carcinoma on sunitinib therapy," *Cancer Chemotherapy and Pharmacology*, vol. 66, no. 2, pp. 409–412, 2010.

[9] Y. Nakahara, T. Fukui, K. Katono et al., "Pneumothorax during Pazopanib Treatment in Patients with Soft-Tissue Sarcoma: Two Case Reports and a Review of the Literature," *Case Reports in Oncology*, vol. 10, no. 1, pp. 333–338, 2017.

[10] T. Iida, T. Yabana, S. Nakagaki, T. Adachi, and Y. Kondo, "A rupture of a lung metastatic lesion of colon cancer, leading to pneumothorax caused by bevacizumab," *Internal Medicine*, vol. 55, no. 21, pp. 3125–3129, 2016.

[11] T. Makino, S. Kudo, and T. Ogata, "Pneumothorax after treatment with bevacizumab-containing chemotherapy for breast cancer - a case report," *Gan To Kagaku Ryoho*, vol. 41, pp. 233–235, 2014.

[12] A. MacDuff, A. Arnold, and J. Harvey, "Management of spontaneous pneumothorax: British Thoracic Society pleural disease guideline 2010," *Thorax*, vol. 65, no. 2, pp. ii18–ii31, 2010.

A Case of Cushing's Syndrome due to Ectopic Adrenocorticotropic Hormone Secretion from Esthesioneuroblastoma with Long Term Follow-Up after Resection

Leslee N. Matheny ⓘ,[1] Sudipa Sarkar,[2] Hanyuan Shi ⓘ,[3] Jiun-Ruey Hu,[4] Hannah Harmsen,[5] Ty W. Abel,[5] Shubhada M. Jagasia,[1] and Shichun Bao ⓘ[1]

[1]Vanderbilt University Medical Center, Division of Endocrinology, Department of Medicine, Vanderbilt University, 1215 21st Avenue South, Nashville, TN 37232, USA

[2]Johns Hopkins University School of Medicine, Division of Endocrinology, Diabetes and Metabolism, 5501 Hopkins Bayview Circle, Baltimore, MD 21224, USA

[3]Vanderbilt University Medical Center, Department of Surgery, Vanderbilt University, 1161 21st Avenue South, Nashville, TN 37232, USA

[4]Vanderbilt University School of Medicine, 2215 Garland Ave, Nashville, TN 37232, USA

[5]Vanderbilt University Medical Center, Department of Pathology, Microbiology and Immunology, 1161 21st Avenue South, Nashville, TN 37232, USA

Correspondence should be addressed to Shichun Bao; shichun.bao@vanderbilt.edu

Academic Editor: Eli Hershkovitz

We present a case of a 52-year-old male who developed Cushing's Syndrome due to ectopic adrenocorticotrophic hormone (ACTH) secretion from a large esthesioneuroblastoma (ENB) of the nasal sinuses. The patient initially presented with polyuria, polydipsia, weakness, and confusion. Computed tomography scan of the head and magnetic resonance imaging showed a 7 cm skull base mass centered in the right cribriform plate without sella involvement. Work-up revealed ACTH-dependent hypercortisolemia, which did not suppress appropriately after high-dose dexamethasone. Subsequent imaging of the chest, abdomen, and pelvis did not reveal other possible ectopic sources of ACTH secretion besides the ENB. His hospital course was complicated by severe hypokalemia and hyperglycemia before successful surgical resection of the tumor, the biopsy of which showed ENB. Postoperatively, his ACTH level dropped below the limit of detection. In the ensuing 4 months, he underwent adjuvant chemoradiation with carboplatin and docetaxel with good response and resolution of hypokalemia and hyperglycemia, with no sign of recurrence as of 30 months postoperatively. His endogenous cortisol production is rising but has not completely recovered.

1. Introduction

Esthesioneuroblastoma (ENB), or olfactory neuroblastoma, is a tumor of the nasal and paranasal sinuses, derived from the olfactory neuroepithelium [1, 2] and represents only 3–6% of all cancers in the nasal cavity and paranasal sinuses [2, 3]. Paraneoplastic ENB is rare and only has been reported in a handful of cases in the literature. One type of paraneoplastic ENB is ectopic adrenocorticotrophic hormone (ACTH) secretion. Ectopic ACTH secretion in ENB is highly unusual and can lead to severe symptoms of Cushing's Syndrome (CS) including persistent hypertension, hypokalemia, hyperglycemia, and opportunistic infections. It is important to be cognizant and recognize the pathophysiology, work-up, and treatment of ACTH-secreting ENB in its varied presentations. We present a case here for that discussion.

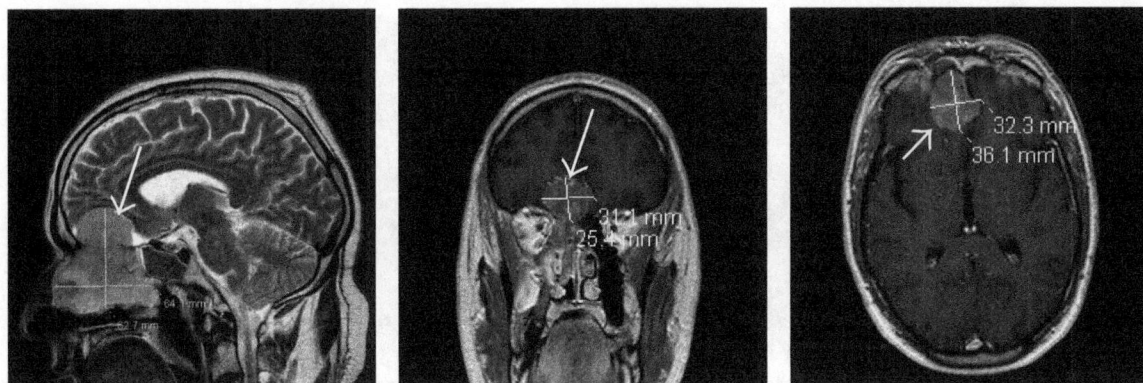

(a) Magnetic resonance imaging scan of the head with contrast, T1, sagittal, coronal, and axial views. These demonstrate a 7.5 × 4.1 × 3.4 cm skull base mass in the right cribriform plate (white arrow)

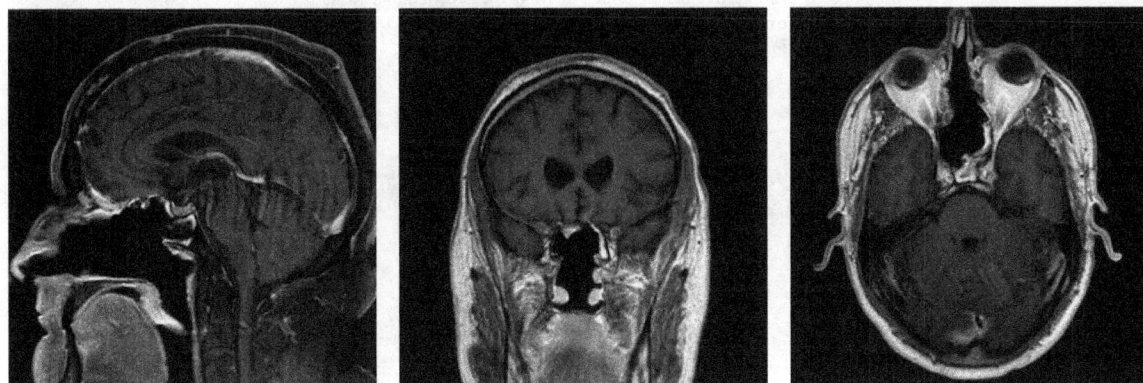

(b) Twenty-eight months later, magnetic resonance imaging scan of the head with contrast and T1 view showing posttreatment changes in anterior cranial fossa with no appreciable change in appearance of dural thickening along cribriform plate and anterior cranial fossa. There is some encephalomalacia and bilateral frontal lobes are unchanged from previous scans

FIGURE 1

2. Case Presentation

A 52-year-old Caucasian male with a past medical history of hypertension presented to our hospital for planned resection of a large skull base mass of the right cribriform plate by the neurosurgery service. He had initially presented at an outside hospital with anosmia and right nasal airway obstruction. He was diagnosed with new onset diabetes mellitus. Computed tomography (CT) scan of the head and magnetic resonance imaging (MRI) of the face revealed a 7.5 × 4.1 × 3.4 cm mass of the right cribriform plate, extending intracranially into the right anterior cranial fossa and displacing the frontal lobe with no sellar involvement. Imaging at our center confirmed the findings (Figure 1(a)). However, on the planned day of procedure, his labs were significant for severe hypokalemia with a potassium of 2.0 mmol/L (normal range: 3.3–4.8) and metabolic alkalosis with arterial pH of 7.64 (7.35–7.45) and serum HCO_3^- of 44 mmol/L (21–29). Surgery was postponed, and the endocrinology service was consulted. It was noted that the patient had been experiencing several weeks of severe weakness, polyuria, and more than 20 pounds of weight loss before the scheduled operation. He was initially treated with oral and intravenous potassium chloride (KCl), but his serum potassium continued to be refractory to acute repletion. In

addition, he had increased insulin requirement to control his serum glucose levels.

As part of his hypokalemia work-up, he was found to have a significantly elevated random plasma cortisol of 1851 nmol/L and plasma ACTH of 152 pmol/L (1.5–11.2). 24-hour urine free cortisol was also grossly elevated at 32,027 nmol/day (<165). His renin and aldosterone levels were normal. His TSH was also normal. Thus, CS was suspected, and imaging was ordered to locate possible sources. CT scan of his chest, abdomen, and pelvis noted bilateral adrenal enlargement, but no distinct nodules and no apparent sources of ACTH secretion were found. This raised the possibility of ENB being the ectopic source. High-dose (8 mg) dexamethasone suppression testing was performed, with the next-day morning cortisol of 1895 nmol/L, which was not suppressed at all, and ACTH was still elevated at 75.7 pmol/L. He continued to be aggressively treated with KCl. Eplerenone, magnesium oxide, and ketoconazole were also added. On day 5, his potassium was stabilized in the low-normal range. He was discharged on day 6, with a plan for a definitive resection of the tumor in 3 weeks, after the Christmas and New Year holidays.

However, the patient was readmitted 3 days later, for confusion, hypotension, and continued hypokalemia

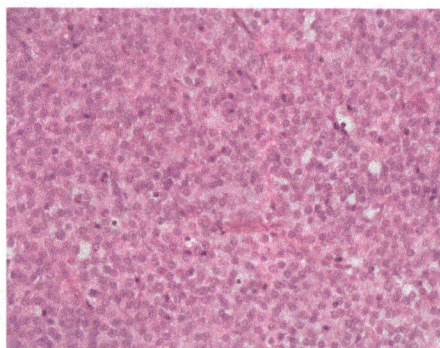

(a) The skull base tumor, measuring 3.5 × 3.0 × 2.0 cm in aggregate. On hematoxylin and eosin (H&E) staining, the tumor is composed of small, round, uniform cells with stippled chromatin and distinct but inconspicuous nucleoli, growing in a diffuse and lobular pattern within a neurofibrillary matrix

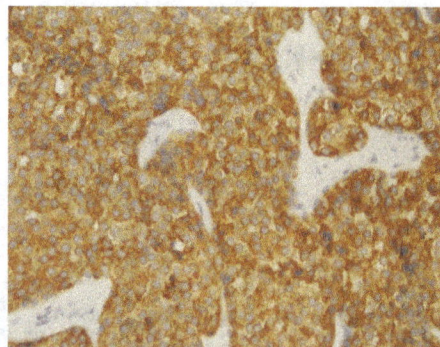

(b) An immunohistochemical stain against synaptophysin, a neuroendocrine marker, shows diffuse, strong cytoplasmic positivity within tumor cells, confirming the neuroendocrine nature of this esthesioneuroblastoma

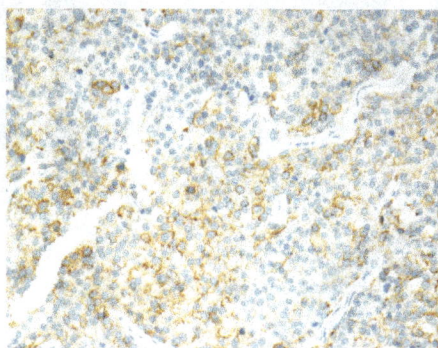

(c) Immunochemistry shows patchy expression of ACTH in the tumor cells (original magnification 400x)

FIGURE 2: Histology staining of tumor.

refractory to his oral potassium medications. He was once again aggressively potassium repleted, and surgery was performed a week later. A bifrontal craniotomy was performed by the neurosurgery team and bilateral maxillary antrostomy, ethmoidectomy, and sphenoidotomy were performed by otolaryngology along with resection of the tumor under endoscopic guidance. The mass was revealed to be a mixed-consistency lesion eroding through the anterior right planum extending through the dura. Intraoperative biopsy showed that the tumor contained lobular growth of small round cells with uniform hyperchromatic chromatin, inconspicuous nucleoli, and scant fibrillary cytoplasm, with rare mitotic figures present (Figure 2(a)). The cells stained positive for chromogranin, synaptophysin, and CD56 on histology, with S100 highlighting the periphery of the clusters (Figure 2(b)). Final confirmation was done with ACTH-staining, which was positive in the tumor cells (Figure 2(c)). The superior septum and anterior inferior septum were involved by tumor, but the tumor was not present on deeper permanent sections.

The postoperative course was uncomplicated, with decreasing daily potassium and insulin requirements and resolution of metabolic alkalosis (Table 1). He no longer required ketoconazole or eplerenone but needed glucocorticoid for central adrenal insufficiency as ACTH dropped to undetectable level at < 1 pmol/L the day after surgery (Table 2). Shortly after, the patient underwent adjuvant chemotherapy with carboplatin and docetaxel as well as intensity-modulated radiation therapy for 7 weeks. He was treated on maintenance doses of dexamethasone 0.5 mg daily and then 0.25 mg daily and eventually tapered down to hydrocortisone 15 mg daily for his adrenal insufficiency. He was tapered off insulin 3 months after surgery, with good diabetes control on metformin 500 mg twice daily alone. He was determined to be in complete remission as of his most recent visit to medical oncology, and MRI scans of the brain and face have been negative for recurrence 28 months after the initial resection (Figure 1(b)). Although his hypokalemia has resolved, his endogenous cortisol production is improving but has not yet recovered completely (Figure 3). ACTH stimulation tests revealed that stimulated cortisol at 60 minutes was 52.4 nmol/L at 3 months, 209.7 nmol/L at 9 months, 234.5 nmol/L at 12 months, 231.7 nmol/L at 16 months, and 364.1 nmol/L at 26 months, with normal cut-off being greater than 500 nmol/L.

TABLE 1: Hospital course.

Laboratory	Day	1	2	3	4	5	6*	9**	10–17	18§	19–26§§
K+ (mmol/L)		2.0	1.9	2.2	2.8	3.4	3.6	2.3	2.5–3.7	3.2	3.1
HCO3– (mmol/L)		44	38	39	32	29	35	35	21–29	31	27
pH		7.64								7.56	7.55
Treatments											
KCl (mEq)		100	200	260	280	200	80	120	(258)	810	(135)
Insulin (Units)		68	111	124	131	153	148	138	(115)	180	(54)
Eplerenone (mg)			25	75	125	150	50				
Ketoconazole (mg)						200	200		(350)		
Dexamethasone (mg)										8	(0.9)

* Patient discharged on day 6 with eplerenone 25 mg twice a day, ketoconazole 200 mg twice a day, KCl 40 mEq four times a day, Lantus 50 units daily, and Lispro 28 units three times a day with meals plus sliding scale. ** Patient readmitted. §Surgical operation (in italic font). §§Patient discharged on day 26, postoperative day 8 on dexamethasone 0.5 mg daily, Lantus 20 units daily, and Lispro 10 units three times a day with meals plus sliding scale. The numbers in parentheses represent the average amount per day over time interval.

TABLE 2: Hormonal changes.

Hormone	Day	2	5	9	19*–26	57	120	214	302	382	495	713	810
Cort-S (60 min)						30	215	243	210	276	235	232	364
Cort-S (30 min)						22	179	229	168	235	204	212	312
Random cortisol		1846	1895	1868		52	141	168	25	160	149	124	141
Plasma ACTH (0–13 pmol/L)		128	76		<1	<1	5	4	1	3	6	6	6
Treatments (per day)													
Hydrocortisone												15 mg →	
Dexamethasone						0.5		0.25 mg					

* Day 19 was postoperative day 1; patient was discharged on day 26. Cort-S = cortisol levels during ACTH stimulation test. Normal stimulated cortisol levels should be >500 nmol/L when measured 60 min after intravenous administration of 0.25 mg ACTH.

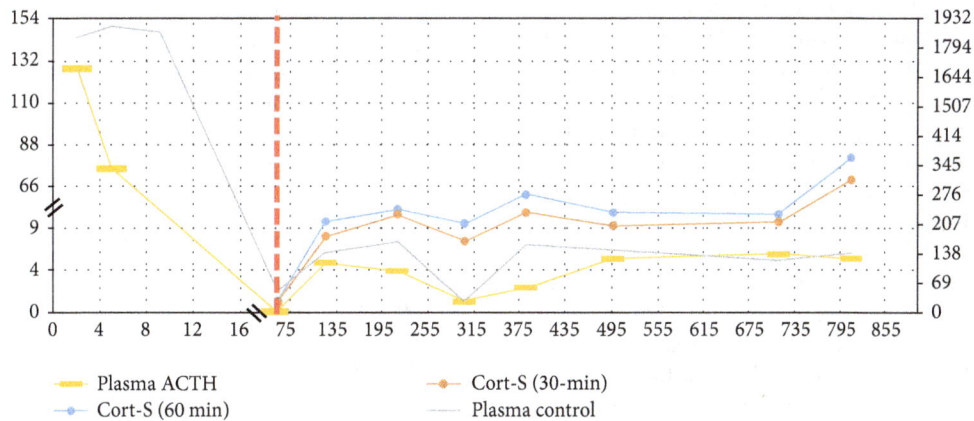

FIGURE 3: Cortisol and ACTH changes before and after operation. The x-axis details the day since initial admission to our hospital. Day 19 or the red line is the resection of the esthesioneuroblastoma. The left y-axis is the level of plasma adrenocorticotropic hormone (ACTH (pmol/L)); the right y-axis is the level of plasma cortisol (Cort-S (nmol/L)). At his outpatient follow-up, 0.25 mg ACTH stimulation tests were done in clinic with assessment of endogenous cortisol production (plasma cortisol level measured at baseline and 30 and 60 minutes after ACTH stimulation).

3. Discussion

This patient was diagnosed with ectopic ACTH syndrome (EAS) based on the preoperative findings of high plasma ACTH concentration, random serum cortisol, and 24-hour urinary cortisol. Other ectopic sources were ruled out by CT scan. At this point, it was strongly suggested that the ENB (Kadish stage B involving two paranasal sinuses) was the source of the ectopic ACTH [4]. Based on these findings and his deteriorating condition, he was emergently taken for resection of the ENB. Pathology of the tumor confirmed synaptophysin positivity on stain, which indicated this was indeed a neuroendocrine neoplasm [5]. This was further confirmed by positive ACTH-staining. Along with the clinical, histological findings and the subsequent improvement in his condition after resection, we confirmed the diagnosis of ectopic ACTH-secreting esthesioneuroblastoma. During his postoperative course, his potassium requirements significantly decreased and he no longer required medication for potassium repletion. Thirty months after resection, the patient still suffers from secondary adrenal insufficiency, but his endogenous cortisol production is improving. He has had no tumor recurrence based on the last surveillance.

Our report demonstrates an unusual presentation of CS due to ectopic ACTH secretion from ENB and adds key data to the literature concerning this rare condition. There are fewer than 25 cases in the literature. We describe an EAS-ENB with comprehensive follow-up up to 30 months after resection, which is one of the longest follow-up periods among studies to date [6, 7]. Our extensive reporting of the initial hospital course and measurements of hypocortisolism after resection has not previously been described.

Our patient required multiple medication dosage adjustments in order to manage his hypokalemia, including oral and intravenous KCl and magnesium, as well as antimineralocorticoid such as eplerenone and steroidogenesis inhibitors such as ketoconazole. These were titrated to give him low-normal potassium levels and to relieve symptoms of muscle weakness and numbness. Other case reports have described usage of metyrapone, etomidate, mitotane, and mifepristone as steroidogenesis inhibitors [8]. As described in our report, this was not enough and he was readmitted to the hospital with severe weakness from electrolyte derangements and altered mental status, where definitive treatment per surgery was emergently performed. In addition, we also saw a significant increase in the patient's insulin requirements that eventually decreased to preadmission units after tumor resection.

The patient was placed on different corticosteroid (dexamethasone and later hydrocortisone) for central adrenal insufficiency the months after tumor resection. Baseline ACTH and cortisol levels remained to be low-normal in our patient. He failed all his ACTH stimulation tests so far (cortisol level <500 nmol/L 60 min after 0.25 mg ACTH stimulation) but has had improvement of stimulated cortisol. The patient does not have clinical symptoms of adrenal insufficiency such as weight loss, cardiovascular collapse, and hypoglycemia. The chronic massive production of ectopic ACTH from EAS has suppressed his endogenous long term cortisol production (over 30 months). Central adrenal insufficiency usually only requires glucocorticoid replacement, not mineralocorticoid, with hydrocortisone preferred as the most physiological option [9].

In conclusion, we report a case of olfactory neuroblastoma with ectopic ACTH secretion that was treated with resection and adjuvant chemoradiation. Given the paucity of this diagnosis, little is known about how best to treat these patients and how best to screen for complications such as adrenal insufficiency and follow-up. Our case adds more data for better understanding of this disease.

Acknowledgments

The authors would like to thank the entire hospital team for their care for this patient and those who continue to support his recovery from this tumor.

References

[1] P. Dulguerov, A. S. Allal, and T. C. Calcaterra, "Esthesioneuroblastoma: a meta-analysis and review," *The Lancet Oncology*, vol. 2, no. 11, pp. 683–690, 2001.

[2] D. Jethanamest, L. G. Morris, A. G. Sikora, and D. I. Kutler, "Esthesioneuroblastoma: a population-based analysis of survival and prognostic factors," *JAMA Otolaryngology–Head & Neck Surgery*, vol. 133, no. 3, pp. 276–280, 2007.

[3] D. M. Mintzer, S. Zheng, M. Nagamine, J. Newman, and M. Benito, "Esthesioneuroblastoma (olfactory neuroblastoma) with ectopic ACTH syndrome: A multidisciplinary case presentation from the Joan Karnell Cancer Center of Pennsylvania Hospital," *The Oncologist*, vol. 15, no. 1, pp. 51–58, 2010.

[4] A. Morita, M. J. Ebersold, K. D. Olsen, R. L. Foote, J. E. Lewis, and L. M. Quast, "Esthesioneuroblastoma: prognosis and management," *Neurosurgery*, vol. 32, no. 5, pp. 706–714, 1993.

[5] B. Wiedenmann, W. W. Franke, C. Kuhn, R. Moll, and V. E. Gould, "Synaptophysin: a marker protein for neuroendocrine cells and neoplasms," *Proceedings of the National Acadamy of Sciences of the United States of America*, vol. 83, no. 10, pp. 3500–3504, 1986.

[6] L. A. Cecenarro, E. T. Rodrigo Fantón, P. Estario et al., "An infrequent presentation of esthesioneuroblastoma with ectopic ACTH syndrome," *Revista argentina de endocrinología y metabolismo*, vol. 51, no. 4, pp. 192–196, 2014.

[7] I. Hodish, T. J. Giordano, M. N. Starkman, and D. E. Schteingart, "Location of ectopic adrenocortical hormone-secreting tumors causing Cushing's syndrome in the paranasal sinuses," *Head & Neck*, vol. 31, no. 5, pp. 699–706, 2009.

[8] B. M. Biller, A. B. Grossman, P. M. Stewart, S. Melmed, X. Bertagna, J. Bertherat et al., "Treatment of adrenocorticotropin-dependent Cushing's syndrome: a consensus statement," *The Journal of Clinical Endocrinology & Metabolism*, vol. 93, no. 7, pp. 2454–2462, 2008.

[9] E. Charmandari, N. C. Nicolaides, and G. P. Chrousos, "Adrenal insufficiency," *The Lancet*, vol. 383, pp. 2152–2167, 2014.

40

A False Positive I-131 Metastatic Survey Caused by Radioactive Iodine Uptake by a Benign Thymic Cyst

Avneet K. Singh,[1] Adina A. Bodolan,[2] and Matthew P. Gilbert[3]

[1]Department of Medicine, The Robert Larner, M.D. College of Medicine at The University of Vermont, Burlington, VT, USA
[2]Department of Pathology and Laboratory Medicine, The Robert Larner, M.D. College of Medicine at The University of Vermont, Burlington, VT, USA
[3]Division of Endocrinology and Diabetes, The Robert Larner, M.D. College of Medicine at The University of Vermont, Burlington, VT, USA

Correspondence should be addressed to Matthew P. Gilbert; matthew.gilbert@vtmednet.org

Academic Editor: Carlo Capella

Thyroid carcinoma is the most common endocrine malignancy in the United States with increasing incidence and diagnosis but stable mortality. Differentiated thyroid cancer rarely presents with distant metastases and is associated with a low risk of morbidity and mortality. Despite this, current protocols recommend remnant ablation with radioactive iodine and evaluation for local and distant metastasis in some patients with higher risk disease. There are several case reports of false positive results of metastatic surveys that are either normal physiologic variants or other pathological findings. Most false positive findings are associated with tissue that has physiologic increased uptake of I-131, such as breast tissue or lung tissue; pathological findings such as thymic cysts are also known to have increased uptake. Our case describes a rare finding of a thymic cyst found on a false positive I-131 metastatic survey. The patient was taken for surgical excision and the final pathology was a benign thymic cyst. Given that pulmonary metastases of differentiated thyroid cancer are rare, thymic cysts, though also rare, must be part of the differential diagnosis for false positive findings on an I-131 survey.

1. Case Description

A 61-year-old female was found to have a palpable thyroid nodule on routine physical examination by her primary care physician. The patient was then referred for a thyroid ultrasound which showed a 2.1 cm, left-sided thyroid nodule. The patient underwent an ultrasound guided fine needle aspiration (FNA) biopsy which revealed a papillary thyroid carcinoma. The patient was referred to ENT and subsequently had a total thyroidectomy. She was referred to our endocrine clinic for postsurgical management of her T1b N1a MX stage 3 papillary thyroid carcinoma 4 weeks after total thyroidectomy. The tumor size was 1.7 cm in maximum diameter and was unifocal. At the time of surgery, the surgical margins were positive and focal lymphovascular invasion was observed with 1 out of 6 dissected lymph nodes positive for metastatic disease. The patient was prepared for radioactive iodine remnant ablation with a low iodine

diet and thyrotropin alfa injections. An initial diagnostic SPECT/CT (Philips Precedence 16P) scan was performed 24 hours after administration of 5.3 mCi of Iodine-123 (I-123). The scan showed uptake in the left posterior thyroid bed and anteriorly at the level of the hyoid bone, both likely representing residual thyroid tissue. Physiologic uptake was also noted in the salivary glands, nasopharyngeal mucosa, and gastrointestinal tract. Additionally, a large (8 cm × 9 cm × 8 cm) heterogeneous left anterior mediastinal mass with mixed solid and cystic architecture was noted. This mass did not demonstrate uptake of the I-123 tracer (Figures 1(a) and 1(b)). A CT-guided biopsy of the mass returned only hemorrhagic material. Serum thyroglobulin tumor marker was found to be low at 0.3 ng/dL and TSH was >125 uIU/mL, which suggested the mass was not metastatic thyroid cancer. Based on these laboratory findings, it was decided to continue with ablation therapy and 157 mCi of Sodium Iodide-131 (I-131) was administered to the patient. Posttreatment

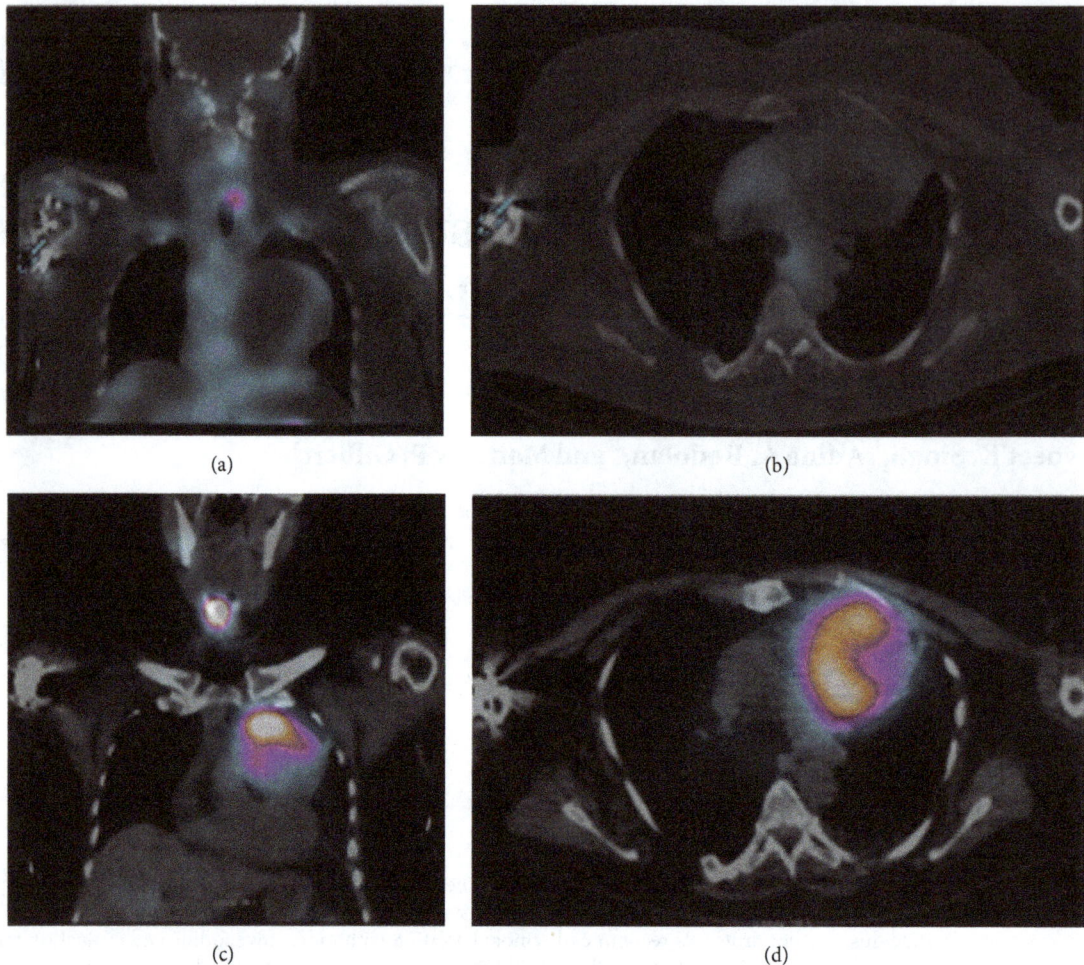

(a)

(b)

(c)

(d)

FIGURE 1: An initial diagnostic SPECT/CT scan was performed 24 hours after administration of 5.3 mCi of Iodine-123. There is uptake in the left, posterior thyroid bed and anteriorly at the level of the hyoid bone. Physiologic uptake was noted in the salivary glands, nasopharyngeal mucosa, and gastrointestinal tract. A large (8 cm × 9 cm × 8 cm) heterogeneous left anterior mediastinal mass with mixed solid and cystic architecture was noted. This mass did not demonstrate uptake of the Iodine-123 tracer ((a), (b)). Posttreatment SPECT/CT one week later showed uptake of radioactive iodine by the mediastinal mass ((c), (d)).

SPECT/CT one week later showed uptake of radioactive iodine by the mediastinal mass (Figures 1(c) and 1(d)). After a repeat CT-guided biopsy was nondiagnostic, the mass was removed via sternotomy.

Surgical pathology sections demonstrated a multiloculated mass composed of cystic spaces lined by a variety of epithelial types, including areas of low-cuboidal (Figure 2(a)), mucinous columnar with goblet cells (Figure 2(b)), ciliated columnar, and keratinizing stratified squamous epithelium. There was no significant cytological atypia or increased mitotic activity. The intervening stroma was densely fibrotic with patchy chronic inflammation, glandular elements, and numerous hemosiderin-laden macrophages—providing evidence of previous hemorrhage (Figure 2(c)). Grossly, the cystic contents ranged from dark brown, likely due to previous hemorrhage, to clear fluid. Adjacent to the cystic spaces, there was a peripheral remnant of normal involuting thymic tissue showing Hassall corpuscles and associated lymphoid tissue (Figure 2(d)). These findings are consistent with a benign multilocular thymic cyst.

2. Discussion

Thyroid carcinoma is a disease of significant interest in American public health given the increasing trend of diagnosis and incidence with relatively stable mortality [1]. Differentiated thyroid cancer (DTC) is associated with a low risk of morbidity and incidence of distant metastasis is relatively uncommon [2]. Recent statistics indicate patients diagnosed with DTC present with distant metastases in approximately 4.2% of cases [3]. As part of the thyroid carcinoma treatment and surveillance algorithm, postthyroidectomy surveillance and assessment for metastases are still commonly accomplished with I-131 metastatic surveys [4]; however, I-123 scans have increased resolution with improved quality of imaging, often characterizing masses missed on I-131 imaging [2].

Uptake of radioiodine by nonthyroid structures can result from normal expression of the sodium-iodide symporter (NIS), presence of metabolized or physiologically retained radioiodine in body fluids, uptake of radioiodine by inflamed tissues, or contamination. Major pathological mechanisms

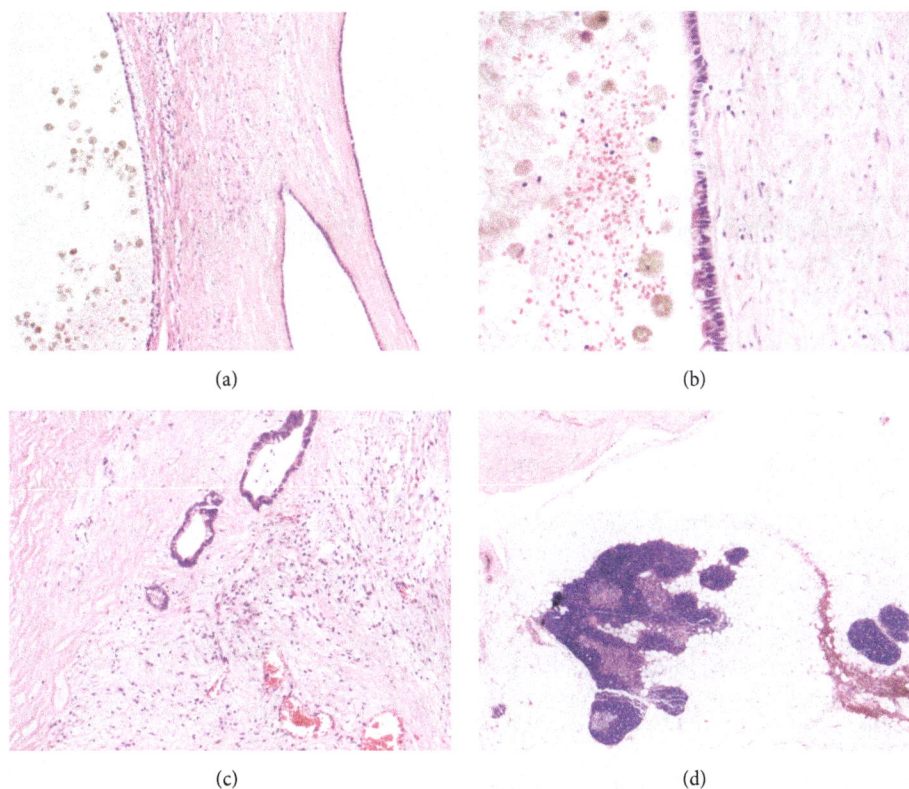

FIGURE 2: Surgical pathology sections of 9.0 cm multilocular thymic cyst. (a) Cyst walls lined by simple low-cuboidal epithelium. (b) Cyst wall lined by simple columnar mucinous epithelium with goblet cells. (c) Fibrous stroma with glandular elements and numerous hemosiderin-laden macrophages. (d) Remnant of normal involuting thymic tissue adjacent to cystic spaces.

of increased I-131 uptake not related to metastases from thyroid carcinoma include those of pathological transudates, inflammation (acute or chronic), and neoplasms of non-thyroid origin [5]; nonpathological variants include tissues with increased secretions in addition to typical expression of NIS and iodine accumulation by lactating breast tissue [2]. Given the complex mechanisms of I-131 uptake, distinguishing between pathological and normal anatomic variants on metastatic survey can prove problematic. Thus, false positive imaging results from I-131 metastatic surveys can and do occur at a rate of 3.85% in patients with DTC [6].

In our case, initial findings on the I-131 posttherapy metastatic survey indicated the presence of possible metastases. However, given the patient's low thyroglobulin tumor marker level following surgery, alternative diagnoses were explored. The initial CT-guided biopsy of the patient's mediastinal mass was an FNA sample. No core biopsies were obtained. In addition, the washout from the FNA was not analyzed for thyroglobulin or PTH. This is a potential limitation of our initial work-up of the patient's abnormal finding on imaging. The patient's serum corrected calcium levels were normal at initial evaluation. The differential diagnoses ranged from acute or chronic inflammatory processes to benign or malignant lesions. Inflammatory lesions localized to the thorax include acute respiratory infections, pulmonary tuberculosis, pulmonary aspergilloma, myocardial infarction, and bronchiectasis. Benign and malignant

lesions include mesothelioma, struma cordis, primary lung cancer, and breast cancer [2]. It is postulated that the pulmonary system is particularly susceptible to false positive I-131 surveys because of the demonstration of iodide secretion into the respiratory tract with elevated blood iodide levels [7].

Functional NIS-mediated radioiodine uptake has been documented in breast tissue, salivary glands, the gastrointestinal tract, and the thymus. There is an association with uptake into serous cavities or cysts such as scrotal hydroceles, lymphoepithelial cysts, ovarian cysts, renal cysts, and pleuropericardial cysts located in the anterior mediastinum [8].

Concentration of radioiodine by the thymus is not commonly observed by whole body scintigraphy, with estimates from a case series in a cohort of 175 female patients suggesting that approximately 1% to 2% of scans may demonstrate thymic uptake [9]. The normal pattern for physiological uptake of radioiodine by the thymus is either diffuse or in a dumbbell shape and is more prevalent in children. Uptake in adults can become more prominent following removal or ablation of the thyroidal tissues and with delayed imaging [2]. Increased thymic uptake has been shown in hyperplasia and carcinoma, but only rarely in cysts [10].

Here we present the rare finding of prominent radioactive iodine uptake by a thymic cyst following total thyroidectomy for papillary thyroid cancer. This patient raises a number of important concepts. First, there are multiple natural sites of radioiodine uptake beyond the thyroid. Second, following excision of a radioiodine avid neoplasm, secondary sites of uptake could represent metastatic disease. Third, there are anatomic variants with iodine avidity that should be considered in the differential diagnosis in cases of aberrant radioiodine uptake. Finally, one must consider the relatively low incidence of pulmonary metastases in DTC. In conclusion, clinicians should consider the array of differential diagnoses for lesions resembling pulmonary metastases from primary differentiated thyroid cancer.

References

[1] L. Davies and H. G. Welch, "Current thyroid cancer trends in the United States," *JAMA Otolaryngology—Head & Neck Surgery*, vol. 140, no. 4, pp. 317–322, 2014.

[2] J. R. Oh and B. C. Ahn, "False-positive uptake on radioiodine whole-body scintigraphy: physiologic and pathologic variants unrelated to thyroid cancer," *American Journal of Nuclear Medicine and Molecular Imaging*, vol. 2, pp. 362–385, 2012.

[3] B. H.-H. Lang, K. P. Wong, C. Y. Cheung, K. Y. Wan, and C.-Y. Lo, "Evaluating the prognostic factors associated with cancer-specific survival of differentiated thyroid carcinoma presenting with distant metastasis," *Annals of Surgical Oncology*, vol. 20, no. 4, pp. 1329–1335, 2013.

[4] M. R. Carlisle, C. Lu, and I. Ross McDougall, "The interpretation of 131I scans in the evaluation of thyroid cancer, with an emphasis on false positive findings," *Nuclear Medicine Communications*, vol. 24, no. 6, pp. 715–735, 2003.

[5] V. Triggiani, V. A. Giagulli, M. Iovino et al., "False positive diagnosis on 131iodine whole-body scintigraphy of differentiated thyroid cancers," *Endocrine Journal*, vol. 53, no. 3, pp. 626–635, 2015.

[6] Q. Jia, Z. Meng, J. Tan et al., "Retrospective imaging study on the diagnosis of pathological false positive iodine-131 scans in patients with thyroid cancer," *Experimental and Therapeutic Medicine*, vol. 10, no. 5, pp. 1995–2001, 2015.

[7] A. J. Fischer, N. J. Lennemann, S. Krishnamurthy et al., "Enhancement of respiratory mucosal antiviral defenses by the oxidation of iodide," *American Journal of Respiratory Cell and Molecular Biology*, vol. 45, no. 4, pp. 874–881, 2011.

[8] B. Shapiro, V. Rufini, A. Jarwan et al., "Artifacts, anatomical and physiological variants, and unrelated diseases that might cause false-positive whole-body 131-I scans in patients with thyroid cancer," *Seminars in Nuclear Medicine*, vol. 30, no. 2, pp. 115–132, 2000.

[9] J. Davidson and I. R. McDougall, "How frequently is the thymus seen on whole-body iodine-131 diagnostic and post-treatment scans?" *European Journal of Nuclear Medicine and Molecular Imaging*, vol. 27, no. 4, pp. 425–430, 2000.

[10] D. Kayano, T. Michigishi, K. Ichiyanagi, A. Inaki, and S. Kinuya, "I-131 uptake in a thymic cyst," *Clinical Nuclear Medicine*, vol. 35, no. 6, pp. 438-439, 2010.

41

Lithium as an Alternative Option in Graves Thyrotoxicosis

Ishita Prakash, Eric Sixtus Nylen, and Sabyasachi Sen

Department of Medicine, Division of Endocrinology & Metabolism, Medical Faculty Associates, The George Washington University, Washington, DC, USA

Correspondence should be addressed to Sabyasachi Sen; ssen1@gwu.edu

Academic Editor: Takeshi Usui

A 67-year-old woman was admitted with signs and symptoms of Graves thyrotoxicosis. Biochemistry results were as follows: TSH was undetectable; FT4 was >6.99 ng/dL (0.7–1.8); FT3 was 18 pg/mL (3–5); TSI was 658% (0–139). Thyroid uptake and scan showed diffusely increased tracer uptake in the thyroid gland. The patient was started on methimazole 40 mg BID, but her LFTs elevated precipitously with features of fulminant hepatitis. Methimazole was determined to be the cause and was stopped. After weighing pros and cons, lithium was initiated to treat her persistent thyrotoxicosis. Lithium 300 mg was given daily with a goal to maintain between 0.4 and 0.6. High dose Hydrocortisone and propranolol were also administered concomitantly. Free thyroid hormone levels decreased and the patient reached a biochemical and clinical euthyroid state in about 8 days. Though definitive RAI was planned, the patient has been maintained on lithium for more than a month to control her hyperthyroidism. Trial removal of lithium results in reemergence of thyrotoxicosis within 24 hours. Patient was maintained on low dose lithium treatment with lithium level just below therapeutic range which was sufficient to maintain euthyroid state for more than a month. There were no signs of lithium toxicity within this time period. *Conclusion.* Lithium has a unique physiologic profile and can be used to treat thyrotoxicosis when thionamides cannot be used while awaiting elective radioablation. Lithium levels need to be monitored; however, levels even at subtherapeutic range may be sufficient to treat thyrotoxicosis.

1. Introduction

Lithium is an alkali metal used to treat bipolar disorder, which has been shown to have significant effects on thyroid function. Lithium carbonate has been used since 1948 to treat manic-depressive states [1], but it was not until the late 1960s and early 1970s that hypothyroidism and goiter were noted as side effects of long-term use of this medication [2, 3]. The rate of hypothyroidism varies from 0 to 47% [4], likely due to differences in definitions, study designs, and duration of lithium treatment. Lithium has been shown to significantly increase TSH as well as TRH-stimulated release of TSH [5]. This leads to hyperplasia of the thyroid gland and a nontender goiter formation. We describe a case of Graves' thyrotoxicosis that was difficult to control due to antithyroidal drug toxicity. In this case, the patient's hyperthyroid state was effectively controlled with lithium for almost two months.

2. Case Report

A 67-year-old female presented with seizures and fever to a different institution. The patient had an extensive medical history, including atypical hemolytic uremic syndrome, seizures, diabetes, and hypertension. Graves' disease was diagnosed during a prior hospitalization approximately 1.5 months earlier. Her TSH was undetectable, and TSI level was 658% (0–139%). Thyroid uptake and scan showed a moderately enlarged gland with diffusely increased tracer uptake at 43% at 24 hours (normal 8–32%). Methimazole and propranolol were started, at the other institution, but the patient developed fulminant hepatitis, which, after extensive workup, was determined to be due to the methimazole. Methimazole was withdrawn when the patient presented to our hospital. She was admitted with history of seizures. She was not tachycardic or hypertensive. She had a temperature of 103.9°F. The Burch-Wartofsky score was 35 [6] and the Glasgow Coma Scale score was 6. She was in normal sinus rhythm and showed no signs or symptoms of heart failure. However, TSH continued to be <0.015 mU/L (0.4–4.7), with elevated FT4 > 6.99 ng/L (0.7–1.8) and FT3 of 18 pg/mL [7–9]. She was started on 300 mg lithium daily which resulted in a serum level of 0.2 mmol/L (therapeutic 0.6–1.2 mmol/L). Other initial labs showed leukocytosis, mild anemia with

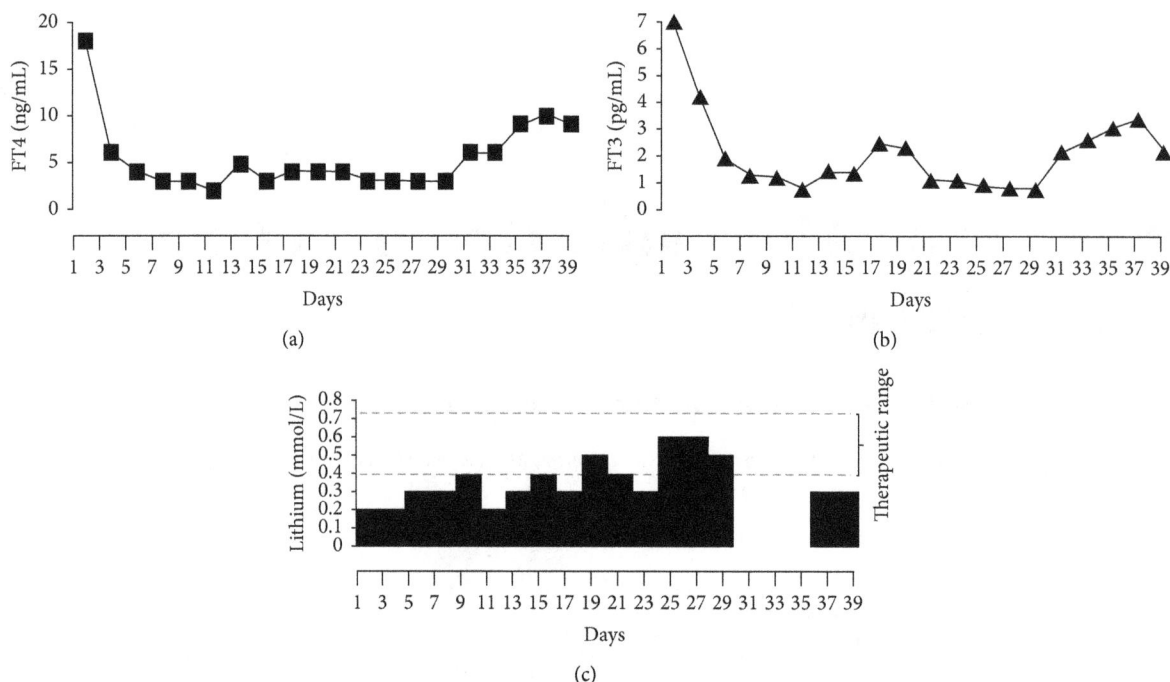

FIGURE 1: Correlation of free thyroid hormone levels and lithium levels over admission period. (a) shows the levels of free T4, followed by the levels of free T3 in (b), and corresponding lithium levels over the period of admission on (c). Note the low lithium level required to maintain *euthyroid* status over the entire course of hospital admission with no side effects.

occasional schistocytes, as well as a mild rise in AST and ALT (transaminitis), indirect bilirubinemia, and elevated lactate dehydrogenase level. The patient was being worked up for recurrent atypical hemolytic anemia and was deemed to be unsuitable to undergo thyroidectomy or to receive radioactive iodine ablation.

After a prolonged debate regarding choice of antithyroid medication we decided to initiate treatment with lithium. We initiated intravenous lithium therapy at 150 mg TID, and the dose was titrated to achieve serum lithium levels in the range of 0.4–0.6 mmol/L.

Over the next 5 days TSH rose to 0.3, FT3 normalized, and FT4 decreased to 1.9 ng/L (Figure 1). We kept following active hormone levels, that is, FT3 and FT4, closely. The patient's mental status improved and she became verbal and coherent and was able to be transferred out of the intensive care unit. High dose glucocorticoids and propranolol, which were started initially, were weaned off and the patient gradually achieved biochemical and clinical euthyroid status. Free hormone levels completely normalized after 8 days of treatment at which time lithium level was 0.3 mmol/L (Figure 1). The lithium dose was stabilized at 300 mg total daily (split into twice daily dosing), to maintain levels between 0.4 and 0.6 mmol/L. The free hormone levels remained normal until 13 days after initial normalization of free hormone level with the lithium levels remaining between 0.4 and 0.6 mmol/L (Figure 1).

At this stage, the patient was moved out of the intensive care unit but remained admitted for observation.

On the 17th day, the patient experienced seizures (11 days after biochemical and clinical stabilization) and required

readmission to intensive care unit with intubation. MRI scan showed features of acute cerebrovascular accident affecting the PCA and ACA territories. Patient remained clinically euthyroid.

We noted increase in FT4 and FT3 levels and at this stage the lithium levels were at 0.3 mmol/L (Figure 1). Lithium dosing was increased to 300 mg in the morning and 150 mg in the evening. On the new higher dose of lithium, the patient achieved biochemical euthyroid status within 4 days, and mental status improved. Patient remained biochemically euthyroid, with lithium level at 0.5–0.6 mmol/L (until 27 days after initial normalization).

On day 28 of admission, lithium was inadvertently stopped in the intensive care unit and patient did not receive lithium for the next 72 hours. Lithium levels reached undetectable levels in plasma and free hormone levels immediately rose again within 24 hours. Lithium was resumed at previous dosing (300 mg in the morning and 150 mg in the evening), with prompt improvement in biochemical thyrotoxicosis.

Over the next few weeks, the patient remained in euthyroid state. The patient was sent to a rehabilitation facility to recover appropriately. While at the center the patient was maintained on twice daily lithium. Her TSH and free T4 remained satisfactory even on a small dose of lithium (at subtherapeutic serum level of lithium) without any fluctuations of her electrolytes and liver enzymes.

3. Discussion

We have described a patient with thyrotoxicosis who developed liver toxicity on thionamide therapy and was subsequently successfully treated with a prolonged low dose of lithium, without any side effects.

Hepatotoxicity due to methimazole tends to be more of a cholestatic process, rather than hepatocellular injury and allergic hepatitis seen with propylthiouracil toxicity [7]. Once hepatotoxicity is established, the medication must be stopped urgently. Generally, an alternative thionamide is not recommended due to the reported cross-reactivity between formulations, which is noted to be as high as 50% [10]. In cases of resistant hyperthyroidism, definitive treatment with radioactive iodine or total thyroidectomy is considered as soon as possible [11]. Plasmapheresis use has been documented in limited case reports of life-threatening, resistant thyrotoxicosis since the 1970s; however there are no randomized trials or guidelines for its use [12].

Other agents such as beta blockers, steroids, iodine, cholestyramine, and lithium have traditionally been used as a temporizing bridge to definitive therapy.

On initial presentation at our center, in our patient, adequate dose of propranolol was used (40 mg three times daily) titrated to heart rate along with 4 mg dexamethasone. Iodine therapy was considered and indeed the initial use of lithium by the outside institution showed hyperthyroid efficacy. However patient on initial presentation was very unstable and we decided to use lithium so as not to prevent the radioiodine option and also the patient had a diagnostic whole body CT scan with contrast few days prior to her admission, which could make further iodine loading redundant. Moreover, our long-term management plan was to utilize the radioiodine concentration ability of lithium to achieve a permanent cure of Graves' disease.

In that scenario lithium appears to be a good alternative. It is highly concentrated in the thyroid follicular cells. It has been shown to inhibit iodine uptake, interfere with tyrosine iodination, change the thyroglobulin structure, and interfere with iodotyrosine synthesis [13]. Lithium is also known to interfere with the sodium-iodide symporter and block iodine uptake into the follicular cell, reducing the substrate needed to create thyroid hormone. Lithium blocks thyroid hormone release from thyroglobulin, which in turn inhibits adenylate cyclase and prevents thyroid stimulating hormone or thyroid stimulating antibody from stimulating the cell via the thyroid hormone receptor [14]. Lastly, lithium inhibits deiodinases in the periphery.

Lithium has been shown to increase the retention of radioactive iodine (RAI) in the thyroid of patients with Graves' thyrotoxicosis [15], in turn, leading to improvement of the efficacy of this therapy. Lithium given before or concomitantly with RAI has been shown to provide more immediate control of hyperthyroidism, by decreasing the release of preformed thyroid hormone, without decreasing the uptake of the RAI [16]. This effect is reminiscent of the Wolff-Chaikoff effect, where increased iodine content inside the follicular cell blocks release of hormone. This effect, much like the effect of iodine, is transient. Older literature notes the similarity of lithium to iodine and recommends its use only for short-term, rapid suppression [17]. However, our case highlights the fact that lithium has several other mechanisms of action that contribute to long-term control of thyrotoxicosis.

There are few cases in the literature that describe use of lithium as a stand-alone drug to treat thyrotoxicosis, without plan for definitive treatment. In one such study, lithium was the only drug used to treat 11 patients with Graves' disease who relapsed after treatment with conventional antithyroid medications, radioiodine treatment, or surgery [18]. Patients were given lithium for 6 months at a dose ranging from 800 to 1200 mg daily, with levels in the blood ranging from 0.5 to 1.5 mmol/L. Eight of the patients studied became clinically euthyroid 2 weeks after starting lithium, with thyroid hormone levels decreasing by a mean of 35%. Another 3 patients took 4–6 weeks to achieve euthyroid state. The important finding was that euthyroid state was maintained after 6 months, and seven patients relapsed into thyrotoxicosis after lithium was stopped for 1–4 weeks.

Lithium reaches peak plasma concentration in 1-2 hours for the immediate release formulation and 4-5 hours for sustained release formulation. A steady state in the body is usually achieved after 4 days [14]. Apart from the effects on the thyroid, reported adverse effects include a spectrum of central nervous system, cardiovascular, and renal side effects. These include confusion, coma, seizures, ventricular irritability, sinus node dysfunction, sinoatrial block, nephrogenic diabetes insipidus, electrolyte imbalance, hypercalcemia, and hypermagnesemia. Studies have shown that lithium doses of 600 mg–1000 mg daily (300 mg every 8 hours), as well as lithium blood levels of 0.6-1.2 mmol/L, are best to control thyrotoxicosis. To avoid toxicity, it is best if serum lithium levels are maintained < 1.0 mmol/L, around 0.5 mmol/L. [14].

Our case illustrates that a low therapeutic level of lithium even around 0.2 mmol/L is sufficient to suppress thyroid overactivity without causing side effects. Lithium at a low dose appears to be an effective antithyroid medication even for a few months.

4. Conclusion

Lithium can be used to treat thyrotoxicosis when other more commonly used therapeutic options are not available, and therapy duration beyond a few weeks is a possibility. Moreover, as shown in this case, lithium doses in the low, subtherapeutic range can still be effective in controlling thyrotoxicosis even over several weeks.

References

[1] J. F. J. Cade, "Lithium salts in the treatment of psychotic excitement," *The Medical Journal of Australia*, vol. 2, no. 10, pp. 349–352, 1949.

[2] M. Schou, A. Amdisen, S. Eskjaer Jensen, and T. Olsen, "Occurrence of goitre during lithium treatment," *British medical journal.*, vol. 3, no. 5620, pp. 710–713, 1968.

[3] J. Candy, "Severe hypothyroidism—an early complication of lithium therapy," *British Medical Journal*, vol. 3, no. 5821, article 277, 1972.

[4] G. Kirov, "Thyroid disorders in lithium-treated patients," *Journal of Affective Disorders*, vol. 50, no. 1, pp. 33–40, 1998.

[5] S. C. Berens, R. S. Bernstein, J. Robbins, and J. Wolff, "Antithyroid effects of lithium," *The Journal of Clinical Investigation*, vol. 49, no. 7, pp. 1357–1367, 1970.

[6] H. B. Burch and L. Wartofsky, "Life-threatening thyrotoxicosis: thyroid storm," *Endocrinology and Metabolism Clinics of North America*, vol. 22, no. 2, pp. 263–277, 1993.

[7] D. S. Cooper, "Antithyroid drugs," *The New England Journal of Medicine*, vol. 352, no. 9, pp. 905–917, 2005.

[8] D. Manna, G. Roy, and G. Mugesh, "Antithyroid drugs and their analogues: synthesis, structure, and mechanism of action," *Accounts of Chemical Research*, vol. 46, no. 11, pp. 2706–2715, 2013.

[9] M. Weiss, D. Hassin, and H. Bank, "Propylthiouracil-induced hepatic damage," *Archives of Internal Medicine*, vol. 140, no. 9, pp. 1184–1185, 1980.

[10] E. Mathieu, O. Fain, M. Sitbon, and M. Thomas, "Systemic adverse effect of antithyroid drugs," *Clinical Rheumatology*, vol. 18, no. 1, pp. 66–68, 1999.

[11] B. Nayak and K. Burman, "Thyrotoxicosis and thyroid storm," *Endocrinology and Metabolism Clinics of North America*, vol. 35, no. 4, pp. 663–686, 2006.

[12] C. Muller, P. Perrin, B. Faller, S. Richter, and F. Chantrel, "Role of plasma exchange in the thyroid storm," *Therapeutic Apheresis and Dialysis*, vol. 15, no. 6, pp. 522–531, 2011.

[13] N. Bagchi, T. R. Brown, and R. E. Mack, "Studies on the mechanism of inhibition of thyroid function by lithium," *Biochimica et Biophysica Acta*, vol. 542, no. 1, pp. 163–169, 1978.

[14] Y. W. Ng, S. C. Tiu, K. L. Choi et al., "Use of lithium in the treatment of thyrotoxicosis," *Hong Kong Medical Journal*, vol. 12, no. 4, pp. 254–259, 2006.

[15] J. G. Turner, B. E. W. Brownlie, and T. G. H. Rogers, "Lithium as an adjunct to radioiodine therapy for thyrotoxicosis," *The Lancet*, vol. 307, no. 7960, pp. 614–615, 1976.

[16] F. Bogazzi, L. Bartalena, A. Campomori et al., "Treatment with lithium prevents serum thyroid hormone increase after thionamide withdrawal and radioiodine therapy in patients with Graves' disease," *The Journal of Clinical Endocrinology & Metabolism*, vol. 87, no. 10, pp. 4490–4495, 2002.

[17] R. Temple, M. Berman, J. Robbins, and J. Wolff, "The use of lithium in the treatment of thyrotoxicosis," *The Journal of Clinical Investigation*, vol. 51, no. 10, pp. 2746–2756, 1972.

[18] J. H. Lazarus, G. M. Addison, A. R. Richards, and G. M. Owen, "Treatment of thyrotoxicosis with lithium carbonate," *The Lancet*, vol. 304, no. 7890, pp. 1160–1163, 1974.

42

Humoral Hypercalcemia of Malignancy with a Parathyroid Hormone-Related Peptide-Secreting Intrahepatic Cholangiocarcinoma Accompanied by a Gastric Cancer

Katsushi Takeda,[1] **Ryosuke Kimura,**[1] **Nobuhiro Nishigaki,**[2] **Shinya Sato,**[3] **Asami Okamoto,**[1] **Kumiko Watanabe,**[1] **and Sachie Yasui**[1]

[1]*Department of Endocrinology and Metabolism, Nagoya City West Medical Center, 1-1-1 Hirate-cho, Kita-ku, Nagoya 462-8508, Japan*
[2]*Department of Gastroenterology, Nagoya City West Medical Center, 1-1-1 Hirate-cho, Kita-ku, Nagoya 462-8508, Japan*
[3]*Department of Experimental Pathology and Tumor Biology, Nagoya City University Graduate School of Medical Sciences, 1 Kawasumi, Mizuho-cho, Mizuho-ku, Nagoya 467-8601, Japan*

Correspondence should be addressed to Katsushi Takeda; k.takeda.51@west-med.jp

Academic Editor: Michael P. Kane

Humoral hypercalcemia of malignancy (HHM) is caused by the oversecretion of parathyroid hormone-related peptide (PTHrP) from malignant tumors. Although any tumor may cause HHM, that induced by intrahepatic cholangiocarcinoma (ICC) or gastric cancer (GC) is rare. We report here a 74-year-old male who displayed HHM with both ICC and GC and showed an elevated serum PTHrP level. Treatment of the hypercalcemia with saline, furosemide, elcatonin, and zoledronic acid corrected his serum calcium level and improved symptoms. Because treatment of ICC should precede that of GC, we chose chemotherapy with cisplatin (CDDP) and gemcitabine (GEM). Chemotherapy reduced the size of the ICC and decreased the serum PTHrP level. One year after diagnosis, the patient was alive in the face of a poor prognosis for an ICC that produced PTHrP. Immunohistochemical staining for PTHrP was positive for the ICC and negative for the GC, leading us to believe that the cause of the HHM was a PTHrP-secreting ICC. In conclusion, immunohistochemical staining for PTHrP may be useful in discovering the cause of HHM in the case of two cancers accompanied by an elevated serum PHTrP level. Chemotherapy with CDDP and GEM may be the most appropriate treatment for a PTHrP-secreting ICC.

1. Introduction

Hypercalcemia is a well-known complication of cancer as seen in the between 20 and 30 percent of cancer patients [1]. Malignant-associated hypercalcemia (MAH) is classified into four groups: humoral hypercalcemia of malignancy (HHM), local osteolytic hypercalcemia (LOH), excess $1,25(OH)_2D$ secretion, and ectopic parathyroid hormone (PTH) secretion. HHM is associated with 80 percent of MAHs and is caused by the effects of the oversecretion of parathyroid hormone-related peptide (PTHrP) [1–3]. Although HHM can essentially be caused by any tumor [1], its induction by cholangiocarcinoma or gastric cancer (GC) is rare [4, 5]. In addition, to date, cases of HHM complicated by two

cancers—cholangiocarcinoma and gastric cancer—have not been reported.

Herein, we report the first case of HHM induced by an intrahepatic cholangiocarcinoma (ICC) that secretes PTHrP, in conjunction with a GC identified by immunohistochemical staining.

2. Case Presentation

A 74-year-old male patient was admitted for hypercalcemia. Over the preceding two months he had suffered from a loss of appetite and had a history of seborrheic keratosis and hypertension. His weight was 47.4 kg, height 153.2 cm, temperature 36.6°C, heart rate 127 beats/minute, and blood pressure 143/92 mmHg. He had tenderness of the right hypochondrium, but an abdominal mass was not palpable.

Laboratory analyses revealed that the patient's corrected serum calcium level was elevated at 14.8 mg/dL. Serum carcinoembryonic antigen (CEA) and carbohydrate antigen (CA) 19-9 were within normal range. Serum alpha fetoprotein (AFP) showed a normal level of 3.8 ng/mL. The serum PTHrP level was elevated at 26.6 pmol/L and the serum intact PTH level was low at 9 pg/mL (Table 1).

Dynamic contrast-enhanced computed tomography (CT) scans revealed a large mass, 76 mm in diameter, and multiple masses in the patient's liver. These masses showed an enhancement of the peripheral zone in the early phase of CT; the inside of such masses gradually became enhanced, suggesting an ICC with intrahepatic metastases (Figure 1(a)). Using fluorodeoxyglucose-positron emission tomography (FDG-PET), the patient's liver tumor showed a SUVmax 7.1 uptake value for FDG. Bone scintigraphy did not reveal any bone metastases. Magnetic resonance imaging (MRI) showed a slightly low signal intensity on a T1-weighted image and a slightly high signal intensity on a T2-weighted image. These tumors showed an enhancement of the peripheral zone in the early phase and low intake of gadolinium ethoxybenzyl diethylenetriamine pentaacetic acid- (Gd-EOB-DTPA-) enhanced MRI in the hepatobiliary phase (Figures 1(b) and 1(c)). Esophagogastroduodenoscopy revealed an infiltrative ulcerative carcinoma in the anterior wall of the antrum of the patient's stomach (Figure 2).

A histological examination of a biopsy specimen from the hepatic tumor revealed an ICC (Figure 3(a)). Immunohistochemically, ICC tumor cells were positive for cytokeratin 7 and PTHrP (Figure 3(d)) and negative for cytokeratin 20, CDX2, and CA19-9. A histological examination of a biopsy specimen from the GC revealed an adenocarcinoma (Figure 3(b)). Immunohistochemically, GC tumor cells were positive for cytokeratin 7, cytokeratin 20, CDX2, and CA19-9 and were negative for PTHrP (Figure 3(e)). These findings indicated that this patient had two cancers, ICC and GC, and that his HHM was induced by the oversecretion of PTHrP from the ICC.

After admission, the patient's hypercalcemia was treated with saline, furosemide, elcatonin, and zoledronic acid. His corrected serum calcium level and symptoms subsequently improved. We used elcatonin only a single time on admission and zoledronic acid five times during the five weeks after admission. Subsequently, his corrected calcium level was kept under 11 mg/dL without using elcatonin and bisphosphonate (Figure 4).

The patient's prognosis was dependent on the ICC since a prognosis for this type of cancer is generally known to be poor and his ICC was complicated by intrahepatic metastasis. Therefore, we treated him with chemotherapy using cisplatin (CDDP) and gemcitabine (GEM). We started chemotherapy on the 30th day after admission, and he was discharged on the 39th day. On the 78th day, his liver tumors were reduced (Figure 5(a)). Moreover, on the 238th day, his liver tumors were smaller than tumors observed on the 78th day (Figure 5(b)). In addition, the volume of his gastric cancer was also decreased on the 273rd day (Figure 6), suggesting

that chemotherapy with CDDP and GEM was also effective for his gastric cancer. His serum PTHrP level had improved to 4.9 pmol/L by the 101st day. A year after diagnosis, the patient was alive.

3. Discussion

HHM is usually caused by the oversecretion of PTHrP by a malignant tumor. Typical tumors causing HHM include

TABLE 1: Laboratory data on admission.

WBC	8900/μL
RBC	$476 \times 10^4/\mu$L
Hb	15.9 g/dL
PLT	$21.7 \times 10^4/\mu$L
TP	6.7 g/dL
Alb	3.6 g/dL
T-Bil.	0.6 mg/dL
D-Bil.	0.2 mg/dL
ALP	515 U/L
GOT	64 U/L
GPT	26 U/L
LDH	190 U/L
Amy	57 U/L
CPK	27 U/L
UA	10.0 mg/dL
BUN	28.5 mg/dL
CRN	1.27 mg/dL
Na	138 mmol/L
K	3.8 mmol/L
Cl	98 mmol/L
Ca	14.4 mg/dL
Corrected Ca	14.8 mg/dL
I-P	2.8 mg/dL
Mg	1.7 mg/dL
CRP	1.5 mg/dL
Glu	129 mg/dL
CEA	1.5 ng/mL (0.0~5.0)*
CA19-9	6.2 U/mL (0.0~37.0)*
AFP	3.8 ng/mL (0.0~10.0)*
HBs antigen	(—)
HCV antibody	(—)
PTH intact	9 pg/mL (10~65)*
PTHrP	26.6 pmol/L (0~1.1)*

*Numbers in parentheses indicate the normal range; WBC: white blood cells; RBC: red blood cells; Hb: hemoglobin; PLT: platelets; TP: total protein; Alb: albumin; T-Bil.: total bilirubin; D-Bil.: direct bilirubin; ALP: alkaline phosphatase; GOT: glutamic oxaloacetic transaminase; GPT: glutamic pyruvic transaminase; LDH: lactate dehydrogenase; Amy: amylase; CPK: creatine phosphokinase; UA: uric acid; BUN: blood urea nitrogen; CRN: creatinine; Na: sodium; K: potassium; Cl: chlorine; Ca: calcium; I-P: inorganic phosphate; Mg: magnesium; CRP: C-reactive protein; Glu: glucose; CEA: carcinoembryonic antigen; CA: carbohydrate antigen; AFP: alpha fetoprotein; HBs: hepatitis B surface; HCV: hepatitis C virus; PTH: parathyroid hormone; PTHrP: parathyroid hormone-related peptide.

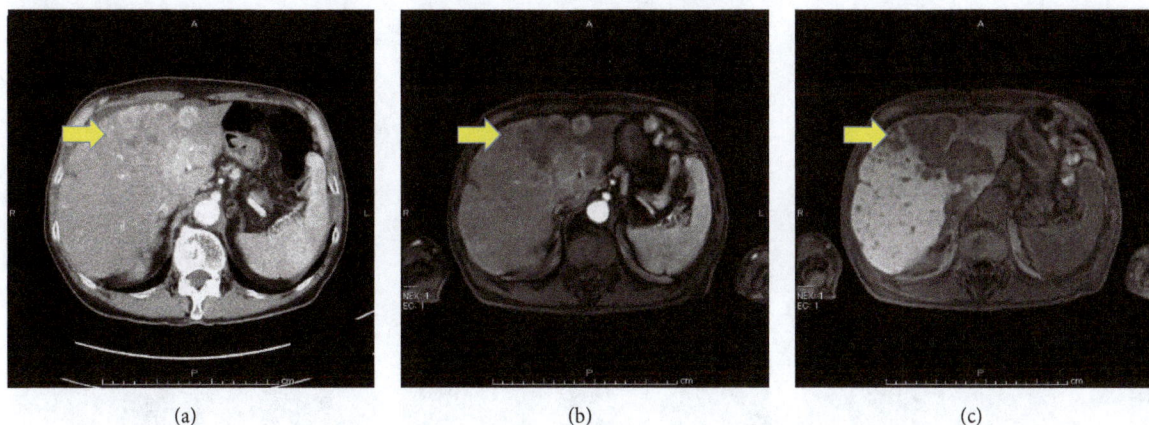

FIGURE 1: Dynamic contrast-enhanced computed tomography (CT) scans showed multiple masses in the patient's liver, suggesting intrahepatic cholangiocarcinoma (ICC; (a), arrow). His liver tumors showed an enhancement of the peripheral zone in the early phase ((b), arrow) and a low intake in the hepatobiliary phase ((c), arrow) in a gadolinium ethoxybenzyl diethylenetriamine pentaacetic acid- (Gd-EOB-DTPA-) enhanced magnetic resonance imaging (MRI).

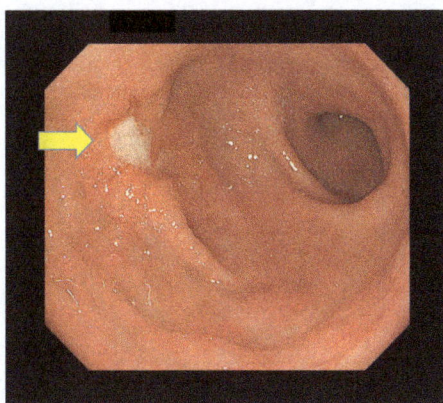

FIGURE 2: Esophagogastroduodenoscopy revealed an infiltrative ulcerative carcinoma (arrow) in the anterior wall of the antrum of the patient's stomach.

various squamous cell carcinomas, renal cancer, ovarian cancer, endometrial cancer, human T-cell lymphotropic virus- (HTLV-) associated lymphoma and breast cancer [1]. The symptoms of HHM are often mild and nonspecific. Nevertheless, HHM is associated with substantial mortality, with about 50% of cancer patients who show hypercalcemia dying within 30 days [2, 6]. Therefore, the early treatment of HHM and control of the serum calcium level are important.

PTHrP has been purified from a human lung cancer cell line [7] and has significant sequence homology with the amino-terminal end of PTH [3, 7–9]. PTHrP is normally synthesized by various tissues and has important physiological roles. For example, in cartilage PTHrP regulates its proliferation and differentiation [10]. It is also produced in the placenta, where it regulates the fetal serum calcium level [11]. However, it is known as a factor responsible for HHM since it enhances the renal retention of calcium and increases

bone resorption [1]. In addition, it has also been recognized as one of the causes of adipose browning and cachexia recently and new treatments of PTHrP may be developed to improve the prognosis of cancer patients in the future [12–14]

ICC accounts for 4.4 percent of primary liver cancers in Japan, so it is relatively rare [15]. ICC is frequently clinically silent in its early stages and is, therefore, often only diagnosed when it develops into an advanced cancer; this is a leading reason for its poor prognosis.

Cholangiocarcinoma is a malignant neoplasm arising from the biliary epithelium and can be anatomically classified into intrahepatic, perihilar, and distal extrahepatic tumors [16]. Surgical resection is the only curative treatment for cholangiocarcinoma; however, most patients with this tumor are not operative candidates [4, 16]. Chemotherapy for cholangiocarcinoma is administered to those patients who are not operative and results have been largely disappointing, especially for cholangiocarcinoma that produces PTHrP [4, 16]. To the best of our knowledge, patients diagnosed with a PTHrP-secreting cholangiocarcinoma who lived for more than six months have been reported in only four instances, including the present case (Table 2) [4, 17, 18]; chemotherapy was performed for each case but surgical resection was not. This suggests the possibility that chemotherapy is one of the effective treatments for a PTHrP-secreting cholangiocarcinoma, like a non-PTHrP-secreting cholangiocarcinoma. However, further reports are needed in order to decide the best therapy for these types of tumors.

Immunohistochemical staining is a widely used technique that demonstrates the expression and distribution of a specific antigen by antigen-antibody immunoreaction. It is often used not only in research, but also in clinical practice, for example, in pathological diagnosis and the determination of molecular-targeted therapy. However, immunohistochemical staining for PTHrP is still uncommon. There are opinions that antibodies for PTHrP may be considered nonspecific.

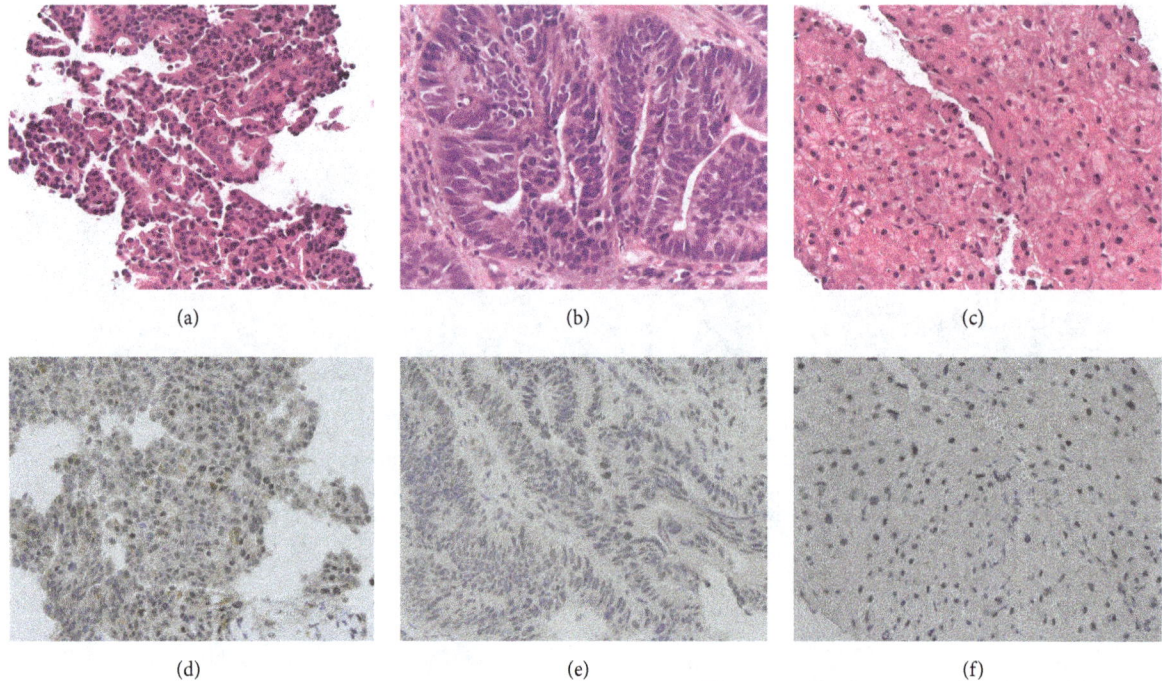

FIGURE 3: Histological examination of an ICC (a, d), gastric cancer (GC; (b, e)), and normal hepatocyte (c, f). Hematoxylin and eosin staining (×400) of an ICC (a), an adenocarcinoma suggesting GC (b), and normal hepatocyte (c). Immunohistochemical staining by anti-PTHrP antibody (H-137; Santa Cruz Biotechnology) in an ICC (d), GC (e), and normal hepatocyte (f).

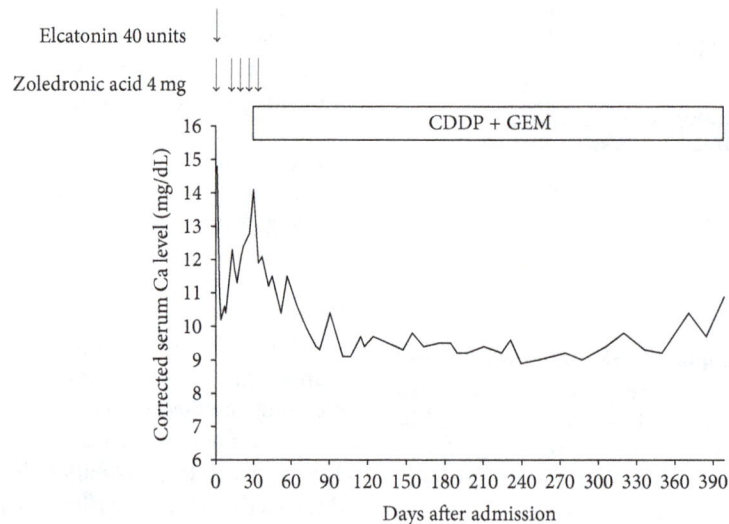

FIGURE 4: The corrected serum Ca level was stable without bisphosphonate after the patient commenced chemotherapy with cisplatin (CDDP) and gemcitabine (GEM).

However, an antibody for PTHrP (H-137; Santa Cruz Biotechnology) is negative for normal hepatocyte which we were able to get when we performed the biopsy (Figure 3(f)), suggesting that this antibody has the specificity for PTHrP. Therefore, our case suggests that immunohistochemical staining by an anti-PTHrP antibody may be useful in the search for the cause of HHM in the case of two cancers accompanied by an elevated serum PTHrP level. Because of an aging society, the occurrence of two cancers together is no longer rare. Therefore, the incidence of HHM with two cancers is also

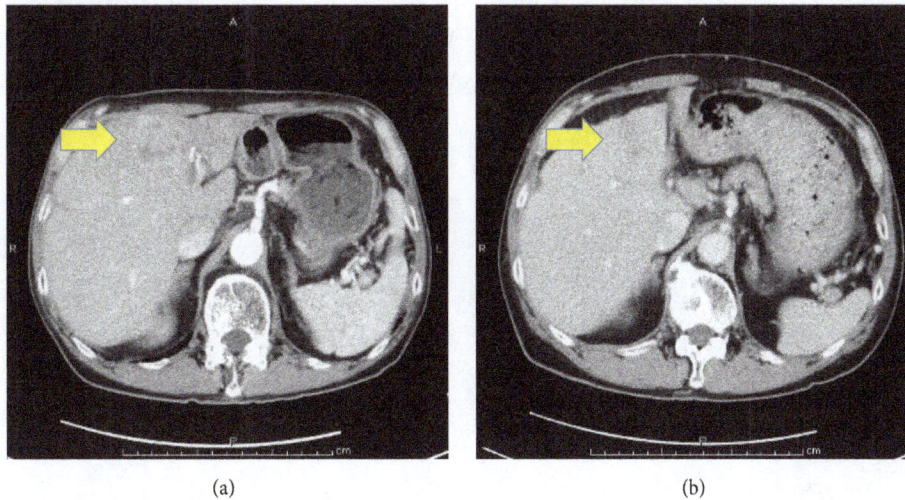

(a)   (b)

FIGURE 5: CT scans showed that the patient's liver tumors (arrows) were reduced by the 78th (a) and 238th day (b) of admission after chemotherapy with CDDP and GEM.

TABLE 2: Reported cases of cholangiocarcinoma secreting PTHrP who are alive for more than half a year.

Number	Authors	Age	Reported year	Sex	Ca level	PTHrP	Therapy	Prognosis
(1)	Davis et al. [17]	54	1994	Male	16.4	5.2	FUDR + 5-FU	Survival (for 6 months)
(2)	Yamada et al. [4]	43	2009	Male	14.4	5.0	TAE + PTPE + GEM + S-1 + Radiation	Died (after 14 months)
(3)	Lim et al. [18]	63	2013	Male	[o]12.1	[x]6.7	CAP + CDDP + Radiation, second-line GEM	Died (after almost 1 year)
(4)	Our case	74	2016	Male	[o]14.8	26.6	CDDP + GEM	Survival (after 1 year)

FUDR: floxuridine; 5-FU: 5-fluorouracil; GEM: gemcitabine; CAP: capecitabine; CDDP: cisplatin; TAE: transcatheter arterial embolization; PTPE: percutaneous transhepatic portal embolization; [x]PTHrP reported by Lim et al. was measured 9 months after an ICC diagnosis; [o]Ca level means corrected Ca.

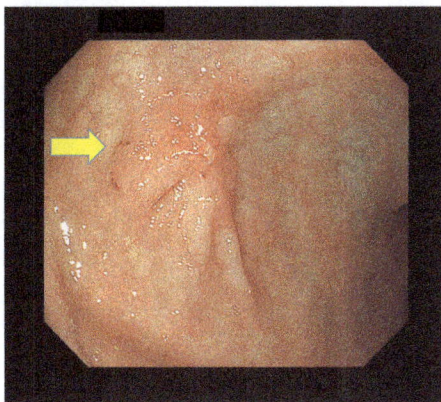

FIGURE 6: Esophagogastroduodenoscopy showed that the patient's gastric cancer (arrow) was reduced on the 273rd day.

expected to increase. The identification of a cancer secreting PTHrP by using immunohistochemical staining will allow the correct prediction of fluctuation of serum calcium level.

In conclusion, we have reported the first case of a patient with a PTHrP-secreting ICC accompanied by GC.

Disclosure

An earlier version of this manuscript was presented as a poster presentation at the 89th annual meeting of the Japan Endocrine Society (April, 2016).

References

[1] A. F. Stewart, "Hypercalcemia associated with cancer," *The New England Journal of Medicine*, vol. 352, no. 4, pp. 373–379, 2005.

[2] J. D. Wright, A. I. Tergas, C. V. Ananth et al., "Quality and Outcomes of Treatment of Hypercalcemia of Malignancy," *Cancer Investigation*, vol. 33, no. 8, pp. 331–339, 2015.

[3] K. Nakajima, M. Tamai, S. Okaniwa et al., "Humoral hypercalcemia associated with gastric carcinoma secreting parathyroid hormone: a case report and review of the literature," *Endocrine Journal*, vol. 60, no. 5, pp. 557–562, 2013.

[4] M. Yamada, H. Shiroeda, S. Shiroeda, K. Sato, T. Arisawa, and M. Tsutsumi, "Cholangiocarcinoma producing parathyroid

hormone-related peptide treated with chemoradiation using gemcitabine and S-1," *Internal Medicine*, vol. 48, no. 24, pp. 2097–2100, 2009.

[5] C. Iino, T. Shimoyama, Y. Akemoto et al., "Humoral hypercalcemia due to gastric carcinoma secreting parathyroid hormone-related protein during chemotherapy: a case report," *Clinical Journal of Gastroenterology*, vol. 9, no. 2, pp. 68–72, 2016.

[6] S. H. Ralston, S. J. Gallacher, U. Patel, J. Campbell, and I. T. Boyle, "Cancer-associated hypercalcemia: morbidity and mortality—clinical experience in 126 treated patients," *Annals of Internal Medicine*, vol. 112, no. 7, pp. 499–504, 1990.

[7] J. M. Moseley, M. Kubota, H. Diefenbach-Jagger et al., "Parathyroid hormone-related protein purified from a human lung cancer cell line," *Proceedings of the National Academy of Sciences of the United States of America*, vol. 84, no. 14, pp. 5048–5052, 1987.

[8] L. J. Suva, G. A. Winslow, R. E. H. Wettenhall et al., "A parathyroid hormone-related protein implicated in malignant hypercalcemia: cloning and expression," *Science*, vol. 237, no. 4817, pp. 893–896, 1987.

[9] A. E. Broadus, M. Mangin, K. Ikeda et al., "Humoral hypercalcemia of cancer: identification of a novel parathyroid hormone-like peptide," *The New England Journal of Medicine*, vol. 319, no. 9, pp. 556–563, 1988.

[10] A. C. Karaplis, A. Luz, J. Glowacki et al., "Lethal skeletal dysplasia from targeted disruption of the parathyroid hormone-related peptide gene," *Genes and Development*, vol. 8, no. 3, pp. 277–289, 1994.

[11] C. P. Rodda, M. Kubota, J. A. Heath et al., "Evidence for a novel parathyroid hormone-related protein in fetal lamb parathyroid glands and sheep placenta: comparisons with a similar protein implicated in humoral hypercalcaemia of malignancy," *Journal of Endocrinology*, vol. 117, no. 2, pp. 261–271, 1988.

[12] S. Kir and B. M. Spiegelman, "Cachexia and brown fat: a burning issue in cancer," *Trends in Cancer*, vol. 2, no. 9, pp. 461–463, 2016.

[13] S. Kir, J. P. White, S. Kleiner et al., "Tumour-derived PTH-related protein triggers adipose tissue browning and cancer cachexia," *Nature*, vol. 513, no. 7516, pp. 100–104, 2014.

[14] A. R. Guntur, C. R. Doucette, and C. J. Rosen, "PTHrp comes full circle in cancer biology," *BoneKEy Reports*, vol. 4, no. 621, 2015.

[15] M. Kudo, N. Izumi, T. Ichida et al., "Report of the 19th follow-up survey of primary liver cancer in Japan," *Hepatology Research*, vol. 46, no. 5, pp. 372–390, 2016.

[16] M. J. Olnes and R. Erlich, "A review and update on cholangio-carcinoma," *Oncology*, vol. 66, no. 3, pp. 167–179, 2004.

[17] J. M. Davis, R. Sadasivan, T. Dwyer, and P. V. Veldhuizen, "Case report: cholangiocarcinoma and hypercalcemia," *The American Journal of the Medical Sciences*, vol. 307, no. 5, pp. 350–352, 1994.

[18] S. Lim, J. Han, K. H. Park et al., "Two cases of humoral hypercalcemia of malignancy in metastatic cholangiocarcinoma," *Cancer Research and Treatment*, vol. 45, no. 2, pp. 145–149, 2013.

43

Identification of a Novel Mutation in a Family with Pseudohypoparathyroidism Type 1a

Adelaide Moutinho ⓘ,[1] **Rosa Carvalho,**[2] **Rita Ferreira Reis,**[3] **and Sandra Tavares**[1]

[1]*Department of Internal Medicine, Hospital de Chaves, Centro Hospitalar de Trás-os-Montes e Alto Douro, Chaves, Portugal*
[2]*Department of Internal Medicine, Hospital de Braga, Braga, Portugal*
[3]*Department of Internal Medicine, Hospital de Lamego, Centro Hospitalar de Trás-os-Montes e Alto Douro, Lamego, Portugal*

Correspondence should be addressed to Adelaide Moutinho; m.adelaide.moutinho@gmail.com

Academic Editor: Toshihiro Kita

Introduction. Pseudohypoparathyroidism type 1a is caused by GNAS mutations leading to target organ resistance to multiple hormones rather than parathyroid hormone, resulting not only in hypocalcemia, but also in Albright's hereditary osteodystrophy phenotype. *Materials and Methods.* DNA sequencing of the GNAS gene identified a novel heterozygous mutation in peripheral blood leukocytes in the family presented in this case report. *Results.* We present a case of a 25-year-old woman with pseudohypoparathyroidism type 1a admitted with seizures, whose family presents an autosomal dominant transmission of a novel heterozygous GNAS mutation (c.524_530+3del). *Conclusion.* Pseudohypoparathyroidism type 1a is mostly caused by inactivating GNAS mutations that have been gradually reported in the literature that lead to a typical and complex clinical phenotype and resistance to multiple hormones. The deletion caused by the mutation identified in the presented case has not been reported previously.

1. Introduction

Pseudohypoparathyroidism (PHP) is a rare disorder characterized by target organ resistance to parathyroid hormone (PTH), resulting in hypocalcemia and hyperphosphatemia [1, 2]. PHP type 1a is due to a heterozygous loss of function of the alpha subunit of a G protein (Gsα), due to a GNAS mutation on the maternal allele of the chromosome 20q13.3, with autosomal dominant inheritance [3, 4]. This intracellular protein is responsible for the production of cyclic AMP (cAMP) in response to PTH, and the reduced G protein activity is the molecular basis for hormone resistance in this disorder [3]. PHP type 1a is characterized by the expression of the Gsα isoform only of the paternal GNAS gene, with resistance to other hormones rather than PTH and by the phenotype of Albright's hereditary osteodystrophy (AHO) with round facies, short stature, obesity, subcutaneous ossifications, brachydactyly, and in some cases mental retardation [3–5].

2. Case Presentation

A 25-year-old woman was admitted to the Emergency Service after a generalized tonic-clonic seizure. She had a history of hypoparathyroidism, hypothyroidism, and mild retardation, being medicated with calcium carbonate 9000 mg plus cholecalciferol 2400 U/day, levothyroxine 0,1 mg/day, and desogestrel/ethinylestradiol 0,15/0,02 mg/day. She had multiple hospital admissions with seizures because of lack of therapeutic compliance and had repeatedly refused further investigation of the underlying disease or regular outpatient follow-up.

Physical examination showed a short stature, obesity (BMI 35 kg/m^2), dental hypoplasia, round facies, and brachydactyly of the fourth and fifth metacarpals (Figure 1) and metatarsals. At admission she was conscious, with Glasgow Coma Scale of 15 points, had normal vitals (blood pressure 120/60 mmHg; heart rate 68 beats per minute; respiratory rate 16 cycles per minute; O$_2$ saturation of 96%; FiO$_2$ 21%), with

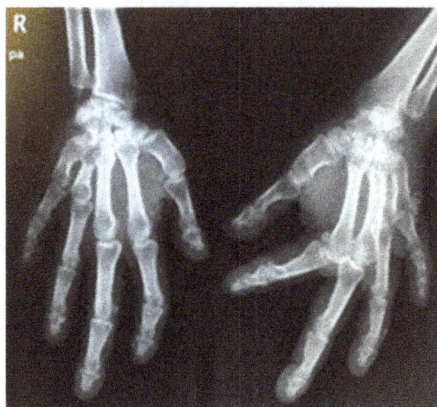

FIGURE 1: Radiography of both hands, revealing brachydactyly of the fourth and fifth metacarpals.

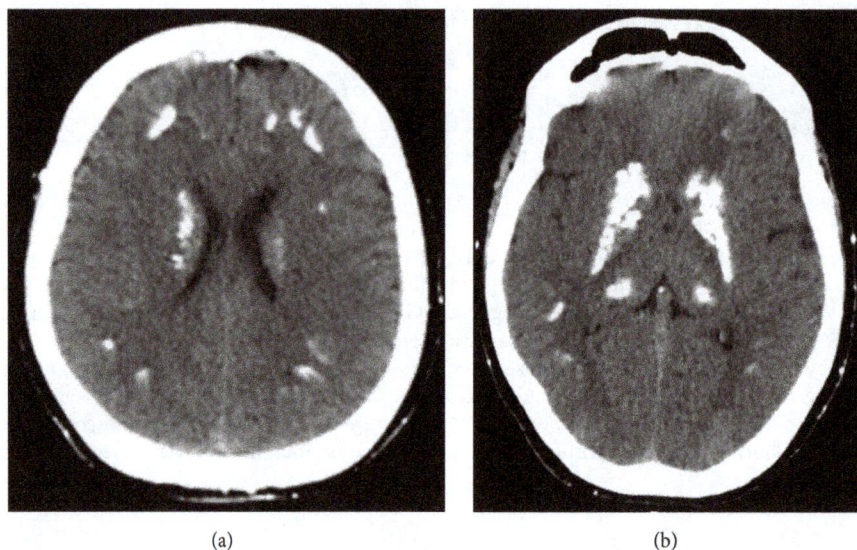

(a)

(b)

FIGURE 2: Axial cuts of CT scan, revealing diffuse subcortical frontoparietal (a) and striatum capsularis and thalamus calcifications (b).

no fever (temperature 36,7°C). She had positive Chovstek and Trousseau signs, without tetany. Her pulmonary and cardiac auscultations were normal. The neurologic examination revealed no focal signs, no photophobia, and negative Kernig's and Brudzinski's signs.

Laboratory tests revealed severe hypocalcemia (serum calcium with albumin correction 5,5 mg/dL; normal range (NR) 8,6–10,0 mg/dL), hyperphosphatemia (6,7 mg/dL; NR 2,7–4,5 mg/dL), and high PTH (160,1 pg/mL; NR 10–65 pg/mL), with normal vitamin D (37 ng/mL; NR 30–100 ng/mL) and low calcium in the 24-hour urine collection (23,9 mg/24 h; NR 100–300 mg/24 h). The thyroid-stimulating hormone (TSH) was normal (4,04 mIU/L; NR 0,27–4,2 mIU/L), with free thyroxine of 16,53 pmol/L (NR 1,17–21,7 pmol/L). The CT scan revealed diffuse subcortical frontoparietotemporal, striatum capsularis, and thalamus calcifications (Figure 2), without other changes.

Her family history revealed an aunt and a sister with clinical diagnosis hypoparathyroidism and AHO, as well as two nephews, without further investigation, and the presence of AHO in her mother, without further investigation; her older brother had a fatal respiratory infection in infancy. Our subject's one-year-old son had AHO and hypoparathyroidism as well. Considering this presentation, we assumed that all individuals should have pseudohypoparathyroidism as well.

Based on the clinical features of AHO plus the pseudohypoparathyroidism with hypocalcemia, hyperphosphatemia, and tissue resistance to the increased level of PTH, she was diagnosed with PHP type 1a. Facing her family history and to support our diagnosis, and after explaining to the patient the implications of the diagnosis for both her and her child, we were able to obtain consent to further investigation that she had refused before. Therefore, we performed a genetic study with DNA analysis of the GNAS gene extracted from peripheral blood leukocytes with identification of the novel mutation c.524_530+3del (p.Gln176Serfs*7) in heterozygosity, in the location 20q13.32-exon 6, both in our patient and in her son. The genogram (Figure 3) suggests an autosomal

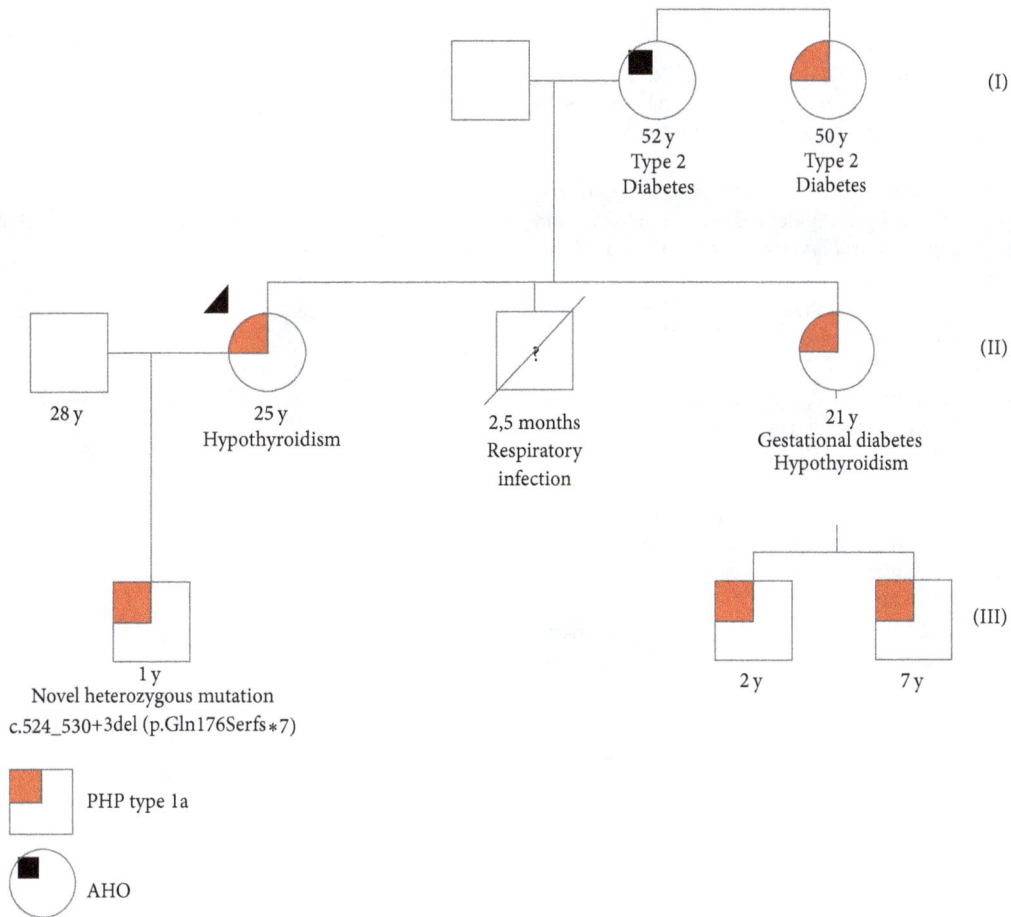

FIGURE 3: Genogram of the subject's family. Our subject is identified by the black arrow-head. y: year(s) old; PHP: pseudohypoparathyroidism; AHO: Albright's hereditary osteodystrophy.

dominant inheritance with maternal derived transmission. We were not able to perform DNA sequencing of the GNAS gene of any other family member.

3. Discussion

PHP type 1a is caused mostly by maternal heterozygous inactivating mutations in the GNAS gene leading to a complex clinical phenotype that includes resistance to multiple hormones, intellectual disability, and AHO [1, 4]. This phenotype is most likely explained by the fact that some tissues (thyroid, pituitary, renal proximal tubules, and gonads) express Gsα predominantly from the maternal allele, while the paternal is silenced through yet unknown mechanisms. In PHP type 1a, inactivating mutations on the maternal allele will result in little or no production of this subunit with haploinsufficiency of Gsα, resulting in multiple hormone resistance within these specific tissues [3]. The resistance to PTH leads to hypocalcemia and hyperphosphatemia, and as calcium plays an essential role in stabilizing the cell membrane, there is an increased risk of seizures, as happened with our patient [2].

Lemos and Thakker [6] identified 343 kindreds with heterozygous Gs-alpha germline mutations in the literature that yielded a total of 176 different germline mutations,

without unknown prevalence, but with some acknowledged mutational hot spots, as exon 1 and codons 189-190 in exon 7. A novel mutation was identified in both our patient and her son in exon 6. The genogram suggests the autosomal dominant maternal transmission to both our patient and her sister. However, we were not able to test our patient's relatives which was a limitation in this case.

In conclusion, there are over 340 reported GNAS mutations leading to PHP type 1a [1], and the identification of the causative mutation in the index case may be useful for screening other family members avoiding late diagnosis or misdiagnosis and for prenatal counseling both to our patient and to her sister and in the future for our patient's son and nephews.

Disclosure

This work was presented at *Jornadas do Médico Interno da Região Autónoma da Madeira* and awarded with the first prize of top posters.

References

[1] M. C. Lemos, P. T. Christie, D. Rodrigues, and R. V. Thakker, "Pseudohypoparathyroidism type 1a due to a novel mutation in the GNAS gene," *Clinical Endocrinology*, vol. 84, no. 3, pp. 463–467, 2016.

[2] L. Underbjerg, T. Sikjaer, L. Mosekilde, and L. Rejnmark, "Pseudohypoparathyroidism—epidemiology, mortality and risk of complications," *Clinical Endocrinology*, vol. 84, no. 6, pp. 904–911, 2016.

[3] O. Tafaj and H. Jüppner, "Pseudohypoparathyroidism: one gene, several syndromes," *Journal of Endocrinological Investigation*, vol. 40, no. 4, pp. 347–356, 2017.

[4] B. L. Clarke, E. M. Brown, M. T. Collins et al., "Epidemiology and diagnosis of hypoparathyroidism," *The Journal of Clinical Endocrinology & Metabolism*, vol. 101, no. 6, pp. 2284–2299, 2016.

[5] M. P. Lopes, B. S. Kliemann, I. B. Bini et al., "Hypoparathyroidism and pseudohypoparathyroidism: etiology, laboratory features and complications," *Archives of Endocrinology and Metabolism*, vol. 60, no. 6, pp. 532–536, 2016.

[6] M. C. Lemos and R. V. Thakker, "GNAS mutations in pseudohypoparathyroidism type 1a and related disorders," *Human Mutation*, vol. 36, no. 1, pp. 11–19, 2015.

44

Psychological Aspects of Androgen Insensitivity Syndrome: Two Cases Illustrating Therapeutical Challenges

Filippa Pritsini,[1,2] **Georgios A. Kanakis,**[1,2] **Ioannis Kyrgios,**[1]
Eleni P. Kotanidou,[1] **Eleni Litou,**[1] **Konstantina Mouzaki,**[1] **Aggeliki Kleisarchaki,**[1]
Dimitrios G. Goulis,[2] **and Assimina Galli-Tsinopoulou**[1]

[1]*Unit of Pediatric Endocrinology, 4th Department of Pediatrics, Medical School, Faculty of Health Sciences,*
 Aristotle University of Thessaloniki, Thessaloniki, Greece
[2]*Unit of Reproductive Endocrinology, 1st Department of Obstetrics and Gynecology, Medical School,*
 Faculty of Health Sciences, Aristotle University of Thessaloniki, Thessaloniki, Greece

Correspondence should be addressed to Assimina Galli-Tsinopoulou; gallitsin@gmail.com

Academic Editor: Eli Hershkovitz

Androgen Insensitivity Syndrome (AIS) and its heterogeneous phenotypes comprise the pieces of a challenging clinical problem. The lack of standardized guidelines results in controversies regarding the proper diagnostic and therapeutic approach, including the time and type of intervention. Due to its variable phenotype, AIS is not diagnosed at the proper age that would allow optimal psychological and medical support to the patient. Therapeutic approaches are not established, mainly due to the rarity of the disease. In addition, various social and ethical consequences may emerge. The aim of this double case report is to outline the difficulties that may rise during diagnostic, therapeutic, and psychological approach of AIS, especially concerning the handling of the relatives' reaction.

1. Introduction

Androgen Insensitivity Syndrome (AIS) is a Disorder of Sexual Differentiation (DSD), characterized by variable target tissue resistance to androgens. It is caused by mutations in the Androgen Receptor (AR) gene, which is located on the long arm of the X chromosome, or by defects of AR signaling, including interacting proteins and coregulatory factors [1–4]. In the majority of the cases, the pattern of inheritance is X-linked recessive; however, occasional de novo mutations have been described. More than 500 mutations have been identified in the AR gene, described in detail in the AR gene mutation database, which is available online at http://androgendb.mcgill.ca/ [accessed 6 September 2016] [5].

As a consequence of AR dysfunction, androgens cannot exert their effects, even since the intrauterine life, resulting in malformations of internal and external genital structures as well as of secondary sexual development and maturation [2]. Depending on the functionality of the AR, the clinical phenotype may vary, ranging from complete feminization to incomplete types with minor degrees of undervirilization or infertility. Accordingly, AIS is classified into three main categories: Complete (CAIS), Partial (PAIS), and Mild (MAIS) (Table 1). Individuals affected by CAIS are born unambiguously female, without any apparent abnormalities. They are usually diagnosed during puberty due to primary amenorrhea. Sexual hair is typically lacking, whereas breast development may be present due to peripheral conversion of excessive testosterone (T) to estrogen. Radiological evaluation reveals the presence of testes in the abdominal cavity, while functioning Sertoli cells prevent the development of Müllerian duct derivatives (uterus, fallopian tubes). Occasionally, a rudimentary prostate gland may be detected. On the contrary, PAIS concludes a heterogeneous group of phenotypes ranging from ambiguous genitalia to mild hypospadias that may be caused by an identifiable AR gene mutation or by an error in AR signaling. Interestingly, identical AR mutations may display a wide spectrum of phenotypes

TABLE 1: Severity of androgen insensitivity.

Grade	Syndrome	Phenotype: genitalia	Phenotype: other
1	MAIS	Male	Infertility
2	PAIS	Male	Mild undermasculinization, hypospadias
3	PAIS	Male	Severe undermasculinization, cryptorchidism, bifid scrotum
4	PAIS	Ambiguous	Severe undermasculinization, phallus between penis and clitoris
5	PAIS	Female	Separate urethral and vaginal orifices, mild clitoridomegaly
6	PAIS	Female	Normal pubic/axillary hair
7	CAIS	Female	Scarce or absent pubic/axillary hair

CAIS: Complete Androgen Insensitivity Syndrome, PAIS: Partial Androgen Insensitivity Syndrome, MAIS: Mild Androgen Insensitivity Syndrome.

[1]. Finally, MAIS may present as isolated impairment of spermatogenesis and infertility [2].

The diagnosis of AIS is based on detailed clinical, laboratory, and radiological evaluation [6]. It is supported by a 46, XY karyotype and by an hormonal profile of elevated T concentrations, accompanied by elevated Luteinizing Hormone (LH) due to impaired feedback of the hypothalamic-pituitary axis. In inconclusive cases, especially in prepubertal children, human Chorionic Gonadotropin (hCG) test can be applied in order to assess androgen production and exclude androgen biosynthetic defects [1]. The diagnosis is confirmed by the documentation of the relevant AR mutation in more than 95% of subjects with CAIS [3, 7]. However, in milder forms of the syndrome this is not the case, as mutation detection frequency varies from 28 to 73%. The underlying cause in cases with negative mutation analysis is speculated to be defects in postreceptor signaling [1, 3, 8]. Last but not least, the psychological aspect of the patient with AIS remains a very sensitive issue, given the lack of widely accepted approaching methods. Unlike previous beliefs, the current trend is that all medical information should be shared with the patient in an age-appropriate way [9]. Despite this "full sharing" approach, there are still challenges that have to be overcome, since the majority of the patients are not aware of their condition. These challenges include the development of effective communication skills by the healthcare team, the successful establishment of a therapeutic relationship, and the final delivery of a patient-centered care, focused on the unique circumstances of each patient. The gender assignment process and the consequent interventions must be accompanied by psychological support of the patient and its family members, as the psychosocial distress may be severe, especially in the case of PAIS. The aim of this double case report is to outline the difficulties that may rise during diagnostic approach of AIS, extending it even to more challenging aspects, including psychological stress that may result from gender assignment process, therapeutic interventions such as genital surgery (if any), and establishment of a solid and trustful communication between the health professionals and the young patient and its family.

2. Case 1

A girl of 11 years and 3 months was referred to our unit due to enlargement of the clitoris associated with obstructive symptoms at micturition. According to her prenatal history, amniocentesis was conducted due to advanced maternal age, revealing a 46, XY karyotype. Pregnancy was otherwise uncomplicated. Cesarean section was performed at the gestational age of 40 weeks and 3 days due to cephalopelvic disproportion and failure to progress. The newborn was a healthy full-term baby, without electrolyte imbalance, presenting with an inadvertent female phenotype. In order to assess the discordance between chromosomal and phenotypical gender, the SRY gene was examined and found to be present, while imaging of the brain, hypothalamus, and pituitary gland was normal. At that time-point, the family decided to take no further action.

Anthropometric characteristics at presentation were in the normal range for girls at the patient's age, while physical examination revealed excessive clitoridomegaly resembling a phallus of 6 cm and a shallow vaginal orifice. No testes were palpable. Pubertal maturation, pubic hair, breast, and axillary hair were of Tanner stage III, I, and II, respectively. Imaging of the lower abdomen with ultrasound and MRI revealed bilateral testicular tissue at the intraperitoneal space near the inner inguinal ring, hypoplastic penile cavernous bodies within a sizable clitoris, and the presence of a rudimentary prostate along with seminal vesicles. Basal hormones assessment showed elevated T (84.0 ng/dl) in the male reference range for the given pubertal stage, accompanied by mildly elevated LH (2.11 mU/mL) and follicular stimulating hormone (FSH) concentrations (18.56 mU/mL). Estradiol (E_2) on the other hand was inappropriately low (14.45 pg/mL). An hCG stimulation test was performed in order to assess synthesis, conversion, and action of T and exclude other causes of 46, XY DSD, using the algorithm proposed elsewhere [7, 10]. The ratio of T to Δ_4-androstenedione (Δ_4A) was >0.8, excluding 17β-hydroxysteroid dehydrogenase-3 (17β-HSD-3) deficiency, while the ratio of T to dihydrotestosterone (DHT) was <20, excluding 5α-reductase deficiency. The high elevation of T concentration (ΔT) after the hCG stimulation (>100 ng/dl) indicated the presence of testicular tissue, excluded gonadal dysgenesis, and supported the diagnosis of AIS (Table 2). Imaging control revealed the presence of bilateral testicular tissue. The combination of almost female phenotype with minimal virilization and proper male gonadal function was supportive for the diagnosis of severe PAIS.

Reasonably, the assignment of female gender was recommended, since the patient had already been raised as a girl and the relevant interventions would be minimal. In addition, the testes that were found during imaging studies had to

TABLE 2: hCG stimulation test in case 1.

Time (days)	Testosterone (ng/dl)	Δ_4-Androstenedione (ng/ml)	Dihydrotestosterone (ng/dl)	Anti-Müllerian hormone (ng/ml)
0	84	2.0	18.6	0.899
1	526	1.8	50.3	—
2	645	2.5	58.9	—
3	532	2.2	60.8	—

hCG: human chorionic gonadotropin.

TABLE 3: hCG stimulation test in case 2.

Time (days)	Testosterone (ng/dl)	Δ_4-Androstenedione (ng/ml)	Dihydrotestosterone (ng/dl)	Anti-Müllerian hormone (ng/ml)
0	<10	0.16	4.1	107.16
1	41	0.19	12	—
2	170	0.25	25	—
3	201	0.30	28	—

hCG: human chorionic gonadotropin.

be removed, as they were atrophic and of increased risk for malignant change. Interestingly, the parents suggested that the child itself should be fully informed and participate in the final decision, and therefore, from the very first beginning, the patient was involved in all discussions made with the attending physicians. It is noteworthy that, being aware of the condition, she stated: "It does not matter if I am female or male, most of all I am a human being and thus gender assignment will not play any significant role in my future life." Eventually, female gender was preferred by both the patient and the parents, and gonadectomy as well as cosmetic surgery of the external genitalia were successfully performed.

3. Case 2

A 3-year-old boy referred to our unit for further evaluation of micropenis, penoscrotal hypospadias, and a history of operated unilateral cryptorchidism. Regarding his perinatal history, progesterone was administered to his mother since 12 weeks of gestation due to placental detachment. Subsequently, intrauterine growth restriction (IUGR) was noticed and amniocentesis was performed, which demonstrated a normal 46, XY karyotype. Due to the persistence of IUGR and fetal circulation redistribution, cesarean section was performed at the gestational age of 33 weeks and 2 days (birth weight: 1130 g, birth length: 38 cm, head circumference: 28 cm) and the newborn was hospitalized in the Neonatal Intensive Care Unit for one month. Apart from the deformities of the external genitalia and right-sided cryptorchidism, the infant was normal at the time of discharge. He was referred for right orchidopexy, which was performed at the age of nine months.

At the time of presentation, somatometric characteristics were within normal range (height: 91 cm, weight: 12.5 kg, 10th to 25th percentile). Regarding external genitalia, microphallus was observed (length 2 cm) with penoscrotal hypospadias; the right testis was palpable in the scrotum, whereas the left one could not be detected. The rest of the physical examination was that of a prepubertal boy. Abdominal ultrasound revealed the left testis at the inner ring of the inguinal canal, while MRI of the hypothalamus-pituitary gland did not reveal any pathology of the sellar region. Basal concentrations of T and gonadotropins were in the prepubertal range. During GnRH stimulation test, a normal prepubertal response was documented. In addition, an hCG stimulation test was performed, showing a T/Δ_4 ratio >0.8, T/DHT ratio < 20, and a ΔT > 100 ng/dl, findings that were indicative of androgen insensitivity (Table 3). Taking under consideration the clinical phenotype of undervirilization, combined with appropriateness for a toddler testicular function, the diagnosis of PAIS grade 3 was set.

What is remarkable in this patient is that undermasculinization of their child was such a stressful situation for the parents, that they subconsciously transferred their anxiety to their toddler. That was particularly evident since, during the few days that he remained hospitalized, the child very often repeatedly said "I am a young man." Taking into consideration this context, the assignment of male gender was recommended. He was prescribed to receive chorionic gonadotropin 1500 units per week intramuscularly and was referred to the surgeons for unilateral orchidopexy as well as surgical repair of hypospadias. However, the follow-up was discontinued early and no further communication with the family was possible.

4. Discussion

The medical approach to AIS should comprise proper and timely diagnosis, gender assignment, a combination of surgical and conservative interventions, and establishment of a strong-based relation with the patient and its family. It demands a long-term management strategy by a multidisciplinary team composed of experienced specialists: pediatric endocrinologist, pediatric surgeon or urologist, gynecologist, clinical geneticist, neonatologist, and/or pediatric psychologist/psychiatrist, according to the needs of each patient [11]. Nevertheless, healthcare professionals that deal with AIS have to overcome several difficulties in order to fulfill the general concepts of care. Proper diagnosis is a challenge, since the majority of patients (especially those with PAIS) do not present a particular phenotypic pattern. In addition, gender assignment is cumbersome and needs to be justified bearing in mind a variety of factors, such as genitalia appearance, surgical options, and views of the family related to cultural, social, and religious beliefs [11].

The cases presented in this study illustrate some of the challenges mentioned above, especially those depending on parental experiences [12]. In the first patient, though being a case of severe PAIS, where female sex assignment and corresponding surgical/medical interventions are strongly recommended, there was a notable delay in the management due to the parents' preference for no intervention at the time when the problem was first recognized. Despite being aware of the discordance between karyotype and phenotype, no medical assistance was sought until the onset of puberty and the development of secondary male characteristics. As a result, they had to choose to involve their child in the gender assignment process, a fact that might increase dramatically the young adolescent's anxiety. Regarding the second case, even though the genital deformities were minimal and congruent with the karyotype, the patient's family was overwhelmingly stressed and avoided regular follow-up of their offspring.

Concerns have been raised on the assimilation of the discordance among chromosomal, phenotypic, and gonadal sex and its complications [8]. Despite the fact that little is known about the criteria of gender assignment in infants with diversity of external masculinization, the options are usually straightforward. Individuals with CAIS are raised as females. They conceptualize their psychosexual development as a female's one and, up to now, there is no observed dissatisfaction with their assigned gender. This might be explained by the effect of androgen unresponsiveness of the brain, in addition to unambiguous female sex of rearing [13]. On the other hand, many patients with PAIS are raised as males, as in case 2; the female gender is preferred only in selected cases with severe PAIS, as in the hereby presented case 1. Being 11 years old, the patient declared no preference to either male or female gender assignment. This is an unusual statement, as these patients are known to have female gender identity. Given the fact that the patient had already been raised as a girl until the time of referral, it is profound that a female gender identity may have already been developed in a subconscious way. A possible explanation for the patient's detached gender assignment declaration may be the parents' approach (the child should be fully informed, involved in all discussions made with the attending physicians, and participating in the final decision). Sex of rearing does not entirely depend on the degree of external masculinization, especially in cases of severe PAIS where there is no precise relationship between genotype and phenotype implying that other factors may influence the decision of the assigned gender. In some countries, the cultural factors define the sex of rearing, like in Asia where male gender is preferred even if the patient is severely undermasculinized. There is a clear need for more research on documenting phenotype, surgical procedures, and outcome criteria that will enhance gender assignment [1]. Unlike CAIS, psychological distress is more often seen in PAIS patients, irrespective of the choice

of gender assignment. Almost 25% of individuals affected by PAIS suffer from identity crisis or dissatisfaction with the decided sex and, sometimes, a gender reassignment may be needed [14, 15]. Psychological support is mandatory. The decision for the assigned gender is made by the medical team and the family, depending on the aforementioned factors. There is also a controversy about the optimal time of gender assignment. Many specialists recommend the assignment to be decided the sooner possible, while others suggest watchful waiting until the age of 3 years, when it is believed that the gender identity begins to develop [3, 11].

Patients who are raised as females will need genitoplasty and gonadectomy (orchiectomy). Orchiectomy is essential, as the ectopically located testes carry a substantial risk of malignancy. This risk is higher in PAIS than in CAIS, with an incidence of 15% and even higher if the testes are located intra-abdominally [3, 7, 8, 11, 14]. Orchiectomy should take place before the onset of puberty, as virilization may take place, as in case 1, and complicate the management. Less severe cases of PAIS will have to undergo hypospadias repair and orchidopexy. The ideal timing is a highly debated topic, with the majority of the experts suggesting that between 6 and 12 months of age [16, 17]. Puberty may be medically induced at the desired timing towards the gender that has been assigned.

Another issue to be addressed is whether it is, from an ethical and psychological point of view, better or not to reveal the underlying condition to the patient himself. In the case of CAIS or severe PAIS, the patient who has been raised as a female has to cope with the fact that she is genetically male and that she will be infertile. In the past, the standard physicians' approach was not to reveal the whole situation either to the patient or to his relatives. Nowadays, according to relevant interview studies [7, 8, 11, 13, 14], the full or partial disclosure constitutes the first-line choice, abandoning the paternalistic approach of the past. Social and cultural factors may be important modifiers in this process, since different societies do not accept this patient-based approach. In any case, although the family has to be informed, the disclosure to the patient depends on both the child's maturity and the social characteristics of the family.

The EuroDSD consortium, the International Disorder of Sex Development (I-DSD) Registry, and the aforementioned AR gene mutation database are great international initiatives that have contributed a lot in this DSD entity, opening a new, promising path for a more holistic management [2, 7, 18, 19]. Nevertheless, longitudinal studies are urgently needed to clarify obscure points in the optimal management of AIS, such as quality of life, sex assignment, and long-term outcomes.

5. Conclusion

In conclusion, these case reports illustrate the obstacles that the healthcare team has to face and overcome when dealing with AIS patients. These two cases highlighted the wide phenotypical spectrum of the syndrome, presented the different procedure for a final assignment (according to age, phenotype, and related circumstances), and underlined the psychological aspect that is strongly affected. More studies need to be conducted in this field so that the provided care and support are more evidence-based.

Additional Points

Limitations. Neither of the cases was genetically tested. Despite the fact that the yield is high in CAIS, it is low in PAIS.

References

[1] A. Deeb, C. Mason, Y. S. Lee, and I. A. Hughes, "Correlation between genotype, phenotype and sex of rearing in 111 patients with partial androgen insensitivity syndrome," *Clinical Endocrinology*, vol. 63, no. 1, pp. 56–62, 2005.

[2] S. Rajender, L. Singh, K. Thangaraj, and W. M. Lee, "Phenotypic heterogeneity of mutations in androgen receptor gene," *Asian Journal of Andrology*, vol. 9, no. 2, pp. 147–179, 2007.

[3] A. Galani, S. Kitsiou-Tzeli, C. Sofokleous, E. Kanavakis, and A. Kalpini-Mavrou, "Androgen insensitivity syndrome: clinical features and molecular defects," *Hormones*, vol. 7, no. 3, pp. 217–229, 2008.

[4] S. Erdoğan, C. Kara, A. Uçaktürk, and M. Aydin, "Etiological classification and clinical assessment of children and adolescents with disorders of sex development," *Journal of Clinical Research in Pediatric Endocrinology*, vol. 3, no. 2, pp. 77–83, 2011.

[5] B. Gottlieb, L. K. Beitel, A. Nadarajah, M. Paliouras, and M. Trifiro, "The androgen receptor gene mutations database: 2012 update," *Human Mutation*, vol. 33, no. 5, pp. 887–894, 2012.

[6] S. F. Ahmed, J. C. Achermann, W. Arlt et al., "Society for Endocrinology UK guidance on the initial evaluation of an infant or an adolescent with a suspected disorder of sex development (Revised 2015)," *Clinical Endocrinology*, vol. 84, no. 5, pp. 771–788, 2016.

[7] I. A. Hughes, J. D. Davies, T. I. Bunch, V. Pasterski, K. Mastroyannopoulou, and J. Macdougall, "Androgen insensitivity syndrome," *The Lancet*, vol. 380, no. 9851, pp. 1419–1428, 2012.

[8] B. Gottlieb, L. K. Beitel, and M. A. Trifiro, "Androgen insensitivity syndrome," in *GeneReviews [Internet]*, R. A. Pagon, M. P. Adam, H. H. Ardinger et al., Eds., University of Washington, Seattle, Wash, USA, 1993–2016.

[9] T. Lundberg, K. Roen, A. L. Hirschberg, and L. Frisén, "'It's part of me, not all of me': young women's experiences of receiving a diagnosis related to diverse sex development," *Journal of Pediatric and Adolescent Gynecology*, vol. 29, no. 4, pp. 338–343, 2016.

[10] M. M. George, M. I. New, S. Ten, C. Sultan, and A. Bhangoo, "The clinical and molecular heterogeneity of 17βHSD-3 enzyme deficiency," *Hormone Research in Paediatrics*, vol. 74, no. 4, pp. 229–240, 2010.

[11] P. A. Lee, C. P. Houk, S. F. Ahmed, I. A. Hughes, and International Consensus Conference on Intersex Organized by the Lawson Wilkins Pediatric Endocrine Society and the European Society for Paediatric Endocrinology, "Consensus statement on management of intersex disorders," *Pediatrics*, vol. 118, no. 2, pp. e488–e500, 2006.

[12] H. P. Crissman, L. Warner, M. Gardner et al., "Children with disorders of sex development: A Qualitative Study Of Early Parental Experience," *International Journal of Pediatric Endocrinology*, vol. 10, 2011.

[13] H. Özbey and S. Etker, "Disorders of sexual development in a cultural context," *Arab Journal of Urology*, vol. 11, no. 1, pp. 33–39, 2013.

[14] C. Gîngu, A. Dick, S. Pătrăşcoiu et al., "Testicular feminization: complete androgen insensitivity syndrome. discussions based on a case report," *Romanian Journal of Morphology and Embryology*, vol. 55, no. 1, pp. 177–181, 2014.

[15] M. El-Sherbiny, "Disorders of sexual differentiation: II. Diagnosis and treatment," *Arab Journal of Urology*, vol. 11, no. 1, pp. 27–32, 2013.

[16] E. Chan, C. Wayne, and A. Nasr, "Ideal timing of orchiopexy: a systematic review," *Pediatric Surgery International*, vol. 30, pp. 87–97, 2014.

[17] A. Bhat, "General considerations in hypospadias surgery," *Indian Journal of Urology*, vol. 24, no. 2, pp. 188–194, 2008.

[18] M. Telles-Silveira, F. Knobloch, and C. E. Kater, "Management framework paradigms for disorders of sex development," *Archives of endocrinology and metabolism*, vol. 59, no. 5, pp. 383–390, 2015.

[19] Z. Kolesinska, S. F. Ahmed, M. Niedziela et al., "Changes over time in sex assignment for disorders of sex development," *Pediatrics*, vol. 134, no. 3, pp. e710–e715, 2014.

45

Mifepristone Improves Octreotide Efficacy in Resistant Ectopic Cushing's Syndrome

Andreas G. Moraitis[1] and Richard J. Auchus[2]

[1]Corcept Therapeutics, 149 Commonwealth Drive, Menlo Park, CA 94025, USA
[2]Division of Metabolism, Diabetes, and Endocrinology, Department of Internal Medicine, University of Michigan, 1150 West Medical Center Drive, Ann Arbor, MI 48109, USA

Correspondence should be addressed to Andreas G. Moraitis; andreas.moraitis@yahoo.com

Academic Editor: Hidetoshi Ikeda

A 30-year-old Caucasian man presented with severe Cushing's syndrome (CS) resulting from ectopic adrenocorticotropin syndrome (EAS) from a metastatic pancreatic neuroendocrine tumor. The patient remained hypercortisolemic despite treatment with steroidogenesis inhibitors, chemotherapy, and octreotide long-acting release (LAR) and was enrolled in a 24-week, phase 3 clinical trial of mifepristone for inoperable hypercortisolemia. After mifepristone was added to ongoing octreotide LAR treatment, EAS symptoms essentially resolved. Cortisol decreased dramatically, despite mifepristone's competitive glucocorticoid receptor antagonist effects. The clinical and biochemical effects reversed upon mifepristone discontinuation despite the continued use of octreotide LAR therapy. Substantial improvement in octreotide LAR efficacy with mifepristone use was noted in this patient with ectopic CS, consistent with upregulation of somatostatin receptors previously downregulated by hypercortisolemia.

1. Introduction

Chronic hypercortisolemia resulting from ectopic adrenocorticotropin hormone secretion (EAS) (nonpituitary) accounts for approximately 10% of all adrenocorticotropin- (ACTH-) dependent Cushing's syndrome (CS) [1, 2]. Although localized primarily in the chest, consisting of mainly bronchial (foregut) neuroendocrine tumors (NETs) and small-cell lung carcinoma, EAS is also associated with medullary thyroid carcinomas, gastrointestinal NETs, and thymic NETs, and, less frequently, other tumor types [2–4]. The primary treatment of EAS is surgical removal of the tumor when possible. If surgical resection is not possible or successful, medical therapy is necessary.

Depending on the etiology, EAS-associated tumors can express multiple somatostatin receptor subtypes (e.g., SST2, SST1, and SST5) [5]. This finding has enabled the use of somatostatin receptor scintigraphy (e.g., [111In]-pentetreo-tide or octreoscan and [68Ga]-octreotide-derivative positron emission tomography) for tumor localization and, in some cases, targeted treatment with somatostatin analog, octreotide [2, 4, 6–9], which has high affinity for SST2 [10]. However, octreotide therapy is frequently ineffective, limiting its utility as a therapeutic and diagnostic agent [11, 12].

Glucocorticoids have been shown to directly downregulate SST2 expression in human NET cells [13], as well as in human and murine corticotrope adenoma cells [14, 15]. The downregulation of SST2 in human neuroendocrine cell lines was found to be reversed with the addition of mifepristone, a glucocorticoid receptor (GR) antagonist [13]. Mifepristone may also directly influence tumoral SST2 expression levels in human NETs [16]. Medical therapy with mifepristone in 2 patients with EAS resulted in increased posttreatment uptake, positive octreoscan, and subsequent tumor localization [16]. In contrast, the capacity of mifepristone to enhance the clinical therapeutic efficacy of somatostatin analogs in reducing ACTH and cortisol production has not yet been demonstrated. We report a case of EAS demonstrating a synergistic effect of mifepristone in combination with octreotide long-acting release (LAR).

TABLE 1: Biochemistry evaluations during treatment with mifepristone[*].

Test (normal range)	Baseline (before MIFE)	Week 6	Week 10	Week 16	Week 24	2-week follow-up (off MIFE)
ACTH, pg/mL (7–50 pg/mL)	345	279	188	250	304	652
UFC, mcg/24 h (2.0–42.4 mcg/24 h)	2250	1536	104	122	434	4716
Serum cortisol, mcg/dL (8 AM, 4.0–22.0 mcg/dL)	46	41	31	31	37	68
Late-night salivary cortisol, mcg/dL (10 PM-11 PM, ≤0.09 mcg/dL)	1.71	2.18	0.56	0.73	1.49	4.91

[*] Patient continued to receive octreotide LAR 30 mg every month throughout the study. ACTH denotes adrenocorticotropin hormone, LAR long-acting release, MIFE mifepristone, and UFC urinary-free cortisol. To convert the values for UFC to nanomoles per 24 h, multiply by 2.76. To convert the values for ACTH to picomoles per liter, multiply by 0.22. To convert the values for serum cortisol and late-night salivary cortisol to nanomoles per liter, multiply by 27.6.

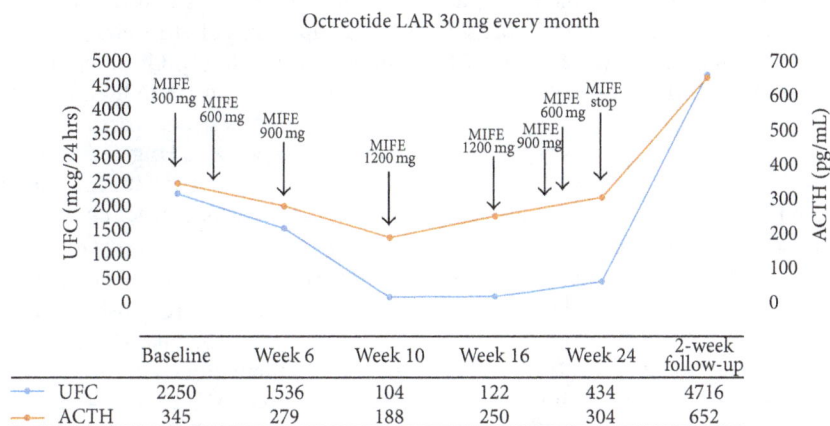

	Baseline	Week 6	Week 10	Week 16	Week 24	2-week follow-up
UFC	2250	1536	104	122	434	4716
ACTH	345	279	188	250	304	652

FIGURE 1: UFC and ACTH concentrations during treatment with mifepristone and octreotide LAR. ACTH denotes adrenocorticotropin hormone, LAR long-acting release, MIFE mifepristone, and UFC urinary-free cortisol. To convert the values for UFC to nanomoles per 24 h, multiply by 2.76. To convert the values for ACTH to picomoles per liter, multiply by 0.22.

2. Case

A 30-year-old man presented with weight gain, hypertension, diabetes, proximal muscle weakness, and nephrolithiasis. He developed moon facies, abdominal striae, and disproportionate supraclavicular and dorsocervical fat pads. Endocrine testing and imaging studies revealed a pancreatic NET with involvement of the inferior vena cava and other local structures. After resection of the tumor, the postoperative ACTH was not suppressed; however, cushingoid features improved significantly. Approximately 2 years later, symptoms of EAS recurred. Ketoconazole and chemotherapy were started but were not successful in resolving hypercortisolemia. Three months later, octreotide LAR was initiated, and the dose was gradually increased to 30 mg every month. A partial biochemical response was noted (ACTH decreased from 517 pg/mL (113.7 pmol/L) to 345 pg/mL (75.9 pmol/L)), but the patient's symptoms of EAS were not controlled. After 3 months of therapy with octreotide LAR, the patient was enrolled in a 24-week, phase 3 clinical trial of mifepristone for inoperable hypercortisolemia (clinicaltrials.gov identifier: NCT00569582 [17]). Prior to the start of mifepristone, baseline urinary-free cortisol (UFC)

was 2250 mcg/24 hours (6207 nmol/24 hours) and ACTH was 345 pg/mL (75.9 pmol/L). Late-night salivary cortisol (1.71 mcg/dL (47.2 nmol/L)) and serum cortisol (46 mcg/dL (1256 nmol/L)) were also elevated (Table 1). At the time of enrollment, the patient had overtly cushingoid features, including moon facies, plethora, and enlarged dorsocervical and supraclavicular fat pads; purple striae; bruising; edema; and proximal muscle weakness that was so severe that he was unable to rise from a chair without use of his hands. He also had ongoing diabetes, depression, and hypertension associated with hypokalemia. Mifepristone was initiated at a daily dose of 300 mg and gradually increased to 1200 mg per protocol. The patient continued to receive octreotide LAR throughout the duration of the trial. By week 4, insulin therapy was discontinued and by week 12, his cushingoid features essentially resolved. In addition to clinical improvement, a dramatic decrease in cortisol and ACTH was noted during therapy with mifepristone and octreotide LAR (Figure 1, Table 1). At week 20, mifepristone was briefly stopped for significant fatigue, low appetite, and nausea. Mifepristone was then resumed at a daily dose of 900 mg and 1 week later reduced to 600 mg; no changes were made to octreotide LAR dose. At week 24, his UFC and ACTH levels were

434 mcg/24 hours (1198.7 nmol/24 hours) and 304 pg/mL (66.9 pmol/L), respectively, and mifepristone was stopped per study protocol. During withdrawal of mifepristone, the cortisol and ACTH rose, and 12 days after mifepristone was stopped, clinical signs and symptoms of EAS returned. After 2 weeks, his UFC and ACTH increased to 4716 mcg/24 hours (13016 nmol/24 hours) and 652 pg/mL (143.4 pmol/L), respectively (Figure 1, Table 1). Mifepristone was resumed for an additional 12-month extension period. Octreotide LAR was discontinued after 2 months and the patient continued with mifepristone for control of his CS-related symptoms. The collection of cortisol and ACTH data was less frequent during the extension study. At the time octreotide was discontinued, the patient's ACTH and serum cortisol were 652 pg/mL (143.4 pmol/L) and 67.8 mcg/dL (1871 nmol/L), respectively. After 12 months in the extension phase, substantial increases in ACTH (3738 pg/mL (822.4 pmol/L)), serum cortisol (135.2 mcg/dL (3732 nmol/L)), and UFC (10716.5 mcg/24 hours (29577.5 nmol/24 hours)) were observed.

3. Discussion

This case describes a patient with pancreatic NET associated with EAS, in whom treatment with the somatostatin analog octreotide became much more effective in controlling cortisol and ACTH after the addition of GR antagonist therapy with mifepristone. Several studies have demonstrated a relationship between GR sensitivity and response to somatostatin analogs [13, 15, 18]. Corticotrope adenomas contain multiple somatostatin receptors, primarily SST5 and lower levels of SST2 [19]. Using murine corticotrope tumor cells, van der Hoek et al. demonstrated a dexamethasone-dependent inhibitory effect of octreotide treatment targeting SST2 that was not found with analogs that targeted primarily SST5 [15]. This result suggests that analogs targeting SST2 are particularly susceptible to glucocorticoid-mediated downregulation, which also might explain the lower SST2 expression found in human corticotrope adenomas and the frequent lack of response to octreotide in patients with Cushing's disease (CD) [14].

Ferrau et al. studied whether a brief treatment with mifepristone modulates the response to acute octreotide administration in 5 patients with CD [18]. This study showed that brief mifepristone pretreatment does not modify ACTH and cortisol response to acute octreotide administration in patients with CD. However, the authors noted that, regardless of mifepristone treatment, decreases in ACTH and cortisol after acute injection of octreotide were observed in patients with lower cortisol levels following dexamethasone suppression testing. Together these results suggest that an intact glucocorticoid signaling pathway within these cells is required for downregulation of SST2.

This model could explain some of the variability in response to SST2 analogs among the various tumor types associated with EAS. In vitro studies in small-cell lung cancer cell lines demonstrated defects in GR function that could lead to glucocorticoid resistance [20, 21]. de Bruin et al. have shown a dexamethasone dose-dependent downregulation of SST2 expression in the human pancreatic NET cell line BON

and the medullary thyroid carcinoma cell line TT, which disappeared after treating these cells with mifepristone [13]. However, the authors reported no glucocorticoid-mediated effects in DMS cells from a small-cell lung cancer line with severe glucocorticoid resistance.

At least 20% to 30% of patients with EAS will suppress plasma and urinary steroids to less than 50% of baseline values during high-dose dexamethasone suppression testing [22]. These patients are clinically and hormonally difficult to differentiate from patients with CD, particularly if the tumor is not localized. With the development of targeting radionuclide diagnostics and therapeutics using somatostatin analogs (theranostics), an additional role of mifepristone might be as a "radiosensitizing" agent. Ejaz et al. reported 2 patients with EAS and occult tumor sources despite multiple imaging attempts whose bronchial NETs were localized via octreotide scintigraphy only after receiving treatment with mifepristone for several weeks [2]. Of note, only 1 of the 2 patients was found to be responsive to high-dose dexamethasone testing. Therefore, additional data are required to determine whether a positive response to 1 mg of dexamethasone in patients with CD or 8 mg in patients with EAS can predict the response to somatostatin analogs targeting the SST2.

In this case, the addition of mifepristone to ongoing octreotide LAR led to a substantial reduction in ACTH and cortisol in our patient with previously resistant EAS associated with severe hypercortisolemia. This effect was lost upon discontinuation of mifepristone after 24 weeks of treatment. Of note, the reduction in ACTH during mifepristone cotreatment was not as pronounced as the observed reduction in cortisol. An assessment of ACTH precursors (proopiomelanocortin and pro-ACTH), which can be markedly elevated in patients with EAS [23, 24], would have provided additional insight. However, measuring precursors and biologically active ACTH would have required separation via chromatography, which was not performed, nor did we have access to patient tumor tissue to assess SST receptor expression. Nonetheless, to our knowledge, this is the first clinical case report that demonstrates a relationship between GR antagonism with mifepristone and increased therapeutic efficacy of the somatostatin analog octreotide, consistent with upregulation of somatostatin receptors previously downregulated by hypercortisolemia.

Disclosure

This paper was prepared according to the International Society for Medical Publication Professionals' "Good Publication Practice for Communicating Company-Sponsored Medical Research: The GPP3 Guidelines" and the International Committee of Medical Journal Editors' "Uniform Requirements for Manuscripts Submitted to Biomedical Journals."

Authors' Contribution

Drs. Moraitis and Auchus conceptualized the case report and drafted and/or critically reviewed the paper. The authors read and approved the final paper.

Acknowledgments

The authors wish to thank Sarah Mizne, PharmD of Med-Val Scientific Information Services, LLC, and Dat Nguyen, PharmD of Corcept Therapeutics, for providing professional writing and editorial assistance. Some of the data for this patient case report came from a clinical trial that was sponsored by Corcept Therapeutics, Menlo Park, CA. Funding to support the preparation of this paper was provided to MedVal Scientific Information Services, LLC, by Corcept Therapeutics.

References

[1] B. L. Wajchenberg, B. B. Mendonca, B. Liberman et al., "Ectopic adrenocorticotropic hormone syndrome," *Endocrine Reviews*, vol. 15, no. 6, pp. 752–787, 1994.

[2] S. Ejaz, R. Vassilopoulou-Sellin, N. L. Busaidy et al., "Cushing syndrome secondary to ectopic adrenocorticotropic hormone secretion: the University of Texas MD Anderson Cancer Center experience," *Cancer*, vol. 117, no. 19, pp. 4381–4389, 2011.

[3] I. Ilias, D. J. Torpy, K. Pacak, N. Mullen, R. A. Wesley, and L. K. Nieman, "Cushing's syndrome due to ectopic corticotropin secretion: twenty years' experience at the National Institutes of Health," *Journal of Clinical Endocrinology and Metabolism*, vol. 90, no. 8, pp. 4955–4962, 2005.

[4] A. M. Isidori, G. A. Kaltsas, C. Pozza et al., "The ectopic adrenocorticotropin syndrome: clinical features, diagnosis, management, and long-term follow-up," *Journal of Clinical Endocrinology and Metabolism*, vol. 91, no. 2, pp. 371–377, 2006.

[5] J. C. Reubi and B. Waser, "Concomitant expression of several peptide receptors in neuroendocrine tumours: molecular basis for in vivo multireceptor tumour targeting," *European Journal of Nuclear Medicine and Molecular Imaging*, vol. 30, no. 5, pp. 781–793, 2003.

[6] K. von Werder, O. A. Muller, and G. K. Stalla, "Somatostatin analogs in ectopic corticotropin production," *Metabolism*, vol. 45, no. 8, supplement 1, pp. 129–131, 1996.

[7] M. Phlipponneau, M. Nocaudie, J. Epelbaum et al., "Somatostatin analogs for the localization and preoperative treatment of an adrenocorticotropin-secreting bronchial carcinoid tumor," *Journal of Clinical Endocrinology and Metabolism*, vol. 78, no. 1, pp. 20–24, 1994.

[8] S. W. Lamberts, W. W. de Herder, E. P. Krenning, and J. C. Reubi, "A role of (labeled) somatostatin analogs in the differential diagnosis and treatment of Cushing's syndrome," *Journal of Clinical Endocrinology and Metabolism*, vol. 78, no. 1, pp. 17–19, 1994.

[9] Z. G. Özkan, S. Kuyumcu, D. Balköse, B. Özkan, and N. Aksakal, "The value of somatostatin receptor imaging with In-111 Octreotide and/or Ga-68 DOTATATE in localizing Ectopic ACTH producing tumors," *Malecular Imaging and Radionuclide Therapy*, vol. 22, no. 2, pp. 49–55, 2013.

[10] S. Grozinsky-Glasberg, I. Shimon, M. Korbonits, and A. B. Grossman, "Somatostatin analogues in the control of neuroendocrine tumours: efficacy and mechanisms," *Endocrine-Related Cancer*, vol. 15, no. 3, pp. 701–720, 2008.

[11] N. W. Cheung and S. C. Boyages, "Failure of somatostatin analogue to control Cushing's syndrome in two cases of ACTH-producing carcinoid tumours," *Clinical Endocrinology*, vol. 36, no. 4, pp. 361–367, 1992.

[12] G. I. Uwaifo, C. A. Koch, B. Hirshberg et al., "Is there a therapeutic role for octreotide in patients with ectopic cushing's syndrome?" *Journal of Endocrinological Investigation*, vol. 26, no. 8, pp. 710–717, 2003.

[13] C. de Bruin, R. A. Feelders, A. M. Waaijers et al., "Differential regulation of human dopamine D2 and somatostatin receptor subtype expression by glucocorticoids *in vitro*," *Journal of Molecular Endocrinology*, vol. 42, no. 1, pp. 47–56, 2009.

[14] G. K. Stalla, S. J. Brockmeier, U. Renner et al., "Octreotide exerts different effects in vivo and in vitro in Cushing's disease," *European Journal of Endocrinology*, vol. 130, no. 2, pp. 125–131, 1994.

[15] J. van der Hoek, M. Waaijers, P. M. van Koetsveld et al., "Distinct functional properties of native somatostatin receptor subtype 5 compared with subtype 2 in the regulation of ACTH release by corticotroph tumor cells," *American Journal of Physiology—Endocrinology and Metabolism*, vol. 289, no. 2, pp. E278–E287, 2005.

[16] C. de Bruin, L. J. Hofland, L. K. Nieman et al., "Mifepristone effects on tumor somatostatin receptor expression in two patients with Cushing's syndrome due to ectopic adrenocorticotropin secretion," *Journal of Clinical Endocrinology and Metabolism*, vol. 97, no. 2, pp. 455–462, 2012.

[17] M. Fleseriu, B. M. K. Biller, J. W. Findling, M. E. Molitch, D. E. Schteingart, and C. Gross, "Mifepristone, a glucocorticoid receptor antagonist, produces clinical and metabolic benefits in patients with Cushing's syndrome," *Journal of Clinical Endocrinology and Metabolism*, vol. 97, no. 6, pp. 2039–2049, 2012.

[18] F. Ferrau, F. Trimarchi, and S. Cannavo, "Adrenocorticotropin responsiveness to acute octreotide administration is not affected by mifepristone premedication in patients with Cushing's disease," *Endocrine*, vol. 47, no. 2, pp. 550–556, 2014.

[19] C. de Bruin, A. M. Pereira, R. A. Feelders et al., "Coexpression of dopamine and somatostatin receptor subtypes in corticotroph adenomas," *Journal of Clinical Endocrinology and Metabolism*, vol. 94, no. 4, pp. 1118–1124, 2009.

[20] D. W. Ray, A. C. Littlewood, A. J. L. Clark, J. R. E. Davis, and A. White, "Human small cell lung cancer cell lines expressing the proopiomelanocortin gene have aberrant glucocorticoid receptor function," *The Journal of Clinical Investigation*, vol. 93, no. 4, pp. 1625–1630, 1994.

[21] D. Gaitan, C. R. DeBold, M. K. Turney, P. Zhou, D. N. Orth, and W. J. Kovacs, "Glucocorticoid receptor structure and function in an adrenocorticotropin-secreting small cell lung cancer," *Molecular Endocrinology*, vol. 9, no. 9, pp. 1193–1201, 1995.

[22] J. W. Findling and J. L. Doppman, "Biochemical and radiologic diagnosis of Cushing's syndrome," *Endocrinology and Metabolism Clinics of North America*, vol. 23, no. 3, pp. 511–537, 1994.

[23] A. White and S. Gibson, "ACTH precursors: biological significance and clinical relevance," *Clinical Endocrinology*, vol. 48, no. 3, pp. 251–255, 1998.

46

Simultaneous Papillary Carcinoma in Thyroglossal Duct Cyst and Thyroid

Gustavo Cancela e Penna,[1,2,3] **Henrique Gomes Mendes,**[1] **Adele O. Kraft,**[4]
Cynthia Koeppel Berenstein,[1,5] **Bernardo Fonseca,**[6] **Wagner José Martorina,**[7]
Andreise Laurian N. R. de Souza,[8] **Gustavo Meyer de Moraes,**[9]
Kamilla Maria Araújo Brandão Rajão,[10] **and Bárbara Érika Caldeira Araújo Sousa**[11]

[1] *Federal University of Minas Gerais (UFMG), Belo Horizonte, MG, Brazil*
[2] *Federal University of Rio de Janeiro, Rio de Janeiro, RJ, Brazil*
[3] *Division of Endocrinology, Hospital Mater Dei, Belo Horizonte, MG, Brazil*
[4] *Department of Pathology, Virginia Commonwealth University, Richmond, VA, USA*
[5] *Division of Pathology, Instituto Roberto Alvarenga, Belo Horizonte, MG, Brazil*
[6] *Division of Radiology, Spectra Institute, Belo Horizonte, MG, Brazil*
[7] *Division of Endocrinology, Hospital Biocor, Belo Horizonte, MG, Brazil*
[8] *Division of Endocrinology, Hospital da Baleia, Belo Horizonte, MG, Brazil*
[9] *Division of Head and Neck Surgery, Hospital das Clinicas, UFMG, Belo Horizonte, MG, Brazil*
[10] *Division of Endocrinology, Hospital das Clinicas, UFMG, Belo Horizonte, MG, Brazil*
[11] *Division of Endocrinology, Hospital Mario Pena, Belo Horizonte, MG, Brazil*

Correspondence should be addressed to Gustavo Cancela e Penna; gustavocpenna@gmail.com

Academic Editor: Thomas Grüning

Thyroglossal duct cyst (TDC) is a cystic expansion of a remnant of the thyroglossal duct tract. Carcinomas in the TDC are extremely rare and are usually an incidental finding after the Sistrunk procedure. In this report, an unusual case of a 36-year-old woman with concurrent papillary thyroid carcinoma arising in the TDC and on the thyroid gland is presented, followed by a discussion of the controversies surrounding the possible origins of a papillary carcinoma in the TDC, as well as the current management options.

1. Background

Thyroglossal duct cyst (TDC) is the most common congenital, benign, midline neck mass, accounting for 7% of midline neck swellings in adults [1]. A TDC arises as a cystic expansion of a remnant of the thyroglossal duct tract and is the most frequent congenital anomaly of the neck [2].

Associated carcinoma is extremely rare, occurring in about 1% of TDC cases [3], with fewer than 300 cases reported since the first description by Brentano in 1911 [4]. The clinical presentation of a TDC carcinoma (TDCCa) is often asymptomatic and very similar to its benign counterpart. Thus, it is difficult to identify the TDCCa on clinical

examination, as well as on ultrasound, scintigraphy, or even at fine needle aspiration biopsy (FNAB) and the diagnosis of the malignancy is generally incidental after surgery [5].

The majority of carcinomas are small (0.2 cm to 1.5 cm) and confined to the cyst, papillary thyroid being the most common histological type [6, 7]. The average patients' age is 40 years old and it is more frequent in females [8]. The finding of a carcinoma in a TDC after adequate excision of the cyst, usually by means of the Sistrunk procedure (SP), is a surprise for both the patient and the physician [5].

It is still debated whether TDCCa originates from the thyroid gland, from the TDC itself (de novo theory) or from both [9–12]. Although the differentiation may be difficult,

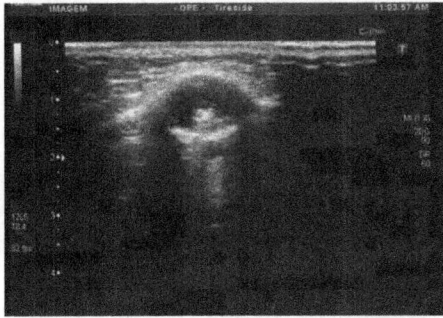

FIGURE 1: Sonography shows an image suggestive of thyroglossal duct cyst containing debris and an eccentric small hyperechoic solid area.

this distinction can play a crucial role in treatment decisions regarding the inclusion of thyroidectomy as part of the treatment strategy versus TDC total resection exclusively [13].

2. Case Presentation

A 36-year-old female patient presented with a slow-growing, painless, midline neck mass. She reported no previous radiation exposure and no signs or symptoms of thyroid abnormalities, hoarseness, breathing difficulty, or dysphagia. Her medical records were reviewed and her medical history was otherwise unremarkable. Physical examination revealed a smooth, well-circumscribed mass along the midline of the neck, overlying the thyrohyoid membrane, mobile with deglutition and protrusion of the tongue. There were no palpable lymph nodes.

3. Investigation

Thyroid function tests were normal. The neck ultrasound revealed a pattern suggestive of a thyroglossal duct cyst: a single, midline, suprahyoid cyst containing debris and an eccentric small hyperechoic solid area. This structure measured $1.6 \, \text{cm}^3$ with absence of flow on Doppler-sonography (Figure 1). The midline neck location and the close relationship between the lesion and the hyoid bone were considered the key to the differential diagnosis of the TDC, which includes branchial cleft cysts and lymph nodes [14]. Because the frequency of thyroglossal cyst carcinoma is very low, in a large percentage of cases the clinicians seldom consider an oncologic diagnosis and therefore do not perform a preoperative fine needle aspiration biopsy, albeit its low sensitivity [15].

After a fully informed written consent, complete excision of thyroglossal duct with central thyroidectomy was performed (standard Sistrunk procedure). The surgical aspect was of that of a thyroglossal duct cyst. The lesion was dissected up to the hyoid bone and then to the base of the tongue. No abnormal findings were observed intraoperatively and there were no intercurrences or complications.

Due to the characteristics observed on the ultrasound and the location of the lesion, it was assumed that it was a thyroglossal cyst. Gross examination showed a 3.0 cm cyst, filled with a gelatinous green material, with a bone fragment

attached to it. The histopathological report revealed a cystic lesion and a tumor characterized by the proliferation of columnar cells in a single layer, mostly arranged in papillae, but also in follicles, supported by a richly vascularized connective tissue. The cells had ovoid, ground glass nuclei ("Orphan Annie" eye), sometimes with grooves and pseudoinclusions (Figures 2(a)–2(h)). The tumor measured 1.4 centimeter. There was minimal infiltration of the adjacent fibroadipose tissue. This histology was compatible with papillary carcinoma in the TDC and it was staged as pT3c N0 M0 [16].

The case was then presented at a multidisciplinary meeting, when all the clinical and radiological data were reviewed.

4. Treatment

A thyroid and cervical lymph node sonography was performed with no abnormalities observed. However, considering the possibility of a concomitant and occult papillary carcinoma in the thyroid, fully informed written consent had been obtained from the patient and total thyroidectomy (TT) with prophylactic bilateral central neck dissection (excision of levels VI and VII lymph nodes) has been performed, once it is the optimal surgical treatment for thyroid carcinoma. No dissected lymph node was macroscopically suggestive of metastasis, as observed intraoperatively.

Considering the American Thyroid Association risk stratification (intermediate risk) [7, 17], it would be necessary to perform RIA therapy. Additionally, the possibility of this tumor being a metastasis from a thyroid cancer supported the rationale of TT.

5. Outcome and Follow-Up

The postthyroidectomy histopathological report revealed a 0.4 cm nonencapsulated papillary thyroid microcarcinoma (mPTC), follicular variant. The neoplastic mass displayed follicular architecture and was composed of cells with ground glass nuclei, nuclear grooves, and pseudoinclusions. No extrathyroidal involvement and vascular or neural invasion were observed. There were no metastasis in the 14 lymph nodes resected, and the surgical margins were free. This absence reinforces the TDCCa diagnosis and makes less likely the differential diagnosis of an occult PTC undergoing conspicuously cystic transformation. The thyroid tumor was staged as pT1a pN0 Mx.

The patient had negative thyroglobulin and antithyroglobulin after surgery. Thyroid remnant ablation was achieved by the administration of 30 mCi of radioactive iodine (RAI-131) and posteriorly a whole-body scintigraphy showed zero uptake of the substance. It was followed by TSH suppression (0.1–0.5 mU/L) and the patient remains disease-free after 9 months of follow-up.

6. Discussion

There is no consensus on the optimal treatment of TDCCa mainly because of the lack of data from larger studies.

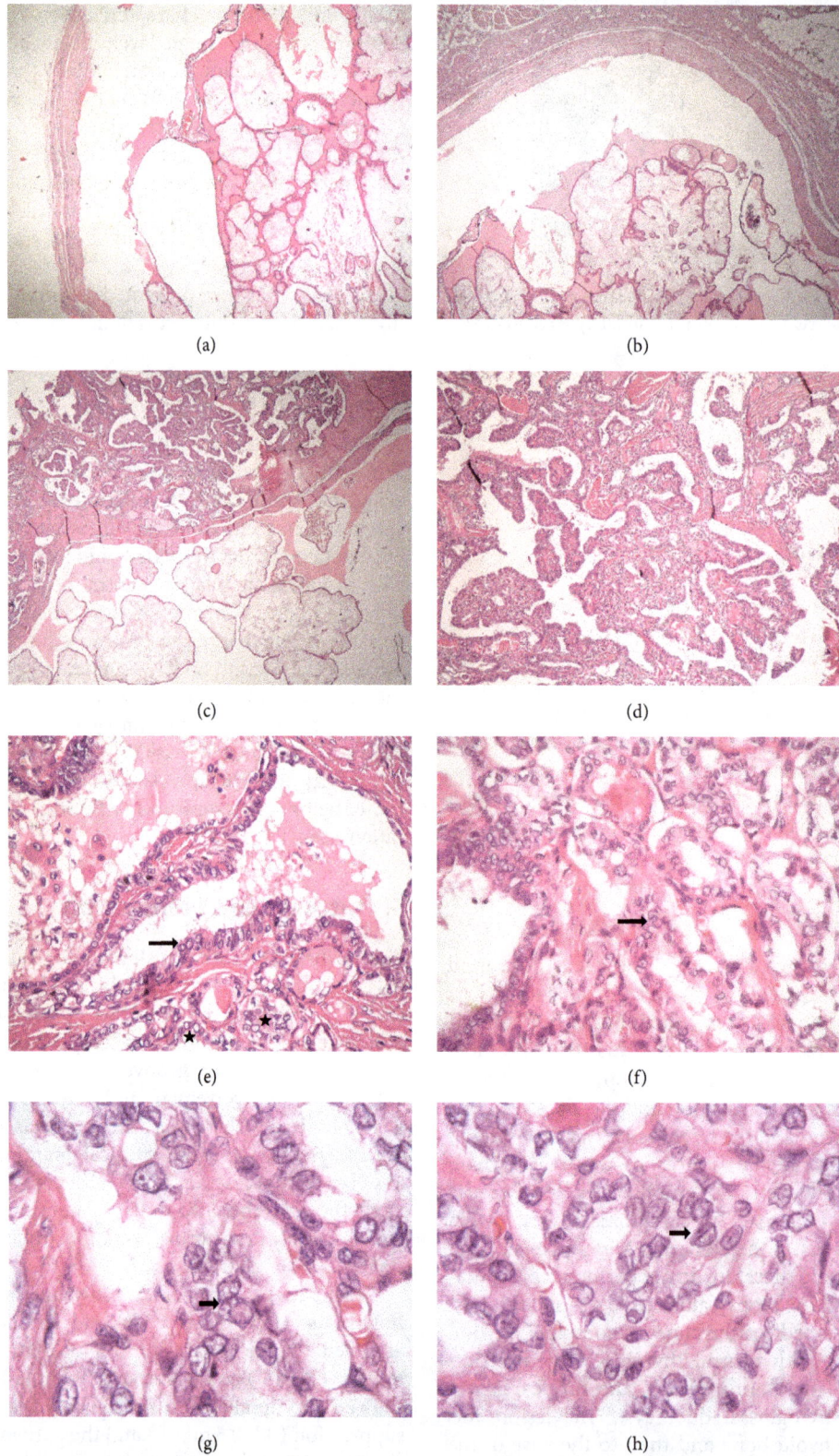

FIGURE 2: Thyroglossal duct cyst carcinoma. (a) and (b) Low power view of the cyst containing the papillary carcinoma (HE, 40x). (c) The papillae were sometimes edematous (HE, 40x). (d) The tumor had papillae, but also some follicles (HE, 100x). (e) Nuclei with pseudoinclusions (arrow) and ground glass appearance (stars) (HE, 400x). (f) Nuclear pseudoinclusion (HE, 400x). (g) Nuclear pseudoinclusion (arrow) (HE, 1000x). (h) Nuclear groove (arrow) (HE, 1000x).

Most authors agree that Sistrunk's procedure (SP), originally described in 1928, a block resection of the TDC along with the hyoid bone and the surrounding soft tissue towards the foramen cecum, is the first-choice surgery for TDCCa [6]. Patel et al. have shown that, in the presence of a clinically normal thyroid gland, the only factor that considerably affected outcome prognosis was the extent of surgery for the thyroglossal cyst itself. Simple cyst excision was inferior to SP (10-year survival rates being 95% and 75%, resp.), and total thyroidectomy was of no additional survival benefit [8].

Recently, total or subtotal thyroidectomy has been recommended if there is cyst wall invasion by the carcinoma or if the TDCCa is larger than 1.0 cm [7]. Although extension to surrounding soft tissue has been reported in 17% to 55% of all TDC malignancies [12, 18, 19], it is not known whether this has any prognostic impact [20]. In our case, it measured 1.4 cm and there was invasion of the capsule.

Prognostic risk group assessment was proposed to identify patients who would benefit from additional TT [7] and TT should be added only to high-risk patients [5]. However, Bakkar et al. reported a 62% rate of concomitant thyroglossal cyst and thyroid carcinomas. Similar high incidence of concomitant thyroid cancers, which may be occult in 25 to 56% of cases, results had been previously observed [20, 21].

Bakkar et al. also reported a 43% risk of missing thyroid malignancy in the setting of a sonographically normal thyroid gland and that the size of the thyroglossal cyst carcinoma could not serve as a predictive factor for the presence or absence of a concomitant thyroid carcinoma. Therefore, they concluded that selecting a subset of patients free of the risk of a concomitant thyroid cancer or free of the need for RAI ablation is a difficult task. Accordingly, they advocated the routine addition of TT to achieve comprehensive loco-regional control [18]. Other authors have this same rationale [19, 20].

Furthermore, TT permits systemic evaluation, treatment, and follow-up using serum markers [21]. Similarly, according to the risk stratification approach [7], a woman presenting a 1.4 cm tumor with cystic wall invasion would not be stated as low risk and would require additional TT.

Regional lymph node metastasis has been reported in up to 88% of TDCCa [22, 23]. This feature supported Hartl et al.'s statement that routine central compartment (level VI) dissection allows more precise lymph node staging, which may modify 131I ablation necessity [23]. It is important to notice that metastasis to the lateral compartment without central compartment involvement is not as rare as it is in thyroid gland cancers.

Despite this clear trend of lateral compartment nodes serving as primary stations for the spread of thyroglossal observed in some studies [12, 23], prophylactic lateral dissection in the absence of detectable nodal metastases has not been routinely recommended by any authors [5, 8, 24], even though regional neck dissection is recommended in high-risk group [7].

Therefore, the basis for a central neck dissection was to follow current guidelines for treatment of differentiated thyroid cancer, as recommended by Hartl et al. [23]. Furthermore, a lateral neck dissection can be performed secondarily if needed without an increase in surgical complications.

Prognosis of TDC papillary thyroid carcinoma seems to be similar to that of papillary carcinoma of the thyroid gland, as well as the long-term follow-up, although the reported follow-up time is short (median time of 12 y) and the number of patients is small. Mortality is low with only a few reported disease-related deaths [24, 25].

We have presented a case of a papillary thyroid carcinoma arising in a thyroglossal duct cyst, a rare condition with few cases published in the literature. There are many controversies about the tumor's origin and the extension of surgery needed, which makes the definition of many aspects related to its management and follow-up difficult. Some characteristics which point to higher recurrence rates can guide treatment. The selection of patients which are likely to have worst prognosis and, consequently, will need a more aggressive treatment is of great importance and an individualized approach is the best option to improve patient outcome.

Additional Points

(i) Thyroglossal duct cyst carcinoma is an extremely rare condition and usually an incidental finding. (ii) Surgery is the mainstay management for thyroglossal cyst carcinoma. However, the optimal surgical strategy remains controversial.

Disclosure

All the designated authors have met all four criteria for authorship defined by the International Committee of Medical Journal Editors.

Acknowledgments

The authors acknowledge the valuable contribution of the Thyroid Study Group (Belo Horizonte, Brazil).

References

[1] P. D. M. Ellis and A. W. P. Van Nostrand, "The applied anatomy of thyroglossal tract remnants," *Laryngoscope*, vol. 87, no. 5, pp. 765–770, 1977.

[2] R. H. B. Allard, "The thyroglossal cyst," *Head and Neck Surgery*, vol. 5, no. 2, pp. 134–146, 1982.

[3] W. C. Boswell, M. Zoller, J. S. Williams, S. A. Lord, and W. Check, "Thyroglossal duct carcinoma," *American Surgeon*, vol. 60, no. 9, pp. 650–655, 1994.

[4] H. Brentano, "Struma aberrata lingual mit druzen metastasen," *Deutsche Medizinische Wochenschrift*, vol. 37, pp. 665–666, 1911.

[5] C. P. Ramírez Plaza, M. E. D. López, C. E.-G. Carrasco, L. M. Meseguer, and A. D. L. F. Perucho, "Management of well-differentiated thyroglossal remnant thyroid carcinoma: time to close the debate? Report of five new cases and proposal of a

definitive algorithm for treatment," *Annals of Surgical Oncology*, vol. 13, no. 5, pp. 745–752, 2006.

[6] W. E. Sistrunk, "Technique of removal of cyst and sinuses of the thyreoglossal duct," *Surgery, Gynecology & Obstetrics*, vol. 46, pp. 109–111, 1928.

[7] M. Tharmabala and R. Kanthan, "Incidental thyroid papillary carcinoma in a thyroglossal duct cyst—management dilemmas," *International Journal of Surgery Case Reports*, vol. 4, no. 1, pp. 58–61, 2013.

[8] S. G. Patel, M. Escrig, A. R. Shaha, B. Singh, and J. P. Shah, "Management of well-differentiated thyroid carcinoma presenting within a thyroglossal duct cyst," *Journal of Surgical Oncology*, vol. 79, no. 3, pp. 134–139, 2002.

[9] T. Baglam, A. Binnetoglu, A. C. Yumusakhuylu, B. Demir, G. Askan, and M. Sari, "Does papillary carcinoma of thyroglossal duct cyst develop de novo?" *Case Reports in Otolaryngology*, vol. 2015, Article ID 382760, 5 pages, 2015.

[10] N. Gupta, A. Dass, M. Bhutani, S. K. Singhal, H. Verma, and R. P. S. Punia, "Papillary carcinoma in thyroglossal duct cyst: an unusual case," *Egyptian Journal of Ear, Nose, Throat and Allied Sciences*, vol. 15, no. 1, pp. 45–47, 2014.

[11] A. W. Hilger, S. D. Thompson, L. A. Smallman, and J. C. Watkinson, "Papillary carcinoma arising in a thyroglossal duct cyst: a case report and literature review," *The Journal of Laryngology & Otology*, vol. 109, no. 11, pp. 1124–1127, 1995.

[12] G. Pellegriti, G. Lumera, P. Malandrino et al., "Thyroid cancer in thyroglossal duct cysts requires a specific approach due to its unpredictable extension," *The Journal of Clinical Endocrinology and Metabolism*, vol. 98, no. 2, pp. 458–465, 2013.

[13] V. Gebbia, C. Di Gregorio, and M. Attard, "Thyroglossal duct cyst carcinoma with concurrent thyroid carcinoma: a case report," *Journal of Medical Case Reports*, vol. 2, article 132, 2008.

[14] N. Kutuya and Y. Kurosaki, "Sonographic assessment of thyroglossal duct cysts in children," *Journal of Ultrasound in Medicine*, vol. 27, no. 8, pp. 1211–1219, 2008.

[15] Y. J. Yang, S. Haghir, J. R. Wanamaker, and C. N. Powers, "Diagnosis of papillary carcinoma in a thyroglossal duct cyst by fine-needle aspiration biopsy," *Archives of Pathology and Laboratory Medicine*, vol. 124, no. 1, pp. 139–142, 2000.

[16] S. B. Edge, D. R. Byrd, C. C. Compton et al., *AJCC Cancer Staging Manual*, vol. 7th, Springer, New York, NY, USA, 2010.

[17] B. R. Haugen, E. K. Alexander, K. C. Bible et al., "2015 american thyroid association management guidelines for adult patients with thyroid nodules and differentiated thyroid cancer: the american thyroid association guidelines task force on thyroid nodules and differentiated thyroid cancer," *Thyroid*, vol. 26, no. 1, pp. 1–133, 2016.

[18] S. Bakkar, M. Biricotti, G. Stefanini, C. E. Ambrosini, G. Materazzi, and P. Miccoli, "The extent of surgery in thyroglossal cyst carcinoma," *Langenbeck's Archives of Surgery*, 2016.

[19] P. Miccoli, M. N. Minuto, D. Galleri, M. Puccini, and P. Berti, "Extent of surgery in thyroglossal duct carcinoma: reflections on a series of eighteen cases," *Thyroid*, vol. 14, no. 2, pp. 121–123, 2004.

[20] S. Basu, T. Shet, and A. M. Borges, "Outcome of primary papillary carcinoma of thyroglossal duct cyst with local infiltration to soft tissues and uninvolved thyroid," *Indian Journal of Cancer*, vol. 46, no. 2, pp. 169–170, 2009.

[21] J. M. Manipadam, M. T. Manipadam, E. M. Thomas et al., "Thyroglossal duct carcinoma: a case series and approach to management," *World Journal of Endocrine Surgery*, vol. 3, no. 2, pp. 59–63, 2011.

[22] R. Dzodic, I. Markovic, B. Stanojevic et al., "Surgical management of primary thyroid carcinoma arising in thyroglossal duct cyst: an experience of a single institution in Serbia," *Endocrine Journal*, vol. 59, no. 6, pp. 517–522, 2012.

[23] D. M. Hartl, A. A. Ghuzlan, L. Chami, S. Leboulleux, M. Schlumberger, and J.-P. Travagli, "High rate of multifocality and occult lymph node metastases in papillary thyroid carcinoma arising in thyroglossal duct cysts," *Annals of Surgical Oncology*, vol. 16, no. 9, pp. 2595–2601, 2009.

[24] W. Kermani, M. Belcadhi, M. Abdelkéfi, and K. Bouzouita, "Papillary carcinoma arising in a thyroglossal duct cyst: case report and discussion of management modalities," *European Archives of Oto-Rhino-Laryngology*, vol. 265, no. 2, pp. 233–236, 2008.

[25] E. Vassilatou, K. Proikas, N. Margari, N. Papadimitriou, D. Hadjidakis, and G. Dimitriadis, "An adolescent with a rare midline neck tumor: thyroid carcinoma in a thyroglossal duct cyst," *Journal of Pediatric Hematology/Oncology*, vol. 36, no. 5, pp. 407–409, 2014.

47

False Positive Findings on I-131 WBS and SPECT/CT in Patients with History of Thyroid Cancer: Case Series

Zeina C. Hannoush,[1] **Juan D. Palacios,**[1] **Russ A. Kuker,**[2] **and Sabina Casula**[1]

[1]*Division of Endocrinology, Diabetes and Metabolism, Department of Medicine, University of Miami Miller School of Medicine, Miami, FL 33136, USA*
[2]*Division of Nuclear Medicine, Department of Radiology, University of Miami Miller School of Medicine, Miami, FL 33136, USA*

Correspondence should be addressed to Sabina Casula; scasula@med.miami.edu

Academic Editor: Suat Simsek

Introduction. Although whole body scan (WBS) with I-131 is a highly sensitive tool for detecting normal thyroid tissue and metastasis of differentiated thyroid cancer (DTC), it is not specific. Additional information, provided by single photon emission computed tomography combined with X-ray computed tomography (SPECT/CT) and by the serum thyroglobulin level, is extremely useful for the interpretation of findings. *Case Presentation.* We report four cases of false positive WBS in patients with DTC: ovarian uptake corresponding to an endometrioma, scrotal uptake due to a spermatocele, rib-cage uptake due to an old fracture, and hepatic and renal uptake secondary to a granuloma and simple cyst, respectively. *Conclusions.* Trapping, organification, and storage of iodine are more prominent in thyroid tissue but not specific. Physiologic sodium-iodine symporter expression in other tissues explains some, but not all, of the WBS false positive cases. Other proposed etiologies are accumulation of radioiodine in inflamed organs, metabolism of radiodinated thyroid hormone, presence of radioiodine in body fluids, and contamination. In our cases nonthyroidal pathologies were suspected since the imaging findings were not corroborated by an elevated thyroglobulin level, which is considered a reliable tumor marker for most well-differentiated thyroid cancers. Clinicians should be aware of the potential pitfalls of WBS in DTC to avoid incorrect management.

1. Introduction

In thyroidectomized patients with history of well-differentiated thyroid cancer (DTC), scintillation scanning of the whole body (WBS) after either a diagnostic or therapeutic dose of radioactive iodine administration is considered the routine method to identify the physical location of local or distant, iodine avid, metastasis [1]. This relies on the fact that most of the DTC cells retain the property, unique to the thyroid epithelial follicular cells, to concentrate, organify, and accumulate iodine through the action of the sodium-iodine symporter (NIS) [2]. Although WBS is highly sensitive for detecting thyroid tissue, it is not very specific; therefore, false positive images can be seen in clinical practice and their recognition is critical for correct management [3, 4].

Single photon emission computed tomography (SPECT) combined with X-ray computed tomography (CT) is a sophisticated adjuvant tool that has shown to be useful for better localization of lesions seen on planar views [5]. Here we describe four clinical cases with positive distant uptake, where SPECT/CT played an essential role in the localization and interpretation of the results seen on WBS. Nonthyroidal pathologies were suspected since the imaging findings were not corroborated by an elevated level of serum thyroglobulin, which in the absence of thyroglobulin antibodies is considered a sensitive and reliable tumor marker for most well-differentiated thyroid cancers. In these clinical scenarios it is essential to avoid exposing the patients to unnecessary additional radioiodine treatment for presumptive metastasis.

2. Case Presentation

Case #1. We present the case of a 46-year-old woman with history of stage T1N0M0 papillary thyroid cancer, mixed

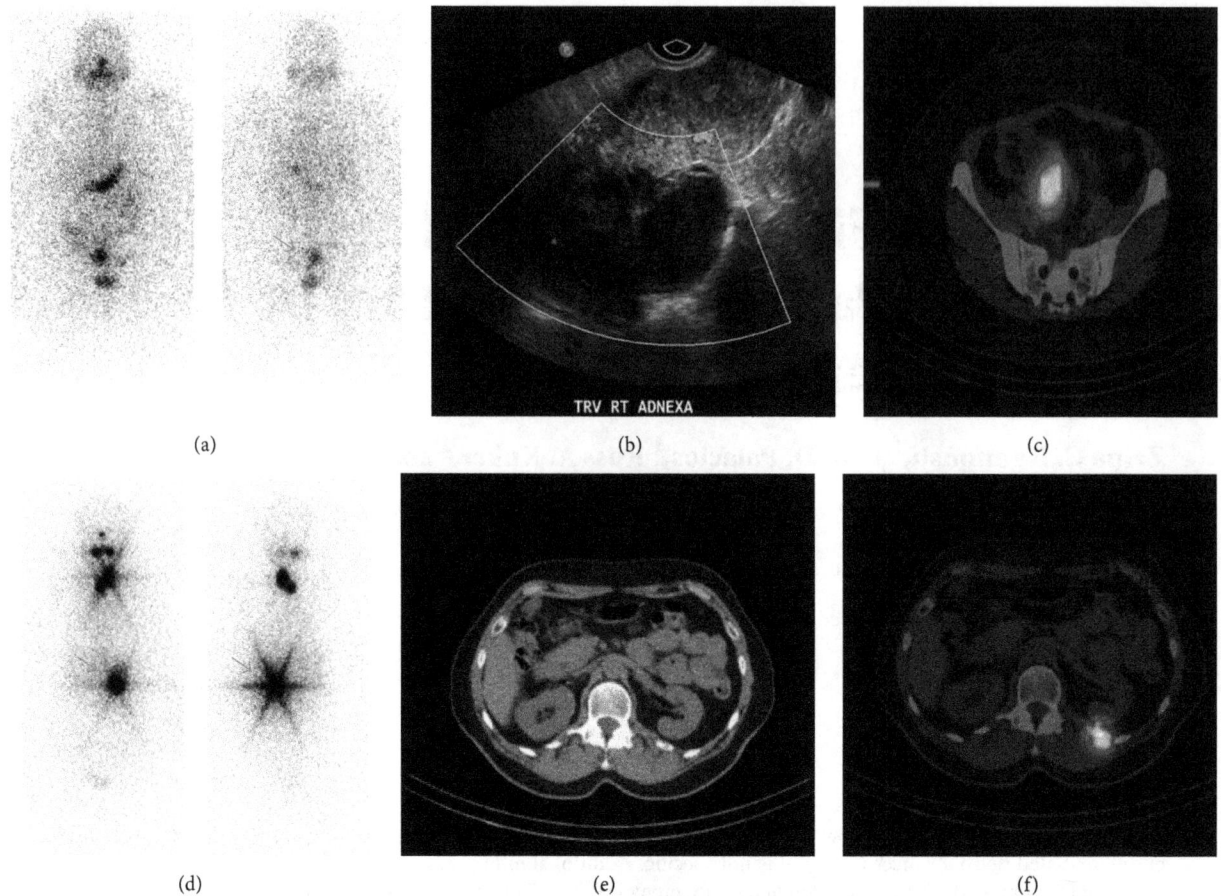

FIGURE 1: (a) Anterior and posterior planar views from a diagnostic I-131 WBS show focal uptake in the right pelvis (arrow). (b) Transverse sonographic image of the right adnexa shows a lobulated complex solid and cystic lesion with internal vascularity. (c) SPECT/CT localizes the area of radioiodine uptake to the right adnexal lesion, which on final pathology after surgical resection showed an endometrioma. (d) Anterior and posterior planar views from a postablation I-131 WBS show expected radiotracer uptake in the neck as well as an incidental focus of intense activity in the left lower thorax (arrow). (e) Axial CT image through the lower thorax shows a nondisplaced fracture of the left twelfth rib. (f) SPECT/CT localizes the area of radioiodine uptake to the left twelfth rib, which was biopsied and showed no evidence of malignancy.

follicular and solid variant status after thyroidectomy followed by radioactive iodine (RAI) ablation therapy with 99 mCi of I-131. Initial WBS showed physiologic uptake in the thyroid bed. On the one-year post-treatment surveillance workup, she was found to be in biochemical remission with a negative stimulated thyroglobulin level and negative thyroglobulin antibodies. However, the I-131 WBS demonstrated an area of iodine accumulation in the pelvis above the urinary bladder, which localized to the right adnexa on SPECT/CT. Pelvic ultrasound revealed an 8 × 8 × 5 cm hypoechoic vascular and lobulated mass in the right adnexal region. For that reason, the patient underwent hysterectomy with right oophorectomy. The pathology was consistent with endometrioma [Figures 1(a)–1(c)].

Case #2. We present the case of a 63-year-old woman with history of stage T1bN1Mx papillary thyroid cancer, follicular and classical variant status after thyroidectomy followed by RAI ablation therapy with 28 mCi of I-131. The post-treatment WBS revealed uptake in the neck, and a separate

focus of intense uptake in the left lower thorax, which localized to the left 12th rib on SPECT/CT. A subsequent bone scan confirmed the presence of an osteoblastic lesion in the left 12th rib suspicious for metastasis. The stimulated thyroglobulin at the time she received her ablation treatment was 7.2 ng/mL with negative thyroglobulin antibodies, more consistent with thyroid remnant than distant metastasis. She underwent biopsy of the suspicious bone lesion and pathology was negative for malignancy. CT scan images revealed a rib fracture at that level (Figures 1(d)–1(f)).

Case #3. We present the case of a 49-year-old man with history of papillary thyroid cancer, classical variant status after thyroidectomy and RAI ablation therapy with 138 mCi of I-131. His thyroglobulin level was unreliable due to the presence of thyroglobulin antibodies. The posttherapy WBS showed uptake in the thyroid bed and in the cervical region compatible with a lymph node. There was an additional focus of iodine uptake in the right lower pelvis that localized above the right testicle on SPECT/CT. A scrotal ultrasound found

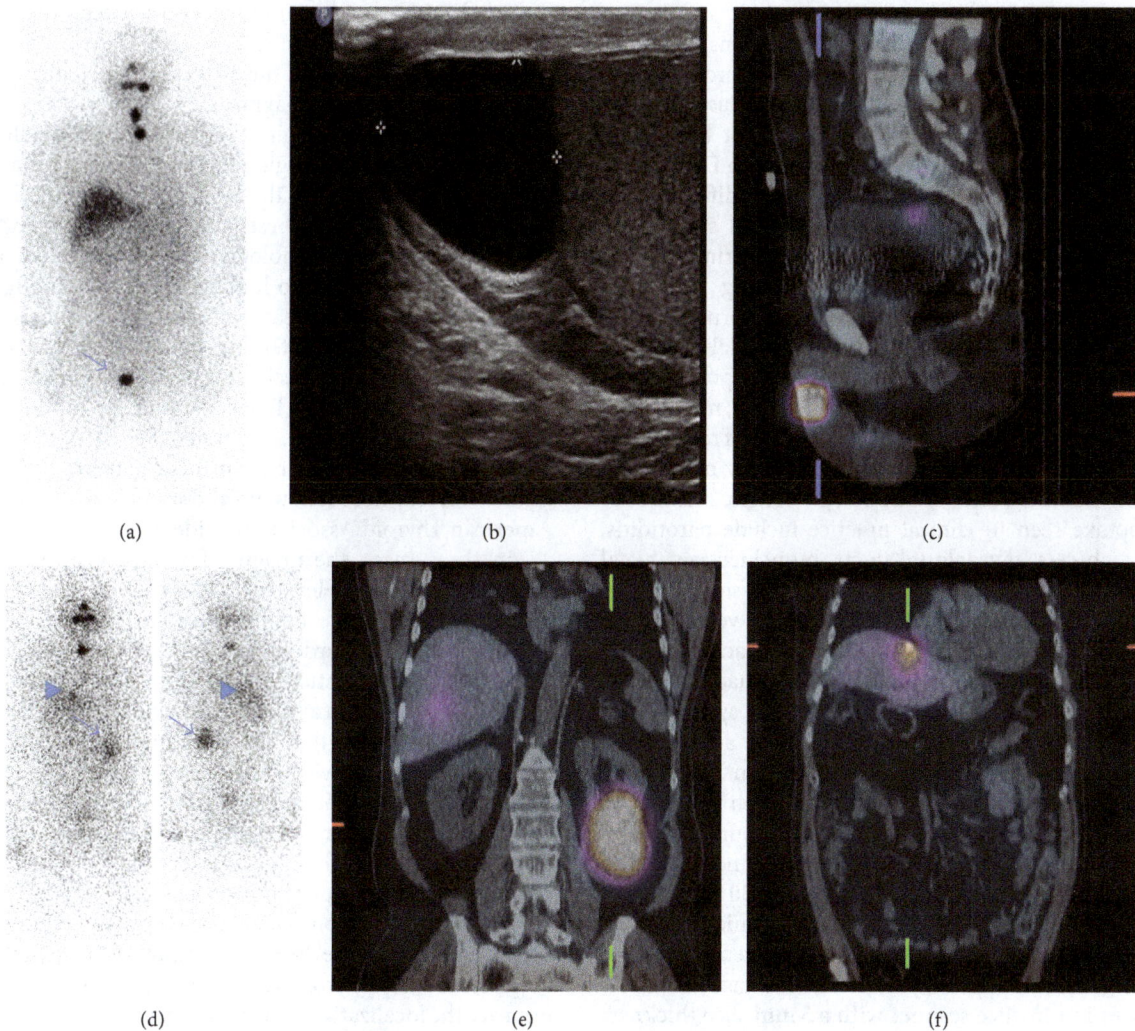

FIGURE 2: (a) Anterior planar view from a postablation I-131 WBS shows satisfactory targeting of radiotracer in the neck with an additional incidental focus of activity in the region of the right scrotum. (b) Sagittal sonographic image of the right scrotum shows a hypoechoic avascular lesion in the right epididymal head likely representing a spermatocele. (c) SPECT/CT localizes the area of radioiodine uptake to the right epididymal lesion. (d) Anterior and posterior planar views from a postablation I-131 WBS show expected radiotracer uptake in the neck as well as two incidental foci projecting over the dome of the liver (arrowhead) and in the left lower quadrant of the abdomen (arrow). (e) SPECT/CT localizes the area of radioiodine uptake to an exophytic cyst arising from the inferior pole of the left kidney. (f) SPECT/CT localizes the second radioiodine avid focus to a calcified granuloma in the dome of the liver.

no evidence of testicular abnormalities, but there was an interval increase in size of a right side spermatocele, which corresponded to the abnormal uptake noted on the nuclear medicine examination (Figures 2(a)–2(c)).

Case #4. We present the case of a 62-year-old man with history of stage T3N1Mx papillary thyroid cancer, classical variant status after thyroidectomy and RAI ablation therapy with 150 mCi of I-131. His stimulated thyroglobulin level was 7.3 ng/mL with negative thyroglobulin antibodies. Post-treatment WBS with SPECT/CT showed physiologic uptake in the area of the thyroid bed as well as focal accumulation of radioiodine in the abdomen likely corresponding to a granuloma in the liver and a simple cyst in the left kidney as demonstrated by a follow-up sonogram. The patient had

negative viral hepatitis serology and normal liver function tests (Figures 2(d)–2(f)).

3. Discussion and Conclusions

Iodine (I), the oxidized form of I^-, is an essential constituent of thyroid hormones which are phenolic rings joined by an ether link iodinated at 3 positions (3,5,3'-tri-iodo-L-thyronine, or T_3) or 4 positions (3,5,3',5'-tetra-iodo-L-thyronine or T_4) [6]. The uptake of iodine through the basolateral membrane of the follicular thyroid cells is a key point in the biosynthesis of thyroid hormone. This process is mediated by the sodium-iodine symporter (NIS), a 13-transmembrane domain glycoprotein that relies on the sodium (Na^+) electrochemical gradient created by the Na^+/K^+ ATPase and allows active concentration of iodine by electrogenic symport of sodium (2 : 1 Na^+ to I^- stoichiometry). Trapping, organification, and storage of iodine are usually more prominent in functioning thyroid tissue than other organs. Based on that principle, radioactive iodine has been used for both diagnostic and therapeutic purposes in patients with DTC [7].

NIS is also expressed in several other differentiated epithelia where it is not regulated by thyroid stimulating hormone (TSH) like salivary glands, thymus, lacrimal glands, gastric mucosa, choroid plexus, and lactating mammary glands [6]. Functional NIS expression in normal tissues can explain some but not all of the cases of false positive results on WBS. Other etiologies that have been proposed are accumulation of radioiodine in inflamed organs, metabolism of radiodinated thyroid hormone, the presence of radioiodine in body fluids, and therefore contamination by physiologic secretions. Common sites of physiologic ectopic radioactive iodine uptake seen in clinical practice include parotiditis, maxillary abscess, thyroglossal ducts, bronchiectasis, hiatal hernia, esophageal retention, and sebaceous cysts [1, 7, 8].

A conventional planar I-131 WBS can be a very sensitive diagnostic tool; however, a lack of anatomical landmarks and the nonspecific uptake of radiotracer somewhat complicate the interpretation of the images [5]. Hybrid systems integrating SPECT with a conventional CT allow a fairly exact overlay of molecular and morphological information and are more accurate for diagnosis and staging than WBS alone [9, 10]. The SPECT/CT images obtained in our case series were performed on Symbia T16 scanner (Siemens Medical Solutions) using a 128×128 pixel matrix and 30 seconds per projection view. Standard reconstruction technique entailed iterative reconstruction with a CT-based attenuation correction algorithm applied to the SPECT images. The CT component is a 16-slice scanner with a 5 mm slice thickness and a pitch of 0.8.

Endometrioma as a cause of false positive WBS findings was first described in 2000 and only a few reported cases exist in the literature [11, 12]. Inflammation has been recognized as a common cause of false positive findings on WBS [1] and our second case is a salient demonstration of how this can be encountered in clinical practice. To the best of our knowledge, radioactive iodine accumulation in a spermatocele causing false positive findings in the pelvis on WBS has not been previously described in the literature.

Diffuse hepatic uptake after I-131 therapy has been previously reported and it is thought to be caused by hepatic metabolism of radioiodinated thyroid hormones released by remnant thyroid tissue. This pattern of activity should be distinguished from focal hepatic uptake [2]. Focal false positive iodine accumulation in the liver has been encountered in patients with biliary duct dilation [13]; this is thought to be due to biliary excretion of radioidinated metabolites. Only a few cases of false positive radioactive iodine accumulation in simple liver cysts, not associated with biliary duct dilation, have been reported and the pathophysiology behind this accumulation is not well understood [14–16]. Many cases of false positive uptake seen in renal cysts have been reported. There are various hypotheses of the pathophysiology behind uptake in renal cysts including an active secretory process by the renal tubules and communication between the cyst and the renal collecting system [17].

Interpreting correctly the WBS can be challenging and often times the final diagnosis requires additional tests including alternative imaging studies and occasionally tissue biopsy. The level of thyroglobulin and the exact location of the uptake determined by the SPECT/CT are helpful tools in the initial assessment of these patients. Based on that knowledge nonthyroidal pathologies were suspected in our patients. It is important to highlight that even though DTC is usually an indolent disease with a good prognosis, distant metastasis is always a potential complication that accounts for most of its disease specific mortality. The most common metastatic sites are in the lungs and bones but brain, breast, liver, kidney, muscle, skin, and other sites of metastasis have been described. For this reason these patients should continue to receive close follow-up and surveillance according to American Thyroid Association guidelines [18].

In three cases, the imaging findings were not corroborated by a reliable elevated level of serum thyroglobulin, which in the absence of thyroglobulin antibodies usually reflects the tumor burden in most cases of DTC [19]. The patient with accumulation of RAI above the right testicle had positive thyroglobulin antibodies known to interfere with the immunometric assay that was used, limiting the interpretation of the test. However, while a case of testicular metastasis from medullary thyroid cancer was previously described [20], to our knowledge, there are no reports of testicular metastasis from DTC. A scrotal ultrasound confirmed that the false positive uptake was due to a spermatocele.

The four cases reported illustrate how the accurate evaluation of radioiodine WBS is critical in the management of patients with thyroid cancer and how SPECT/CT can improve the localization and characterization of lesions. Clinicians involved in the management of DTC should be aware of the potential pitfalls of radioiodine scans and of the possible mechanisms involved to avoid incorrect management.

Disclosure

All figures are original.

References

[1] Y. B. Garger, M. Winfeld, K. Friedman, and M. Blum, "In thyroidectomized thyroid cancer patients, false-positive I-131 whole body scans are often caused by inflammation rather than thyroid cancer," *Journal of Investigative Medicine High Impact Case Reports*, vol. 4, no. 1, 2016.

[2] D. I. Glazer, R. K. J. Brown, K. K. Wong, H. Savas, M. D. Gross, and A. M. Avram, "SPECT/CT evaluation of unusual physiologic radioiodine biodistributions: pearls and pitfalls in image interpretation," *Radiographics*, vol. 33, no. 2, pp. 397–418, 2013.

[3] V. Triggiani, V. A. Giagulli, M. Iovino et al., "False positive diagnosis on 131iodine whole-body scintigraphy of differentiated thyroid cancers," *Endocrine*, vol. 53, no. 3, pp. 626–635, 2015.

[4] P. O. Kara, E. C. Gunay, and A. Erdogan, "Radioiodine contamination artifacts and unusual patterns of accumulation in whole-body I-131 imaging: a case series," *International Journal of Endocrinology and Metabolism*, vol. 12, no. 1, Article ID e9329, 2014.

[5] Y. Xue, Z. Qiu, H. Song, and Q. Luo, "Value of 131I SPECT/CT for the evaluation of differentiated thyroid cancer: a systematic review of the literature," *European Journal of Nuclear Medicine and Molecular Imaging*, vol. 40, no. 5, pp. 768–778, 2013.

[6] C. Portulano, M. Paroder-Belenitsky, and N. Carrasco, "The Na$^+$/I$^-$ symporter (NIS): mechanism and medical impact," *Endocrine Reviews*, vol. 35, no. 1, pp. 106–149, 2014.

[7] J. R. Oh and B. C. Ahn, "False-positive uptake on radioiodine whole-body scintigraphy: physiologic and pathologic variants unrelated to thyroid cancer," *American Journal of Nuclear Medicine and Molecular Imaging*, vol. 2, no. 3, pp. 362–385, 2012.

[8] V. Triggiani, M. Moschetta, V. A. Giagulli, B. Licchelli, and E. Guastamacchia, "Diffuse 131I lung uptake in bronchiectasis: a potential pitfall in the follow-up of differentiated thyroid carcinoma," *Thyroid*, vol. 22, no. 12, pp. 1287–1290, 2012.

[9] S. Kohlfuerst, I. Igerc, M. Lobnig et al., "Posttherapeutic 131I SPECT-CT offers high diagnostic accuracy when the findings on conventional planar imaging are inconclusive and allows a tailored patient treatment regimen," *European Journal of Nuclear Medicine and Molecular Imaging*, vol. 36, no. 6, pp. 886–893, 2009.

[10] A. Spanu, M. E. Solinas, F. Chessa, D. Sanna, S. Nuvoli, and G. Madeddu, " ^{131}I SPECT/CT in the follow-up of differentiated thyroid carcinoma: incremental value versus planar imaging," *Journal of Nuclear Medicine*, vol. 50, no. 2, pp. 184–190, 2009.

[11] T.-L. Chuang, C.-S. Hsu, and Y.-F. Wang, "(131)I SPECT/CT demonstrated ovarian endometrioma," *Clinical Nuclear Medicine*, vol. 39, no. 2, pp. 193–195, 2014.

[12] M. Lungo, F. Tenenbaum, P. Chaumerliac et al., "Ovarian endometriosis cyst with iodine 131 uptake: first case of false positive in the follow up for differentiated thyroid carcinoma," *Annales d'Endocrinologie*, vol. 61, no. 2, pp. 147–150, 2000.

[13] D.-L. You, K.-Y. Tzen, J.-F. Chen, P.-F. Kao, and M.-F. Tsai, "False-positive whole-body iodine-131 scan due to intrahepatic duct dilatation," *Journal of Nuclear Medicine*, vol. 38, no. 12, pp. 1977–1979, 1997.

[14] C. Okuyama, Y. Ushijima, M. Kikkawa et al., "False-positive I-131 accumulation in a liver cyst in a patient with thyroid carcinoma," *Clinical Nuclear Medicine*, vol. 26, no. 3, pp. 198–201, 2001.

[15] D. H. Gunawardana, A. G. Pitman, and M. Lichtenstein, "Benign hepatic Cyst mimicking a functional thyroid carcinoma metastasis on whole-body I-131 imaging," *Clinical Nuclear Medicine*, vol. 28, no. 6, pp. 527–528, 2003.

[16] R. Ranade, S. Pawar, A. Mahajan, and S. Basu, "Unusual false positive radioiodine uptake on ^{131} I whole body scintigraphy in three unrelated organs with different pathologies in patients of differentiated thyroid carcinoma: a case series," *World Journal of Nuclear Medicine*, vol. 15, no. 2, pp. 137–141, 2016.

[17] A. Campennì, R. M. Ruggeri, S. Giovinazzo, A. Sindoni, D. Santoro, and S. Baldari, "Radioiodine uptake in a renal cyst mimicking a metastasis in a patient affected by differentiated thyroid cancer: case report and review of the literature," *Annals of Nuclear Medicine*, vol. 28, no. 5, pp. 472–476, 2014.

[18] H.-J. Song, Y.-L. Xue, Y.-H. Xu, Z.-L. Qiu, and Q.-Y. Luo, "Rare metastases of differentiated thyroid carcinoma: pictorial review," *Endocrine-Related Cancer*, vol. 18, no. 5, pp. R165–R174, 2011.

[19] C. A. Spencer, J. S. LoPresti, S. Fatemi, and J. T. Nicoloff, "Detection of residual and recurrent differentiated thyroid carcinoma by serum thyroglobulin measurement," *Thyroid*, vol. 9, no. 5, pp. 435–441, 1999.

[20] M. Appetecchia, A. Barnabei, V. Pompeo et al., "Testicular and inguinal lymph node metastases of medullary thyroid cancer: a case report and review of the literature," *BMC Endocrine Disorders*, vol. 14, article no. 84, 2014.

48

A Rare Complication following Thyroid Percutaneous Ethanol Injection: Plummer Adenoma

Roberto Cesareo,[1] Anda Mihaela Naciu,[2] Valerio Pasqualini,[3] Giuseppe Pelle,[3] Silvia Manfrini,[2] Gaia Tabacco,[2] Angelo Lauria Pantano,[2] Alessandro Casini,[1] Roberto Cianni,[3] and Andrea Palermo[2]

[1]Department of Internal Medicine, "S. M. Goretti" Hospital, Latina, Italy
[2]Department of Endocrinology, University Campus Bio-Medico, Rome, Italy
[3]Department of Radiology, "S. M. Goretti" Hospital, Latina, Italy

Correspondence should be addressed to Andrea Palermo; a.palermo@unicampus.it

Academic Editor: Osamu Isozaki

Percutaneous ethanol injection (PEI) is a technique used only for benign thyroid nodules, cystic or mixed cystic-solid with a large fluid component. It is a quite low-cost, safe, and outpatient method of treatment. Rare and severe complications have been described after PEI: jugular vein thrombosis and severe ethanol toxic necrosis of the larynx combined with necrotic dermatitis. Moreover, only four thyrotoxicosis cases due to Graves' disease have been reported. We report a case of 58-year-old female with a voluminous thyroid cystic nodule, occupying almost the entire left thyroid lobe. Our patient had already performed surgical visit and intervention of thyroidectomy had been proposed to her, which she refused. At baseline, our patient has a normal thyroid function with negative autoantibodies. According to the nodular structure, intervention of PEI has been performed with a significant improvement of compressive symptoms and cosmetic disorders. About 30 days after treatment, there was a significant volume reduction, but patient developed an acclaimed symptomatic thyrotoxicosis. After ruling out several causes of hyperthyroidism and according to the thyroid scintigraphy findings, we made the diagnosis of Plummer adenoma. To our knowledge, our patient is the first case of Plummer adenoma following PEI treatment of nontoxic thyroid nodule.

1. Introduction

Thyroid nodules disease is one of the most common clinical endocrine disorders, mainly in iodine lacking regions. Thyroid nodules are characterized by undue growth of structure, functional transformation, and/or cystic degeneration of one or more zones inside the gland. Thyroid nodules are frequently incidental findings, following noninvasive methods such as thyroid ultrasound or radionuclide thyroid scans [1–4].

The progression and management of thyroid nodules are still controversial. If surgery is refused or contraindicated, there are currently a lot of alternative approaches including radioiodine treatment, levothyroxine therapy, percutaneous laser ablation (PLA), percutaneous radiofrequency ablation (RFA), and percutaneous ethanol injection (PEI) [5].

PEI under ultrasonography guidance has been used for more than ten years in solitary hot, toxic, and even cold thyroid nodules, but the most convincing effect was seen in solitary thyroid cysts. Presently, PEI is used only for benign thyroid nodules and cystic or mixed cystic-solids with large fluid components [5, 6]. PEI is quite a low-cost, safe, and outpatient method of treatment.

However, like other mini-invasive procedures, PEI may have partial efficacy, possible adverse effects, and, typically, mild complications [5]. In the related literature, cases of thyrotoxicosis due to Graves' disease have been identified subsequent to PEI. To our knowledge, our case is the first

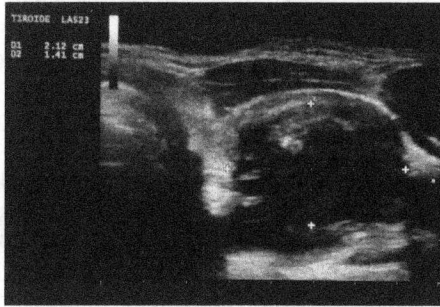

FIGURE 1: Left side nodule before PEI.

thyrotoxicosis caused by Plummer's adenoma following treatment with PEI.

2. Case Presentation

We report a case of a 58-year-old female presented to our center with a voluminous thyroid nodule overall size of 40 × 33 × 26 mm (volume of 17.9 ml), occupying almost the entire left thyroid lobe (Figure 1). Our patient had already had a surgical visit and an intervention of thyroidectomy had been proposed to her, which she refused. A thyroid function test demonstrated TSH 0.8 mIU/l, FT3: 3.77 pg/ml, and FT4: 1.37 ng/dL (normal values for TSH: 0.3–3.74 mIU/l; FT3: 2.2–4.2 pg/ml, and FT4: 0.8–1.7 ng/dL), peroxidase antibodies (TPOAb) 31.2 IU/ml and thyroglobulin antibodies (TgAb) 18 IU/ml (normal values for TPOAb: 0–60 UI/ml; TgAb: 0–60 UI/ml). After evaluation, symptom score and cosmetic score were positive. A thyroid ultrasound demonstrated a right lobe with a normal volume and a left lobe with increased volume (right volume 6.1 ml, left volume 22.2 ml), with normal echogenicity and moderately inhomogeneous echotexture. Due to the nodular structure, intervention of PEI was proposed to which she expressed favorable consensus.

Before PEI, our patient had been submitted to fine needle aspiration on this mixed cystic-solid thyroid nodule, with a cytological diagnosis of Thy2: nonneoplastic. With the patient in a supine position, a total dose of 5 ml of 95% sterile ethanol was injected slowly via a 22 gauge needle under real time ultrasound guidance [7]. We monitored the injection as a hyperechogenic region and completed the procedure in five minutes. After a successful PEI procedure, color Doppler examination showed complete disappearance of intranodular hypervascularization.

Following PEI treatment, the patient detected immediate improvement of compressive symptoms and cosmetic disorders. About 30 days after the treatment there was a significant volume reduction (5.9 ml versus baseline volume of 17.9 ml, volume reduction rate of 67%) but the patient complained of dyspnea, tremors and tachycardia. The cardiorespiratory function parameters were as follows: blood pressure 150/85 mmHg, heart rate 112/min with an ECG highlighted sinus tachycardia, breath frequency 20/min, and oxygen saturation 96%. Thyroid hormone tests showed a framework of

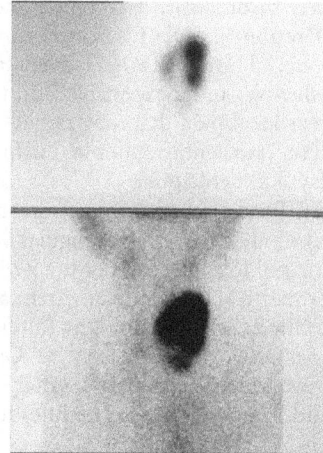

FIGURE 2: Thyroid technetium 99m scintigraphy showing hyperactive nodule on the left lobe and full suppression in the remainder of the gland.

acclaimed thyrotoxicosis TSH < 0.01 mIU/l; FT3: 5.8 pg/ml, FT4 19.1 ng/dL (normal values for TSH: 0.3–3.74 mIU/l; FT3: 2.2–4.2 pg/ml; and FT4: 0.8–1.7 ng/dL). Autoantibodies measurements were performed (TRAb, TPOAb, and TgAb) to investigate the cause of thyrotoxicosis. These autoantibodies were undetectable and we ruled out the diagnosis of Graves' disease and hashitoxicosis. The lack of neck pain and the normality of acute inflammation parameters (erythrocyte sedimentation rate (ESR) and PCR) allowed us to exclude the diagnosis of subacute thyroiditis. The patient was therefore submitted to thyroid scintigraphy which showed a left nodule under complete functional autonomy, corresponding to the nodule treated with PEI (Figure 2). Based upon clinical, laboratory, and imagistic findings, a diagnosis of Plummer adenoma was made. *After thyrostatic treatment (methimazole 15 mg/day for 3 months) and beta-blockers (Propranolol 40 mg 1 cpr every 8 hours for 3 months), the patient has been treated with radioiodine therapy (131I), achieving a euthyroid status.*

3. Discussion

PEI is a nonsurgical option of therapy for cystic or mixed cystic-solid benign thyroid nodules, with an important quote of liquid, with efficacy ranging from 38 to 85% [8]. It was proposed for the first time by Livraghi et al., for treating autonomously functioning thyroid nodules [9], but is no longer used for solid nodules. In addition to its favorable outcomes, PEI has the benefit of not affecting extranodular thyroid tissue as occurs when using I131 therapy, which exposes the surrounding thyroid tissue to significant radiation doses [7].

Injection of ethanol causes reduction in the volume of cystic thyroid nodules by causing cellular dehydration and protein denaturation, leading to reactive fibrosis, as documented in a few papers with thyroid histopathology following PEI treatment [10]. A histopathological investigation after an intranodular ethanol injection shows local injury associated with small vessels thrombosis, a complex and irreversible hemorrhagic infarction, coagulative necrosis, and fibrosis on areas outside the nodule [11]. PEI is a relatively safe technique, well-tolerated, effective, and inexpensive [12], with common side effects such as local pain that may radiate to the jaw or retroauricular area, transient dysphonia, flushing, dizziness, fever lasting a day, and hematoma.

In the related literature, severe but rare complications have been described after PEI, such as jugular vein thrombosis and severe ethanol toxic necrosis of the larynx combined with necrotic dermatitis [13]. Moreover, three cases of Graves' disease without Graves' ophthalmopathy (after treatment of toxic thyroid adenomas) and one case of Graves' disease with severe Graves' ophthalmopathy (after treatment of mixed cystic-solid, nontoxic thyroid nodule) have been also reported [5].

Graves' disease is a complication that can be expected after PEI, probably due to the extensively damaged follicular thyroid cells. The mechanism for causality between the PEI and Graves' disease is not completely known. Regalbuto et al. issued a theory that contended that the destruction of thyroid tissue after injection of ethanol, among subjects genetically predisposed to autoimmune reactions, could release a large quantity of antigenic material (including TSHr protein) from follicular thyroid cells that may trigger an autoimmune inflammatory response throughout thyroid and orbital soft tissues [5].

Usually, there is a transient elevation in serum concentration of thyroid hormones resulting in the sudden release of stored thyroid hormones after follicular destruction produced by an ethanol injection.

This phenomenon does not lead to any clinical and biochemical consequences in nontoxic nodules because free thyroid hormones' concentrations are constantly within limits. Among patients with toxic nodules, a moderate worsening of symptoms could appear [14].

Our patient was a female with no family history of autoimmune disease, with TSH and free thyroid hormones within limits and with no clinical signs of hyperthyroidism before PEI, even if her TSH was at the lower limit of the normal range. All autoantibodies were measured before and after PEI, with normal values, which allowed us to rule out the theory speculated by Regalbuto et al. Unfortunately, thyroid scintigraphy before PEI was not performed because there was no reason in the absence of any signs or symptoms. Therefore, a preexistent form of subclinical Plummer adenoma cannot be ruled out.

To our knowledge, our patient is the first case of Plummer adenoma following PEI treatment of nontoxic thyroid nodule.

4. Conclusions

In spite of the fact that severe complications after PEI treatment are rare, they should be considered in subjects who have indication to this kind of treatment.

Authors' Contributions

Drafting of the manuscript was done by Roberto Cesareo, Anda Mihaela Naciu, Valerio Pasqualini, Giuseppe Pelle, Silvia Manfrini, Gaia Tabacco, Angelo Lauria Pantano, Alessandro Casini, Roberto Cianni, and Andrea Palermo. Critical revision of the manuscript for important intellectual content was done by Roberto Cesareo, Anda Mihaela Naciu, and Andrea Palermo. Clinical management of the patient was done by Roberto Cesareo, Anda Mihaela Naciu, Valerio Pasqualini, Giuseppe Pelle, Silvia Manfrini, Gaia Tabacco, Angelo Lauria Pantano, Alessandro Casini, Roberto Cianni, and Andrea Palermo.

References

[1] B. R. Haugen, "2015 American Thyroid Association Management Guidelines for Adult Patients with Thyroid Nodules and Differentiated Thyroid Cancer: what is new and what has changed?" *Cancer*, vol. 123, no. 3, pp. 372–381, 2017.

[2] A. Gülhan, O. Muhyettin, P. Murat et al., "Cutaneous sinus formation is a rare complication of thyroid fine needle aspiration biopsy," *Case Reports in Endocrinology*, vol. 2014, Article ID 923438, 3 pages, 2014.

[3] S. Ezzat, D. A. Sarti, D. R. Cain, and G. D. Braunstein, "Thyroid incidentalomas," *Archives of Internal Medicine*, vol. 154, no. 16, pp. 1838–1840, 1994.

[4] M. C. Ferreira, C. Piaia, and A. C. Cadore, "Percutaneous ethanol injection versus conservative treatment for benign cystic and mixed thyroid nodules," *Archives of Endocrinology and Metabolism*, vol. 60, no. 3, pp. 211–216, 2016.

[5] C. Regalbuto, R. Le Moli, V. Muscia, M. Russo, R. Vigneri, and V. Pezzino, "Severe graves' ophthalmopathy after percutaneous ethanol injection in a nontoxic thyroid nodule," *Thyroid*, vol. 22, no. 2, pp. 210–213, 2012.

[6] S. J. Bonnema, V. E. Nielsen, and L. Hegedüs, "Radioiodine therapy in non-toxic multinodular goitre. The possibility of effect-amplification with recombinant human TSH (rhTSH)," *Acta Oncologica*, vol. 45, no. 8, pp. 1051–1058, 2006.

[7] J. S. Felício, A. M. Conceição, F. M. Santos et al., "Ultrasound-guided percutaneous ethanol injection protocol to treat solid and mixed thyroid nodules," *Frontiers in Endocrinology*, vol. 7, article 52, 2016.

[8] N. Basu, D. Dutta, I. Maisnam et al., "Percutaneous ethanol ablation in managing predominantly cystic thyroid nodules: an eastern India perspective," *Indian Journal of Endocrinology and Metabolism*, vol. 18, no. 5, pp. 662–668, 2014.

[9] T. Livraghi, A. Paracchi, C. Ferrari et al., "Treatment of autonomous thyroid nodules with percutaneous ethanol injection: preliminary results. Work in progress," *Radiology*, vol. 175, no. 3, pp. 827–829, 1990.

[10] A. Crescenzi, E. Papini, C. M. Pacella et al., "Morphological changes in a hyperfunctioning thyroid adenoma after percutaneous ethanol injection: histological, enzymatic and submicroscopical alterations," *Journal of Endocrinological Investigation*, vol. 19, no. 6, pp. 371–376, 1996.

[11] L. Pomorski and M. Bartos, "Histologic changes in thyroid nodules after percutaneous ethanol injection in patients subsequently operated on due to new focal thyroid lesions," *Acta Pathologica, Microbiologica et Immunologica Scandinavica*, vol. 110, no. 2, pp. 172–176, 2002.

[12] L. Tarantino, G. Francica, I. Sordelli et al., "Percutaneous ethanol injection of hyperfunctioning thyroid nodules: long-term follow-up in 125 patients," *American Journal of Roentgenology*, vol. 190, no. 3, pp. 800–808, 2008.

[13] P.-S. Mauz, M. M. Maassen, B. Braun, and S. Brosch, "How safe is percutaneous ethanol injection for treatment of thyroid nodule? Report of a case of severe toxic necrosis of the larynx and adjacent skin," *Acta Oto-Laryngologica*, vol. 124, no. 10, pp. 1226–1230, 2004.

[14] S. Can, "Percutaneous ethanol injection in thyroid nodules: preliminary results," *Turkish Journal of Endocrinology and Metabolism*, vol. 1, pp. 27–31, 2000.

49

Normalization of Bilateral Adrenal Gland Enlargement after Treatment for Cryptococcosis

Yuka Muraoka,[1] Shintaro Iwama,[1,2] and Hiroshi Arima[1]

[1]Department of Endocrinology and Diabetes, Nagoya University Graduate School of Medicine, Nagoya 466-8550, Japan
[2]Research Center of Health, Physical Fitness and Sports, Nagoya University, Nagoya 464-8601, Japan

Correspondence should be addressed to Shintaro Iwama; siwama@med.nagoya-u.ac.jp

Academic Editor: Takeshi Usui

Cryptococcosis usually occurs in immunocompromised patients and can cause enlargement of the adrenal glands, although the morphologic changes after treatment have not been reported in detail. We report the case of 24-year-old man with fevers, headaches, and impaired consciousness who had been treated with glucocorticoids for a protein-losing gastroenteropathy. The cerebrospinal fluid analysis revealed cryptococcal meningitis. Computed tomography showed bilateral adrenal enlargement. A retrospective analysis revealed that the enlargement had been detected 5 months before admission and gradually increased. The enlargement was improved with antifungal therapy and normalized 6 months later. This is the first report describing morphological changes in the adrenal glands associated with cryptococcal meningitis. Adrenal enlargement by cryptococcosis can be improved without any abnormal findings, including calcifications, which may be a unique characteristic from other diseases, including tuberculosis.

1. Introduction

Cryptococcosis is a fatal fungal disease caused by infections with *Cryptococcus* species. Immunocompromised patients, such as those treated with immunosuppressants (including glucocorticoids), often develop cryptococcosis [1]. Although the lungs are commonly involved in cryptococcal infections, disseminated cryptococcosis can also affect the adrenal glands. Adrenal infections with *Cryptococcus* can cause bilateral enlargement of the glands [2] but the morphologic changes after treatment have not been described in detail. Herein we report a case involving an immunocompromised patient with cryptococcal meningitis, including the morphologic findings of the adrenal glands before and after antifungal treatment.

2. Case Presentation

A 24-year-old man with a protein-losing gastroenteropathy due to an intestinal lymphangiectasia was treated with glucocorticoids (prednisolone, 7.5 mg/day) and developed low-grade fevers 7 months before admission. He did not have any remarkable life histories. Five months before admission,

the man complained of headaches, fatigue, and a hearing abnormality. Then, he experienced nausea, diarrhea, and drowsiness for 6 days and subsequently sought evaluation at our hospital. The physical examination at the time of admission revealed that he was slow to respond (Japan Coma Scale 1-1). The following measurements were obtained: height, 161.2 cm; weight, 51.0 kg; BMI, 19.6 kg/m^2; blood pressure, 119/78 mmHg; heart rate, 62 bpm; and body temperature, 37.4°C. The remainder of the examination findings were normal, without any signs of meningitis.

The initial laboratory data showed a white blood cell count of 11700/μL, with 87.0% neutrophils (86% segmented and 1% band neutrophils), 2.0% lymphocytes, 10% monocytes, 0% eosinophils, 1% metamyelocytes, hemoglobin = 15.7 g/dL, and a platelet count of 157,000/μL. The serum C-reactive protein level was slightly elevated (0.80 mg/dL). Although the serum sodium level was slightly decreased (130 mEq/L), the potassium (4.6 mEq/L), chloride (97 mEq/L), creatinine (0.59 mg/dL), fasting glucose (85 mEq/L), and HbA1c (5.1%) concentrations were normal.

An abdominal computed tomography (CT) showed bilateral adrenal enlargement (right, 10.0 × 20.0 mm; left, 29.0 × 29.0 mm). A retrospective analysis of the CT images revealed

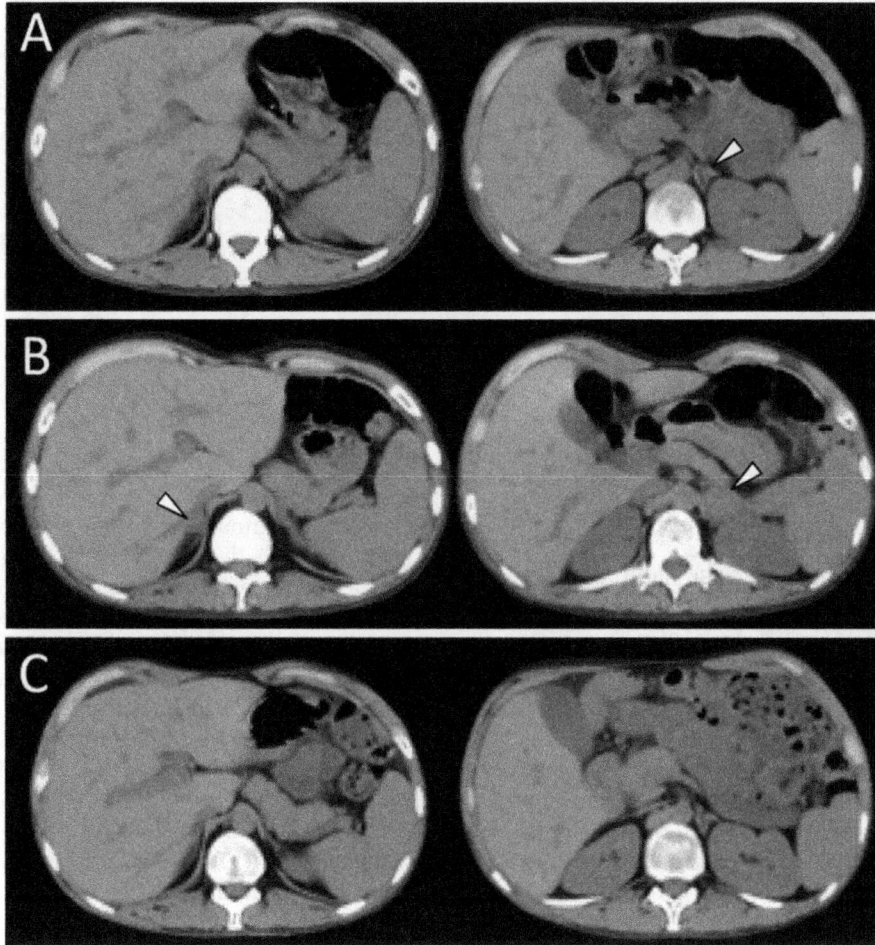

FIGURE 1: Computed tomography showing the time-course changes in the enlarged adrenal glands. Computed tomography showing gradual exacerbation of the bilaterally enlarged adrenal glands (arrowheads) evaluated at 5 months (A) and day 0 (B) before treatment and improvement at 6 months (C) after initiation of treatment.

that the enlargement in the left adrenal gland developed 5 months before admission (Figure 1(A)), which coincided with the onset of fevers and headaches. Subsequently, the bilateral adrenal enlargement progressed (Figure 1(B)). The differential diagnosis of adrenal enlargement includes metastatic carcinoma, bilateral adrenal hyperplasia, tuberculosis, and fungal infections. A whole-body examination failed to find a primary malignant lesion. The QuantiFERON-TB test and HIV antibody titer were negative. Although there were no signs of meningeal irritation, a diagnostic lumbar puncture was performed. The cerebrospinal fluid revealed an increased white blood cell count (240/μL), a normal protein level, a decreased glucose level (0.10 g/l), and a positive cryptococcal antigen titer. The pathologic specimen showed the presence of yeast-like organisms, such as *Cryptococcus* spp. on Alcian blue staining, which was subsequently determined to be *Cryptococcus neoformans*.

Although the level of serum adrenocorticotropic hormone (ACTH) was elevated (131.3 pg/mL; normal range, 7.2–63.3 pg/mL) at the time of the diagnosis of cryptococcosis (Table 1), cortisol release in response to ACTH (Cortrosyn), which was evaluated 1 day after prednisolone cessation, was

increased (Table 2). Oral prednisolone (7.5 mg/day) was then resumed as treatment for the protein-losing gastroenteropathy. The other endocrinological data of adrenal gland ruled out the possibility of pheochromocytoma and aldosterone-secreting tumors in this patient (Table 2).

Amphotericin B (250 mg/day) was initiated, followed by the addition of fluconazole (400 mg/day). The symptoms improved gradually after beginning antifungal treatment. Fluconazole alone was continued after discharge. After the initiation of antifungal treatment, the elevated ACTH levels were decreased and varied during the treatment (Table 1), suggesting a stressed condition with infection at the diagnosis and unstable absorption of prednisolone due to the protein-losing gastroenteropathy. Mild hyponatremia probably due to relative adrenal insufficiency was improved to the normal range (138 mEq/L) one month after the initiation of the antifungal treatment.

An abdominal CT, which was routinely obtained during follow-up, showed that the size of the adrenal glands decreased following antifungal therapy and became normal without any abnormal findings, including calcifications, 6 months after starting treatment (Figure 1(C)).

TABLE 1: Endocrinological data of the patient during antifungal treatments.

	Time of the diagnosis	Time after initiation of antifungal treatments		
		2 months	4 months	6 months
ACTH (pg/mL)	131.3	4.6	28.1	1.9
Cortisol (μg/dl)	38.4	16.9	14.1	6.7
Dehydroepiandrosterone-sulfate (DHEA-s) (μg/dL)	482			
Epinephrine (ng/ml)	0.332	0.015		
Norepinephrine (ng/ml)	0.487	0.089		
Dopamine (ng/ml)	0.027	0.012		
Urine metanephrine (ng/mg Cr)	328	119		
Urine normetanephrine (ng/mg Cr)	63	176		
Plasma renin activity (ng/mL/hr)	3.2			
Aldosterone (pg/mL)	202.0			

TABLE 2: Rapid ACTH test.

Time	0 min	30 min	60 min
Cortisol (μg/dl)	23.5	32.0	36.6

3. Discussion

Cryptococcal infections usually involve the lungs and central nervous system [3] and sometimes cause disseminated lesions, including the adrenal glands [2]. Adrenal cryptococcosis, first reported in 1948 [4], often accompanies bilateral enlargement of the adrenal glands and adrenal insufficiency. In the patient presented herein, the size of adrenal glands gradually increased before treatment but decreased after antifungal therapy. The data herein suggest that the adrenal glands were infected with *Cryptococcus*. As the enlargement was detected 5 months before admission, it is possible that the adrenal infection with *Cryptococcus* was present at that time.

Although there are several reports showing enlargement of the adrenal glands in patients with cryptococcosis, the time-course changes in the morphology of the adrenal glands after antifungal treatment have not been precisely described. In most of the reports, the enlargement was mentioned [5–8] at the diagnosis or did not change, even after the antifungal treatment was effective [9–14]. There is only one report which shows a decrease in adrenal gland enlargement after treatment with amphotericin B [15]; however, the images obtained after treatment clearly showed adrenal gland enlargement. This is the first report of a dynamic change in the size of adrenal glands infected with *Cryptococcus* from the exacerbation to recovery phase. Although it is well known that adrenal tuberculosis often causes calcifications of the adrenal glands [2], the morphology of the adrenal glands in our patient improved without any abnormalities, including calcifications. While further follow-up is necessary, our case may suggest a unique feature of adrenal cryptococcosis.

There are several reports showing histopathological features of the surgical specimens or biopsy samples in adrenal cryptococcosis. The infected glands showed caseating necrosis [5, 6, 10, 13, 16] or necrotizing granuloma [6, 14], accompanied by yeast-like organism, chronic inflammation with giant cells, multinucleated histiocytes, and a few lymphocytes. Although there were no histological data from the adrenal glands in this patient, infiltration of inflammatory cells into the adrenal glands could cause the enlargement. Then, the enlargement was decreased in association with the improvement of cryptococcal infection. It is well known that calcification occurs in the inflamed lesion in tuberculosis. Although the precise mechanisms remain unclear, several possibilities have been reported, including hypercalcemia in patients with tuberculosis [17, 18] or overproduction of vitamin D from inflammatory cells [19, 20]. Given the normal serum calcium levels (4.6 mEq/L) and the improvement of the enlarged adrenal glands without calcification, it is possible that there is a different process between tuberculosis and cryptococcosis in calcification.

Despite the long-term use of prednisolone (7.5 mg/day), the basal ACTH level was elevated and cortisol release was increased in response to ACTH injection in our patient. These data suggest that (1) prednisolone administered orally was not absorbed enough to suppress the ACTH release due to the protein-losing gastroenteropathy, (2) the patient was in a stressed condition with the disease, and/or (3) he had partial adrenal insufficiency. There are several case reports which have shown the development of adrenal insufficiency in patients with adrenal cryptococcosis, especially when accompanied by meningoencephalitis [5, 6, 11, 13, 21]. It is thus important to follow adrenal function serially in our patient, although he must continue prednisolone therapy for the underlying disease. The finding that the morphology of the adrenal glands infected with *Cryptococcus* improved completely after treatment in our patient, together with the possibility that cryptococcosis can cause adrenal insufficiency, suggests that we should consider previous adrenal cryptococcosis as a possible cause of adrenal insufficiency, even if the adrenal glands are morphologically normal. In addition, since the enlargement showed slow progression, adrenal cryptococcosis may be considered as a differential diagnosis when the bilateral enlargement is present especially in immunocompromised patients. In conclusion, adrenal enlargement by *Cryptococcus* is completely reversible without any abnormality after antifungal treatment, which may be a unique characteristic from other diseases, including tuberculosis.

Authors' Contributions

All authors were concerned with the treatment, drafted the manuscript, and read and approved the final manuscript.

References

[1] M. Chayakulkeeree and J. R. Perfect, "Cryptococcosis," *Infectious Disease Clinics of North America*, vol. 20, no. 3, pp. 507–544, 2006.

[2] W. F. Paolo Jr. and J. D. Nosanchuk, "Adrenal infections," *International Journal of Infectious Diseases*, vol. 10, no. 5, pp. 343–353, 2006.

[3] H. E. Bowman and J. O. Ritchey, "Cryptococcosis (torulosis) involving the brain, adrenal and prostate," *The Journal of Urology*, vol. 71, no. 3, pp. 373–378, 1954.

[4] A. J. Rawson, L. H. Collins Jr., and J. L. Grant, "Histoplasmosis and torulosis as causes of adrenal insufficiency," *The American Journal of the Medical Sciences*, vol. 215, no. 4, pp. 363–371, 1948.

[5] B. F. Walker, C. J. Gunthel, J. A. Bryan, N. B. Watts, and R. V. Clark, "Disseminated cryptococcosis in an apparently normal host presenting as primary adrenal insufficiency: diagnosis by fine needle aspiration," *The American Journal of Medicine*, vol. 86, pp. 715–717, 1989.

[6] B. Shah, H. C. Taylor, I. Pillay, M. Chung-Park, and R. Dobrinich, "Adrenal insufficiency due to cryptococcosis," *The Journal of the American Medical Association*, vol. 256, no. 23, pp. 3247–3249, 1986.

[7] Y.-C. Liu, D.-L. Cheng, C.-Y. Liu, M.-Y. Yen, and R.-S. Wang, "Isolated cryptococcosis of the adrenal gland," *Journal of Internal Medicine*, vol. 230, no. 3, pp. 285–287, 1991.

[8] C. N. Powers, G. M. Rupp, S. J. Maygarden, and W. J. Frable, "Fine-needle aspiration cytology of adrenal cryptococcosis: a case report," *Diagnostic Cytopathology*, vol. 7, no. 1, pp. 88–91, 1991.

[9] R. Cocker, S. A. McNair, L. Kahn et al., "Isolated adrenal cryptococcosis, diagnosed by fine-needle aspiration biopsy: a case report," *Diagnostic Cytopathology*, vol. 42, no. 10, pp. 899–901, 2014.

[10] Z.-S. Hung, Y.-H. Lai, Y.-H. Hsu, C.-H. Wang, T.-C. Fang, and B.-G. Hsu, "Disseminated cryptococcosis causes adrenal insufficiency in an immunocompetent individual," *Internal Medicine*, vol. 49, no. 11, pp. 1023–1026, 2010.

[11] A. Takeshita, H. Nakazawa, H. Akiyama et al., "Disseminated cryptococcosis presenting with adrenal insufficiency and menigitis: resistant to prolonged antifungal therapy but responding to bilateral adrenalectomy," *Internal Medicine*, vol. 31, no. 12, pp. 1401–1405, 1992.

[12] H.-M. Cheng, A. S.-B. Chou, K.-H. Chiang, H.-W. Huang, P.-Y. Chang, and P.-S. Yen, "Primary adrenal insufficiency in isolated cryptococcosis of the adrenal gland: CT and MR imaging appearances," *European Journal of Radiology Extra*, vol. 75, no. 3, pp. e111–e113, 2010.

[13] M. Kawamura, S. Miyazaki, S. Mashiko et al., "Disseminated cryptococcosis associated with adrenal masses and insufficiency," *American Journal of the Medical Sciences*, vol. 316, no. 1, pp. 60–64, 1998.

[14] Y. Matsuda, H. Kawate, Y. Okishige et al., "Successful management of cryptococcosis of the bilateral adrenal glands and liver by unilateral adrenalectomy with antifungal agents: a case report," *BMC Infectious Diseases*, vol. 11, article 340, 2011.

[15] P. Ranjan, M. Jana, S. Krishnan, D. Nath, and R. Sood, "Disseminated cryptococcosis with adrenal and lung involvement in an immunocompetent patient," *Journal of Clinical and Diagnostic Research*, vol. 9, no. 4, pp. OD04–OD05, 2015.

[16] P. Benešová, V. Buchta, J. Cerman, and P. Žá, "Cryptococcosis—a review of 13 autopsy cases from a 54-year period in a large hospital," *APMIS*, vol. 115, no. 3, pp. 177–183, 2007.

[17] A. Roussos, I. Lagogianni, A. Gonis et al., "Hypercalcaemia in Greek patients with tuberculosis before the initiation of anti-tuberculosis treatment," *Respiratory Medicine*, vol. 95, no. 3, pp. 187–190, 2001.

[18] F. Shai, R. K. Baker, J. R. Addrizzo, and S. Wallach, "Hypercalcemia in mycobacterial infection," *Journal of Clinical Endocrinology and Metabolism*, vol. 34, no. 2, pp. 251–256, 1972.

[19] J. Cadranel, A. J. Hance, B. Milleron, F. Paillard, G. M. Akoun, and M. Garabedian, "Vitamin D metabolism in tuberculosis. Production of $1,25(OH)_2D_3$ by cells recovered by bronchoalveolar lavage and the role of this metabolite in calcium homeostasis," *American Review of Respiratory Disease*, vol. 138, no. 4, pp. 984–989, 1988.

[20] J. Cadranel, M. Garabedian, B. Milleron, H. Guillozo, G. Akoun, and A. J. Hance, "1,25(OH)2D3 production by T lymphocytes and alveolar macrophages recovered by lavage from normocalcemic patients with tuberculosis," *Journal of Clinical Investigation*, vol. 85, no. 5, pp. 1588–1593, 1990.

[21] W. R. Salyer, C. L. Moravec, D. C. Salyer, and P. F. Guerin, "Adrenal involvement in cryptococcosis," *American Journal of Clinical Pathology*, vol. 60, no. 4, pp. 559–561, 1973.

50

A Novel RET D898Y Germline Mutation in a Patient with Pheochromocytoma

Jin Wook Yi [iD],[1,2] Hye In Kang,[1] Su-jin Kim [iD],[1,2] Chan Yong Seong,[1] Young Jun Chai,[3] June Young Choi [iD],[4] Moon-Woo Seong,[5] Kyu Eun Lee [iD],[1,2] and Sung Sup Park[5]

[1]Department of Surgery, Seoul National University Hospital and College of Medicine, 101 Daehak-ro, Jongno-gu, Seoul 110-744, Republic of Korea
[2]Cancer Research Institute, Seoul National University College of Medicine, 101 Daehak-ro, Jongno-gu, Seoul 110-744, Republic of Korea
[3]Department of Surgery, Seoul National University Boramae Medical Center, 20 Boramae-ro 5-gil, Dongjak-gu, Seoul 156-70, Republic of Korea
[4]Department of Surgery, Seoul National University Bundang Hospital, Seoul National University College of Medicine, Seongnam, Republic of Korea
[5]Department of Laboratory Medicine, Seoul National University Hospital and College of Medicine, 101 Daehak-ro, Jongno-gu, Seoul 110-744, Republic of Korea

Correspondence should be addressed to Su-jin Kim; su.jin.kim.md@gmail.com and Kyu Eun Lee; kyueunlee@snu.ac.kr

Academic Editor: Eli Hershkovitz

Pheochromocytoma and paraganglioma are tumors of neuroectoderm origin. Up to 40% of patients with these tumors have germline mutations in known susceptibility genes. We report a novel *RET* germline mutation (exon 15; c.2692G>T (D898Y)) in a pheochromocytoma patient, as well as in her two asymptomatic sons and older sister. A 49-year-old female came to our clinic presenting with a right adrenal gland mass detected during a healthcare examination. Her mother and two sisters had previously undergone thyroidectomy for papillary thyroid carcinomas. The levels of vanillylmandelic acid and other catecholamines were elevated in 24-hour urine, and an imaging study revealed a right adrenal mass. She underwent laparoscopic adrenalectomy and the final pathologic diagnosis was pheochromocytoma. Mutation screening detected a *RET* p.D898Y mutation, both in the patient and in the patient's two sons and older sister. This is the first description of a *RET* D898Y mutation in a pheochromocytoma patient and her family. The mutation should be categorized as a variant of unknown significance because no RET gene related disorders were detected in this family. Long term follow-up will be required to determine the clinical significance of the *RET* D898Y mutation.

1. Introduction

Pheochromocytomas (PCCs) and paragangliomas (PGLs) are chromaffin cell origin neuroendocrine tumors. PCCs arise from the adrenal medulla and produce catecholamines, whereas paragangliomas occur in the thoracoabdominal sympathetic or parasympathetic ganglia and may, or may not, be associated with catecholamine secretion [1]. World Health Organization tumor classification (2004) defined PCC as an intra-adrenal paraganglioma, due to evidence for shared genetic predisposition to these tumors [2]. With the advancement of molecular pathogenesis, germline mutations

in pheochromocytoma and/or paraganglioma (PPGL) susceptibility genes, such as *NF1*, *RET*, *VHL*, *SDHD*, *SDHC*, *SDHB*, *SDHAF2*, *SDHA*, *TMEM127*, *MAX*, *EPAS1*, and *FH*, have been identified during the past 15 years. The total incidence of germline mutations in both familial and sporadic PPGL is up to 40% [3–6].

Among the many PPGL susceptibility genes, *RET* is a well-known protooncogene, germline mutations of which cause multiple endocrine neoplasia type 2 (MEN2), which is characterized by medullary thyroid carcinoma (MTC), PCC, and hyperparathyroidism [7, 8]. Almost 100% of MEN2 patients will develop MTC, and there is a 50% risk of PCC penetrance in their lifetime [9–12]. To date (2018), over 100 genetic alterations in *RET* have been reported and registered in the "*RET* protooncogene database" [13], and the penetrance of *RET* mutation-related diseases varies depending on the site of the *RET* mutation [10]. In patients with some *RET* gene mutation types, the occurrence of PCC as an initial clinical manifestation is more frequent than the occurrence of MTC [14–18]. For this reason, mutation screening of *RET* in PPGL patients and their families is important for the establishment of appropriate treatment management plans [10, 11].

In the present study, a novel germline *RET* gene mutation (c.2692G>T, p.Asp898Tyr) of unknown significance was identified in a patient with PCC and her family members at the Seoul National University Hospital, South Korea. We evaluated the genomic features and familial characteristics of the mutation using a computational biology tool. This study was approved by the Institutional Review Board of Seoul National University Hospital (IRB number: H-1677-006-772).

2. Methods

2.1. Case Presentation. In November 2012, a 49-year-old Korean woman was referred to the Department of Endocrine Surgery due to a right adrenal mass, identified by abdominal sonography during a routine healthcare checkup. She had been suffering from headache, tachycardia, palpitations, and cold sweats for 5 years but had not previously undergone adrenal disease related diagnostic tests. Her mother and two sisters had a history of thyroidectomy as treatment for papillary thyroid cancer. Twenty-four-hour urine collection revealed elevated vanillyl mandelic acid (VMA; 11.7 mg/day, reference: 2–7 mg/day), metanephrine (1625.6 μg/day, reference: 52–341 μg/day), normetanephrine (5459.5 μg/day, reference: 88–444 μg/day), epinephrine (256.4 μg/day, reference: 0.20 μg/day), and norepinephrine (153.2 μg/day, reference: 15–80 μg/day). An abdominal computed tomography (CT) scan revealed a heterogeneous right adrenal mass of approximately 4.7×3.5 cm (Figure 1(a)). Metaiodobenzylguanidine scintigraphy and single-photon emission CT showed increased uptake in the right adrenal gland (Figure 1(b)). The patient underwent right adrenalectomy using the posterior retroperitoneoscopic approach. The final pathologic diagnosis was a PCC with a size of $6.0 \times 4.0 \times 3.0$ cm and a high risk of malignancy with a "PCC of the adrenal gland scaled score" of 13.

During the 65-month follow-up after adrenalectomy, the levels of urine VMA, catecholamine, serum calcitonin, calcium, carcinoembryonic antigen, and parathyroid hormone remained within normal ranges. There was no evidence of malignant thyroid nodules on neck ultrasound examination. Genetic counseling was performed by a specialist nurse. Due to the family history of thyroid cancer, we suggested germline mutation screening of the *RET* gene to the patient and her family members. The index patient and her two sons, two younger brothers, one younger sister, and mother agreed to the germline mutation test and provided informed consent. The informed consent statement contained a statement concerning the sharing of results as follows: "The research, which was conducted for your information or human tissue samples,

can be shared with other researchers through congress. We can publish the results so that other interested people can learn from this study."

2.2. Mutation Analysis. Genomic DNA was extracted from peripheral blood samples from the index patient and her family members. For the index patient, mutation testing included *RET* gene exons 8, 10, 11, 13, 14, 15, and 16 and their flanking regions using PCR and direct sequencing of DNA. For the family members, direct sequencing was performed only for *RET* exon 15. The GenBank reference sequence used to analyze data generated by direct sequencing was NM_020975.4. The Ensembl VEP (variant effect predictor, http://www.ensembl.org/info/docs/tools/vep/index.html) program was used to predict the biological effect of single nucleotide variants. To predict the impact of amino acid changes on protein structure and function, we used the SIFT (http://sift.jcvi.org/) and PolyPhen (http://genetics.bwh.harvard.edu/pph2/bgi.shtml) prediction tools. The ExAC database (http://exac.broadinstitute.org/) was used to identify the frequency of novel single nucleotide variants in the general population. To evaluate the clinical significance of previously reported *RET* gene variants, we exploited the dbSNP (https://www.ncbi.nlm.nih.gov/SNP/) and ClinVar (https://www.ncbi.nlm.nih.gov/clinvar/) databases.

3. Results

A germline mutation in the *RET* gene was identified in the index patient, her two sons, and her older sister. It was not identified in the mother or two younger brothers and one sister of the patient (Figure 2). Sanger sequencing revealed that the *RET* gene mutation was a c.2692G>T substitution (chromosome 10:43120165, reference sequence, GRCh38.p5), (Figure 3(a)). VEP analysis indicated that the mutation alters a GAT codon to TAT, resulting in a change in codon 898 (p.D898Y, Figure 3(b)). The score of the change according to the SIFT tool was 0, indicating that it is predicted to be "deleterious." The PolyPhen score was 1, indicating that it is predicted as "probably damaging." The frequency of the mutant allele in the population, estimated using the ExAC database, was $1.648e - 05$, indicating that this is an extremely rare allele. Her sister and two sons, who also carried the mutation, did not develop any tumors during the 65-month surveillance period, although her sister had a history of thyroid cancer (Figure 2).

4. Discussion

The *RET* protooncogene is a member of the cadherin superfamily and encodes the RET transmembrane tyrosine kinase protein. *RET* maps to chromosome 10q11.2 and consists of 55,000 base pairs including 21 exons [19]. Mutations of *RET* are associated with MEN types 2A and 2B and familial MTC [7]. Hundreds of *RET* mutations have been identified, and the penetrance and aggressiveness of MEN related tumors vary according to the specific mutations [20]. For example, mutation of *RET* codon 634 is the most frequently identified mutation in western countries and is

(a)   (b)

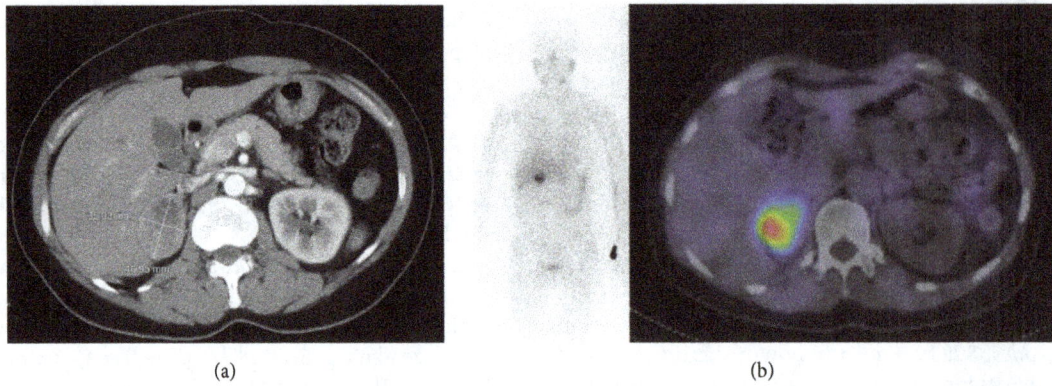

FIGURE 1: (a) Abdominal computed tomography showing a heterogeneous enhanced mass in the right adrenal gland. (b) Image generated by scintigraphy and single-photon emission computed tomography showing the right adrenal mass and demonstrating increased uptake of metaiodobenzylguanidine.

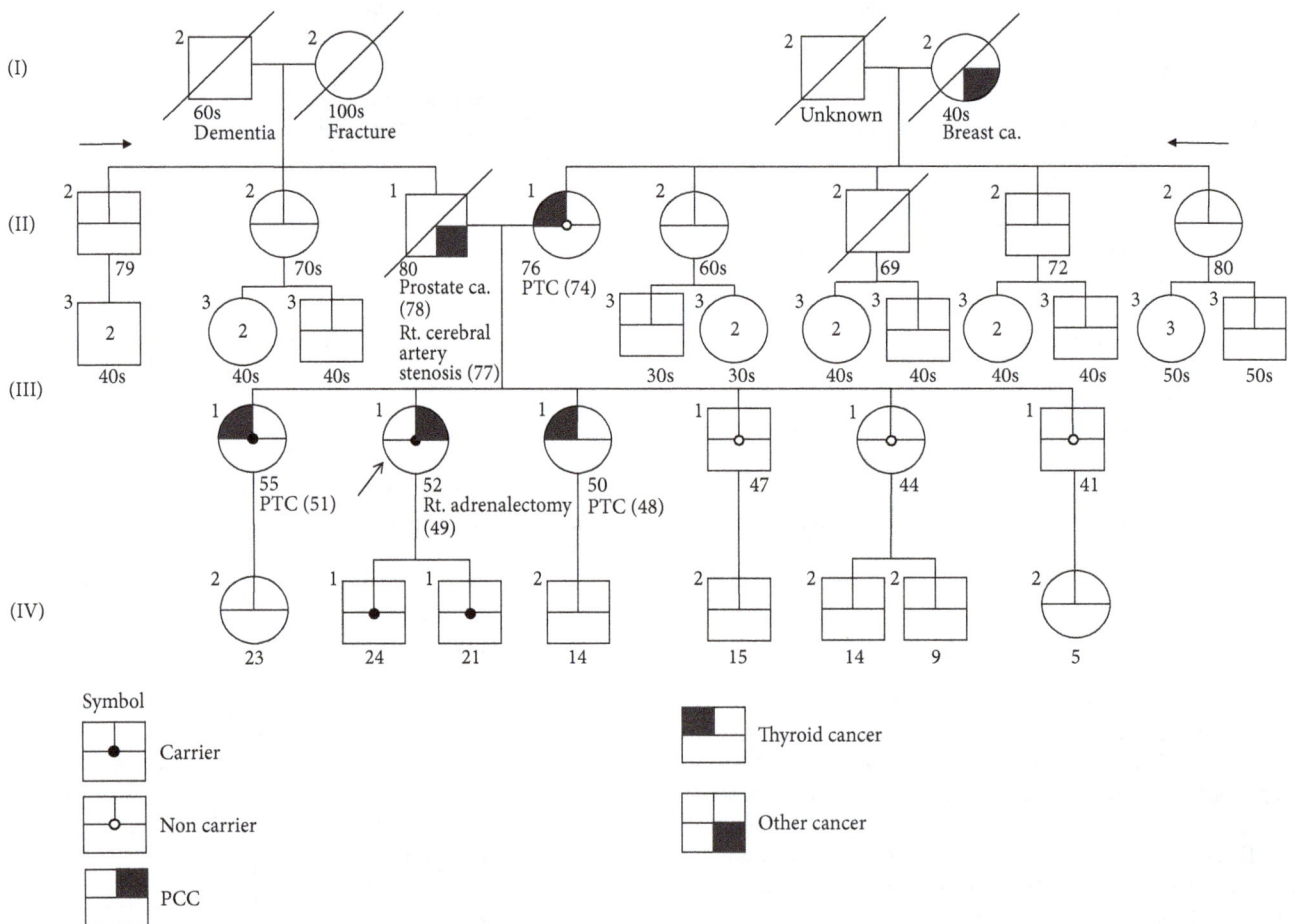

FIGURE 2: Pedigree of the index patient (arrow) and her family. The *RET* D898Y germline mutation was detected in the index patient, her two sons, and her older sister.

associated with increased aggressiveness and younger onset of MTC compared with other *RET* mutations. Prophylactic thyroidectomy is recommended for children under 5 years old carrying the *RET* 634 mutation [21, 22]. The American Thyroid Association guidelines (2015) for managing MTC list the relationships between important *RET* gene mutations

and aggressiveness of MTC and incidence of PCC and other related tumors, in order to provide clinical guidance on the management of MEN patients [10].

Here, we describe the first *RET* D898Y germline mutation identified in a PCC patient and her two first-degree relatives. The *RET* D898Y mutation was previously reported once

NM_020975.3(*RET*): c.2692G>T, p.Asp898Tyr, heterozygote

(a)

(b)

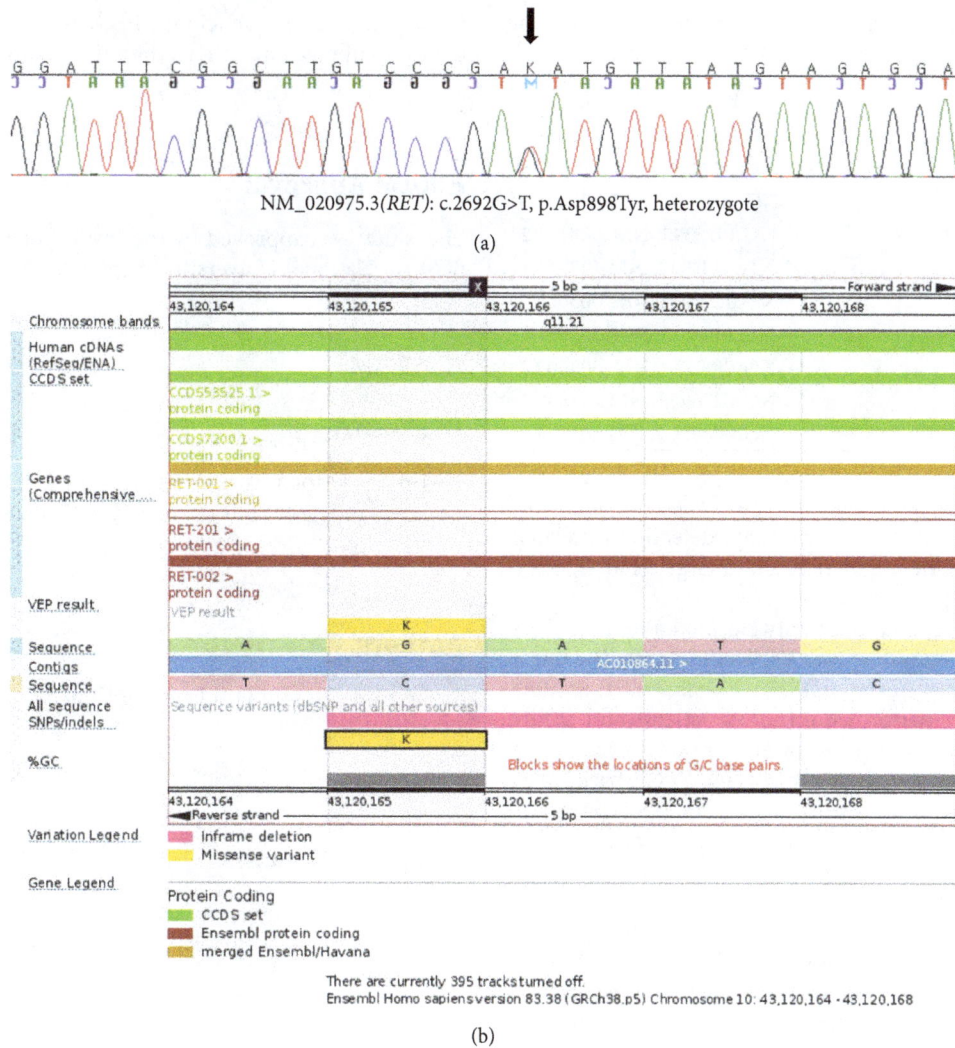

FIGURE 3: (a) Sanger sequencing revealed a *RET* mutation (c.2692G>T, p.Asp898Tyr) (chromosome 10:43120165). (b) Detailed information on the RET c.2692G>T, p.Asp898Tyr mutation generated by variant effect predictor (http://www.ensembl.org/info/docs/tools/vep/index.html).

in dbSNP (rs587780810) and once in the ClinVar database (RCV000123314.1) as a variant of uncertain significance. There is no other clinical reports describing the *RET* D898Y mutation in the literature. Judging from the pedigree and sequencing results (Figures 2 and 3), this mutation has an autosomal dominant inheritance pattern with heterozygosity, although the index patient and family members did not show diagnostic features characteristic of MEN or MEN related diseases. PCC was also found in the index patient. The genotype-phenotype correlation and penetrance of MEN related tumors or PCC have not been proven. We suggest that this mutation be classified as a novel germ line mutation of unknown significance. Long term surveillance of this patient and her relatives will be needed to reveal genotype-phenotype correlations of this mutation. A follow-up plan for the index patient and her family members carrying *RET* D898Y should consist of yearly checkups, including assaying for parathyroid hormone, carcinoembryonic antigen, calcitonin, 24-hour urine catecholamine, and VMA levels, as well as screening using thyroid ultrasound to detect PCC, MTC, or hyperparathyroidism.

The prevalence of germline mutations in PPGL is reported as approximately 40%, and recent genomic studies report that the incidence of overall germline plus somatic mutation in PPGL is as high as 60% [3–6]. Using next generation sequencing and transcriptome analysis, researchers have identified many PPGL susceptibility genes, which are classified into two clusters: cluster 1 (the angiogenic cluster) consists of *EGLN1*, *PHD2*, *VHL*, *SDHX*, *IDH*, *HIF2A*, *EPAS1*, *FH*, and *MDH2*, while cluster 2 (the kinase signaling cluster) includes *KIF1B*, *RET*, *NF1*, *TMEM127*, *MAX*, and *MEN1* [4, 23]. For these reasons, genetic counseling and mutation screening tests of all PPGL patients are essential for proper management of multiple endocrine tumors and can modulate

TABLE 1: Paraganglioma/pheochromocytoma genetic mutational panel screened in the rare disease control program in Korea.

Gene	Reference sequence
MAX	NG_029830.1, NM_002382.4
NF1	NG_009018.1, NM_000267.3
RET	NG_007489.1, NM_020975.4
SDHA	NG_012339.1, NM_004168.2
SDHAF2	NG_023393.1, NM_017841.2
SDHB	NG_012340.1, NM_003000.2
SDHC	NG_012767.1, NM_003001.3
SDHD	NG_012337.2, NM_003002.2
TMEM127	NG_027695.1, NM_017849.3
VHL	NG_008212.3, NM_000551.3

surgical treatment plans and early stage detection of related tumors and allow the use of medication targeted for specific mutations [24, 25].

In the Seoul National University Hospital, PPGL patients undergo genetic counseling with a specialist nurse. The nurse takes their family histories and draws pedigrees. Germline mutation tests are performed on index patients and family members with their informed consent. At present (2018), we operate a mutation panel test for specific PPGL patients as part of a nationalized rare disease diagnosis support program. Patients who have one of the following criteria can enroll in this program: age under 50 years, family history of PPGL, and multiple or bilateral tumors, recurrent PPGL, or malignant tumors diagnosed by pathology. Targeted sequencing of ten PPGL susceptibility genes, *MAX, NF1, RET, SDHA, SDHAF2, SDHB, SDHC, SDHD, TMEM127,* and *VHL*, is performed with the support of funds from a national budget (Table 1).

Recent advances in next generation sequencing technology have produced a cost-effective method to discover novel mutations responsible for hereditary disease. Whole exome sequencing or targeted next generation sequencing has a faster sequencing time and lower cost than conventional Sanger sequencing when performing analysis of multiple candidate genes, such as that required for PPGL [26–28]. Another analytic platform, RNA sequencing, can not only detect novel sequence alterations (single nucleotide variants, indels, and chromosomal rearrangements), but can also quantify gene expression through analysis of read alignment counts, allowing more comprehensive analysis [26]. However, analysis of whole exome sequence or targeted next generation sequencing data requires more complex analytic pipelines and bioinformatics expertise than direct sequencing analysis.

5. Conclusions

We identified a D898Y mutation in the *RET* gene with autosomal dominant inheritance in a PCC patient and her first-degree relatives. Monitoring the development of PPGL and MTC in the patient and carrier family members is ongoing; hence the penetrance of tumors is unknown. Mutational screening using targeted sequencing is important for proper management of PPGL patients and their families.

Next generation sequencing is likely to be more helpful for detection of novel mutations than classic direct sequencing.

Ethical Approval

This study was approved by the Institutional Review Board of Seoul National University Hospital (IRB no. H-1677-006-772).

Disclosure

This manuscript was presented as an abstract in the 68th Congress of Korean Surgical Society, November 3–5, 2016.

Authors' Contributions

Su-jin Kim and Kyu Eun Lee contributed equally to the work in this paper.

Acknowledgments

This study was supported by research grants from Seoul National University Hospital (no. 04-2017-3050).

References

[1] J. W. M. Lenders, G. Eisenhofer, M. Mannelli, and K. Pacak, "Phaeochromocytoma," *The Lancet*, vol. 366, no. 9486, pp. 665–675, 2005.

[2] K. Pacak, G. Eisenhofer, H. Ahlman et al., "Pheochromocytoma: Recommendations for clinical practice from the First International Symposium," *Nature Clinical Practice Endocrinology & Metabolism*, vol. 3, no. 2, pp. 92–102, 2007.

[3] J. Favier, L. Amar, and A.-P. Gimenez-Roqueplo, "Paraganglioma and phaeochromocytoma: from genetics to personalized medicine," *Nature Reviews Endocrinology*, vol. 11, no. 2, pp. 101–111, 2015.

[4] S. Pillai, V. Gopalan, R. A. Smith, and A. K.-Y. Lam, "Updates on the genetics and the clinical impacts on phaeochromocytoma and paraganglioma in the new era," *Critical Review in Oncology/Hematology*, vol. 100, pp. 190–208, 2016.

[5] A.-P. Gimenez-Roqueplo, P. L. Dahia, and M. Robledo, "An update on the genetics of paraganglioma, pheochromocytoma, and associated hereditary syndromes," *Hormone and Metabolic Research*, vol. 44, no. 5, pp. 328–333, 2012.

[6] H. P. Neumann, B. Bausch, and S. R. McWhinney, "Germline mutations in nonsyndromic pheochromocytoma," *The New England Journal of Medicine*, vol. 346, no. 19, pp. 1459–1466, 2002.

[7] L. M. Mulligan, J. B. J. Kwok, C. S. Healey et al., "Germ-line mutations of the RET proto-oncogene in multiple endocrine neoplasia type 2A," *Nature*, vol. 363, no. 6428, pp. 458–460, 1993.

[8] C. Eng, "Seminars in medicine of the Beth Israel Hospital, Boston: The RET proto- oncogene in multiple endocrine neoplasia type 2 and Hirschsprung's disease," *The New England Journal of Medicine*, vol. 335, no. 13, pp. 943–951, 1996.

[9] J. R. Howe, J. A. Norton, and S. A. Wells, "Prevalence of pheochromocytoma and hyperparathyroidism in multiple endocrine neoplasia type 2A: Results of long-term follow-up," *Surgery*, vol. 114, no. 6, pp. 1070–1077, 1993.

[10] S. A. Wells, S. L. Asa, H. Dralle et al., "Revised American thyroid association guidelines for the management of medullary thyroid carcinoma the American thyroid association guidelines task force on medullary thyroid carcinoma," *Thyroid*, vol. 25, no. 6, pp. 567–610, 2015.

[11] J. W. M. Lenders, Q.-Y. Duh, and G. Eisenhofer, "Pheochromocytoma and paraganglioma : an endocrine society clinical practice guideline," *The Journal of Clinical Endocrinology & Metabolism*, vol. 99, no. 6, pp. 1915–1942, 2014.

[12] C. Romei, E. Pardi, F. Cetani, and R. Elisei, "Genetic and clinical features of multiple endocrine neoplasia types 1 and 2," *Journal of Oncology*, vol. 2012, Article ID 705036, 15 pages, 2012.

[13] R. L. Margraf, D. K. Crockett, P. M. F. Krautscheid et al., "Multiple endocrine neoplasia type 2 RET protooncogene database: Repository of MEN2-associated RET sequence variation and reference for genotype/phenotype correlations," *Human Mutation*, vol. 30, no. 4, pp. 548–556, 2009.

[14] M. S. Elston, G. Y. Meyer-Rochow, I. Holdaway, and J. V. Conaglen, "Patients with RET D631Y mutations most commonly present with pheochromocytoma and not medullary thyroid carcinoma," *Hormone and Metabolic Research*, vol. 44, no. 5, pp. 339–342, 2012.

[15] P. Santos, T. Pimenta, and A. Taveira-Gomes, "Hereditary pheochromocytoma," *International Journal of Surgical Pathology*, vol. 22, no. 5, pp. 393–400, 2014.

[16] R. A. Toledo, S. M. Wagner, F. L. Coutinho, D. M. Lourenço Jr, J. A. Azevedo, and V. C. Longuini, "High penetrance of pheochromocytoma associated with the novel C634Y/Y791F double germline mutation in the RET protooncogene," *The Journal of Clinical Endocrinology and Metabolism*, vol. 95, no. 3, pp. 1318–1327, 2010.

[17] J. W. Min, Y. J. Park, H. J. Kim, and M.-C. Chang, "Bilateral adrenal pheochromocytoma with a germline L790F mutation in the RET oncogene," *Journal of the Korean Surgical Society*, vol. 82, no. 3, pp. 185–189, 2012.

[18] C. Scollo, M. Russo, L. De Gregorio et al., "A novel RET gene mutation in a patient with apparently sporadic pheochromocytoma," *Endocrine Journal*, vol. 63, no. 1, pp. 87–91, 2016.

[19] B. Pasini, R. M. W. Hofstra, L. Yin et al., "The physical map of the human RET proto-oncogene," *Oncogene*, vol. 11, no. 9, pp. 1737–1743, 1995.

[20] J. W. B. de Groot, T. P. Links, J. T. M. Plukker, C. J. M. Lips, and R. M. W. Hofstra, "RET as a diagnostic and therapeutic target in sporadic and hereditary endocrine tumors," *Endocrine Reviews*, vol. 27, no. 5, pp. 535–560, 2006.

[21] C. Romei, A. Tacito, E. Molinaro et al., "Twenty years of lesson learning: how does the *RET* genetic screening test impact the clinical management of medullary thyroid cancer?" *Clinical Endocrinology*, vol. 82, no. 6, pp. 892–899, 2015.

[22] F. Raue and K. Frank-Raue, "Genotype-phenotype correlation in multiple endocrine neoplasia type 2," *Clinics*, vol. 67, pp. 69–75, 2012.

[23] P. L. M. Dahia, "Pheochromocytoma and paraganglioma pathogenesis: learning from genetic heterogeneity," *Nature Reviews Cancer*, vol. 14, no. 2, pp. 108–119, 2014.

[24] L. Fishbein, S. Merrill, D. L. Fraker, D. L. Cohen, and K. L. Nathanson, "Inherited mutations in pheochromocytoma and paraganglioma: why all patients should be offered genetic testing," *Annals of Surgical Oncology*, vol. 20, no. 5, pp. 1444–1450, 2013.

[25] M. Jafri and E. R. Maher, "The genetics of phaeochromocytoma: using clinical features to guide genetic testing," *European Journal of Endocrinology*, vol. 166, no. 2, pp. 151–158, 2012.

[26] R. A. Toledo and P. L. M. Dahia, "Next-generation sequencing for the diagnosis of hereditary pheochromocytoma and paraganglioma syndromes," *Current Opinion in Endocrinology, Diabetes and Obesity*, vol. 22, no. 3, pp. 169–179, 2015.

[27] A. M. McInerney-Leo, M. S. Marshall, B. Gardiner et al., "Whole exome sequencing is an efficient and sensitive method for detection of germline mutations in patients with phaeochromocytomas and paragangliomas," *Clinical Endocrinology*, vol. 80, no. 1, pp. 25–33, 2014.

[28] J. Welander, A. Andreasson, C. C. Juhlin et al., "Rare germline mutations identified by targeted next-generation sequencing of susceptibility genes in pheochromocytoma and paraganglioma," *The Journal of Clinical Endocrinology & Metabolism*, vol. 99, no. 7, pp. E1352–E1360, 2014.

51

An Atypical HNF4A Mutation Which Does Not Conform to the Classic Presentation of HNF4A-MODY

Andrew J. Spiro ⓘ,[1] **Katherine N. Vu,**[2,3] **and Alicia Lynn Warnock** ⓘ[2,3]

[1]Department of Internal Medicine, Walter Reed National Military Medical Center, Bethesda, MD, USA
[2]Department of Endocrinology, Metabolism and Diabetes, Walter Reed National Military Medical Center, Bethesda, MD, USA
[3]Uniformed Services University of Health Sciences, Bethesda, MD, USA

Correspondence should be addressed to Andrew J. Spiro; andrewspiro22@gmail.com

Academic Editor: Michael P. Kane

Objective. To present the case of an atypical Hepatocyte Nuclear Factor 4 Alpha *(HNF4A)* mutation that is not consistent with the classically published presentation of *HNF4A*-Mature Onset Diabetes of the Young (MODY). *Methods*. Clinical presentation and literature review. *Results*. A 43-year-old nonobese man was referred to the endocrinology clinic for evaluation of elevated fasting blood glucose (FBG) measurements. Laboratory review revealed prediabetes and hypertriglyceridemia for the previous decade. Testing of autoantibodies for type 1 diabetes was negative. Genetic testing showed an autosomal dominant, heterozygous missense mutation (c.991C>T; p.Arg331Cys) in the *HNF4A* gene, which is correlated with *HNF4A*-MODY. Phenotypically, patients with an *HNF4A*-MODY tend to have early-onset diabetes, microvascular complications, low triglyceride levels, increased birth weight, fetal macrosomia, and less commonly neonatal hyperinsulinemic hypoglycemia. The patient did not demonstrate any of these features but instead presented with late-onset diabetes, an elevated triglyceride level, and a normal birth weight. *Conclusion*. Our patient likely represents an atypical variant of *HNF4A*-MODY with a milder clinical presentation. Patients with atypical, less-severe presentations of *HNF4A*-MODY may be largely undiagnosed or misdiagnosed, but identification is important due to implications for treatment, pregnancy, and screening of family members.

1. Introduction

MODY describes a cluster of monogenic disorders that are inherited in an autosomal dominant manner. The classic depiction of MODY is diabetes that presents before the age of 25 years, is not insulin-dependent, and shows no evidence of autoimmune pathology or insulin resistance. While MODY is only responsible for 1% of all cases of diabetes, it is the cause for 5% of people diagnosed before 45 years [1]. To date, several MODY-causing genes have been identified but the most common are glucokinase (*GCK*), *HNF1A*, and *HNF4A* [1]. The *HNF4A*-MODY (MODY 1) and *HNF1A*-MODY (MODY 3) phenotypes resemble one another, producing significant pancreatic *β*-cell dysfunction which results in hyperglycemia and microvascular complications, whereas *GCK*-MODY (MODY 2) produces a mild hyperglycemia, which often does not require treatment [1] (see Table 1). A recent large-scale study in the United Kingdom showed that

HNF4A-MODY (MODY 1), *GCK*-MODY (MODY 2), and *HNF1A*-MODY (MODY 3) represent 10%, 32%, and 52% of MODY cases in that population [2]. The prevalence of different MODY mutations varies from one country to another. In countries like France, Italy, and Spain, where asymptomatic glucose testing is common, *GCK*-MODY (MODY 2) is the most common subtype. *HNF1A*-MODY (MODY 3) is the most common subtype in countries where random glucose testing is less routine [3]. We describe a patient with a heterozygous missense mutation in *HNF4A* whose clinical presentation does not conform to the classically described features of the *HNF4A*-MODY.

2. Case Report

A 43-year-old nonobese man was referred to the endocrinology clinic for evaluation of elevated FBG measurements. His FBG and hemoglobin A1C (HbA1C) had been in the

TABLE 1: Comparison of patient phenotype with the common MODY subtypes.

	Patient (*HNF4A* mutation)	*HNF4A*-MODY (MODY 1)	*HNF1A*-MODY (MODY 3)	*GCK*-MODY (MODY 2)
Frequency[*]	–	≤10%	~30–50%	~30–50%
Age of Diagnosis	41 y/o	<25 y/o	<25 y/o	Usually age when blood glucose levels first measured
Pathophysiology	–	Transcription factor, decreased insulin secretion	Transcription factor, Decreased insulin secretion	Decreased glucose sensitivity, decreased glycogen storage
Characteristics	No current evidence of microvascular complications Managed with lifestyle modifications Hypertriglyceridemia, mildly elevated LDL and VLDL Normal Apo-B, Apo-A1	Microvascular complications Sensitive to sulfonylureas Low TG, high LDL, low HDL Low Apo A-II, C-III, B Fetal Macrosomia Neonatal hypoglycemia	Microvascular complications Sensitive to sulfonylureas Normal or high HDL Glycosuria	No microvascular complications Mild, generally does not require treatment

[*]Percentage of occurrence among MODY patient with a genetic diagnosis. MODY = Mature Onset Diabetes of the Young; HNF = Hepatocyte Nuclear Factor; GCK = glucokinase; TG = triglyceride; LDL = low density lipoprotein; HDL = high density lipoprotein; VLDL = very low density lipoprotein; Apo = apolipoprotein. See reference [1].

TABLE 2: Patient laboratory data over time.

Age (years)	36.96	37.01	41.24	41.43	43.20	43.27	43.29	43.35
HbA1C (%)		5.7	6.7	6.3		6.2		
FBG (mg/dL)	123	113			131	198	115	188
C-peptide (ng/mL)								7.0
Fasting Insulin (mcU/mL)							14.7	
Glucose, 2 hr Post 75 gm Oral Glucose Load							178	
Total Cholesterol (mg/dL)	213	250	215	154	153			
HDL	52	47	37	39	38			
TG	277	342	397	165	144			
LDL	106	142	107	81	88			
BMI (kg/m^2)		25.1	25.6	24.4		24.8		

HbA1C = hemoglobin A1C; FBG = fasting blood glucose; HDL = high density lipoprotein cholesterol; TG = triglyceride; LDL = low density lipoprotein cholesterol; BMI = body mass index; normal reference ranges for laboratory: (1) insulin (mcU/mL): (2.6–24.9); (2) C-peptide (ng/mL): (1.1–4.4). *Note.* For the duration listed, the patient was taking a moderate-intensity statin and not taking any medication for treatment of diabetes.

prediabetic range for the past decade, except for one elevated HbA1C of 6.7% (50 mmol/mol) two years prior (see Table 2). The patient denied any classic symptoms of diabetes. His medical history was notable for gout, hyperlipidemia, and hypertriglyceridemia. The patient was taking allopurinol and had been taking a moderate-intensity-statin for the previous 10 years. His mother had premature coronary artery disease (CAD) and type 2 diabetes (T2DM), controlled with oral medication. Physical exam showed a healthy, lean, and muscularly fit individual with a body mass index of 24.8 kg/m^2. His latest HbA1C was 6.2% (44 mmol/mol) and recent FBG measurements were 131, 198, 115, and 188 mg/dL. An oral glucose tolerance test showed a result in the prediabetic range (178 mg/dL). Autoantibodies (Glutamate Decarboxylase 65 Ab, Pancreatic Islet Cell Ab, Islet Cells Ab 512, and Insulin Ab) were negative. His fasting insulin level was within normal limits while a C-peptide level was mildly elevated; however, these levels were checked at different time points and do not directly correlate with one another (see Table 2). Initially, his

presentation was attributed to early well-controlled T2DM with elements of metabolic syndrome; however, due to his atypical physical appearance, he was referred for genetic testing for MODY. Testing revealed an autosomal dominant, heterozygous missense mutation (c.991C>T; p.Arg331Cys) in the *HNF4A* gene.

3. Discussion

As noted above, *HNF4A*-MODY (MODY 1) and *HNF1A*-MODY (MODY 3) are generally associated with the classic MODY features while *GCK*-MODY (MODY 2) has been recognized as a milder variant. The clinical manifestation of our patient's *HNF4A* mutation was atypical for multiple reasons. The primary atypical feature was that he did not meet laboratory criteria for diabetes diagnosis until the age of 41 (HbA1C = 6.7%; 50 mmol/mol), after which he was able to maintain his HbA1C levels in the prediabetic range with only lifestyle modification. Recent data showed that 71%

of individuals with pathogenic *HNF4A* mutations developed diabetes by age of 30, with mean age of diagnosis in the early 20s. This data did not include the p.R114W mutation [4]. While uncommon, presentations later in life are not exceedingly rare. Another recent study reported approximately 82% penetrance of mutations at age of 40 years [5]. Aside from early-onset diabetes, *HNF4A* mutations have been associated with increased birth weight and macrosomia [6]. In one study, 56% of mutation carriers met criteria for macrosomia and carriers demonstrated a 790 g average increase in birth weight compared to noncarrier family members [7]. Our patient reported a birth weight between 6 and 7 lbs and had no history of macrosomia. Examination of the lipid profiles in *HNF4A*-MODY has revealed decreased serum triglycerides and Apo AII [6]. Evidence has also shown high LDL, low HDL, low apo CIII, and low apo B [1]. In contrast, our patient demonstrated consistent hypertriglyceridemia and normal-to-high levels of HDL and LDL. Apo B and Apo A-I were within the normal range.

The variance between our patient's clinical presentation and that of classic *HNF4A*-MODY can be explored by examining the function of the HNF4A protein. HNF4A is a transcription factor that is primarily expressed in the liver, in addition to the kidneys and pancreas [8]. It is not completely understood how *HNF4A* mutations result in impaired β-cell function and insulin secretion or alter the lipid profile. It is known though that HNF4A regulates expression of genes involved in glucose transport (GLUT2), glycolysis (aldolase B, liver pyruvate kinase), and lipid metabolism (Apo AII, apoB, and apoCIII) [8]. It has been proposed that low triglyceride concentrations found in typical *HNF4A*-MODY could result from the decreased transcriptional activity of the mutated HNF4A leading to less expression of apoB and apoCIII [8]. In our patient, the delayed and less-severe presentation of diabetes supports a milder impairment of β-cell function and insulin secretion in the pancreas. His elevated triglyceride level supports that expression of apoCIII and apoB has not been altered in the liver in the typical manner. It must be considered though that a definitive conclusion cannot be drawn based on a single patient. Other predisposing or protective factors should be weighed. Our patient's elevated triglyceride levels may not be related to his *HNF4A* mutation but instead due to a distinct and separate condition. With consideration of his mother's reported history of CAD and T2DM, he may have a separate predisposition to hypertriglyceridemia or metabolic syndrome.

There are more than 103 *HNF4A*-MODY mutations in 173 families and there is great variation in the types of mutations (i.e., missense, frameshift, and nonsense) [6]. Thus, there is potential for a spectrum of phenotypes. Our patient likely represents a variant of *HNF4A*-MODY with a milder clinical presentation than the classic picture. A recent study which described the (p.R114W) mutation presented an *HNF4A*-MODY variant with a less-severe presentation of diabetes, noting a pathogenic penetrance of only 54% by age of 30 [4]. Patients with less-severe *HNF4A*-MODY variants, like those with the (p.R114W) mutation, present a particularly difficult population to diagnose and they may in fact be largely misdiagnosed. In the United Kingdom, it is estimated that >80% of MODY is misdiagnosed [2]. The milder degree of β-cell impairment and the delayed age of diagnosis can strongly mimic T2DM; however, clinical suspicion for MODY should increase in diabetics with negative autoimmune markers who do not demonstrate obesity and the metabolic syndrome [1]. Distinguishing *HNF4A*-MODY from T2DM has important implications for management. Sensitivity to sulfonylureas is well-established in *HNF4A*-MODY [6]. Use of sulfonylureas in *HNF4A*-MODY and *HNF1A*-MODY has been shown to improve glycemic control and can improve a patient's quality of life by avoiding insulin therapy [1]. Further, *HNF4A* mutations can have important ramifications during pregnancy. If either the mother or the father is known to be a mutation carrier, then there is increased risk of complications due to macrosomia, while the neonates who inherit the mutation are at risk of neonatal hypoglycemia [6]. Lastly, identifying an *HNF4A* mutation allows family members to be screened for carrier status and receive appropriate counselling. Genetic screening is recommended for all diabetic family members and genetic counselling is recommended for all nondiabetic members [1].

4. Conclusion

Our patient exhibited an atypical clinical presentation of an *HNF4A* mutation which likely represents a less-severe variant of *HNF4A*-MODY. Features of this milder variant include late-onset diabetes, hypertriglyceridemia, and a normal birth weight. There is great variation in the types of *HNF4A* mutations and potential for a spectrum of resultant phenotypes. Diagnosis of individuals who present with atypical, less-severe presentations of *HNF4A*-MODY is difficult, and they may be largely misdiagnosed. Identification of these patients is important due to implications for treatment, pregnancy, and the screening of family members.

Disclosure

The views expressed in this manuscript are those of the authors and do not reflect the official policy of the Department of the Navy, the Department of Defense or the United States Government. One or more of the authors are military service members (or employee of the U.S. Government). This work was prepared as part of the authors' official duties. Title 17 U.S.C. 105 provides the "Copyright protection under this title is not available for any work of the United States Government." Title 17 U.S.C. 101 defines a U.S. Government work as a work prepared by a military service member or employee of the U.S. Government as part of that person's official duties. The authors certify that all individuals who qualify as authors have been listed; each has participated in the conception and design of this work, the analysis of data (when applicable), the writing of the document, and/or the approval of the submission of this version; the document represents valid work; if we used information derived from another source, we obtained all necessary approvals to use it and made appropriate acknowledgements in the document; and each takes public responsibility for it.

References

[1] A. Anik, G. Çatli, A. Abaci, and E. Böber, "Maturity-onset diabetes of the young (MODY): an update," *Journal of Pediatric Endocrinology and Metabolism*, vol. 28, no. 3-4, pp. 251–263, 2015.

[2] B. M. Shields, S. Hicks, M. H. Shepherd, K. Colclough, A. T. Hattersley, and S. Ellard, "Maturity-onset diabetes of the young (MODY): how many cases are we missing?" *Diabetologia*, vol. 53, no. 12, pp. 2504–2508, 2010.

[3] G. Thanabalasingham and K. R. Owen, "Diagnosis and management of maturity onset diabetes of the young (MODY)," *BMJ*, vol. 343, no. 7828, Article ID d6044, 2011.

[4] T. W. Laver, K. Colclough, M. Shepherd et al., "The common p.R114W HNF4A mutation causes a distinct clinical subtype of monogenic diabetes," *Diabetes*, vol. 65, no. 10, pp. 3212–3217, 2016.

[5] K. A. Patel, J. Kettunen, M. Laakso et al., "Heterozygous RFX6 protein truncating variants are associated with MODY with reduced penetrance," *Nature Communications*, vol. 8, no. 1, p. 888, 2017.

[6] K. Colclough, C. Bellanne-Chantelot, C. Saint-Martin, S. E. Flanagan, and S. Ellard, "Mutations in the genes encoding the transcription factors hepatocyte nuclear factor 1 alpha and 4 alpha in maturity-onset diabetes of the young and hyperinsulinemic hypoglycemia," *Human Mutation*, vol. 34, no. 5, pp. 669–685, 2013.

[7] E. R. Pearson, S. F. Boj, A. M. Steele et al., "Macrosomia and Hyperinsulinaemic Hypoglycaemia in Patients with Heterozygous Mutations in the HNF4A Gene," *PLoS Medicine*, vol. 4, pp. 760–769, 2007.

[8] M. Lehto, P.-O. Bitzén, B. Isomaa et al., "Mutation in the HNF-4α gene affects insulin secretion and triglyceride metabolism," *Diabetes*, vol. 48, no. 2, pp. 423–425, 1999.

52

Asymptomatic Congenital Hyperinsulinism due to a Glucokinase-Activating Mutation, Treated as Adrenal Insufficiency for Twelve Years

Kae Morishita, Chika Kyo, Takako Yonemoto, Rieko Kosugi, Tatsuo Ogawa, and Tatsuhide Inoue

Center for Diabetes, Endocrinology and Metabolism, Shizuoka General Hospital, No. 4-27-1, Kita-Ando, Aoi-ku, Shizuoka, Shizuoka 420-8527, Japan

Correspondence should be addressed to Takako Yonemoto; takakoi@kuhp.kyoto-u.ac.jp

Academic Editor: John Broom

Congenital hyperinsulinism (CHI) caused by a glucokinase- (GCK-) activating mutation shows autosomal dominant inheritance, and its severity ranges from mild to severe. A 43-year-old female with asymptomatic hypoglycemia (47 mg/dL) was diagnosed as partial adrenal insufficiency and the administration of hydrocortisone (10 mg/day) was initiated. Twelve years later, her 8-month-old grandchild was diagnosed with CHI. Heterozygosity of exon 6 c.590T>C (p.M197T) was identified in a gene analysis of GCK, which was also detected in her son and herself. The identification of GCK-activating mutations in hyperinsulinemic hypoglycemia patients may be useful for a deeper understanding of the pathophysiology involved and preventing unnecessary glucocorticoid therapy.

1. Introduction

Congenital hyperinsulinism (CHI) is a condition that leads to recurrent hypoglycemia due to the inappropriate secretion of insulin by pancreatic islet β cells. Recent developments in gene analyses of CHI-related hypoglycemia have provided detailed information on each mutation detected [1]. Mutations are most frequently detected in the ABCC8 and KCNJ11 genes, which code for the two KATP-channel subunits SUR1 and Kir6.2, respectively [2, 3]. Mutations in the glucokinase (GCK), glutamate dehydrogenase (GLUD1), insulin receptor (INSR), hepatocyte nuclear factor 4a (HNF4A), and monocarboxylate transporter 1 (SLC16A1) genes have less commonly been reported to cause CHI and similar syndromes featuring hyperinsulinemic hypoglycemia [4–8].

Glucokinase (GCK), an enzyme that facilitates the phosphorylation of glucose to glucose-6-phosphate, is an important regulator of glucose homeostasis. GCK has been detected in the pancreas, liver, gut, and brain. In each of these organs, GCK plays an important role in the regulation of carbohydrate metabolism by acting as a glucose sensor in pancreatic β cells and promoting the synthesis of glycogen and triglycerides within the liver. A mutation in GCK leads to an inappropriate threshold for glucose-stimulated insulin secretion. Inactivating mutations have been shown to cause maturity-onset diabetes of the young (MODY), whereas activating mutations cause CHI-related hypoglycemia. The activation of glucokinase mutations increases the affinity of glucokinase for glucose and resets the threshold for glucose-stimulated insulin secretion. Thus, insulin continues to be produced at lower blood glucose levels. There appears to be little correlation between specific genotypes and the phenotype of GCK-activating mutations; although some case reports have claimed a relationship between severity of the hyperinsulinism and higher relative activity index of the expressed mutant enzyme, the glucose "set point" for most cases appears to be quite stable in a plasma glucose range of 55–65 mg/dL [9]. Information on the prevalence, natural history, and endocrinological effects of chronic hypoglycemia from GCK mutations is currently limited.

Here we describe the clinical course of GCK-activating mutation, especially focusing on the endocrinological aspects

TABLE 1: Data of the patient.

	First visit	12 years later
Age (years)	44	56
Body weight (kg)	51	54.8
Height (cm)	148	148
BMI	23.2	24.8
Blood pressure (mmHg)	112/72	149/88
Fasting plasma glucose	52 mg/dL (2.8 mmol/L)	65 mg/dL (3.6 mmol/L)
Fasting serum insulin (μIU/mL)	2.0	7.5
HbA1c (%)	4.1	4.6
Total cholesterol (mg/dL)	179	224
Cortisol (μg/dL) (at 8:00 AM)	6.9–7.9	4.5–8.8
ACTH (pg/mL) (at 8:00 AM)	23.8–25.2	15.0–21.3

of chronic hypoglycemia. Identification of this mutation may be essential for preventing erroneous diagnosis, avoiding unnecessary glucocorticoid therapy, and having deeper understanding of the pathophysiology of hyperinsulinemic hypoglycemia.

2. Case Reports

The patient was a 56-year-old female. When she was 44 years old, she was referred to our hospital due to asymptomatic hypoglycemia with a plasma glucose level of 47 mg/dL, which was detected in a periodic health examination. Her glucose level at hospitalization was approximately 60 mg/dL and HbA1c level was 4.1% (Tables 1 and 2(a)). Neither reactive hypoglycemia nor hyperinsulinemia was detected by the oral glucose tolerance test (OGTT) (Table 2(b)). In the 18-hour fasting test, plasma glucose and immunoreactive insulin were 55 mg/dL and 3.0 μIU/mL, respectively, suggesting that insulinoma was unlikely. The insulin tolerance test revealed the suppression of C-peptide as well as the poor responses of ACTH and cortisol (Table 2(c)). Although a circadian variation was maintained in plasma cortisol, her cortisol level in the early morning was slightly low (6.9 μg/dL) (Table 2(d)). The response of cortisol in the rapid ACTH (250 μg) stimulation test was at the lower limit of normal (cortisol peaked at 18.4 $\geq$ 18 μg/dL) [10], while its response in the CRH stimulation test was relatively poor (cortisol peaked at 12.2 μg/dL) (Tables 2(e) and 2(f)). The excretion of 17-hydroxycorticosteroids (17-OHCS) and 17-keto steroids (17-KS) in urine was 2.4 mg/day and 2.5 mg/day, respectively, both of which were below the normal ranges (2.6–7.8 mg/day and 3.1–8.8 mg/day, resp.). No morphological abnormalities were detected in the adrenal glands, liver, or pancreas on enhanced dynamic CT images. She was diagnosed with hypoglycemia due to partial adrenal insufficiency, and so the administration of hydrocortisone (10 mg/day) was initiated. Steroid supplementation slightly increased her fasting plasma glucose levels from 52 mg/dL to 65 mg/dL and HbA1c levels from 4.1% to 4.6%. These levels then plateaued for 12 years

(Table 1). Further examinations were not conducted at that time.

Twelve years later, her 8-month-old grandchild was found to be hypoglycemic (46 mg/dL) while being treated for gastroenteritis. The grandchild's father, the son of our patient, was also diagnosed with asymptomatic hypoglycemia (below 60 mg/dL) in a health examination. A family history of asymptomatic hypoglycemia in three generations made the attending doctor of the grandchild suspect GCK-activating mutations. The DNA of her grandchild was analyzed by direct sequencing of the entire coding region and exon-intron boundaries of GCK in Osaka City General Hospital. The heterozygosity of exon 6 c.590T>C (p.M197T), a novel GCK mutation which has already been reported to be an activating mutation in vitro study [11], was identified in her grandson and her son.

CHI due to the same gene mutation was suspected in our patient, and she was hospitalized for a detailed examination when she was 56 years old. Reassessment of glucose diurnal rhythm revealed that her plasma glucose level was 59–83 mg/dL during the intake of 10 mg of hydrocortisone (Table 3(a)). When our patient decreased and discontinued oral hydrocortisone, her plasma glucose level was definitely lower (48 mg/dL) but no symptoms were observed (Table 3(a)). The circadian variation in cortisol was maintained without any intake of hydrocortisone (Table 3(b)). Although her basal cortisol level was relatively low (4.5–8.8 μg/dL), cortisol responses to the ACTH and CRH stimulation tests were within the normal ranges; peaks in serum cortisol were observed at 24.5 μg/dL and 15.8 μg/dL, respectively (Tables 3(c) and 3(d)).

After obtaining written informed consent, a GCK gene analysis was conducted. The sequencing of exon 6 in her DNA revealed the same mutation as her son and grandchild, and she was diagnosed with congenital hyperinsulinemic hypoglycemia (Figure 1). Since there seems to be no correlation between genotype and phenotype of GCK mutation, we were unable to estimate the severity of hypoglycemia according to the mutation site [9, 12]. However, the severity of hypoglycemia was classified as mild based on her physical and mental states at the age of 43 in the absence of any treatment. Therefore, we decided to stop prescribing hydrocortisone. A favorable course has been followed for several years after the discontinuation of oral hydrocortisone.

3. Discussion

We encountered a family with CHI due to a novel mutation in GCK, with an 8-month-old infant as the index case. This GCK mutation itself has already been reported previously as a case report of the grandson [13]. We demonstrated here endocrinological aspects before and after steroid treatment in the patient with GCK-activating mutation, suggesting when and how we should suspect the GCK mutation as differential diagnoses of hypoglycemia.

Glucokinase-activating mutations result in hyperinsulinemic hypoglycemia. The diagnosis and treatment of hyperinsulinemic hypoglycemia have markedly advanced in recent

TABLE 2: Results of examinations at first visit.

(a) Glucose diurnal rhythm.

Clock time	7:30	10:00	11:30	14:00	17:30	20:00	23:00
Plasma glucose							
(mg/dL)	57	59	62	64	61	84	64
(mmol/L)	3.1	3.2	3.4	3.5	3.3	4.6	3.5

(b) OGTT (oral glucose tolerance test) performed with 75 g glucose.

Time (min)	0	30	60	90	120
Plasma glucose					
(mg/dL)	62	119	120	84	75
(mmol/L)	3.4	6.6	6.6	4.6	4.1
Insulin (μU/mL)	2.0	24.3	45.5	38	17.9

(c) Plasma glucose, c-peptide, glucagon, cortisol, and ACTH responses to insulin tolerance test (0.05 U/kg BW of Humulin R).

Time (min)	0	15	30	45	60	75	90	120
Plasma glucose								
(mg/dL)	53	36	30	48	55	53	52	53
(mmol/L)	2.9	2.0	1.6	2.6	3.0	2.9	2.8	2.9
C-peptide (ng/mL)	1.2	0.7	0.5	0.5	0.5	0.4	0.4	0.5
Glucagon (pg/mL)	213	230	297	232	207	174		174
ACTH (pg/mL)	40	32.8	41.3	42.4	29.5	24.4	17.2	20.1
Cortisol (μg/dL)	6.6	13.2	12	15	12.8	11.9	11.2	8.4

Normal values.
Glucagon 70–174 (pg/mL), ACTH: 7.2–63.3 (pg/mL), and cortisol: 8.0–18.0 (μg/dL).
Interpretation of results.
The normal peak ACTH value poststimulation should be an increment no less than 50 pg/mL at 60'. Baseline cortisol values <5 μg/dL are diagnostic of adrenal insufficiency. The normal peak cortisol value poststimulation should be an increment no less than 7 μg/dL and a maximal level >20 μg/dL at 30'.

(d) Circadian variation in cortisol.

Clock time	8:00	17:00	23:00
ACTH (pg/mL)	23.8	14.3	14.5
Cortisol (μg/dL)	6.9	2.0	>1.0

(e) Cortisol response to the rapid ACTH stimulation test (250 μg, intravenous bolus).

Time (min)	0	30	60
Cortisol (μg/dL)	7.9	16.5	18.4

Interpretation of results.
The normal peak cortisol value poststimulation should be an increment no less than 18 μg/dL.

(f) Cortisol and ACTH responses to the CRH stimulation test (100 μg, intravenous bolus).

Time (min)	0	15	30	60	90	120
ACTH (pg/mL)	35.2	49.3	54.6	54	45.9	37.8
Cortisol (μg/dL)	10.4	11.4	12.2	12.2	11.6	11.4

Interpretation of results.
The normal peak ACTH value poststimulation should be an increment no less than 20 pg/mL. Cortisol should be an increment no less than 5 μg/dL.

years [14]. Severe hypoglycemia in infancy causes neurological dysfunctions and requires appropriate management. On the other hand, some cases of congenital hyperinsulinism are mild and overlooked until adulthood [15]. CHI related to a GCK-activating mutation was suspected in this case due to the presence of autosomal dominant inheritance and hyperinsulinism, with her blood glucose level being relatively low without symptoms. Difficulties are often associated with diagnosing CHI because, as in this case, some cases not accompanied by hyperinsulinemic hypoglycemia even though GCK gene mutations are present [12].

Glucokinase is a key regulatory enzyme in pancreatic β-cells. It phosphorylates glucose as a second substrate to form glucose-6-phosphate (G6P) as a first step in the glycolytic pathway. Since it plays a crucial role in the regulation of insulin secretion and is termed the glucose sensor in pancreatic β-cells, it is understandable that a mutation in GCK leads to an inappropriate threshold for

TABLE 3: Results of examinations on the patient after 12 years.

(a) Glucose diurnal rhythm.

Clock time	7:30	11:30	17:30	20:00	23:00
Plasma glucose					
10 mg hydrocortisone (8:00)					
(mg/dL)	63	80	59	83	81
(mmol/L)	3.5	4.4	3.2	4.6	4.5
5 mg hydrocortisone (8:00)					
(mg/dL)	58	68	67	84	80
(mmol/L)	3.2	3.7	3.7	4.6	4.4
no hydrocortisone					
(mg/dL)	48	64	57	77	67
(mmol/L)	2.6	3.5	3.1	4.2	3.7

(b) Circadian variation in cortisol.

Clock Time	8:00	17:00	23:00
ACTH (pg/mL)	21.3	10.2	8.3
Cortisol (μg/dL)	8.8	2.8	1.1

(c) Cortisol response to the ACTH rapid stimulation test (250 μg, intravenous bolus).

Time (min)	0	30	60
Cortisol (μg/dL)	6.8	22.2	24.5

Interpretation of results.
The normal peak cortisol value poststimulation should be an increment no less than 18 μg/dL.

(d) Cortisol and ACTH responses to the CRH stimulation test (100 μg, intravenous bolus).

Time (min)	0	15	30	60	90	120
ACTH (pg/mL)	15	62.8	75.3	53.6	38	33.8
Cortisol (μg/dL)	4.5	9	15.8	15.5	13	12.6

Interpretation of results.
The normal peak ACTH value poststimulation should be an increment no less than 20 pg/mL. Cortisol should be an increment no less than 5 μg/dL.

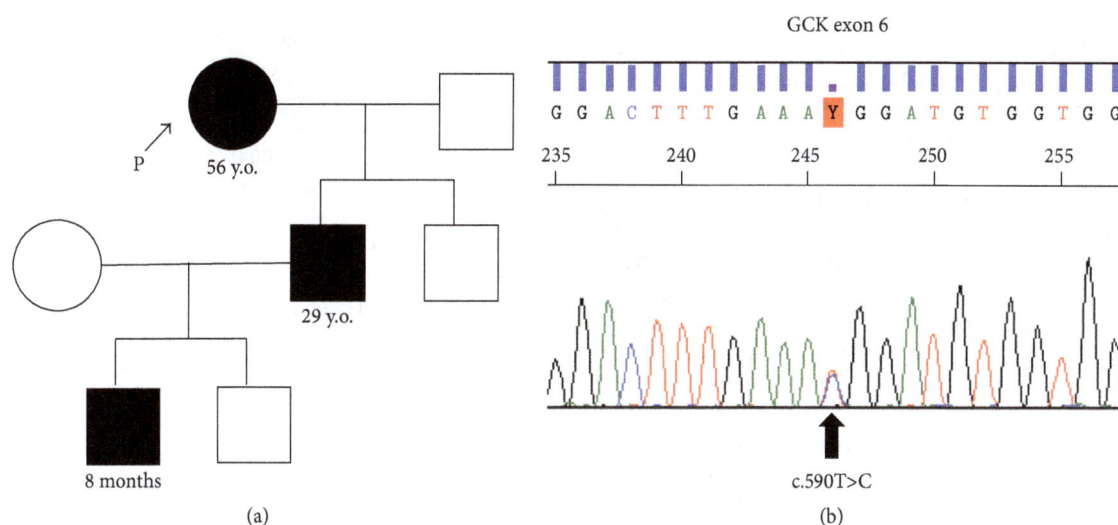

FIGURE 1: (a) Pedigree tree of the patient. (b) GCK gene analysis of the patient (grandmother). The heterozygosity of exon 6 c.590T>C (p.M197T), a novel GCK-activating mutation, was identified.

glucose-stimulated insulin secretion. A glucokinase-activating mutation is one of the rare variants of congenital hyperinsulinism (CHI), and only 12 activating GCK mutations have been described and identified in 8 families and 7 individuals to date [12]. GCK gene mutations have been associated with various grades of symptoms such that many mild cases may be left undiagnosed until adulthood [16]. No criteria currently exist for the treatment of asymptomatic CHI.

A gene analysis involving GCK needs to be conducted when hypoglycemia with an unknown etiology is encountered. Although a family history is very important, there may be cases of new unnoticed-familial mutations. Information on genetic mutations, except for GCK, generally assists in predicting prognoses and responses to CHI treatments. In contrast, since the GCK mutation in the same family had a variety of phenotypes, we were unable to estimate the severity of hypoglycemia based on the mutation site [12]. It should be noted that our patient did not have any difficulties with stressful events, such as the delivery of her son, without any treatment. Therefore, the lower set point of hypoglycemia in our patient was not expected to become a serious problem throughout the rest of her life.

Our patient had been taking hydrocortisone for 12 years based on her poor response to the CRH stimulation test. According to previous findings on patients not only with diabetes [17, 18], but also without diabetes [19], hypoglycemia attenuated sympathoadrenal responses to declining plasma glucose concentrations, leading to hypoglycemia-associated autonomic failure (HAAF). Chronic hypoglycemia due to a GCK mutation may influence cortisol responses. Recent studies suggested that glucokinase in the hypothalamus and hindbrain participated in the activation of the norepinephrine and epinephrine neurons needed for the counterregulatory response [20, 21]. We speculated that not only HAAF but also a glucose sensing abnormality due to the activation of glucokinase in neuronal cells accounted for the counterregulatory hormone levels (basal and responses) of our patient.

An overdose of steroids is associated with a risk of side effects, including weight gain, hypertension, hyperlipidemia, and, sometimes, suppression of the HPA axis. Actually, her body weight increased by 3.8 kg (BMI: from 23.2 to 24.8) and blood pressure elevated (112/72 mmHg to 149/88 mmHg) during the 12-year treatment (Table 1). Two months after discontinuation of steroids, she had lost 1.8 kg in weight and her blood pressure decreased to 125/80 mmHg. Though 10 mg of oral hydrocortisone is within the physiological range, her circadian variation of cortisol must have been unnatural [22]. Considering these facts, 10 mg of oral hydrocortisone probably bears some responsibility with weight gain and hypertension.

In conclusion, the identification of GCK-activating mutations in hyperinsulinemic hypoglycemia patients may be useful for a deeper understanding of the pathophysiology involved and preventing unnecessary glucocorticoid therapy. More precise interpretations are needed while treating hypoglycemia and adrenal dysfunction.

Authors' Contributions

Kae Morishita and Chika Kyo contributed equally to this work.

Acknowledgments

The authors sincerely thank Dr. Tohru Yorifuji (Department of Pediatric Endocrinology and Metabolism, Children's Medical Center, Osaka City General Hospital, Osaka, Japan) for analyzing the GCK mutation. The authors also thank Dr. Kenji Nanao (Department of Pediatrics, Hino Municipal Hospital, Tokyo, Japan), the doctor of the subject's grandchild, for his kind advice.

References

[1] C. A. Stanley, "Perspective on the genetics and diagnosis of congenital hyperinsulinism disorders," *Journal of Clinical Endocrinology and Metabolism*, vol. 101, no. 3, pp. 815–826, 2016.

[2] P. M. Thomas, G. J. Cote, N. Wohllk et al., "Mutations in the sulfonylurea receptor gene in familial persistent hyperinsulinemic hypoglycemia of infancy," *Science*, vol. 268, no. 5209, pp. 426–429, 1995.

[3] P. Thomas, Y. Ye, and E. Lightner, "Mutation of the pancreatic islet inward rectifier Kir6.2 also leads to familial persistent hyperinsulinemic hypoglycemia of infancy," *Human Molecular Genetics*, vol. 5, no. 11, pp. 1809–1812, 1996.

[4] B. Glaser, P. Kesavan, M. Heyman et al., "Familial hyperinsulinism caused by an activating glucokinase mutation," *New England Journal of Medicine*, vol. 338, no. 4, pp. 226–230, 1998.

[5] C. A. Stanley, Y. K. Lieu, B. Y. L. Hsu et al., "Hyperinsulinism and hyperammonemia in infants with regulatory mutations of the glutamate dehydrogenase gene," *New England Journal of Medicine*, vol. 338, no. 19, pp. 1352–1357, 1998.

[6] K. Højlund, T. Hansen, M. Lajer et al., "A novel syndrome of autosomal-dominant hyperinsulinemic hypoglycemia linked to a mutation in the human insulin receptor gene," *Diabetes*, vol. 53, no. 6, pp. 1592–1598, 2004.

[7] E. R. Pearson, S. F. Boj, A. M. Steele et al., "Macrosomia and hyperinsulinaemic hypoglycaemia in patients with heterozygous mutations in the HNF4A gene," *PLoS Medicine*, vol. 4, no. 4, article no. e118, 2007.

[8] T. Otonkoski, H. Jiao, N. Kaminen-Ahola et al., "Physical exercise-induced hypoglycemia caused by failed silencing of monocarboxylate transporter 1 in pancreatic β cells," *The American Journal of Human Genetics*, vol. 81, no. 3, pp. 467–474, 2007.

[9] D. D. Deleon and C. A. Stanley, Eds., *Monogenic Hyperinsulinemic Hypoglycemia Disorders. Frontiers in Diabetes*, Karger, Geneva, Swizerland, 2012.

[10] The Japan Endocrine Society, "Guideline of management and treatment of adrenal insufficiency," 2014 (Japanese), http://square.umin.ac.jp/endocrine/hottopics/20140311sinryousisin.pdf.

[11] S. Sayed, D. R. Langdon, S. Odili et al., "Extremes of clinical and enzymatic phenotypes in children with hyperinsulinism caused by glucokinase activating mutations," *Diabetes*, vol. 58, no. 6, pp. 1419–1427, 2009.

[12] T. Meissner, J. Marquard, N. Cobo-Vuilleumier et al., "Diagnostic difficulties in glucokinase hyperinsulinism," *Hormone and Metabolic Research*, vol. 41, no. 4, pp. 320–326, 2009.

[13] K. Nanao, T. Yorifuji, T. Kamimaki et al., "Congenital hyperinsulinism in a Japanese family with a novel heterozygous GCK mutation," *Clinical Endocrinology*, vol. 59, pp. 1049–1051, 2011 (Japanese).

[14] T. Yorifuji, M. Masue, and H. Nishibori, "Congenital hyperinsulinism: global and Japanese perspectives," *Pediatrics International*, vol. 56, no. 4, pp. 467–476, 2014.

[15] K. K. Osbak, K. Colclough, C. Saint-Martin et al., "Update on mutations in glucokinase (*GCK*), which cause maturity-onset diabetes of the young, permanent neonatal diabetes, and hyperinsulinemic hypoglycemia," *Human Mutation*, vol. 30, no. 11, pp. 1512–1526, 2009.

[16] J. Marquard, A. A. Palladino, C. A. Stanley, E. Mayatepek, and T. Meissner, "Rare forms of congenital hyperinsulinism," *Seminars in Pediatric Surgery*, vol. 20, no. 1, pp. 38–44, 2011.

[17] A. L. Cuesta-Muñoz, H. Huopio, T. Otonkoski et al., "Severe persistent hyperinsulinemic hypoglycemia due to a de novo glucokinase mutation," *Diabetes*, vol. 53, no. 8, pp. 2164–2168, 2004.

[18] P. E. Cryer, "Mechanisms of hypoglycemia-associated autonomic failure in diabetes," *New England Journal of Medicine*, vol. 369, no. 4, pp. 362–372, 2013.

[19] S. Mathur, J. Boparai, S. N. Mediwala et al., "Reversible Adrenal insufficiency in three patients with Post-Roux-en-Y gastric bypass noninsulinoma pancreatogenous hypoglycemia syndrome," *Journal of Investigative Medicine High Impact Case Reports*, pp. 1–6, 2014.

[20] L. Zhou, C.-Y. Yueh, D. D. Lam et al., "Glucokinase inhibitor glucosamine stimulates feeding and activates hypothalamic neuropeptide Y and orexin neurons," *Behavioural Brain Research*, vol. 222, no. 1, pp. 274–278, 2011.

[21] J. Zhou, D. S. Roane, X. Xi et al., "Short-term food restriction and refeeding alter expression of genes likely involved in brain glucosensing," *Experimental Biology and Medicine*, vol. 228, no. 8, pp. 943–950, 2003.

[22] S. Hahner and B. Allolio, "Management of adrenal insufficiency in different clinical settings," *Expert Opinion on Pharmacotherapy*, vol. 6, no. 14, pp. 2407–2417, 2005.

53

A Case Report of Dramatically Increased Thyroglobulin after Lymph Node Biopsy in Thyroid Carcinoma after Total Thyroidectomy and Radioiodine

Mandana Moosavi[1] and Stuart Kreisman[2]

[1]*Vancouver Coastal Health, Canada*
[2]*Division of Endocrinology, St. Paul's Hospital, 1081 Burrard Street, Vancouver, BC, Canada V6Z 1Y6*

Correspondence should be addressed to Mandana Moosavi; mandana.moosavi@mail.mcgill.ca

Academic Editor: Osamu Isozaki

Thyroglobulin (Tg) is an important modality for monitoring patients with thyroid cancers, especially after thyroidectomy followed by radioiodine (RAI). It is also used as a marker for burden of thyroid tissue whether malignant or benign. Although there have been several reports of rising serum Tg transiently after thyroid biopsy in intact glands and following palpation or trauma, there are no reports in the literature of elevation in Tg after biopsy of suspicious lesions in thyroidectomized patients. In this paper we report a fascinating case of a considerable and initially worrying, although ultimately transient, rise in Tg in a patient 2 years after total thyroidectomy and RAI ablation after fine needle aspiration (FNA) of a suspicious thyroid bed nodule that was proven positive.

1. Background

Tg is a storage form for thyroxine and triiodothyronine. It is synthesized only by follicular thyroid cells. Due to its cellular specificity, Tg is an excellent marker that has long been used for surveillance after thyroidectomy and after RAI ablation in thyroid cancer patients. The American Thyroid Association Guidelines recommend routine measurement of Tg along with neck ultrasounds as the principal modalities of patient follow-up [1]. If Tg levels are elevated, ultrasound followed by biopsy of growing or suspicious nodules is recommended; however there are no guidelines on timing of biopsy with respect to Tg measurements [1]. Tg is known to increase with benign thyroid swelling, after trauma and surgery as well as with FNA of the intact thyroid gland itself [1]. It is thus potentially important to know when to check serum Tg and how to properly interpret the result as it can cause significant concern for the physician and the patient, suggesting not only cancer recurrence, but also disease acceleration.

There have been several reports of Tg rising after FNA of nodules and normalizing within a few days. The half-life of circulating Tg is 65 hours [2]. In one study, 12 patients with a solitary cold nodule or multinodular goitre had serum Tg measured before and 5–60 minutes after FNA. Seven of them had statistically significant increases in serum thyroglobulin ranging from 35.4 ng/mL to 58 ng/mL with an increase of 305% being seen in one patient with follicular carcinoma [2]. This study, although in a small sample, suggested a greater rise in Tg in malignant nodules. In another study, an increase in Tg ranging from 35% to 341% was also seen 5 minutes to 3 hours after FNA irrespective of whether the biopsied nodule was benign or malignant. The Tg values normalized 2 weeks after FNA in all the subjects. There was no change in thyroid-stimulating hormone, total thyroxine, free thyroxine, or free triiodothyronine with FNA [3]. A similar rise of 35–77% in Tg was also seen in 22 out of 25 patients measured before and 60 minutes after FNA in a third study where the Tg rise persisted for up to 15 days [4]. There have not been any reports of a rise in serum Tg or Tg antibody in patients who have been thyroidectomized with or without radioiodine and are undergoing biopsies for possible recurrence. In this paper we aim to discuss a case of Tg rise after biopsy in a patient after thyroidectomy and RAI.

2. Patient

We report a case of a patient who had increase in Tg after biopsy for assessment of a suspicious ultrasound finding after thyroidectomy and radioiodine for thyroid cancer. She is a 46-year-old woman originally from Ukraine who was exposed to the Chernobyl disaster. Her family history was negative for thyroid cancer. On an ultrasound done for follow-up of her multinodular goiter, there was a suspicious nodule of 7 mm, with biopsy consistent with papillary thyroid carcinoma. Left thyroid lobectomy showed that her tumor had positive margins with no lymphatic or vascular invasion. She underwent completion thyroidectomy 8 months later, which showed two additional foci of 2 and 1 mm of papillary carcinoma in the right lobe, with clear margins. Histology report revealed conventional papillary carcinoma with enlarged nuclei. She initially did not have any RAI therapy, but her Tg started to rise without stimulation to 6 and 8 from previous values of 1 for both cases (see Table 1) and a subsequent biopsy of a left thyroid bed nodule returned positive. Modified neck exploration was performed and histology showed metastases in 4 of 12 lymph nodes. She was then treated with 100 mCi of radioiodine by thyroid hormone withdrawal (her TSH was 111 with Tg of 6 ng/mL at the time). The 7-day posttreatment scan showed some activity in the thyroid bed but no evidence of distant metastases. Part of the reason she was investigated so intensely was due to her extreme anxiety and concern about her prognosis, despite reassurance. One year after her third surgery (the neck exploration), ultrasound in the left thyroid bed showed two hypoechoic nodules of 10 mm and 4 mm. Biopsy of both nodules was again positive for papillary thyroid carcinoma. One month before biopsy her TSH was 11.2 and Tg was 0.9 ng/mL, at which point her thyroxine dose was increased. Another Tg was ordered around the time of biopsy and by chance was done after biopsy by the patient. To our surprise her thyroglobulin increased to 39 ng/mL, 3 days after biopsy (time zero in Table 1). Given patient's already anxious mindset, this finding led to even more anguish. Because of this and a hypothesis that the rise may have been biopsy related, Tg was repeated six days later and had already fallen to 10.3 ng/mL and rapidly came back down to 0.9 ng/mL six weeks after (see Table 1). Her second neck exploration occurred 3 weeks after second biopsy that also showed four nodes positive for papillary thyroid carcinoma. She then had 150 mCi MBq of RAI followed by a whole body scan a week later, which showed neither residual activity in the thyroid bed nor evidence of functioning thyroid metastases. In our hospital, the surgical approach in patients with lymph node metastasis involves total thyroidectomy with central compartment lymphadenectomy and modified neck dissection. Her last two thyroid ultrasounds were after second lymph node excision, both of which did not demonstrate any suspicious findings. One year after her second neck exploration, for the first time she had undetectable Tg and Tg antibody. Her most recent Tg was <0.1 ng/mL and TSH was 0.03 two years after biopsy.

3. Discussion

American Thyroid Association Guidelines recommend any suspicious nodules be investigated with ultrasound and possible biopsy, while routine measurement of Tg is not part of the standard work-up of nodules prior to cancer diagnosis. It is known that Tg can be elevated postsurgically as well as in association with benign and malignant thyroid tissue. However, although there have been several reports of rising Tg after FNA, there have not yet been any reports of Tg rise after FNA in thyroidectomized patients regardless of radioiodine or lymph node status. In our case, Tg transiently rose to 39 ng/mL and at the time there was nothing in literature to help interpret this finding. Although this was hypothesized to be biopsy related, it could also have represented an ominous marker of accelerating disease, leading to much anxiety for the patient. Interassay variation can be significant, often due to variation in antithyroglobulin antibodies used, or the heterogeneity of Tg itself due to alternative processing. With intra-assay variation, small fluctuations can be expected in the same patient [5], but not such high values as in our case.

It is important to know the significance of findings on both ultrasound and biopsy as well as values of Tg and anti-Tg antibody. As reported in the case above, an increase in Tg can cause extreme concern for both the patient and the physician; thus it is important to both know when to check Tg values and interpret them in the appropriate clinical context in order to avoid unnecessary investigations. Current guidelines do not address the timing of Tg with respect to biopsy, and we had previously never given any instructions to our patients in this regard. In general, unless stimulated, Tg rise in recurrent thyroid cancer is slow and steady and the rapid rise in this case led to concern of the disease somehow having become more aggressive. In this case biopsy effect was hypothesized as being the more likely explanation from the outset and confirmed when Tg dropped shortly after. Hence it is our recommendation that future guidelines should instruct on timing Tg measurement before any planned biopsy. On the other hand, if interpreted carefully thyroglobulin after biopsy may have some diagnostic utility. While the lack of any rise in a nondiagnostic biopsy would be reassuring, presumably biopsy of benign residual after surgical thyroid bed tissue would also lead to some rise in Tg. Whether the magnitude of such rise differs from that following biopsy of malignant lesions could be worth investigating.

Abbreviations

Tg: Thyroglobulin
FNA: Fine needle aspiration
RAI: Radioiodine.

TABLE 1: Summary of thyroglobulin levels and thyroglobulin antibodies in patient discussed (day zero is biopsy date). Tg: thyroglobulin in ng/mL; Tg-Ab: thyroglobulin antibody.

	After total thyroidectomy: 4 yr	After total thyroidectomy: 3 yr	After total thyroidectomy: 3 yr	After total thyroidectomy: 3 yr	After neck dissection: 1yr	After RAIl: 30 days	Day 3	Day 6	Day 42	Day 365	Day 730
Tg (ng/mL)	1	6	7	8	6 (stimulated Tg with TSH 111)	0.9 (one year after RA ablation)	39	10.3	0.9	<0.1	<0.1
Tg-Ab	<10	<10	<10	<10	<10	<10	<10	<10	<10	<10	<10

Authors' Contribution

Dr. Mandana Moosavi wrote the paper and Dr. Stuart Kreisman edited and reviewed the paper.

Acknowledgments

The authors would like to thank Genzyme and UBC Department of Endocrinology for funding the paper.

References

[1] B. R. Haugen, E. K. Alexander, K. C. Bible et al., "2015 American Thyroid Association management guidelines for adult patients with thyroid nodules and differentiated thyroid cancer: The American Thyroid Association guidelines task force on thyroid nodules and differentiated thyroid cancer," *Thyroid*, vol. 26, no. 1, pp. 1–133, 2016.

[2] M. Bayraktar, M. Ergin, A. Boyacioglu, and S. Demir, "A preliminary report of thyroglobulin release after fine needle aspiration biopsy of thyroid nodules," *The Journal of International Medical Research*, vol. 18, no. 3, pp. 253–255, 1990.

[3] S. A. Polyzos and A. D. Anastasilakis, "Alterations in serum thyroid-related constituents after thyroid fine-needle biopsy: a systematic review," *Thyroid*, vol. 20, no. 3, pp. 265–271, 2010.

[4] R. Luboshitzky, I. Lavi, and A. Ishay, "Serum thyroglobulin levels after fine-needle aspiration of thyroid nodules," *Endocrine Practice*, vol. 12, no. 3, pp. 264–269, 2006.

[5] D. R. Weightman, U. K. Mallick, J. D. Fenwick, and P. Perros, "Discordant serum thyroglobulin results generated by two classes of assay in patients with thyroid carcinoma: correlation with clinical outcome after 3 years of follow-up," *Cancer*, vol. 98, no. 1, pp. 41–47, 2003.

54

Atypical Parathyroid Adenoma Complicated with Protracted Hungry Bone Syndrome after Surgery

Óscar Alfredo Juárez-León,[1] **Miguel Ángel Gómez-Sámano,**[1] **Daniel Cuevas-Ramos,**[1] **Paloma Almeda-Valdés,**[1] **Manuel Alejandro López-Flores A La Torre,**[2] **Alfredo Adolfo Reza-Albarrán,**[1] **and Francisco Javier Gómez-Pérez**[1]

[1]*Endocrinology and Metabolism Department, Instituto Nacional de Ciencias Médicas y Nutrición Salvador Zubirán, 14080 Mexico City, Mexico*
[2]*School of Medicine, Universidad Panamericana, 03920 Mexico City, Mexico*

Correspondence should be addressed to Francisco Javier Gómez-Pérez; gomezperezfco@gmail.com

Academic Editor: Hidetoshi Ikeda

Hungry Bone Syndrome refers to the severe and prolonged hypocalcemia and hypophosphatemia, following parathyroidectomy in patients with hyperparathyroidism. We present the case of an eighteen-year-old woman with a four-year history of hyporexia, polydipsia, weight loss, growth retardation, and poor academic performance. The diagnostic work-up demonstrated primary hyperparathyroidism with hypercalcemia of 13.36 mg/dL, a PTH level of 2551 pg/mL, bone brown tumors, and microcalcifications within pancreas and kidneys. Neck ultrasonography revealed a parathyroid adenoma of $33 \times 14 \times 14$ mm, also identified on ^{99}Tc-sestamibi scan. Bone densitometry showed decreased Z-Score values (total lumbar Z-Score of −4.2). A right hemithyroidectomy and right lower parathyroidectomy were performed. Pathological examination showed an atypical parathyroid adenoma, of 3.8 g of weight and 2.8 cm in diameter. After surgery she developed hypocalcemia with tetany and QTc interval prolongation. The patient required 3 months of oral and intravenous calcium supplementation due to Hungry Bone Syndrome (HBS). After 42 months, she is still under oral calcium. Usually HBS lasts less than 12 months. Therefore we propose the term "Protracted HBS" in patients with particularly long recovery of 1 year. We present a literature review of the diagnosis, pathophysiology, and treatment of HBS.

1. Introduction

The Hungry Bone Syndrome (HBS) was first described by Albright and Reifenstein in 1950, in patients with hyperparathyroidism with a severe and prolonged hypocalcemia after parathyroidectomy [1].

Most HBS definitions consider clinical manifestations of hypocalcemia and biochemical variables including hyperparathyroidism requiring surgery, hypophosphatemia, and hypomagnesemia. Some authors denote HBS when patients develop postoperative hypocalcemia (<8.5 mg/dL), a simultaneous inorganic phosphate value of <3.0 mg/dL [2], and hypocalcemia longer than 4 days requiring calcium supplementation, despite optimization of supportive therapy with normal vitamin D levels [3, 4].

Parathyroid hormone (PTH) and calcitriol $(1\alpha,25[OH]_2D_3)$ regulate calcium and phosphate homeostasis. PTH is secreted in response to hypocalcemia after being sensed by the parathyroid calcium-sensing receptor (CaSR) [5]. PTH receptors are mainly present in kidney and bone tissue [6], and when activated, they increase bone calcium efflux and decrease renal excretion to maintain normal serum calcium concentrations. The HBS pathophysiology begins with elevated PTH production (primary, secondary, or tertiary hyperparathyroidism) which augments bone metabolism and calcium turnover, leading to increased

TABLE 1: Laboratory findings at hospital admission and at last outpatient follow-up visit.

	Hospitalization [February 2010]	Follow-up [November 2013]	Reference values
Serum calcium [mg/dL]	12.1	8.9	8.6–9.9
Corrected serum calcium [mg/dL]*	12.6	7.9	
Serum phosphate [mg/dL]	2.7	3	2.7–4.5
Serum magnesium [mg/dL]	1.3	2	1.9–2.7
Serum albumin [g/dL]	3.4	5.2	3.5–5.7
Serum creatinine [mg/dL]	4.83	1.05	0.42–1.09
Creatinine clearance [ml/min/1.73 m^2]	12	76	≥90
PTH [pg/mL]	2551	91.7	12–88
25-OH vitamin D [ng/mL]	13	25.9	30–100
Alkaline phosphatase [IU/L]	4410	126	34–104
Urinary calcium [mg/day]	213	22	100–300
Urinary phosphorus [mg/day]	413	524	<1000
Prolactin [ng/mL]	12.6	—	2.64–13.13
FSH [mIU/mL]	4.4	—	3.85–8.78$^{\text{(follicular phase)}}$
LH [mIU/mL]	17	—	2.12–10.89$^{\text{(follicular phase)}}$
Estradiol [pg/mL]	36.13	—	12–40$^{\text{(follicular phase)}}$
T3 [nmol/L]	1.78	—	0.64–1.81
T4 [nmol/L]	69.33	—	66–181
TSH [μUI/mL]	1.85	—	0.3–5
Thyroglobulin [ng/mL]	5.7	—	0–36.8
ACTH [pg/mL]	19	—	10–100
Morning cortisol [μg/dL]	15.76		6.7–22.6

PTH parathyroid hormone.
*Corrected calcium with albumin using the following formula: $Ca^{2+}_{corrected} = Ca^{2+}_{measured} + 0.8 \times [4 - albumin_{measured}]$.

serum calcium levels. Treatment of primary hyperparathyroidism often requires surgical resection of an adenoma, causing a sudden halt in bone turnover. Consequently, a marked depletion of serum circulating calcium, phosphate, and magnesium is seen due to bone remineralization [2].

The most common etiologies associated with HBS are secondary and primary hyperparathyroidism [3, 7, 8]. Other less frequent causes are parathyroid carcinoma, drugs, multiple endocrine neoplasia, and metastatic prostate cancer [9–14].

Here we present a clinical case of an unusual longlasting HBS developed in a female patient with primary hyperparathyroidism after surgical treatment of an atypical adenoma.

2. Case Presentation

An 18-year-old previously healthy woman presented at our institution after a four-year history of hyporexia, polydipsia, weight loss, growth retardation, and poor academic performance. One month prior to presentation, outpatient laboratory analysis revealed increased serum calcium and parathyroid hormone (PTH). She did not have any other significant personal or family history.

She was admitted to our hospital in February 2010. On physical examination her height was 1.40 m and weight was 30 kg. Her vital signs were within normal limits. She presented with a marked cervical kyphosis.

Relevant laboratory results showed hypercalcemia (13.36 mg/dL, normal 8.6–9.9 mg/dL), elevated PTH (2551 pg/mL, normal 12–88 pg/mL), elevated alkaline phosphatase level (4410 IU/L, normal 34–104 IU/L), hypercalciuria (urinary calcium of 213 mg/24 H, normal 100–250 mg/24 H), low creatinine clearance (25.84 mL/min/1.73 m^2, normal ≥90 mL/min/1.73 m^2), and low 25[OH]D$_3$ circulating level (13 ng/mL, normal 30–100 ng/mL). The laboratory findings at hospital admission and last follow-up visit are summarized in Table 1. Biochemical approach was further completed with prolactin 12.6 ng/mL, FSH 4.4 mIU/mL, LH 17 mIU/mL, estradiol 36.13 pg/mL, T3 1.78 nmol/L, T4 69.33 nmol/L, TSH 1.85 μUI/mL, thyroglobulin 5.7 ng/mL, ACTH 19 pg/mL, and morning cortisol 15.76 μg/dL, all within normal limits.

Skeletal X-rays showed skull with "salt and pepper" lesions, vertebral compression fractures, brown tumors within the left humerus, and profuse calcifications within the pancreas and kidneys (Figure 1). The patient did not refer to abdominal pain, nor any symptomatology related to endocrine and exocrine pancreatic insufficiency. The electrocardiogram was unremarkable. Abdominal ultrasound revealed kidney stones causing bilateral dilation of the renal pelvis. Neck ultrasonography showed microcalcifications within a large echogenic mass, posterior to the right lobe of

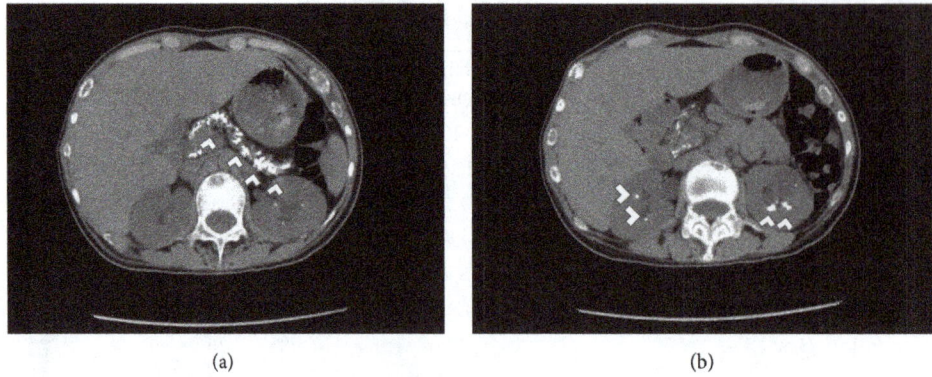

(a)   (b)

FIGURE 1: Abdominal computed tomography (CT) on admission. (a) Diffuse pancreatic calcifications; (b) bilateral kidney calcifications on axial computed tomography. Findings are marked with white arrow heads.

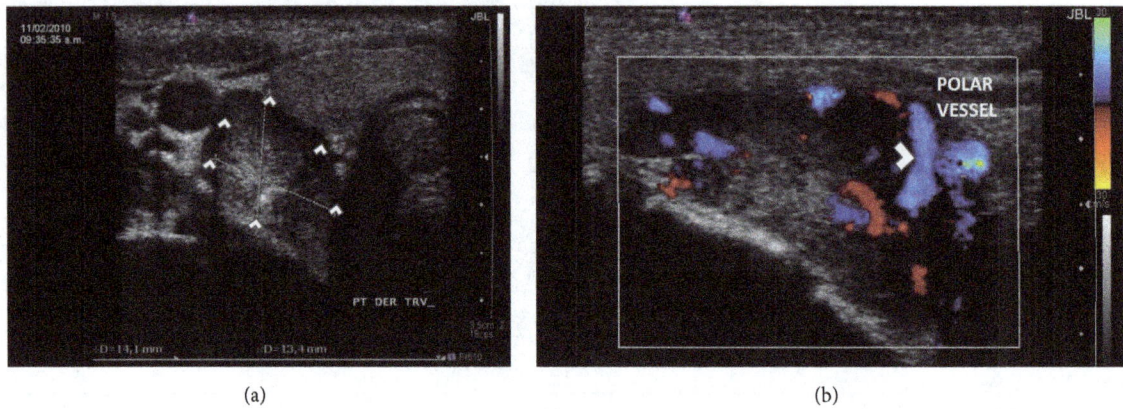

(a)   (b)

FIGURE 2: Neck ultrasonography on admission. (a) Large echogenic mass dorsal to the right lobe of the thyroid gland. (b) Doppler effect showing polar vessel finding, present in most adenomas. Findings are marked with white arrow heads.

the thyroid gland of $33 \times 14 \times 14$ mm, Figure 2. A 25 mCi ^{99}Tc-sestamibi scintigraphy reported persistence of the radionuclide material at 120 minutes in the right inferior parathyroid gland at the same location of the mass shown in the US, Figure 3. Bone densitometry showed decreased Z-Score values (total lumbar Z-Score of -4.2), Table 2. Primary hyperparathyroidism secondary to a large parathyroid tumor was diagnosed.

For HBS prophylaxis, before surgery, she received a 400,000 IU of vitamin D2 (Drisdol) (ergocalciferol) and 1 mg of calcitriol. Right hemithyroidectomy with right lower parathyroidectomy was performed. A tumor of 2.8 cm with 3.8 g of weight was resected. Pathological revision reported a focal lesion containing parathyroid tissue; it infiltrated the nodule capsule, without trespassing it, and the diagnosis was consistent with an atypical parathyroid adenoma. Two lymph nodes demonstrated follicular hyperplasia. Despite the administration of vitamin D (50,000 per week) and calcitriol 0.75 mg per day after surgery, the 25-hydroxyvitamin D levels never reached a value above 30. 1,25-dihydroxy vitamin D was not measured.

Postsurgical laboratory analysis showed PTH values of 31.3 pg/mL, serum calcium of 8.5 mg/dL, phosphate of 1.9 mg/dL, and magnesium of 1.8 mg/dL; on physical examination

TABLE 2: Densitometry values on admission and at the last follow-up visit as an outpatient. The most affected segment is presented.[*]

	Hospitalization [February 2010]		Follow-up [November 2013]	
Lumbar BMD	L1	Total	L1	Total
[g/cm^2]	0.53	0.551	1.061	1.07
Z-Score	—	−4.2	1.4	0.4
T score	−3.6	−4.5	1.2	0.2
Hip BMD	Neck	Total	Neck	Total
[g/cm^2]	0.41	0.481	0.939	0.998
Z-Score[*]	—	—	0.6	0.4
T score	−3.9	−3.6	0.5	0.3

Osteoporosis is diagnosed in young adults when both Z-score <-2.0 and fractures are present.
[*] Due to the age of presentation, baseline Z-scores could not be obtained with the equipment used in our patient.

she presented upper extremity distal contractures, oromandibular dystonia, Chvostek and Trousseau signs, and QTc interval prolongation. PTH levels reached up to 48.6 pg/mL after 1 month, coexisting with hypophosphatemia of 2.7 mg/dL. At last follow-up, PTH serum levels were between 80

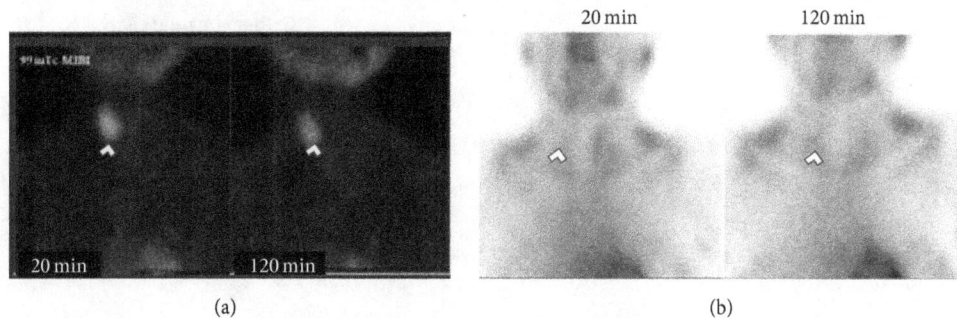

FIGURE 3: Neck scintigraphies with 25 mCi of ^{99}Tc-sestamibi with $0'$ and $120'$ wash-out sequences. (a) 2010 Admission Scintigraphy. $120'$ washout sequence shows residual capitation from right lower thyroid lobe suggesting a parathyroid adenoma. (b) 2013 postparathyroidectomy control scintigraphy. $120'$ wash-out sequence shows no apparent residual captation. Findings are marked with white arrow heads.

and 90 pg/mL, Table 2. She developed a prolonged and severe HBS that required 3 months with oral and intravenous calcium supplementation. The calcium IV infusion was stopped three months later. High PTH levels with hypocalcemia but also hypophosphatemia ruled out hypoparathyroidism. "Protracted" HBS was therefore diagnosed. During her hospitalization she underwent two episodes of lithotripsy as treatment for the kidney stones. Serum calcium, phosphate, and magnesium levels during hospitalization and follow-up are shown in Figure 4.

After 42 months of treatment, bone densitometry scores improved within normal limits, Table 2. As an outpatient since 2010 she has been receiving an average of 1197 mg of oral elemental calcium, 1600 units of vitamin D, and 3 grams of magnesium sulfate per day. She was kept under close medical evaluation as an outpatient. Unfortunately in November 2013 the patient stopped coming to our institution with no clear reason, Table 1.

3. Discussion

We described a case of "Protracted" HBS in a female patient following parathyroidectomy for primary hyperparathyroidism caused by an atypical parathyroid adenoma. The primary hyperparathyroidism remained undiagnosed for at least 4 years and was complicated by the occurrence of brown tumors, severe osteoporosis, nephrocalcinosis, and short stature.

Postoperative hypocalcemia following parathyroidectomy could be associated with numerous causes. Some common causes are transient hypoparathyroidism due to extensive surgical removal of parathyroid glands, disruption of blood supply to remnant parathyroid glands, radical neck exploration, and major remineralization of bone such as in HBS [2, 7, 15]. The main features that favor the diagnosis of hypoparathyroidism versus HBS are the extent of surgery, bilateral neck exploration, or prior neck surgery. Also hypoparathyroidism usually presents with hypocalcemia and hyperphosphatemia [2, 16]. HBS is associated with high and long term requirements of calcium and vitamin D supplementation with normal or high PTH levels [2, 7].

The lack of consensus for the definition of HBS hinders the comparison of reported cases, validation of risk factors,

determination of severity and prognosis predictors, proposal of prophylaxis regimens, and delineation of treatment goals, as well as resolution criteria [4, 7].

Clinical and laboratory risk factors for HBS are older age, weight and volume of resected parathyroid glands, elevated alkaline phosphatase, evidence of significant bone disease, and blood urea nitrogen [2, 7]. The length of hospitalization has been associated with severity of hypocalcemia [2].

In order to prevent HBS, some authors suggest treatment with bisphosphonates in primary [17] and secondary hyperparathyroidism [18]; however, this approach may delay bone remodeling [19].

The lesion resected from our patient was compatible with atypical adenoma, because it presented capsule invasion without trespassing its boundaries, the rest of the surgical piece was analyzed finding normal thyroid and lymph nodes without invasion. According to the World Health Organization criteria (WHO, 2004) [20] an atypical adenoma refers to large glands with either excess mitotic cells and tumor capsule invasion without exceeding its boundaries, or with marked fibrotic divisions pattern. It is associated with neither spontaneous tumor necrosis, nor vascular invasion to surrounding tissues [21, 22]. These pathology characteristics have been usually associated with a benign course in terms of survival. Parathyroid carcinoma specimens have been associated with the development of HBS [8, 10–12].

Due to the sporadic nature, severity of symptoms, and young age at presentation, genetic abnormalities could be suspected as the cause of this clinical presentation, such as gain of function of protooncogenes (e. gr. cyclinD1/PRAD1), or inactivation of tumor suppressor genes (e. gr. MEN1, multiple endocrine neoplasia 1).

Primary hyperparathyroidism (PHPT) is the most common feature of MEN1 and presents in approximately 90% of MEN1 patients [23, 24]. The PHPT main manifestations reported as part of MEN1 syndrome are earlier age at onset (20 to 25 yrs *versus* 55 yrs), demineralization, and/or recurrent kidney stones [24], findings consistent with the presentation of our patient. Normal laboratory analysis ruled out functional pituitary adenoma at this time; however, she will continue to be under close observation.

Since the patient did not refer to any symptomatology for the suspicion of a functional pancreatic/gastrointestinal (GI)

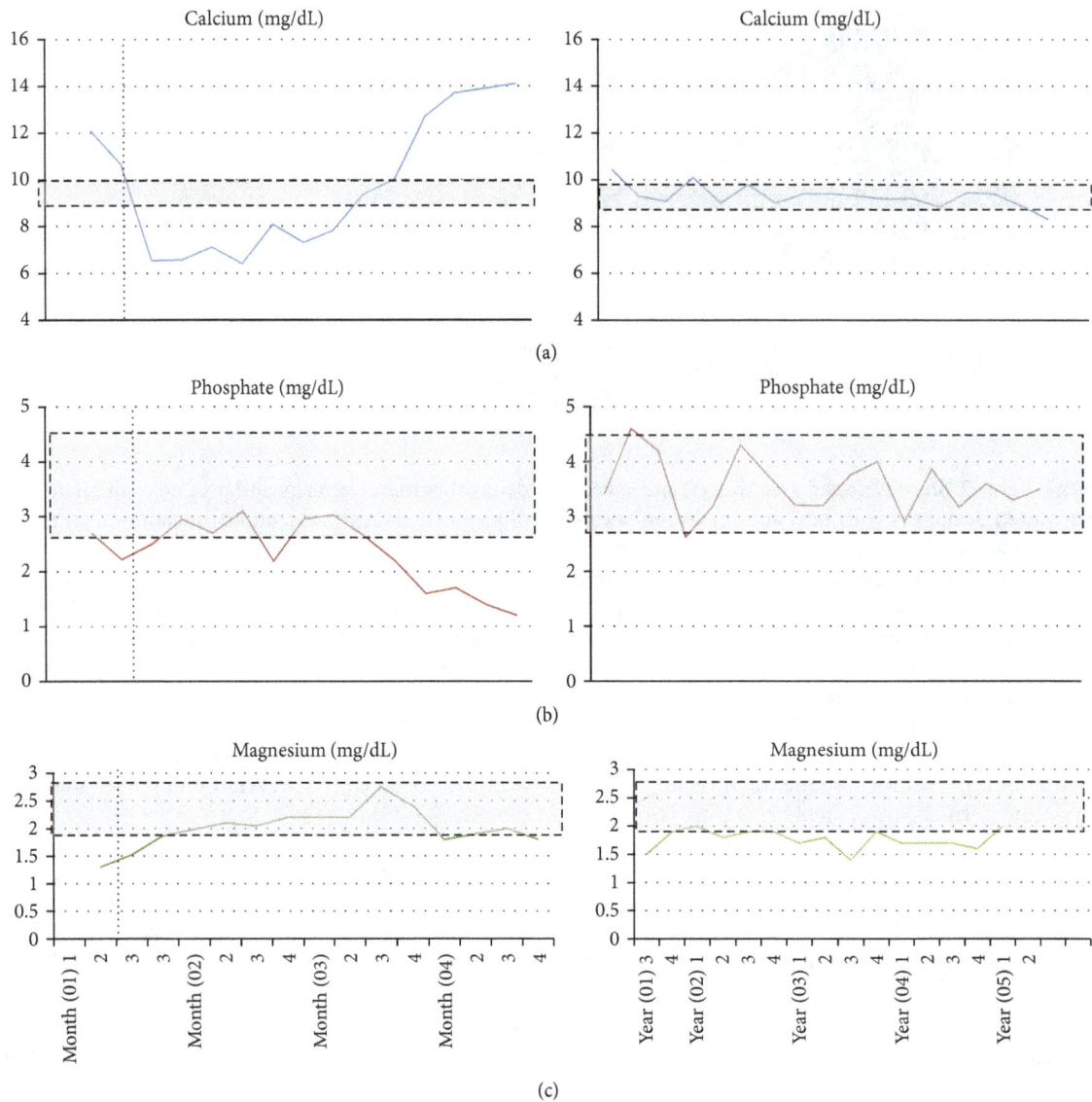

FIGURE 4: (a) Corrected serum calcium during hospitalization and as outpatient. (b) Serum phosphate values during hospitalization and as outpatient. (c) Serum magnesium values during hospitalization and as outpatient. *Gray area represents reference values. **Vertical dotted line represents treatment beginning, which continued beyond last medical assessment at our institution.

adenoma, no additional biochemical analyses were carried out. No apparent pancreatic tumors were found on the abdominal CT.

Clinical manifestations of hypocalcemia in HBS range from relative benign symptoms such as weakness, headache, paresthesias, ileus, malabsorption, and muscle cramps to life threatening features such as arrhythmias, seizures, laryngeal stridor, tetany, and overt severe heart failure [4, 7, 25]. Our patient presented mainly musculoskeletal manifestations.

In patients with HBS, serum electrolytes, such as calcium, phosphate, and magnesium, should be cautiously monitored over the first postoperative hours and days, as severe electrolytes disturbances may develop [2, 3]. During hospitalization the patient required up to 1289 mg of elemental calcium IV per day or 42.9 mg/kg of elemental calcium IV. Treatment of hypocalcemia is based on oral and intravenous calcium

replacement. Reported daily requirements of calcium in patients with severe hypocalcemia range from 6 to 16 g of elemental calcium per day [7, 10, 26–28].

The preferred calcium administration route depends on signs and symptoms severity, promptness of the onset of manifestations, and serum calcium levels [29, 30]. Oral calcium supplementation could be reasonably used in patients with mild symptoms and serum calcium concentrations greater than 7.5 mg/dL. Intravenous treatment is required for patients with calcium below this level or prolonged QTc interval on electrocardiogram and may be necessary for those cases who are currently unable to swallow or absorb oral calcium [30–32].

Intravenous calcium gluconate is preferred over calcium chloride due to its lower association with local irritation. For acute hypocalcemia management, one or two 10 mL ampoules of 10% calcium gluconate (10 mL of a 10% solution = 93 mg elemental Ca or 1 ampule) should be diluted in 50–100 mL of 5% dextrose or saline in order to infuse it over 10 minutes [10, 31, 33]. After the patient is stable, a calcium infusion is continued adding 10 ampoules of calcium gluconate (100 mL of 10% calcium gluconate) to 1000 mL normal saline or 5% dextrose making up a solution containing 1 mg/mL of elemental calcium [33]. Typical patient requirements are 0.5 to 1.5 mg/kg of elemental calcium per hour [30]. Throughout hospitalization the patient required up to 43,113.6 mg of elemental calcium orally per day (equivalent to 108 tablets of 1 g of calcium carbonate; each tablet contains approximately 400 mg of elemental calcium).

In HBS, once the hyperparathyroid state is resolved, it is important to assess serum magnesium and phosphate circulating concentrations. Significant hypomagnesaemia and hypophosphatemia may develop and perpetuate hypocalcemia [34, 35]. Even though mild hypomagnesaemia habitually is asymptomatic, chronic deficiency may be associated with diverse comorbid situations, such as arrhythmias, hypertension, and an increase in progression of kidney disease [34]. Magnesium levels after parathyroidectomy may decrease secondary to increased bone mineralization, causing a lower PTH secretion and a relative tissue specific resistance, increasing risk of severe hypocalcemia. Therefore, magnesium should be also supplemented [36].

Hypophosphatemia in HBS is probably due to an increase in bone uptake to facilitate matrix remineralization [6]. The administration of phosphate in patients with HBS is generally avoided because phosphate can precipitate with calcium, decreasing even further the circulating calcium concentration. Phosphate administration is reserved to those patients with less than 1.0 mg/dL and severe symptoms such as muscle weakness or heart failure [5]. Phosphate availability increases secondary to the intestinal action of vitamin D.

HBS duration has been defined as the time taken to remineralize the skeleton and/or cessation of additional calcium supplementation [7], evidenced by normalization of bone turnover markers, healing of radiological features of osteitis fibrosa cystica and brown tumours, and significant gain in bone mass. Due to the lack of consensus on definitions for HBS length, we take into account two of the most cited terms found in HBS related literature: bone mineral density (BMD) recovery and calcium supplementation length.

Considering HBS resolution with BMD normalization criteria, HBS lasted from 4.5 to 16 months with a median of 10 months [2, 13, 37–40] (Table 3). Calcium replenishment has been reported throughout 0.5 months to 12 months, with a median of 5.1 months. [3, 10, 13, 26, 41, 42]. Using this information, HBS lasts between 10 and 12 months. We therefore propose the term of "Protracted Hungry Bone Syndrome" to refer to those cases with a particularly long recovery taking more than one year.

In a case series of patients with HBS, parathyroidectomy improved femoral neck bone mineral density (BMD) scores from 35 to 131% in 1 year after surgery, considering basal BMD values ranging from 0.234 to 0.564 g/cm^2, and 1 year follow-up values of 0.541–0.942 g/cm^2 [43]. The significant recovery

TABLE 3

Time to reach normal bone density values	Time required of calcium replenishment	References
4.5 months	—	[2]
—	5 months	[41]
8 months	—	[37]
—	5.2 months	[26]
—	6 months	[10]
16 months	3 months	[13]
	0.5 months	[3]
12 months		[7]
(i) 8 months		[38]
(ii) 12 months		[39]
(iii) 12 months		[40]
—	12 months	[42]
Median (months): 10	Median (months): 5.1	—

from baseline pathologic findings to the value above normal found in our patient is consistent with previously reported BMD recovery (Table 3). Bone densitometries were only done at hospital admission and three years after surgery as outpatient (Table 2). The factors that contribute to this impressive BMD improvement in our case were the resolution of primary hyperparathyroidism and the high amounts of calcium and vitamin D administered for over 42 months to treat the HBS.

To the best of our knowledge, the case presented here is one of the longest HBS reported. In spite of the HBS criteria described that requires recovery of bone remineralization, we believe that our patient still has HBS, based on the fact that she continues with oral calcium and magnesium supplementation to maintain normal serum levels, normal circulating vitamin D, and normal high PTH levels.

4. Conclusion

HBS is a consequence of hyperparathyroidism following parathyroidectomy. It is an infrequent cause of hypocalcemia, hypophosphatemia, and hypomagnesemia that requires adequate therapy to avoid complications in the acute and chronic scenarios. We propose the term of "Protracted Hungry Bone Syndrome" to refer to those cases with a particularly prolonged course of recovery that takes more than one year.

Authors' Contribution

Óscar Alfredo Juárez-León and Miguel Ángel Gómez-Sámano contributed equally to this work.

Acknowledgments

Óscar Alfredo Juárez-León wants to acknowledge Gabriel Juarez and Guadalupe Leon for their support. Miguel Ángel Gómez-Sámano wants to acknowledge Luz del Carmen Abascal Olascoaga for her support.

References

[1] "The parathyroid glands and metabolic bone disease," *Ulster Medical Journal*, vol. 19, no. 1, pp. 130–131, 1950.

[2] A. R. Brasier and S. R. Nussbaum, "Hungry bone syndrome: clinical and biochemical predictors of its occurrence after parathyroid surgery," *The American Journal of Medicine*, vol. 84, no. 4, pp. 654–660, 1988.

[3] J. Latus, M. Roesel, P. Fritz et al., "Incidence of and risk factors for hungry bone syndrome in 84 patients with secondary hyperparathyroidism," *International Journal of Nephrology and Renovascular Disease*, vol. 6, pp. 131–137, 2013.

[4] M. Goldfarb, S. S. Gondek, S. M. Lim, J. C. Farra, V. Nose, and J. I. Lew, "Postoperative hungry bone syndrome in patients with secondary hyperparathyroidism of renal origin," *World Journal of Surgery*, vol. 36, no. 6, pp. 1314–1319, 2012.

[5] M. Filopanti, S. Corbetta, A. M. Barbieri, and A. Spada, "Pharmacology of the calcium sensing receptor," *Clinical Cases in Mineral and Bone Metabolism*, vol. 10, no. 3, pp. 162–165, 2013.

[6] R. Dunlay and K. Hruska, "PTH receptor coupling to phospholipase C is an alternate pathway of signal transduction in bone and kidney," *The American Journal of Physiology—Renal Fluid and Electrolyte Physiology*, vol. 258, no. 2, pp. F223–F231, 1990.

[7] J. E. Witteveen, S. van Thiel, J. A. Romijn, and N. A. Hamdy, "Hungry bone syndrome: still a challenge in the post-operative management of primary hyperparathyroidism: a systematic review of the literature," *European Journal of Endocrinology/ European Federation of Endocrine Societies*, vol. 168, no. 3, pp. R45–R53, 2013.

[8] R. Varma, Y. J. Kim, K. Garjian, and D. Barank, "Hyperparathyroidism and hungry bone syndrome revisited," *Clinical Nuclear Medicine*, vol. 39, no. 8, pp. 704–706, 2014.

[9] R. K. Crowley, M. Kilbane, T. F. J. King, M. Morrin, M. O'Keane, and M. J. McKenna, "Hungry bone syndrome and normalisation of renal phosphorus threshold after total parathyroidectomy for tertiary hyperparathyroidism in X-linked hypophosphataemia: a case report," *Journal of Medical Case Reports*, vol. 8, article 84, 2014.

[10] M. S. Rathi, R. Ajjan, and S. M. Orme, "A case of parathyroid carcinoma with severe hungry bone syndrome and review of literature," *Experimental and Clinical Endocrinology & Diabetes*, vol. 116, no. 8, pp. 487–490, 2008.

[11] M. N. Ohe, R. O. Santos, F. Hojaij et al., "Parathyroid carcinoma and hungry bone syndrome," *Arquivos Brasileiros de Endocrinologia & Metabologia*, vol. 57, no. 1, pp. 79–86, 2013.

[12] K.-M. Kim, J.-B. Park, K.-S. Bae, and S.-J. Kang, "Hungry bone syndrome after parathyroidectomy of a minimally invasive parathyroid carcinoma," *Journal of the Korean Surgical Society*, vol. 81, no. 5, pp. 344–349, 2011.

[13] S. Tachibana, S. Sato, T. Yokoi et al., "Severe hypocalcemia complicated by postsurgical hypoparathyroidism and hungry bone syndrome in a patient with primary hyperparathyroidism, Graves' disease, and acromegaly," *Internal Medicine*, vol. 51, no. 14, pp. 1869–1873, 2012.

[14] S. A. Vogelgesang and J. M. McMillin, "Hypocalcemia associated with estrogen therapy for metastatic adenocarcinoma of the prostate," *The Journal of Urology*, vol. 140, no. 5, pp. 1025–1027, 1988.

[15] D. Shoback, "Hypoparathyroidism," *The New England Journal of Medicine*, vol. 359, no. 4, pp. 391–403, 2008.

[16] J. P. Bilezikian, A. Khan, J. T. Potts Jr. et al., "Hypoparathyroidism in the adult: epidemiology, diagnosis, pathophysiology, target-organ involvement, treatment, and challenges for future research," *Journal of Bone and Mineral Research*, vol. 26, no. 10, pp. 2317–2337, 2011.

[17] I.-T. Lee, W. H.-H. Sheu, S.-T. Tu, S.-W. Kuo, and D. Pei, "Bisphosphonate pretreatment attenuates hungry bone syndrome postoperatively in subjects with primary hyperparathyroidism," *Journal of Bone and Mineral Metabolism*, vol. 24, no. 3, pp. 255–258, 2006.

[18] A. Davenport and M. P. Stearns, "Administration of pamidronate helps prevent immediate postparathyroidectomy hungry bone syndrome," *Nephrology*, vol. 12, no. 4, pp. 386–390, 2007.

[19] M. Coco, D. Glicklich, M. C. Faugere et al., "Prevention of bone loss in renal transplant recipients: a prospective, randomized trial of intravenous pamidronate," *Journal of the American Society of Nephrology*, vol. 14, no. 10, pp. 2669–2676, 2003.

[20] R. A. DeLellis, *Pathology and Genetics of Tumours of Endocrine Organs*, IARC, Lyon, France, 2004.

[21] Z. W. Baloch and V. A. LiVolsi, "Pathology of the parathyroid glands in hyperparathyroidism," *Seminars in Diagnostic Pathology*, vol. 30, no. 3, pp. 165–177, 2013.

[22] G. G. Fernandez-Ranvier, E. Khanafshar, K. Jensen et al., "Parathyroid carcinoma, atypical parathyroid adenoma, or parathyromatosis?" *Cancer*, vol. 110, no. 2, pp. 255–264, 2007.

[23] R. V. Thakker, P. J. Newey, G. V. Walls et al., "Clinical practice guidelines for multiple endocrine neoplasia type 1 (MEN1)," *The Journal of Clinical Endocrinology and Metabolism*, vol. 97, no. 9, pp. 2990–3011, 2012.

[24] P. Grzegorz, C. Jerzy, and W. Andrzej, "Primary hyperparathyroidism in patients with multiple endocrine neoplasia type 1," *International Journal of Endocrinology*, vol. 2010, Article ID 928383, 6 pages, 2010.

[25] E. Mallet, "Hypocalcemia: clinical signs and mechanisms," *Archives de Pédiatrie*, vol. 15, no. 5, pp. 642–644, 2008.

[26] H. Demirci, E. Suyani, A. Karakoc et al., "A longstanding hungry bone syndrome," *The Endocrinologist*, vol. 17, no. 1, pp. 10–12, 2007.

[27] O. Laitinen, "Bone, calcium, and hydroxyproline metabolism in hyperparathyroidism and after removal of parathyroid adenoma," *Acta Medica Scandinavica*, vol. 202, no. 1-2, pp. 39–42, 1977.

[28] S. M. Corsello, R. M. Paragliola, P. Locantore et al., "Postsurgery severe hypocalcemia in primary hyperparathyroidism preoperatively treated with zoledronic acid," *Hormones*, vol. 9, no. 4, pp. 338–342, 2010.

[29] J. F. Tohme and J. P. Bilezikian, "Hypocalcemic emergencies," *Endocrinology and Metabolism Clinics of North America*, vol. 22, no. 2, pp. 363–375, 1993.

[30] J. Fong and A. Khan, "Hypocalcemia: updates in diagnosis and management for primary care," *Canadian Family Physician Médecin de Famille Canadien*, vol. 58, no. 2, pp. 158–162, 2012.

[31] M. S. Cooper and N. J. Gittoes, "Diagnosis and management of hypocalcaemia," *The British Medical Journal*, vol. 336, no. 7656, pp. 1298–1302, 2008.

[32] J.-J. Body and R. Bouillon, "Emergencies of calcium homeostasis," *Reviews in Endocrine & Metabolic Disorders*, vol. 4, no. 2, pp. 167–175, 2003.

[33] D. Shoback, "Hypocalcemia: definition, etiology, pathogenesis, diagnosis, and management," in *Primer on the Metabolic Bone Diseases and Disorders of Mineral Metabolism*, chapter 68, John Wiley & Sons, Hoboken, NJ, USA, 2009.

[34] J. H. F. de Baaij, J. G. J. Hoenderop, and R. J. M. Bindels, "Magnesium in man: implications for health and disease," *Physiological Reviews*, vol. 95, no. 1, pp. 1–46, 2015.

[35] F. M. Hannan and R. V. Thakker, "Investigating hypocalcaemia," *British Medical Journal*, vol. 346, no. 7911, Article ID f2213, 2013.

[36] Z. S. Agus, "Hypomagnesemia," *Journal of the American Society of Nephrology*, vol. 10, no. 7, pp. 1616–1622, 1999.

[37] F. Ghanaat and J. A. Tayek, "Hungry bone syndrome: a case report and review of the literature," *Nutrition Research*, vol. 24, no. 8, pp. 633–638, 2004.

[38] K. Natsui, K. Tanaka, M. Suda et al., "Oxyphil parathyroid adenoma associated with primary hyperparathyroidism and marked post-operative hungry bone syndrome," *Internal Medicine*, vol. 35, no. 7, pp. 545–549, 1996.

[39] T. Y. Yong and J. Y. Z. Li, "Mediastinal parathyroid carcinoma presenting with severe skeletal manifestations," *Journal of Bone and Mineral Metabolism*, vol. 28, no. 5, pp. 591–594, 2010.

[40] T. França, L. Griz, J. Pinho et al., "Bisphosphonates can reduce bone hunger after parathyroidectomy in patients with primary hyperparathyroidism and osteitis fibrosa cystica," *Revista Brasileira de Reumatologia*, vol. 51, no. 2, pp. 131–137, 2011.

[41] C. Campusano and J. López, "Complete recovery of hungry bone syndrome using intravenous calcium infusion. Report of one case," *Revista Medica de Chile*, vol. 131, no. 7, pp. 779–784, 2003.

[42] G. Ghilardi and L. De Pasquale, "Hungry bone syndrome after parathyroidectomy for primary hyperthyroidism," *Surgery: Current Research*, vol. 4, article 168, 2014.

[43] T. C. P. T. de França, L. Griz, J. Pinho et al., "Bisphosphonates can reduce bone hunger after parathyroidectomy in patients with primary hyperparathyroidism and osteitis fibrosa cystica," *Revista Brasileira de Reumatologia*, vol. 51, no. 2, pp. 131–137, 2011.

55

Calcitonin-Secreting Neuroendocrine Carcinoma of Larynx with Metastasis to Thyroid

Lauren LaBryer,[1,2] Ravindranauth Sawh,[2,3] Colby McLaurin,[2,4] and R. Hal Scofield[1,2,5]

[1]*Division of Endocrinology, Department of Internal Medicine, University of Oklahoma Health Sciences Center, Oklahoma City, OK 73104, USA*
[2]*Oklahoma City VA Health Care Systems, Oklahoma City, OK 73104, USA*
[3]*Department of Pathology, University of Oklahoma Health Sciences Center, Oklahoma City, OK 73104, USA*
[4]*Department of Otolaryngology, University of Oklahoma Health Sciences Center, Oklahoma City, OK 73104, USA*
[5]*Oklahoma Medical Research Foundation, Oklahoma City, OK 73104, USA*

Correspondence should be addressed to R. Hal Scofield; scofieldh@omrf.org

Academic Editor: Osamu Isozaki

Primary neuroendocrine tumors of the larynx are rare, with moderately differentiated neuroendocrine carcinoma (MDNC) being the most frequent histologic type. We report a MDNC in a 57-year-old gentleman with an enlarging right-sided neck mass. Flexible fiberoptic exam revealed a right arytenoid lesion. Histology from excisional biopsy was concerning for medullary thyroid carcinoma (MTC) versus NET of the larynx. Immunohistochemistry was diffusely positive for calcitonin and CEA and focally positive for TTF-1. Serum calcitonin was elevated. Thyroid ultrasound was unremarkable. The patient underwent laryngectomy, thyroidectomy, and neck dissection. Pathology showed neuroendocrine carcinoma of right arytenoid with positive cervical lymph nodes. A 4 mm deposit of NET was present in right thyroid with adjacent intravascular tumor consistent with thyroidal metastasis from a primary laryngeal NET (MDNC). MDNC and MTC can be microscopically indistinguishable. Both tumors can stain positively for calcitonin and CEA. TTF-1 staining has been useful to help distinguish these tumors as it is strongly and diffusely positive in MTC, but usually negative (or only focally positive) in MDNC. We report the fourth case of primary neuroendocrine carcinoma of the larynx associated with elevated serum calcitonin level and the first such case associated with metastasis to the thyroid.

1. Introduction

Neuroendocrine tumors of the larynx are rare, accounting for ~0.6% of laryngeal neoplasms [1]. Four types of neuroendocrine tumors of the larynx have been identified by the WHO: well-differentiated neuroendocrine carcinoma (typical carcinoid), moderately differentiated neuroendocrine carcinoma (atypical carcinoid), poorly differentiated neuroendocrine carcinoma (small cell carcinoma, neuroendocrine type), and paraganglioma [2]. Moderately differentiated neuroendocrine carcinoma (MDNC) is the most frequent type of all neuroendocrine tumors of the larynx [2, 3].

MDNC of the larynx and medullary thyroid carcinoma (MTC) demonstrate similar morphological features and can be microscopically indistinguishable, particularly when presenting as metastasis [4]. Both tumors stain positively for calcitonin and CEA. TTF-1 staining has been useful to help distinguish these tumors as it is strongly and diffusely positive in medullary thyroid carcinoma, but usually negative (or only focally positive) in MDNC [2, 4]. To the best of our knowledge, only 3 cases of neuroendocrine carcinoma of the larynx with elevated serum calcitonin have been reported [5–7]. We report the fourth case of primary calcitonin-producing neuroendocrine tumor of the larynx. There are <20 cases of neuroendocrine tumors metastasizing to the thyroid [8–10]. This is the first case reported of a neuroendocrine tumor of larynx with suspected metastasis to the thyroid.

2. Case Presentation

A 57-year-old gentleman presented with 1-year history of an enlarging right-sided neck mass. The patient noted significant pain/tenderness around the mass with associated right-sided otalgia, odynophagia, and hoarseness. He was a former smoker and alcoholic with no other significant past medical history. There was no family history of cancer or endocrinopathy. Physical exam was remarkable for a 2.5 cm × 1.5 cm mass palpable in the right side of his neck. Flexible fiberoptic exam of the larynx showed a right medial arytenoid lesion of approximately 1 cm in size, mucosally covered with central ulceration. The patient underwent FNA of the palpable right neck mass. Initial pathology was concerning for metastatic carcinoma, favoring poorly differentiated adenocarcinoma of likely primary lung origin. Both PET scan and CT thorax failed to reveal significant lung pathology but rather redemonstrated the laryngeal lesion. The patient then underwent microlaryngoscopy with excisional biopsy of the right arytenoid mass en bloc with the superior aspect of the arytenoid cartilage. Immunohistochemistry was diffusely positive for calcitonin, polyclonal CEA, synaptophysin, chromogranin, and cytokeratin and focally positive for TTF-1. Pathology was concerning for medullary thyroid carcinoma versus neuroendocrine tumor of the larynx. Serum calcitonin was elevated at 157 pg/mL (ref 0–8 pg/mL). Serum CEA was normal. Thyroid ultrasound revealed no abnormalities of the thyroid. Ki-67 staining was 15%, consistent with a moderately differentiated neuroendocrine carcinoma. The case was discussed at our head and neck tumor board with recommendations for total laryngectomy and bilateral neck dissection given the diagnosis of MDNC with evidence of regional lymph node metastasis but no distant metastasis on PET scan. Total thyroidectomy was also recommended given the remaining question on pathology of MDNC versus MTC. The patient subsequently underwent total laryngectomy, bilateral neck dissection, and total thyroidectomy for suspected neuroendocrine tumor.

Pathology showed calcitonin-positive neuroendocrine carcinoma of right arytenoid with 7 positive cervical lymph nodes (5/5 positive right level IIA, 1/3 positive right level III, and 1/5 positive left level IV). A 4 mm calcitonin-positive deposit of neuroendocrine carcinoma was present in right upper pole of the thyroid with adjacent intravascular tumor consistent with thyroidal metastasis from a primary laryngeal NET (moderately differentiated neuroendocrine tumor). Initial pathology did not report C-cell hyperplasia. However, on re-review of the images, it was felt that the calcitonin stain was less than ideal. Repeat staining was conducted and it is believed that there may be bilateral C-cell hyperplasia in the thyroid in addition to the tumor focus. RET mutation testing has been requested on one of the large metastatic tumor deposits in the lymph nodes.

While serum calcitonin level remained elevated, it did significantly decrease to 35 pg/mL postoperatively. The patient subsequently underwent adjuvant radiation therapy to the operative site delivered by intensity-modulated radiation therapy (IMRT). At 2-month follow-up, serum calcitonin had increased to 55 pg/mL, but without palpable recurrence on examination. At 6-month follow-up, serum calcitonin level had increased to 320 pg/mL. CEA remained normal. The patient complained of development of multiple subcutaneous nodules on chest, back, and forearm. These nodules were palpable on exam but had no associated overlying skin changes. PET scan showed interval development of multiple FDG avid nodules in subcutaneous tissue corresponding to the palpable nodules. There was no evidence of recurrence in the neck. Fine needle aspiration of one of the subcutaneous nodules was consistent with metastatic neuroendocrine carcinoma (positive for both calcitonin and synaptophysin). The patient was discussed at a multidisciplinary tumor board and it was determined that his disease was incurable given his distant metastasis (M1 stage). He was offered palliative chemotherapy and radiation; however the patient elected for no further treatment and is currently on hospice care.

3. Discussion

Neuroendocrine tumors of the larynx are rare, with just over 500 cases recorded in the literature since initially described by Goldman et al. in 1969 [11]. MDNC is the most common of the neuroendocrine tumors of the larynx [3]. MDNC is the second most common primary laryngeal malignancy following only squamous cell carcinoma. This tumor occurs 2-3 times more commonly in men and usually in heavy smokers. The average age at presentation is 61. Clinically, patients present with hoarseness, dysphagia, throat pain, and/or a neck mass [2]. Over 90% arise in the supraglottic larynx, in vicinity of the aryepiglottic fold, arytenoid, or false vocal cord [2]. Most thyroid carcinomas, on the other hand, invade the subglottis or trachea, sparing the supraglottis [12].

Medullary carcinoma of the thyroid (MCT) is another rare tumor of neuroendocrine origin. It accounts for ~3–5% of all thyroid gland cancers [13]. MTC arises from the C-cells of the thyroid gland which secrete calcitonin. The majority of the cases are sporadic (75%), although approximately 25% of MTC is hereditary due to germline mutation of the RET protooncogene, as seen in multiple endocrine neoplasias (MEN) 2A and 2B [13]. Sporadic MTC most commonly occurs in the 4th and 6th decade of life [14] and is slightly more common in females [13]. The classic presentation is a palpable solitary thyroid nodule. As C-cells are predominately located in the superior portion of the thyroid gland, the majority of MTC localize to the upper third of a lobe [13, 14].

Histologically, MDNC of the larynx and MTC have overlapping features, including epithelioid to spindle cells with moderate amounts of pale eosinophilic cytoplasm, an architectural arrangement in cords, nests, and solid sheets, characteristic nuclei with stippled neuroendocrine-type chromatin, scattered mitoses, and prominent vascular network [4]. Separating MDNC from MTC may be challenging since both tumors also stain positively for synaptophysin, calcitonin, and CEA [2]. TTF-1 has been useful in that it is strongly and diffusely positive in MTC but usually negative or only focally weakly positive in MDNC [2, 4]. Serum CEA is almost universally elevated in MTC. However, it has not been reported to be elevated in MDNC [2, 15]. Serum calcitonin is also almost invariably elevated in MTC. While many neuroendocrine tumors have been reported to secrete calcitonin, including paragangliomas, pheochromocytomas, gastric carcinomas, small cell pulmonary tumors, VIPomas,

Table 1: Comparison of reported MDNC of larynx with hypercalcitoninemia.

	Sweeney et al. (1981) [6]	Smets et al. (1990) [5]	Insabato et al. (1993) [7]	LaBryer et al. (present study)
Age/sex	54-year-old man	55-year-old man	69-year-old man	57-year-old man
Symptomatology	Hoarseness	Hoarseness and dysphagia	Hoarseness	Hoarseness, otalgia, odynophagia
Location of tumor	Left arytenoid, 3 cervical lymph nodes	Epiglottis, 3 submandibular lymph nodes	Right arytenoid, 1 cervical lymph node	Right arytenoid, 7 cervical lymph nodes
Immunostaining	Calcitonin+ CEA+ TTF-1 – no report	Calcitonin+ CEA+ TTF-1 – no report Cytokeratin+ Chromogranin A+ NSE+	Calcitonin+ CEA – no report TTF-1 – no report Cytokeratin+ Chromogranin A+ NSE+	Calcitonin+ CEA+ TTF-1+ (focally) Cytokeratin+ Chromogranin A+ NSE – not done
Serum calcitonin	1200 ng/L (ref < 200)	3790 pg/L (ref < 100)	970 pg/mL (ref < 300)	157 pg/mL (ref < 8)
Thyroidectomy specimen	Negative for MTC	Negative for MTC	Diffuse goiter, negative for MTC	4 mm focus of tumor with adjacent intravascular tumor

CEA = carcinoembryonic antigen; TTF-1 = thyroid transcription factor-1; NSE = neuron specific enolase; MTC = medullary thyroid carcinoma.

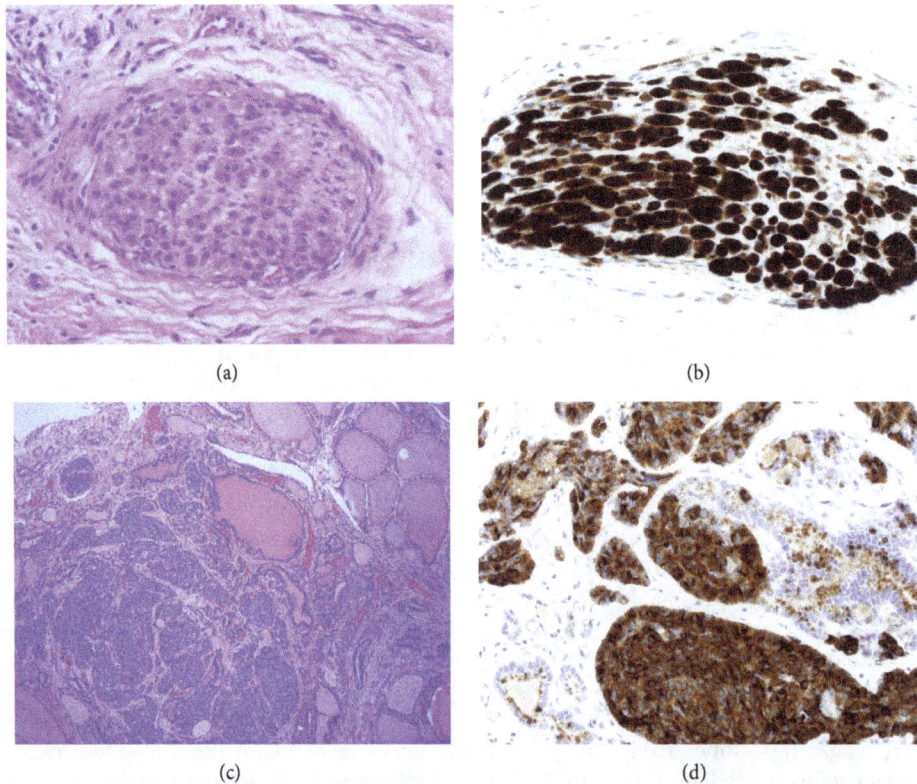

(a)

(b)

(c)

(d)

Figure 1: Tumor bed of laryngectomy and thyroid tumor, H&E stain and calcitonin immunostains. (a) H&E stain ×400: tumor bed, laryngectomy: solitary nerve twig infiltrated by plump epithelioid tumor cells. (b) Calcitonin immunostain ×400: tumor bed, laryngectomy: the infiltrating tumor cells are strongly immunoreactive for calcitonin. (c) H&E stain ×100: thyroid, right lobe nodule: 4 mm tumor nodule (left) adjacent to pink colloid-filled thyroid follicles (right). (d) Calcitonin immunostain ×400: thyroid: tumor cells are strongly reactive for calcitonin and can be seen focally invading into benign thyroid follicles.

TABLE 2: Features favoring diagnosis of MDNC of larynx.

Features favoring diagnosis of MDNC of larynx	Features disfavoring MDNC of larynx
Age & sex	Bilateral C-cell hyperplasia of thyroid*
Smoking history	
Clinical presentation of neck mass, hoarseness, and odynophagia	
Supraglottic location of primary tumor	
Normal serum CEA	
Serum calcitonin level compared to tumor volume	
Bilateral lateral cervical lymph node involvement	
Extensive lymph-vascular space invasion by tumor in lymph nodes	
Only focally positive TTF-1 staining in primary tumor and thyroid tumor	
Subcutaneous nodule metastases without overlying skin changes	
Negative amyloid stains of thyroid tumor and lymph node metastasis	

*RET mutation testing pending.

insulinomas, and enteropancreatic endocrine tumors [16], only 3 prior reports of hypercalcitoninemia have been reported in MDNC of the larynx.

Sweeney et al. [5] reported the first case of a neuroendocrine tumor of the larynx metastatic to cervical lymph nodes with an elevated serum calcitonin in 1981. This was followed by two additional patients reported by Smets et al. [6] and Insabato et al. [7]. In all three, thyroidectomy failed to disclose a primary thyroid neoplasm. Table 1 compares our patient with the previous three.

As in the previous three reports, the significantly elevated serum calcitonin level in our patient raised initial concerns for possible medullary thyroid carcinoma despite the supraglottic location of primary tumor. Additionally, in our patient, total thyroidectomy revealed 4 mm focus of tumor within the right lobe of the thyroid. Figure 1 demonstrates H&E and calcitonin stains of tumor bed of laryngectomy and the 4 mm thyroid tumor. However, (1) the relatively small size of the thyroid tumor, (2) location of tumor in right arytenoid region (uncommon for MTC metastasis), (3) predominantly lateral cervical distribution of lymph node involvement (more typical for laryngeal than thyroid primary tumor), (4) extensive lymph-vascular space invasion by tumor present in cervical lymph nodes, and particularly (5) the presence of intravascular tumor adjacent to the right thyroid lobe nodule (Figure 2) were more consistent with the diagnosis of thyroidal metastasis from a primary laryngeal neuroendocrine carcinoma. MTC is associated with amyloid deposition in surrounding tissues. Congo red stains performed on both the thyroid tumor and one of the lymph node metastases were negative for demonstrable amyloid. The degree of calcitonin elevation in MTC correlates well with tumor volume [17]. Given our patient's tumor mass, a higher level of calcitonin would be expected for MTC. While more aggressive MTC may secrete less calcitonin, these tumors tend to have significantly elevated CEA levels [17]. Our patient's normal serum CEA level and focally positive TTF-1 stain are most consistent with MDNC. TTF-1 staining pattern in both the thyroid tumor and laryngeal tumor was similar to weak nuclear staining of tumor cells. This was in contrast to the strong nuclear staining of normal thyroid

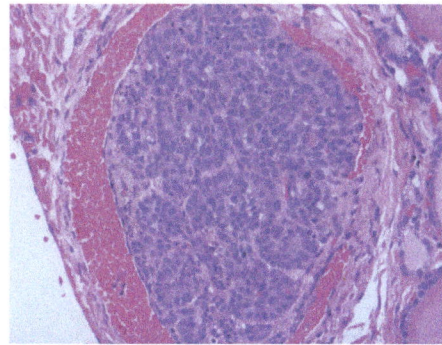

FIGURE 2: H&E stain ×400. Intravascular tumor adjacent to the right thyroid lobe nodule consistent with the diagnosis of intrathyroidal metastasis from a primary laryngeal neuroendocrine carcinoma.

epithelium (Figure 3). To our knowledge, this is the first report of a laryngeal neuroendocrine tumor metastatic to the thyroid. We must acknowledge that the bilateral C-cell hyperplasia raises the possibility that the metastasis is actually a micro-MTC. RET testing is currently pending. But, autopsy studies have shown that a substantial proportion (up to 33%) of the normal adult population could have C-cell hyperplasia [18, 19].

Cutaneous metastatic carcinoma is a rare clinical finding. The overall incidence of cutaneous metastases for all types of carcinomas has been estimated to be 5.3% [20]. Skin metastasis of MTC is very rare, with only 16 cases reported in English literature to date [21, 22]. These metastases usually present as flesh-colored nodules that are tender and most commonly located on the scalp. However, laryngeal neuroendocrine tumors are known to metastasize to the skin and subcutaneous tissue. In a review by Woodruff and Senie of 127 published cases of laryngeal MDNC, 22% had metastasis to the skin or subcutaneous sites [23]. Thus, the skin involvement is another factor favoring a diagnosis of MDNC of the larynx. Table 2 recaps the features favoring and disfavoring the diagnosis of MDNC of the larynx with metastasis to the thyroid.

(a)

(b)

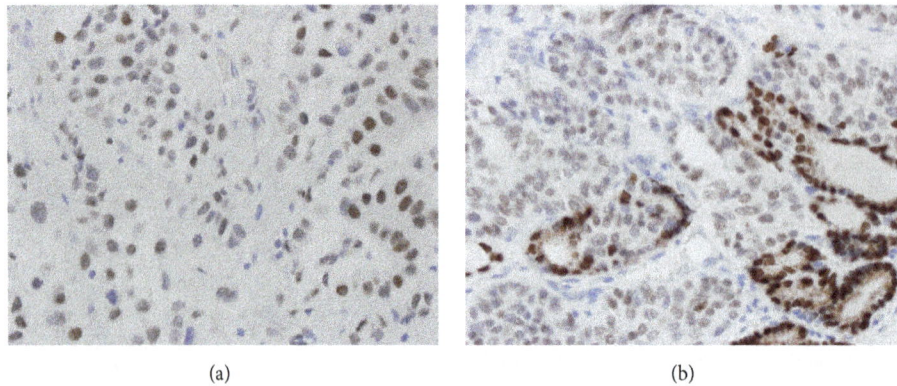

FIGURE 3: (a) Larynx, TTF-1 stain ×400: weak (light brown) nuclear staining of tumor cells. (b) Thyroid, TTF-1 stain ×400: weak (light brown) nuclear staining of tumor cells with strong (dark brown) nuclear staining of normal thyroid epithelium.

In conclusion, the differential diagnosis in a patient with head/neck cancer and hypercalcitoninemia must include not only medullary thyroid cancer, but neuroendocrine tumors as well. Due to significant overlap in features, even pathological diagnosis may be difficult. Serum CEA levels and staining pattern for TTF-1 may be useful in distinguishing these two tumor types. While skin metastases are rare, this complication is more likely to occur in MDNC than MTC.

References

[1] G. Giordano, L. Corcione, D. Giordano, T. D'Adda, L. Gnetti, and T. Ferri, "Primary moderately differentiated neuroendocrine carcinoma (atypical carcinoid) of the larynx: a case report with immunohistochemical and molecular study," *Auris Nasus Larynx*, vol. 36, no. 2, pp. 228–231, 2009.

[2] L. Barnes, J. W. Eveson, P. Reichart, and D. Sidransky, Eds., *World Health Organization Classification of Tumours, Pathology and Genetics of Head and Neck Tumours*, IARC Press, Lyon, France, 2005.

[3] A. Gillenwater, J. Lewin, D. Roberts, and A. El-Naggar, "Moderately differentiated neuroendocrine carcinoma (atypical carcinoid) of the larynx: a clinically aggressive tumor," *Laryngoscope*, vol. 115, no. 7, pp. 1191–1195, 2005.

[4] M. S. Hirsch, W. C. Faquin, and J. F. Krane, "Thyroid transcription factor-1, but not p53, is helpful in distinguishing moderately differentiated neuroendocrine carcinoma of the larynx from medullary carcinoma of the thyroid," *Modern Pathology*, vol. 17, no. 6, pp. 631–636, 2004.

[5] G. Smets, F. Warson, M.-F. Dehou et al., "Metastasizing neuroendocrine carcinoma of the larynx with calcitonin and somatostatin secretion and CEA production, resembling medullary thyroid carcinoma," *Virchows Archiv A Pathological Anatomy and Histopathology*, vol. 416, no. 6, pp. 539–543, 1990.

[6] E. C. Sweeney, L. McDonnell, and C. O'Brien, "Medullary carcinoma of the thyroid presenting as tumors of the pharynx and larynx," *Histopathology*, vol. 5, no. 3, pp. 263–275, 1981.

[7] L. Insabato, G. de Rosa, L. M. Terracciano, G. Lupoli, D. Montedoro, and C. Ravetto, "A calcitonin-producing neuroendocrine tumor of the larynx: a case report," *Tumori*, vol. 79, no. 3, pp. 227–230, 1993.

[8] E. Sivrikoz, N. C. Ozbey, B. Kaya et al., "Neuroendocrine tumors presenting with thyroid gland metastasis: a case series," *Journal of Medical Case Reports*, vol. 6, article 73, 2012.

[9] N. Tsoukalas, M. Zoulamoglou, M. Tolia, E. Bournakis, E. Ronne, and V. Barbounis, "Submerged goiter proven to be metastatic infiltration of a neuro-endocrine Merkel cell carcinoma," *SpringerPlus*, vol. 3, no. 1, pp. 1–5, 2014.

[10] G. Aydogdu, D. Ece, D. Yilmazbayhan et al., "Carcinoid tumour metastatic to the thyroid gland diagnosed by fine needle aspiration: a report of 2 cases," in *Proceedings of the 36th European Congress of Cytology*, Istanbul, Turkey, September 2011.

[11] N. C. Goldman, C. I. Hood, and G. T. Singleton, "Carcinoid of the larynx," *Archives of Otolaryngology*, vol. 90, no. 1, pp. 64–67, 1969.

[12] A. Machens, H.-J. Holzhausen, and H. Dralle, "Minimally invasive surgery for recurrent neuroendocrine carcinoma of the supraglottic larynx," *European Archives of Oto-Rhino-Laryngology*, vol. 256, no. 5, pp. 242–246, 1999.

[13] F. K. Azar, S. L. Lee, and J. E. Rosen, "Medullary thyroid cancer: an update for surgeons," *The American Surgeon*, vol. 81, no. 1, pp. 1–8, 2015.

[14] S. Leboulleux, E. Baudin, J.-P. Travagli, and M. Schlumberger, "Medullary thyroid carcinoma," *Clinical Endocrinology*, vol. 61, no. 3, pp. 299–310, 2004.

[15] M. P. Pusztaszeri, M. Bongiovanni, and W. C. Faquin, "Update on the cytologic and molecular features of medullary thyroid carcinoma," *Advances in Anatomic Pathology*, vol. 21, no. 1, pp. 26–33, 2014.

[16] S. P. A. Toledo, D. M. Lourenço Jr., M. A. Santos, M. R. Tavares, R. A. Toledo, and J. E. D. M. Correia-DeurI, "Hypercalcitoninemia is not pathognomonic of medullary thyroid carcinoma," *Clinics*, vol. 64, no. 7, pp. 699–706, 2009.

[17] R. S. Sippel, M. Kunnimalaiyaan, and H. Chen, "Current management of medullary thyroid cancer," *The Oncologist*, vol. 13, no. 5, pp. 539–547, 2008.

[18] S. Guyétant, M.-C. Rousselet, M. Durigon et al., "Sex-related C cell hyperplasia in the normal human thyroid: a quantitative autopsy study," *The Journal of Clinical Endocrinology & Metabolism*, vol. 82, no. 1, pp. 42–47, 1997.

[19] S. Guyétant, N. Josselin, F. Savagner, V. Rohmer, S. Michalak, and J.-P. Saint-André, "C-cell hyperplasia and medullary thyroid carcinoma: clinicopathological and genetic correlations in 66 consecutive patients," *Modern Pathology*, vol. 16, no. 8, pp. 756–763, 2003.

[20] G. Nava, K. Greer, J. Patterson, and K. Y. Lin, "Metastatic cutaneous breast carcinoma: a case report and review of the literature," *Canadian Journal of Plastic Surgery*, vol. 17, no. 1, pp. 25–27, 2009.

[21] P. R. Dahl, D. G. Brodland, J. R. Goellner, and I. D. Hay, "Thyroid carcinoma metastatic to the skin: a cutaneous manifestation of a widely disseminated malignancy," *Journal of the American Academy of Dermatology*, vol. 36, no. 4, pp. 531–537, 1997.

[22] A. Ghanadan, "Asynchronous cutaneous metastases of medullary thyroid carcinoma," *South Asian Journal of Cancer*, vol. 4, no. 2, pp. 103–104, 2015.

[23] J. M. Woodruff and R. T. Senie, "Atypical carcinoid tumor of the larynx. A critical review of the literature," *ORL*, vol. 53, no. 4, pp. 194–209, 1991.

56

Early Onset Primary Hyperparathyroidism Associated with a Novel Germline Mutation in *CDKN1B*

Marianne S. Elston,[1,2] Goswin Y. Meyer-Rochow,[2,3] Michael Dray,[4] Michael Swarbrick,[5] and John V. Conaglen[2]

[1]*Department of Endocrinology, Waikato Hospital, Private Bag 3200, Hamilton 3240, New Zealand*
[2]*Faculty of Medicine and Health Sciences, University of Auckland, Waikato Clinical Campus, Private Bag 3200, Hamilton 3240, New Zealand*
[3]*Department of Surgery, Waikato Hospital, Private Bag 3200, Hamilton 3240, New Zealand*
[4]*Department of Pathology, Waikato Hospital, Private Bag 3200, Hamilton 3240, New Zealand*
[5]*Department of Radiology, Waikato Hospital, Private Bag 3200, Hamilton 3240, New Zealand*

Correspondence should be addressed to Marianne S. Elston; marianne.elston@waikatodhb.health.nz

Academic Editor: Hidetoshi Ikeda

Individuals presenting with primary hyperparathyroidism (PHPT) at a young age commonly have an underlying germline gene mutation in one of the following genes: *MEN1*, *CASR*, or *CDC73*. A small number of families with primary hyperparathyroidism have been identified with germline mutations in *CDKN1B* and those patients with primary hyperparathyroidism have almost exclusively been women who present in middle age suggesting that the age of onset of PHPT in MEN4 may be later than that of MEN1. We present a case of apparently sporadic PHPT presenting in adolescence with single gland disease associated with a novel *CDKN1B* germline mutation (heterozygote for a missense mutation in exon 1 of the *CDKN1B* gene (c.378G>C) (p.E126D)). The implication from this case is that *CDKN1B* germline mutations may be associated with PHPT at an earlier age than previously thought.

1. Introduction

Primary hyperparathyroidism (PHPT) is a relatively common endocrine disorder with a prevalence of approximately 6.7/1000 in the adult population [1]. PHPT is more common in women and is typically diagnosed between the ages of 40 and 75 years [1, 2]. Most cases of PHPT are sporadic, that is, not familial or part of a syndrome. Primary hyperparathyroidism presenting at a young age is uncommon and needs to be differentiated from familial hypocalciuric hypercalcaemia (FHH) in order to avoid unnecessary surgery for the latter disorder. Young patients with PHPT are more likely to have an underlying germline mutation in genes such as *MEN1*, *CASR*, *RET*, or *CDC73* [3]. Germline mutations in cyclin-dependent kinase inhibitor 1B (*CDKN1B*) have also recently been identified to be associated with a Multiple Endocrine Neoplasia (MEN) syndrome which may include

PHPT, termed MEN4 (OMIM number 610755) [4]. In MEN1 syndrome, tumours occur in the parathyroid glands, pancreas, and pituitary and less commonly elsewhere, whereas in the very rare MEN4 syndrome a broader spectrum of organ pathology including PHPT, pituitary, and pancreatic tumours occurs, with neuroendocrine tumours also described at a variety of other sites (e.g., cervix, bronchus, and stomach) [5–9]. *CDKN1B* encodes p27(kip1), a cyclin-dependent kinase 2 inhibitor involved with the control of the cell cycle at G1 [10]. To date, only a small number of families have been identified with germline mutations in *CDKN1B* and of those cohorts, patients with primary hyperparathyroidism have almost exclusively been women who present in middle age [4–9, 11, 12]. This suggests that the age of onset of PHPT in MEN4 may be later than that of MEN1 [5]. The questions are raised as to at what age screening for PHPT in *CDKN1B* carriers should start and whether assessment of germline mutations in *CDKN1B* should be considered in patients with familial or young onset PHPT in the absence of other gene mutations predisposing to PHPT.

We report a case of primary hyperparathyroidism presenting with renal stones at age 15 associated with a novel germline heterozygous missense mutation in *CDKN1B*.

2. Case Presentation

A previously fit and well 15-year-old girl presented with recurrent renal calculi. Her serum calcium was elevated at 2.9 mmol/L (reference range (RR) 2.1–2.55 mmol/L), with a reduced phosphate of 0.63 mmol/L (RR 0.7–1.5 mmol/L) and increased PTH at 11.6 pmol/L (RR 1.3–6.8 pmol/L). Twenty-four-hour urine calcium was elevated at 16.3 mmol/d (RR 2.5–7.5 mmol/d) and urine calcium/creatinine clearance ratio was 0.025, consistent with primary hyperparathyroidism. There was no clinical or biochemical evidence of any other endocrinopathy. There was no family history of calcium or other endocrine disorders and both of her parents had a normal serum calcium level.

Initial sestamibi imaging suggested an enlarged left lower parathyroid gland but at surgery only brown fat was present in this location and four-gland exploration failed to identify a parathyroid adenoma or the left inferior parathyroid. The other parathyroid glands appeared normal. Additional imaging studies, including 4D CT scanning, repeat sestamibi, and MRI, were inconclusive. Selective venous sampling demonstrated markedly elevated levels of PTH in the thymic vein consistent with an adenoma in the anterior mediastinum. This was unable to be removed by a cervical approach and was resected via an upper hemisternotomy resulting in normalization of her calcium and parathyroid hormone status. Histology demonstrated a parathyroid adenoma surrounded by normal thymic parenchyma. Parafibromin staining of the adenoma was positive and PGP9.5 negative making a *CDC73* germline mutation unlikely.

Despite the lack of a family history of calcium disorders, given her young age genetic testing was offered to determine whether there was a predisposing germline mutation. PCR and Sanger sequencing of leukocyte DNA for the *MEN1*, *CASR* (all coding regions and flanking intronic regions), and *RET* (exons 10–16 including splice junctions) genes did not identify a mutation. However she was found to be heterozygote for a novel missense mutation in exon 1 of the *CDKN1B* gene (c.378G>C) resulting in an amino acid substitution (p.E126D). Her mother (aged 46) and maternal grandfather (aged 74 years) also carried the same missense mutation but both were normocalcemic with normal PTH levels. The immunohistochemical staining pattern of the adenoma for p27 (mouse monoclonal antibody clone SX53G8, Cell Marque) demonstrated normal nuclear staining (Figure 1).

3. Discussion

We present a case of apparently sporadic PHPT presenting in adolescence with single gland disease and a novel *CDKN1B* germline mutation.

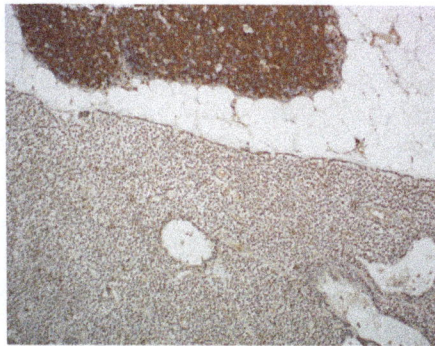

FIGURE 1: Immunohistochemical staining for p27 (original magnification ×100). Positive nuclear staining for parathyroid adenoma in lower half and positive nuclear staining for thymic lymphocytes in upper half.

Primary hyperparathyroidism is rare in children and adolescents. In a Scottish epidemiological study in which adults aged 20+ years with probable or definite PHPT were identified from community biochemistry data, based on an elevated serum calcium level with inappropriately normal or elevated PTH levels, only 1.4% of PHPT occurred in patients under the age of 30 years [1]. In that study, patients aged <20 years were excluded because of the increased likelihood of FHH; however, FHH was not excluded in those patients aged between 20 and 30 years [1]. As not all patients in that study had confirmed PHPT based on detailed clinical assessment and surgical outcomes, the true rate of definite PHPT is likely to be less than the 1.4% reported. In a large American study of surgically treated patients with PHPT only 0.86% (88/10190) of patients were aged <20 years [2]. A higher rate of 2.1% of patients <20 years with PHPT (21/1000) was found in another US study of surgically treated PHPT but the authors reported that this proportion was probably falsely increased due to referral bias [13]. As such, it is likely that if patients with FHH are excluded, <2% of cases of PHPT occur in patients <30 years. Interestingly, young patients who do develop PHPT are reported to be more liable to be symptomatic than their adult counterparts, that is, more likely to have renal stones, fatigue, depression, and weakness [13].

PHPT may be sporadic (accounting for the vast majority of cases) or occur as part of a familial syndrome associated with a germline mutation in one of the predisposing genes such as *MEN1*, *RET*, *CASR*, *CDC73*, or *CDKN1B*. Young onset PHPT has been reported to be more frequently associated with an underlying germline mutation [3]. In a recent study patients who had undergone parathyroid surgery and were aged <45 years at the time of surgery were offered germline mutation testing of *MEN1*, *RET*, *CDC73*, and *CASR* [3]. Of the 102 patients, 16 patients had familial PHPT identified either preoperatively or as part of the work-up (11 MEN1, 4 MEN2a, and 1 HPT-JT). Of the remaining 86 patients who had nonsyndromic, apparently sporadic disease 8 further patients were identified as having relevant germline mutations (4 *MEN1*, 3 *CASR*, and 1 *CDC73*). Overall, in that cohort of patients aged <45 years at the time of surgery, 24% of those tested had an underlying germline mutation identified [3].

Conversely, in a study from a different unit of surgically treated young PHPT patients aged <20 years, 18/21 had single gland disease and of the 3 patients with multigland disease only 1 was identified as having an underlying germline mutation (*MEN1*) [13]. However, it is unclear from this paper as to whether all patients underwent germline testing and which genes were assessed [13]. In a Northern Finnish cohort where testing for *MEN1*, *CDC73*, *CASR*, *CDKN1B*, and *AIP* genes was offered to all patients presenting with PHPT aged <40 years or with multigland or recurrent disease or family history of PHPT or MEN1 only 1/29 had a mutation detected (which was in *MEN1*) [14].

Guidelines from the Proceedings of the Fourth International Workshop on Asymptomatic PHPT recommend testing those who present at a young age (although the age is not specified), the presence of multigland disease, parathyroid carcinoma, or atypical adenoma, and those with a family history or evidence of syndromic disease [15]. In the absence of syndromic features the recommended guidelines for sequence of gene testing based on order of likely frequency are *MEN1*, *CASR*, *AP2S1*, *GNA11*, *CDC73*, and *CDKN1A/1B/2C* genes, *RET*, and *PTH* [15]. Screening is useful in identifying carriers who can continue to be monitored for both PHPT and other tumours associated with the syndrome for which they carry a gene mutation. Investigating family members for specific gene mutations also allows those who do not carry the germline mutation to be reassured and avoids the expense of ongoing assessment and testing of these individuals.

In our unit, due to financial constraint, in the absence of familial or syndromic features we offer genetic testing only to those with an onset of PHPT aged <30 years (*MEN1*, *RET*, *CDKN1B*, *CASR*, and *CDC73* (with germline mutation testing for the latter being guided by parafibromin staining of the parathyroid lesion [16])). Until more clinical data is available to suggest a different approach, we also limit testing for *AP2S1* and *GNA11* to those with an FHH phenotype. This practice is likely to miss some cases in which the penetrance is low or if a detailed family history is not available.

Germline *CDKN1B* mutations are associated with MEN4 [4]. To date, only a few families have been reported [4–9, 11, 12]. Based on the limited published data, the penetrance of primary hyperparathyroidism in MEN4 is assumed to be fairly high, although there remains a lack of large well-documented families to confirm this concept. Interestingly, the diagnosis of primary hyperparathyroidism in MEN4 appears to occur later than MEN1 and predominantly in women with the average age reported being 56 years compared to 20–25 years for MEN1 [5]. In our case, we have identified early onset primary hyperparathyroidism, with its associated complications (renal stones) present at age 15 associated with a germline *CDKN1B* variant but no other features of MEN4. If the E126D *CDKN1B* variant is pathogenic, it would suggest that *CDKN1B* mutations may need to be considered in young patients presenting with PHPT when other mutations are not identified. Detailed assessment of the family we describe has not yet revealed any other endocrinopathies in affected members or their untested relatives suggesting that the disease

penetrance for this particular missense mutation may be low.

The missense mutation identified in the proband (c.378G>C) has not previously been reported. The base change results in an amino acid substitution of glutamic acid to aspartic acid at position 126 (E126D) in exon 1. The region in which this change occurs is a highly conserved area in a c-Jun activation domain-binding protein-1 (JAB1) binding domain. JAB1 is important in shuttling p27 from the nucleus to the cytoplasm and in p27 degradation [17]. PolyPhen-2, a predictive software tool which predicts the possible impact of an amino acid substitution on the structure and function of a human gene [18], predicts the E126D variant as probably damaging (score 0.996, sensitivity 0.55, and specificity 0.98). In this case normal p27 immunohistochemical staining was present in the parathyroid adenoma. *CDKN1B* is somewhat atypical for a tumour suppressor gene as, rather than two "hits" being necessary for the development of disease [19], haploinsufficiency is thought to potentially be sufficient [20]. A limitation of this paper is that functional studies have not been performed to confirm that this variant is pathological; however despite extensive testing no other cause for the patient's PHPT was identified making it possible that this germline variant was a predisposing factor.

4. Conclusions

Young onset PHPT (aged <30 years) is uncommon and even in the absence of syndromic features and multigland disease an underlying germline mutation in one of the PHPT predisposing genes should be considered. This case suggests that *CDKN1B* mutations may be associated with early onset PHPT.

Acknowledgments

The authors would like to thank Associate Professor Anthony Gill for performing parafibromin staining of the parathyroid adenoma and Drs. Carolyn Tysoe and Martina Owens for performing genetic testing. Immunohistochemistry for p27 staining was funded by an Auckland University PBRF grant (awarded to Marianne S. Elston).

References

[1] N. Yu, P. T. Donnan, M. J. Murphy, and G. P. Leese, "Epidemiology of primary hyperparathyroidism in Tayside, Scotland, UK," *Clinical Endocrinology*, vol. 71, no. 4, pp. 485–493, 2009.

[2] B. S. Miller, J. Dimick, R. Wainess, and R. E. Burney, "Age- and sex-related incidence of surgically treated primary hyperparathyroidism," *World Journal of Surgery*, vol. 32, no. 5, pp. 795–799, 2008.

[3] L. F. Starker, T. Åkerström, W. D. Long et al., "Frequent germline mutations of the MEN1, CASR, and HRPT2/CDC73 genes

in young patients with clinically non-familial primary hyperparathyroidism," *Hormones & Cancer*, vol. 3, no. 1-2, pp. 44–51, 2012.

[4] N. S. Pellegata, L. Quintanilla-Martinez, H. Siggelkow et al., "Germ-line mutations in p27Kip1 cause a multiple endocrine neoplasia syndrome in rats and humans," *Proceedings of the National Academy of Sciences of the United States of America*, vol. 103, no. 42, pp. 15558–15563, 2006.

[5] F. Tonelli, F. Giudici, F. Giusti et al., "A heterozygous frameshift mutation in exon 1 of CDKN1B gene in a patient affected by MEN4 syndrome," *European Journal of Endocrinology*, vol. 171, no. 2, pp. K7–K17, 2014.

[6] M. Georgitsi, A. Raitila, A. Karhu et al., "Germline CDKN1B/p27Kip1 mutation in multiple endocrine neoplasia," *Journal of Clinical Endocrinology and Metabolism*, vol. 92, no. 8, pp. 3321–3325, 2007.

[7] S. K. Agarwal, C. M. Mateo, and S. J. Marx, "Rare germline mutations in cyclin-dependent kinase inhibitor genes in multiple endocrine neoplasia type 1 and related states," *Journal of Clinical Endocrinology and Metabolism*, vol. 94, no. 5, pp. 1826–1834, 2009.

[8] S. Molatore, I. Marinoni, M. Lee et al., "A novel germline CDKN1B mutation causing multiple endocrine tumors: clinical, genetic and functional characterization," *Human Mutation*, vol. 31, no. 11, pp. E1825–E1835, 2010.

[9] G. Occhi, D. Regazzo, G. Trivellin et al., "A novel mutation in the upstream open reading frame of the CDKN1B gene causes a MEN4 phenotyp," *PLoS Genetics*, vol. 9, no. 3, Article ID e1003350, 2013.

[10] K. Polyak, J.-Y. Kato, M. J. Solomon et al., "P27Kip1, a cyclin-Cdk inhibitor, links transforming growth factor-β and contact inhibition to cell cycle arrest," *Genes and Development*, vol. 8, no. 1, pp. 9–22, 1994.

[11] J. Costa-Guda, I. Marinoni, S. Molatore, N. S. Pellegata, and A. Arnold, "Somatic mutation and germline sequence abnormalities in CDKN1B, encoding p27Kip1, in sporadic parathyroid adenomas," *Journal of Clinical Endocrinology and Metabolism*, vol. 96, no. 4, pp. E701–E706, 2011.

[12] D. Malanga, S. De Gisi, M. Riccardi et al., "Functional characterization of a rare germline mutation in the gene encoding the cyclin-dependent kinase inhibitor p27Kip1 (CDKN1B) in a Spanish patient with multiple endocrine neoplasia-like phenotype," *European Journal of Endocrinology*, vol. 166, no. 3, pp. 551–560, 2012.

[13] I. Pashtan, R. H. Grogan, S. P. Kaplan et al., "Primary hyperparathyroidism in adolescents: the same but different," *Pediatric Surgery International*, vol. 29, no. 3, pp. 275–279, 2013.

[14] O. Vierimaa, A. Villablanca, A. Alimov et al., "Mutation analysis of MEN1, HRPT2, CASR, CDKN1B, and AIP genes in primary hyperparathyroidism patients with features of genetic predisposition," *Journal of Endocrinological Investigation*, vol. 32, no. 6, pp. 512–518, 2009.

[15] R. Eastell, M. L. Brandi, A. G. Costa, P. D'Amour, D. M. Shoback, and R. V. Thakker, "Diagnosis of asymptomatic primary hyperparathyroidism: proceedings of the fourth international workshop," *Journal of Clinical Endocrinology and Metabolism*, vol. 99, no. 10, pp. 3570–3579, 2014.

[16] A. J. Gill, A. Clarkson, O. Gimm et al., "Loss of nuclear expression of parafibromin distinguishes parathyroid carcinomas and hyperparathyroidism-jaw tumor (HPT-JT) syndrome-related adenomas from sporadic parathyroid adenomas and hyperplasias," *The American Journal of Surgical Pathology*, vol. 30, no. 9, pp. 1140–1149, 2006.

[17] K. Tomoda, Y. Kubota, and J.-Y. Kato, "Degradation of the cyclin-dependent-kinase inhibitor p27Kip1 is instigated by Jab1," *Nature*, vol. 398, no. 6723, pp. 160–165, 1999.

[18] I. A. Adzhubei, S. Schmidt, L. Peshkin et al., "A method and server for predicting damaging missense mutations," *Nature Methods*, vol. 7, no. 4, pp. 248–249, 2010.

[19] A. G. Knudson Jr., "Mutation and cancer: statistical study of retinoblastoma," *Proceedings of the National Academy of Sciences of the United States of America*, vol. 68, no. 4, pp. 820–823, 1971.

[20] M. L. Fero, E. Randel, K. E. Gurley, J. M. Roberts, and C. J. Kemp, "The murine gene p27Kip1 is haplo-insufficient for tumour suppression," *Nature*, vol. 396, no. 6707, pp. 177–180, 1998.

A Rare Presentation of Transfusional Hemochromatosis: Hypogonadotropic Hypogonadism

Rifki Ucler,[1] **Erdal Kara,**[2] **Murat Atmaca,**[1] **Sehmus Olmez,**[3] **Murat Alay,**[1] **Yaren Dirik,**[4] **and Aydin Bora**[5]

[1]*Department of Endocrinology and Metabolism, Medical Faculty, Yuzuncu Yil University, 65080 Van, Turkey*
[2]*Department of Hematology, Medical Faculty, Yuzuncu Yil University, 65080 Van, Turkey*
[3]*Department of Gastroenterology, Medical Faculty, Yuzuncu Yil University, 65080 Van, Turkey*
[4]*Department of Internal Medicine, Medical Faculty, Yuzuncu Yil University, 65080 Van, Turkey*
[5]*Department of Radiology, Medical Faculty, Yuzuncu Yil University, 65080 Van, Turkey*

Correspondence should be addressed to Rifki Ucler; rifkiucler@gmail.com

Academic Editor: Gianluca Aimaretti

Hemochromatosis is a disease caused by extraordinary iron deposition in parenchymal cells leading to cellular damage and organ dysfunction. β-thalassemia major is one of the causes of secondary hemochromatosis due to regular transfusional treatment for maintaining adequate levels of hemoglobin. Hypogonadism is one of the potential complications of hemochromatosis, usually seen in patients with a severe iron overload, and it shows an association with diabetes and cirrhosis in adult patients. We describe a patient with mild transfusional hemochromatosis due to β-thalassemia major, presenting with central hypogonadism in the absence of cirrhosis or diabetes. Our case showed an atypical presentation with hypogonadotropic hypogonadism without severe hyperferritinemia, cirrhosis, or diabetes. With this case, we aim to raise awareness of hypogonadotropic hypogonadism in patients with intensive transfused thalassemia major even if not severe hemochromatosis so that hypogonadism related complications, such as osteoporosis, anergia, weakness, sexual dysfunction, and infertility, could be more effectively managed in these patients.

1. Introduction

Hemochromatosis is a disease caused by extraordinary iron deposition in parenchymal cells leading to cellular damage and organ dysfunction. The disorder has two classifications: genetic (or primary) hemochromatosis and secondary (or acquired) hemochromatosis [1]. β-thalassemia major is one of the causes of secondary hemochromatosis with adoption of an intensive transfusional regimen to maintain adequate levels of hemoglobin. In these patients, increased absorption of iron from the gastrointestinal tract as a consequence of ineffective erythropoiesis and chronic transfusion therapy causes iron accumulation, which can be decreased by adequate iron chelation therapy [2–4]. When serum levels are elevated, iron is preliminarily deposited in the reticuloendothelial cells; however, when their capacity is saturated, the excess iron is deposited in parenchymal cells of the liver,

spleen, pancreas, and bone marrow in a crystalline form as ferritin and hemosiderin [5]. Thus, cirrhosis and diabetes are known clinical manifestations in patients with transfusional hemochromatosis. Moreover, as iron storage continues to increase, there is deposition in the skin, heart, gonads, and endocrine glands [1, 6, 7].

Hypogonadism, secondary to pituitary dysfunction, is thought to be due to iron-induced cellular damage to pituitary gonadotrophs [6–8]. Patients without hepatic cirrhosis, diabetes mellitus, or markedly elevated serum ferritin levels are unlikely to have hypogonadism [9]. In contrast to the known situation, our case presented hypogonadotropic hypogonadism without expected organ involvement in hemochromatosis. With this case, we aim to raise awareness of hypogonadotropic hypogonadism in patients with intensive transfused thalassemia major even if not severe hemochromatosis.

2. Case Report

A 26-year-old female patient was referred to our clinic with a 3 yr history of amenorrhea. Medical history showed a diagnosis of β-thalassemia major since the age of one and treatment with regular blood transfusions (once a month until the age of seven, thereafter twice a month) to maintain adequate levels of hemoglobin. She had also undergone splenectomy due to hypersplenism and massive splenomegaly at eight years old. She received iron chelation therapy with deferasirox (500 mg t.i.d.) for the last 6 years, having had irregular desferroxamine treatment before this. Her menarche was at the age of 13 years. She had a regular menstrual cycle over the next 10 years. There were no other possible causes of functional hypothalamic amenorrhea such as weight loss, eating disorders, excessive exercise, and psychosocial stress. Her blood pressure was 110/65 mmHg, she was 168 cm tall, and she weighed 53 kg. Stages of female breast and pubic hair development, according to Marshall and Tanner, were stages B-4 and P-5, respectively. There were no pathological findings except for skin hyperpigmentation on physical examination. The patient had low LH and FSH levels in association with the low estradiol levels. A bolus of 100 g synthetic LHRH was administered intravenously, and serum samples for gonadotropin measurements were drawn 0, 30, 60, 90, and 120 minutes after LHRH injection. Even after stimulation with LHRH, pituitary response was subnormal, consistent with hypogonadotropic hypogonadism. Peak levels of growth hormone and cortisol with insulin tolerance test were 11.6 ng/mL and 26.3 μg/dL, respectively. Her serum ferritin was 887 ng/mL (normal range 4.6–204) and transferrin saturation was 66.4%. Other laboratory test results were normal except for the anemia and thrombocytosis (Table 1). Abdominal magnetic resonance imaging was unremarkable except for asplenia. Magnetic resonance imaging (MRI) showed decreased signal intensity of the pituitary gland on T2-weighted images (Figure 1). With these findings, the patient was accepted as isolated gonadotropin deficiency resulting from iron deposition in the pituitary gland. Additionally, bone densitometry (BMD) showed osteopenia, with a Z score of −1.8 in the femur and −2.1 in the spine. Combined estrogen/progesterone replacement therapy and calcium/vitamin D supplementation therapy were then prescribed for hypogonadism and osteopenia.

3. Discussion

Diabetes and hepatic cirrhosis are the usual complications of hemochromatosis. The main pathophysiological mechanism leading to these diseases in haemochromatosis is thought to involve beta-cell and hepatocyte dysfunction, with iron deposition directly damaging the pancreatic islets and hepatocytes [1, 8, 10]. Despite its relatively low prevalence, hypogonadism is an important complication of hemochromatosis. Other pituitary axes are generally normal in pituitary insufficiency due to hemochromatosis, indicating an affinity of iron for gonadotropic cells [2, 6–8]. Identification of hypogonadism is very crucial, since its presence may be associated with significant long-term morbidity, including osteoporosis,

TABLE 1: Laboratory results of the case.

		Reference range
CBC parameters		
WBC ($10^3/\mu$L)	11.8	4.8–10.8
Hb (g/dL)	8.9	12–16
HCT (%)	27.3	37–47
RBC ($10^3/\mu$L)	3.05	4.2–5.4
MCV (fL)	89.5	(80–94)
MCH (g/dL)	29.4	32–36
RDW (%)	17.4	10–20
PLT ($10^3/\mu$L)	1239	130–400
Hormonal measurements		
FSH (μIU/mL)	1.39	3.03–8.08[*]
LH (μIU/mL)	0.75	2.39–6.6[*]
Estradiol (pg/mL)	<10	21–251[*]
Progesterone (mg/mL)	0.2	0–0.3[*]
GH (ng/mL)	2.53	(0–8)
Somatomedin-C (ng/mL)	151	(90–271)[**]
ACTH (pg/mL)	43.2	(0–46)
Cortisol (μg/dL)	15.9	(3.7–19.4)
Prolactin (mg/mL)	9.29	(5.2–26.5)
sT3 (pg/mL)	3.64	1.71–3.71
sT4 (ng/dL)	1.21	0.7–1.48
TSH (μIU/mL)	1.38	0.35–4.94
PTH (pg/mL)	95.7	15–68.3
25-OH-vitamin D (ng/mL)	11.9	15–60
Biochemical measurements		
Glucose (mg/dL)	81	65–95
Cre (mg/dL)	0.63	0.7–1.3
AST (U/L)	18	0–31
ALT (U/L)	15	0–31
GGT (U/L)	16.3	5–36
ALP (U/L)	245	0–270
T. bil (mg/dL)	2.8	0.2–1.2
D. bil (mg/dL)	0.44	0–0.5
T. prot (g/dL)	7.5	6.6–8.7
Alb (g/dL)	5	3.5–5.2
Ca (mg/dL)	9.7	8.5–10.5
Iron (μg/dL)	239	37–145
Ferritin (ng/mL)	887	4.6–204
TIBC (μg/dL)	357	215–480

Dynamic tests
LHRH stimulation test (0, 30, 60, 90, and 120 min):
    FSH (μIU/mL): 1.14–1.33–1.41–1.72
    LH (μIU/mL): 0.75–0.75–0.80–0.91
Insulin tolerance test:
    Peak GH: 11.6 ng/mL
    Peak cortisol: 26.3 μg/dL

[*] For follicular phase.
[**] For age 26–30.

anergia, weakness, sexual dysfunction, and infertility. Hormone replacement therapy can significantly improve the quality of life of these patients by restoring sexual function [11].

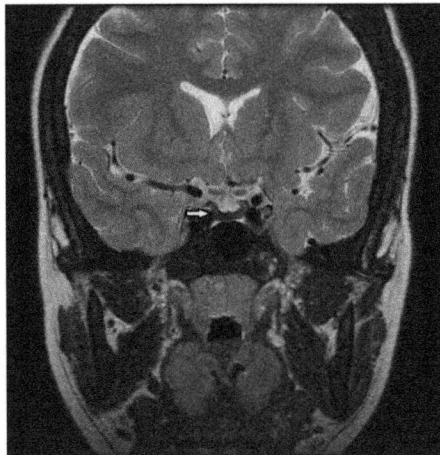

FIGURE 1: T2-weighted MRI showed decreased signal intensity of the pituitary gland, compatible with iron deposition.

MRI [6, 7]. T2-weighted MR images showed decreased signal intensity of the pituitary gland, compatible with iron deposition, which enabled us to rule out other causes in our patient (Figure 1).

In conclusion, our case has shown that hypogonadism is an important complication in transfusional hemochromatosis without overt signs of severe iron accumulation. Careful clinical, hormonal, and radiological assessment for hypogonadism should constitute an essential part of the evaluation of patients with thalassemia major even if not severe hemochromatosis. Additionally, T2-weighted MR images must be considered in evaluating such patients. Thus, management of hypogonadism related complications such as osteoporosis, anergia, weakness, sexual dysfunction, and infertility could be more effective in patients with hemochromatosis.

In our case, the endocrine profile was consistent with hypogonadotropic hypogonadism, but there was no evidence of liver damage or diabetes mellitus. This situation was exceptional for hypogonadism associated with hemochromatosis, with the absence of severe hyperferritinemia, hepatic cirrhosis, or diabetes [9]. In furtherance of this association, Lu et al. [12] reported a 23-year-old man with beta-thalassemia major and transfusional hemochromatosis, which manifested as diabetic ketoacidosis and hypogonadotropic hypogonadism. Magnetic resonance imaging of the abdomen showed decreased signal intensity in the liver, spleen, and pancreas in their case. In our case, MR imaging of abdomen was unremarkable. In addition, the pituitary gland also showed heterogeneous low signal intensity in these cases like our case.

We did not perform a liver biopsy in this case, because of The American Association for the Study of Liver Disease advisory that liver biopsy is not necessary in patients less than 40 years of age in whom liver blood tests are normal and in whom serum ferritin is less than 1000 ng/mL [13]. Additionally, genetic causes of isolated hypogonadotropic hypogonadism such as KAL1, FGFR1/FGF8, PROKR2/PROK2, CHD7, or GNRH1 gene mutations [14] have not been studied because the patient had a normal puberty and regular menstruation before the amenorrhea.

Bone changes and osteoporosis may also influence the functional prognosis and quality of life of patients with hemochromatosis [15, 16]. In our case, the reduction in BMD was consistent with osteopenia. We found low vitamin D status and high parathormone (PTH) levels in our patient. The combination of estradiol deficiency, direct iron toxicity to osteoblasts, and vitamin D deficiency probably contributed to the low bone mass in our patient.

Magnetic resonance imaging can be used as a noninvasive method to provide identification of pituitary iron overload to support clinical and laboratory data in patients with transfusional hemochromatosis. The best predictor of pituitary iron overload is the detection of decreased signal intensity of the anterior lobe of the pituitary gland on T2-weighted

References

[1] S. R. Hollán, "Transfusion-associated iron overload," *Current Opinion in Hematology*, vol. 4, no. 6, pp. 436–441, 1997.

[2] M. Toumba, A. Sergis, C. Kanaris, and N. Skordis, "Endocrine complications in patients with Thalassaemia major," *Pediatric Endocrinology Reviews*, vol. 5, no. 2, pp. 642–648, 2007.

[3] I. Stoppelli, S. Dessole, S. Milia, and C. Firinu, "Hypogonadotropic hypogonadism in a patient with thalassemia major. Case report," *Panminerva Medica*, vol. 25, no. 1, pp. 27–29, 1983.

[4] P. C. J. L. Santos, R. D. Cançado, A. C. Pereira, C. S. Chiattone, J. E. Krieger, and E. M. Guerra-Shinohara, "HJV hemochromatosis, iron overload, and hypogonadism in a Brazilian man: treatment with phlebotomy and deferasirox," *Acta Haematologica*, vol. 124, no. 4, pp. 204–205, 2010.

[5] E. S. Siegelman, D. G. Mitchell, R. Rubin et al., "Parenchymal versus reticuloendothelial iron overload in the liver: distinction with MR imaging," *Radiology*, vol. 179, no. 2, pp. 361–366, 1991.

[6] G. Sparacia, M. Midiri, P. D'Angelo, and R. Lagalla, "Magnetic resonance imaging of the pituitary gland in patients with secondary hypogonadism due to transfusional hemochromatosis," *Magnetic Resonance Materials in Physics, Biology and Medicine*, vol. 8, no. 2, pp. 87–90, 1999.

[7] G. Sparacia, A. Iaia, A. Banco, P. D'Angelo, and R. Lagalla, "Transfusional hemochromatosis: quantitative relation of MR imaging pituitary signal intensity reduction to hypogonadotropic hypogonadism," *Radiology*, vol. 215, no. 3, pp. 818–823, 2000.

[8] M. K. Kim, J. W. Lee, K. H. Baek et al., "Endocrinopathies in transfusion-associated iron overload," *Clinical Endocrinology*, vol. 78, no. 2, pp. 271–277, 2013.

[9] J. H. McDermott and C. H. Walsh, "Hypogonadism in hereditary hemochromatosis," *The Journal of Clinical Endocrinology & Metabolism*, vol. 90, no. 4, pp. 2451–2455, 2005.

[10] A. Jacobs, "Iron overload—clinical and pathologic aspects," *Seminars in Hematology*, vol. 14, no. 1, pp. 89–113, 1977.

[11] R. T. Chung, J. Misdraji, and D. V. Sahani, "Case 33-2006: a 43-year-old man with diabetes, hypogonadism, cirrhosis, arthralgias, and fatigue," *The New England Journal of Medicine*, vol. 355, no. 17, pp. 1812–1819, 2006.

[12] J. Y. Lu, C. C. Chang, H. C. Tsai, K. S. Lin, Y. M. Tsang, and K. M. Huang, "Diabetic ketoacidosis and hypogonadotropic hypogonadism in association with transfusional hemochromatosis in a man with beta-thalassemia major," *Journal of the Formosan Medical Association*, vol. 100, no. 7, pp. 492–496, 2001.

[13] A. S. Tavill, "Diagnosis and management of hemochromatosis," *Hepatology*, vol. 33, no. 5, pp. 1321–1328, 2001.

[14] K. Beate, N. Joseph, D. R. Nicolas, and K. Wolfram, "Genetics of isolated hypogonadotropic hypogonadism: role of GnRH receptor and other genes," *International Journal of Endocrinology*, vol. 2012, Article ID 147893, 9 pages, 2012.

[15] N. G. Angelopoulos, A. K. Goula, G. Papanikolaou, and G. Tolis, "Osteoporosis in HFE2 juvenile hemochromatosis. A case report and review of the literature," *Osteoporosis International*, vol. 17, no. 1, pp. 150–155, 2006.

[16] P. Guggenbuhl, Y. Deugnier, J. F. Boisdet et al., "Bone mineral density in men with genetic hemochromatosis and HFE gene mutation," *Osteoporosis International*, vol. 16, no. 12, pp. 1809–1814, 2005.

Permissions

All chapters in this book were first published in CRE, by Hindawi Publishing Corporation; hereby published with permission under the Creative Commons Attribution License or equivalent. Every chapter published in this book has been scrutinized by our experts. Their significance has been extensively debated. The topics covered herein carry significant findings which will fuel the growth of the discipline. They may even be implemented as practical applications or may be referred to as a beginning point for another development.

The contributors of this book come from diverse backgrounds, making this book a truly international effort. This book will bring forth new frontiers with its revolutionizing research information and detailed analysis of the nascent developments around the world.

We would like to thank all the contributing authors for lending their expertise to make the book truly unique. They have played a crucial role in the development of this book. Without their invaluable contributions this book wouldn't have been possible. They have made vital efforts to compile up to date information on the varied aspects of this subject to make this book a valuable addition to the collection of many professionals and students.

This book was conceptualized with the vision of imparting up-to-date information and advanced data in this field. To ensure the same, a matchless editorial board was set up. Every individual on the board went through rigorous rounds of assessment to prove their worth. After which they invested a large part of their time researching and compiling the most relevant data for our readers.

The editorial board has been involved in producing this book since its inception. They have spent rigorous hours researching and exploring the diverse topics which have resulted in the successful publishing of this book. They have passed on their knowledge of decades through this book. To expedite this challenging task, the publisher supported the team at every step. A small team of assistant editors was also appointed to further simplify the editing procedure and attain best results for the readers.

Apart from the editorial board, the designing team has also invested a significant amount of their time in understanding the subject and creating the most relevant covers. They scrutinized every image to scout for the most suitable representation of the subject and create an appropriate cover for the book.

The publishing team has been an ardent support to the editorial, designing and production team. Their endless efforts to recruit the best for this project, has resulted in the accomplishment of this book. They are a veteran in the field of academics and their pool of knowledge is as vast as their experience in printing. Their expertise and guidance has proved useful at every step. Their uncompromising quality standards have made this book an exceptional effort. Their encouragement from time to time has been an inspiration for everyone.

The publisher and the editorial board hope that this book will prove to be a valuable piece of knowledge for researchers, students, practitioners and scholars across the globe.

List of Contributors

Cem Sahin and Mustafa Levent
Department of Internal Medicine, School of Medicine, Mugla Sıtkı Kocman University, Orhaniye Mahallesi, İsmet Catak Caddesi, 48000 Mugla, Turkey

Gulhan Akbaba
Department of Endocrinology, School of Medicine, Mugla Sıtkı Kocman University, Orhaniye Mahallesi, İsmet Catak Caddesi, 48000 Mugla, Turkey

Bilge Kara
Department of Psychiatry, School of Medicine, Mugla Sıtkı Kocman University, Orhaniye Mahallesi, Ismet Catak Caddesi, 48000 Mugla, Turkey

Emine Nese Yeniceri and Betul Battaloglu Inanc
Department of Family Medicine, Faculty of Medicine, Mugla Sıtkı Kocman University, Orhaniye Mahallesi, Ismet Catak Caddesi, 48000 Mugla, Turkey

Shraddha Narechania, Amrita Bath, Laleh Ghassemi, Chetan Lokhande, Abdo Haddad, AliMir Yousuf, Jessica Marquard and K. V. Gopalakrishna
Internal Medicine Residency, Fairview Hospital, Cleveland, OH 44111, USA

Chetan Lokhande
Anesthesia Department, Fairview Hospital, Cleveland, OH 44111, USA

Abdo Haddad
Cleveland Clinic Taussig Cancer Institute, Fairview Hospital, Cleveland, OH 44111, USA

Ali Mir Yousuf
Strongsville Family Health and Surgery Center, 16761 Southpark Center, Strongsville, OH 44136, USA

Jessica Marquard
Genomic Medicine Institute, 9500 Euclid Avenue NE5, Cleveland, OH 44195, USA

Anahita Shahrrava, Sunnan Moinuddin and Prajwal Boddu
Department of Internal Medicine, Advocate Illinois Masonic Medical Center, 836 West Wellington Avenue, Chicago, IL 60657, USA

Rohan Shah
Department of Radiology, Advocate Illinois Masonic Medical Center, 836 West Wellington Avenue, Chicago, IL 60657, USA

Resmi Premji, Nira Roopnarinesingh, Joshua Cohen and Sabyasachi Sen
Division of Endocrinology, Diabetes and Metabolism, George Washington University, Washington, DC 20037, USA

Giampaolo Papi
Endocrinology Unit of the Northern Area, Azienda USL di Modena, Modena, Italy
Unit of Endocrinology, Universit`a Cattolica del Sacro Cuore and Fondazione Policlinico Universitario Agostino Gemelli, Rome, Italy

Carlo Di Donato
Endocrinology Unit of the Northern Area, Azienda USL di Modena, Modena, Italy
Department of Internal Medicine, Azienda USL Modena, Modena, Italy

Rosa Maria Paragliola, Alfredo Pontecorvi and Salvatore Maria Corsello
Unit of Endocrinology, Universitá Cattolica del Sacro Cuore and Fondazione Policlinico Universitario Agostino Gemelli, Rome, Italy

Paola Concolino
Laboratory of Molecular Biology, Institute of Biochemistry and Clinical Biochemistry, Catholic University of Sacred Heart, Rome, Italy

Maria Susana Mallea-Gil and Carolina Ballarino
Servicio de Endocrinologıa, Hospital Militar Central, 726 Luis María Campos Avenue, 1425 Buenos Aires, Argentina

Ignacio Bernabeu and Lourdes Loidi
Endocrinology Division and Fundacion Publica Galega de Medicina Xenomica (Unidad de Medicina Molecular), Complejo Hospitalario Universitario de Santiago de Compostela, Universidad de Santiago de Compostela, Travesia Choupana s/n, Santiago de Compostela, 15706 La Coru ña, Spain

Adriana Spiraquis
Servicio de Gastroenterologıa, Hospital Militar Central, 726 Luis María Campos Avenue, 1425 Buenos Aires, Argentina

Alejandra Avangina
Departamento de Anatomıa Patologica, Hospital de Clínicas, Universidad de Buenos Aires, 2351 C´ordoba Avenue, 1120 Buenos Aires, Argentina

Umal Azmat and Fadi Nabhan
Division of Endocrinology, Diabetes and Metabolism, The Ohio State University, Columbus, OH, USA

David Liebner
Division of Medical Oncology and Department of Biomedical Informatics, The Ohio State University, Columbus, OH, USA

Amy Joehlin-Price
Department of Pathology, The Ohio State University, Columbus, OH, USA

Amit Agrawal
Department of Otolaryngology, Head and Neck Surgery, The Ohio State University, Columbus, OH, USA

Ann Miller
Department of Medicine, University of Maryland Medical Center, Baltimore, MD, USA

Lauren K. Brooks, Silpa Poola-Kella and Rana Malek
Department of Medicine, Division of Endocrinology, Diabetes and Nutrition, University of Maryland Medical Center, Baltimore, MD, USA

Kentaro Fujii, Kazutoshi Miyashita, Isao Kurihara, Ken Hiratsuka, Seiji Sato, Kenichi Yokota, Sakiko Kobayashi and Hiroshi Itoh
Department of Internal Medicine, School of Medicine, Keio University, 35 Shinanomachi, Shinjuku-ku, Tokyo 160-8582, Japan

Hirotaka Shibata
Department of Endocrinology, Metabolism, Rheumatology and Nephrology, Faculty of Medicine, Oita University, 700 Dannoharu, Oita 870-1192, Japan

Adele Latina, Elena Castellano, Micaela Pellegrino and Giorgio Borretta
Division of Endocrinology, Diabetology and Metabolism, Santa Croce e Carle Hospital, Via M. Coppino 26, 12100 Cuneo, Italy

Massimo Terzolo, Anna Pia and Giuseppe Reimondo
Internal Medicine 1, Department of Clinical and Biological Sciences, University of Turin, San Luigi Gonzaga Hospital, Regione Gonzole 10, Orbassano, 10043 Turin, Italy

Suheyla Gorar
Department of Endocrinology and Metabolism, Antalya Education and Research Hospital, 07100 Antalya, Turkey

Doga Turkkahraman
Department of Pediatric Endocrinology, Antalya Education and Research Hospital, 07100 Antalya, Turkey

Kanay Yararbas
Department of Medical Genetics, Acibadem Mehmet Ali Aydinlar University, 34752 Istanbul, Turkey

Ana Misir Krpan
Department of Oncology, University Hospital Center Zagreb, Kispaticeva 12, 10000 Zagreb, Croatia

Tina Dusek and Darko Kastelan
Zagreb University School of Medicine, Department of Endocrinology, University Hospital Center Zagreb, Kispaticeva 12, 10000 Zagreb, Croatia

Mirsala Solak and Ivana Kraljevic
Department of Endocrinology, University Hospital Center Zagreb, Kispaticeva 12, 10000 Za greb, Croatia

Vesna Bisof
Osijek University School of Medicine, Department of Oncology, University Hospital Center Zagreb, Kispaticeva 12, 10000 Zagreb, Croatia

David Ozretic
Department of Radiology, University Hospital Center Zagreb, Kispaticeva 12, 10000 Zagreb, Croatia

Cheng Cheng, Jose Kuzhively and Sanford Baim
Division of Endocrinology and Metabolism, Rush University Medical Center, Chicago, IL, USA

Kelly Wentworth, Alyssa Hsing, Ashley Urrutia and Edward C. Hsiao
Division of Endocrinology, Diabetes, and Metabolism andb The Institute for Human Genetics, Department of Medicine, University of California, San Francisco, San Francisco, CA 94143, USA

Yan Zhu and Murat Bastepe
Endocrine Unit, Massachusetts General Hospital and Harvard Medical School, Boston, MA 02114, USA

Andrew E. Horvai
Departments of Pathology and Laboratory Medicine, University of California, San Francisco, San Francisco, CA 94143, USA

Konstantinos Segkos and Fadi Nabhan
Endocrinology, Diabetes and Metabolism, The Ohio State University Wexner Medical Center, 5th Floor McCampbell Hall, 1581 Dodd Drive, Columbus, OH 43210, USA

Carl Schmidt
Surgical Oncology, The Ohio State University Wexner Medical Center, N-924 Doan Hall, 410W. 10th Avenue, Columbus, OH 43210, USA

C. A. Simões, M. R. Tavares, N. M. M. Andrade, T. M. Uehara, R. A. Dedivitis, and C. R. Cernea
Department of Head and Neck Surgery, Hospital das Cl´inicas, School of Medicine, University of São Paulo, São Paulo, SP, Brazil

Anukrati Shukla, Syeda Alqadri, Premkumar Nattanmai and Christopher R. Newey
Department of Neurology, University of Missouri, Columbia, MO, USA

Ashley Ausmus
Department of Pharmacy, University of Missouri, Columbia, MO, USA

Robert Bell
Department of Neurosurgery, University of Missouri, Columbia, MO, USA

Fatma Dilek Dellal and Gulfem Kaya
Department of Endocrinology and Metabolism, Ataturk Training and Research Hospital, 06800 Ankara, Turkey

Didem Ozdemir, Cevdet Aydin, Reyhan Ersoy and Bekir Cakir
Department of Endocrinology and Metabolism, Faculty of Medicine, Yildirim Beyazit University, 06800 Ankara, Turkey

Yan Ren, Xi Li, Haoming Tian, Zhenmei An and Tao Chen
Department of Endocrinology and Metabolism, West China Hospital of Sichuan University, Chengdu, China

Sihao Yang
Department of Endocrinology and Metabolism, West China Hospital of Sichuan University, Chengdu, China Department of Chinese Traditional Medicine, The Second People's Hospital of Yibin, Yibin, China

Thomas Dacruz
University Hospital of Wales, Cardiff, UK

Atul Kalhan
Department of Diabetes and Endocrinology, Royal Glamorgan Hospital, Mid Glamorgan CF72 8XR, UK

Majid Rashid and Kofi Obuobie
Royal Gwent Hospital, Newport, UK

Gerson Geovany Andino-Ríos, Lesly Portocarrero-Ortiz, Carlos Rojas-Guerrero and Alejandro Terrones-Lozano
Neuroendocrinology Department, Instituto Nacional de Neurologíay Neurocirugía Manuel Velasco Suárez, Ciudad de Mèxico, Mexico

Alma Ortiz-Plata
Experimental Neuropathology Laboratory, Instituto Nacional de Neurologíay Neurocirugía Manuel Velasco Súarez, Ciudad de México, Mexico

Alfredo Adolfo Reza-Albarrán
Endocrinology and Metabolism Department, Instituto Nacional de Ciencias Mèdicasy Nutrición Salvador Zubirán, Ciudad de Mèxico, Mexico

Xiao Lin, Xiaoyu Miao, Pengli Zhu, and Fan Lin
Department of VIP, Fujian Provincial Hospital, Fujian Medical University, 134 East Street, Fuzhou 350001, China

Gil A. Geva
The Hebrew University Hadassah Medical School, Hadassah-Hebrew University Medical Center, Jerusalem, Israel

David J. Gross
Endocrinology and Metabolism Service, Hadassah-Hebrew University Medical Center, Jerusalem, Israel

Haggi Mazeh
Department of General Surgery, Hadassah-Hebrew University Medical Center, Jerusalem, Israel

Karine Atlan
Department of Pathology, Hadassah-Hebrew University Medical Center, Jerusalem, Israel

Iddo Z. Ben-Dov
Nephrology and Hypertension Services, Hadassah-Hebrew University Medical Center, Jerusalem, Israel

Matan Fischer
Department of Internal Medicine, Hadassah-Hebrew University Medical Center, Jerusalem, Israel

Sebahattin Destek
Department of General Surgery, Bezmialem Vakıf University School of Medicine, Istanbul, Turkey

Vahit Onur Gul
General Surgery Department, Edremit Government Hospital, Edremit, 10300 Balikesir, Turkey

Serkan Ahioglu
Biochemistry Department, Edremit State Hospital, Edremit, 10300 Balikesir, Turkey

Kursat Rahmi Serin
General Surgery Department, Liv Hospital, Ulus, Istanbul, Turkey

Vishnu Garla, Karthik Kovvuru, Shradha Ahuja, Venkatataman Palabindala, Bharat Malhotra and Sohail Abdul Salim
Department of Internal Medicine, University of Mississippi Medical Center, Jackson, MS, USA

Neil Tolley
Department of Surgery, Hammersmith Hospital, Imperial College Healthcare NHS Trust, London, UK

Darren K. Patten
Department of Surgery, Hammersmith Hospital, Imperial College Healthcare NHS Trust, London, UK
Department of Surgery and Cancer, The Imperial Centre for Translational and Experimental Medicine, Imperial College London, Hammersmith Campus, London, UK

Alia Ahmed
Department of General Medicine, Wexham Park Hospital, NHS Frimley Health Foundation Trust, London, UK

Owain Greaves
Department of Life Sciences, Imperial College London, London, UK

Roberto Dina and Rashpal Flora
Department of Histopathology, Hammersmith Hospital, Imperial College Healthcare NHS Trust, London, UK

Regina Belokovskaya
Internal Medicine Department, Mount Sinai St. Luke's and Roosevelt Hospitals, Icahn School of Medicine at Mount Sinai, 1111 Amsterdam Avenue, New York, NY 10025, USA

Alice C. Levine
Division of Endocrinology, Metabolism and Bone Diseases, Icahn School of Medicine at Mount Sinai, 1 Gustave L. Levy Place, P.O. Box 1055, New York, NY 10029, USA

Eon Ju Jeon, Ho Sang Shon and Eui Dal Jung
Department of Internal Medicine, Catholic University of Daegu, School of Medicine, Daegu 42472, Republic of Korea

Stefano Benedini, Giorgia Grassi, Carmen Aresta and Livio Luzi
Department of Biomedical Sciences for Health, Universitá degli Studi di Milano, Milan, Italy

Antonietta Tufano
Endocrinology Unit, IRCCS Policlinico San Donato, San Donato Milanese, Italy

Luca Fabio Carmignani
Urology Department, IRCCS Policlinico San Donato, San Donato Milanese, Italy

Barbara Rubino
Pathology Department, IRCCS Policlinico San Donato, San Donato Milanese, Italy

Sabrina Corbetta
Endocrinology Service, Department of Biomedical Sciences for Health, University of Milan, IRCCS Istituto Ortopedico Galeazzi, Milan, Italy

Jien Shim and Run Yu
Division of Endocrinology, Diabetes, and Metabolism, Department of Medicine, University of California, Los Angeles, David Geffen School of Medicine, Los Angeles, CA 90095, USA

Jianyu Rao
Department of Pathology and Laboratory Medicine, University of California, Los Angeles, David Geffen School of Medicine, Los Angeles, CA 90095, USA

R. H. Bishay and R. C. Y. Chen
Department of Endocrinology and Metabolism, Concord Repatriation General Hospital, Concord, NSW2139, Australia
Concord Clinical School, Sydney Medical School, University of Sydney, Sydney, NSW2005, Australia

Ashley Schaffer, Vidya Puthenpura and Ian Marshall
Department of Pediatrics, Rutgers-RobertWood Johnson Medical School, 89 French Street, New Brunswick, NJ 08901, USA

Ramesh Sharma Poudel and Sushma Bhandari
Hospital Pharmacy, Chitwan Medical College Teaching Hospital, Chitwan, Nepal

Shakti Shrestha
Department of Pharmacy, Shree Medical and Technical College, Chitwan, Nepal

Rano Mal Piryani and Shital Adhikari
Department of Internal Medicine, Chitwan Medical College Teaching Hospital, Chitwan, Nepal

Habib G. Zalzal and Jeffson Chung
Department of Otolaryngology-Head and Neck Surgery, West Virginia University School of Medicine, Morgantown, WV, USA

Jessica A. Perini
Section of Endocrinology, Department of Internal Medicine, West Virginia University School of Medicine, Morgantown, WV, USA

Tansit Saengkaew, Taninee Sahakitrungruang, Suttipong Wacharasindhu and Vichit Supornsilchai
Division of Endocrinology, Department of Pediatrics, Faculty of Medicine, Chulalongkorn University, Bangkok 10330, Thailand

Hui Jin, Huanhuan Yan, Miao Zheng, Chaojie Wu and Jun Liu
Shanghai General Hospital of Nanjing Medical University, Shanghai 201620, China
Department of Breast-Thyroid-Vascular Surgery, Shanghai General Hospital, Shanghai Jiaotong University, Shanghai 201620, China

Huamei Tang
Pathological Center of School of Medicine, Shanghai Jiaotong University, Shanghai 201620, China

Anthony Liberatore and Ronald M. Lechan
Department of Medicine, Division of Endocrinology, Diabetes and Metabolism, Tupper Research Institute, Tufts Medical Center, Boston, MA 02111, USA

Haruhiko Yamazaki, Hiroyuki Iwasaki, Toshinari Yamashita, Tatsuya Yoshida, Nobuyasu Suganuma and Takashi Yamanaka
Department of Breast and Endocrine Surgery, Kanagawa Cancer Center, Yokohama, Japan

Katsuhiko Masudo
Department of Breast andThyroid Surgery, Yokohama City University Medical Center, Yokohama, Japan

Hirotaka Nakayama, Kaori Kohagura, Yasushi Rino and Munetaka Masuda
Department of Surgery, Yokohama City University School of Medicine, Yokohama, Japan

Leslee N. Matheny, Shubhada M. Jagasia and Shichun Bao
Vanderbilt University Medical Center, Division of Endocrinology, Department of Medicine, Vanderbilt University, 1215 21st Avenue South, Nashville, TN 37232, USA

Sudipa Sarkar
Johns Hopkins University School of Medicine, Division of Endocrinology, Diabetes and Metabolism, 5501 Hopkins Bayview Circle, Baltimore, MD 21224, USA

Hanyuan Shi
Vanderbilt University Medical Center, Department of Surgery, Vanderbilt University, 1161 21st Avenue South, Nashville, TN 37232, USA

Jiun-Ruey Hu
Vanderbilt University School of Medicine, 2215 Garland Ave, Nashville, TN 37232, USA

Hannah Harmsen and Ty W. Abel
Vanderbilt University Medical Center, Department of Pathology, Microbiology and Immunology, 1161 21st Avenue South, Nashville, TN 37232, USA

Avneet K. Singh
Department of Medicine, The Robert Larner, M.D. College of Medicine at The University of Vermont, Burlington, VT, USA

Adina A. Bodolan
Department of Pathology and Laboratory Medicine, The Robert Larner, M.D. College of Medicine at The University of Vermont, Burlington, VT, USA

Matthew P. Gilbert
Division of Endocrinology and Diabetes, The Robert Larner, M.D. College of Medicine atThe University of Vermont, Burlington, VT, USA

Ishita Prakash, Eric Sixtus Nylen and Sabyasachi Sen
Department of Medicine, Division of Endocrinology and Metabolism, Medical Faculty Associates, The George Washington University, Washington, DC, USA

Katsushi Takeda, Ryosuke Kimura, Asami Okamoto, Kumiko Watanabe and Sachie Yasui
Department of Endocrinology andMetabolism, Nagoya CityWestMedical Center, 1-1-1 Hirate-cho, Kita-ku, Nagoya 462-8508, Japan

Nobuhiro Nishigaki
Department of Gastroenterology, Nagoya CityWest Medical Center, 1-1-1 Hirate-cho, Kita-ku, Nagoya 462-8508, Japan

Shinya Sato
Department of Experimental Pathology and Tumor Biology, Nagoya City University Graduate School of Medical Sciences, 1 Kawasumi, Mizuho-cho, Mizuho-ku, Nagoya 467-8601, Japan

Adelaide Moutinho and Sandra Tavares
Department of Internal Medicine, Hospital de Chaves, Centro Hospitalar de Trás-os-Montes e Alto Douro, Chaves, Portugal

Rosa Carvalho
Department of Internal Medicine, Hospital de Braga, Braga, Portugal

Rita Ferreira Reis
Department of Internal Medicine, Hospital de Lamego, Centro Hospitalar de Trás-os-Montes e Alto Douro, Lamego, Portugal

Ioannis Kyrgios, Eleni P. Kotanidou, Eleni Litou, Konstantina Mouzaki, Aggeliki Kleisarchaki and Assimina Galli-Tsinopoulou
Unit of Pediatric Endocrinology, 4th Department of Pediatrics, Medical School, Faculty of Health Sciences, Aristotle University of Thessaloniki, Thessaloniki, Greece

Filippa Pritsini and Georgios A. Kanakis
Unit of Pediatric Endocrinology, 4th Department of Pediatrics, Medical School, Faculty of Health Sciences, Aristotle University of Thessaloniki, Thessaloniki, Greece
Unit of Reproductive Endocrinology, 1st Department of Obstetrics and Gynecology, Medical School, Faculty of Health Sciences, Aristotle University of Thessaloniki, Thessaloniki, Greece

Dimitrios G. Goulis
Unit of Reproductive Endocrinology, 1st Department of Obstetrics and Gynecology, Medical School, Faculty of Health Sciences, Aristotle University ofThessaloniki, Thessaloniki, Greece

Andreas G.Moraitis
CorceptTherapeutics, 149 Commonwealth Drive, Menlo Park, CA 94025, USA

Richard J. Auchus
Division of Metabolism, Diabetes, and Endocrinology, Department of Internal Medicine, University of Michigan, 1150West Medical Center Drive, Ann Arbor, MI 48109, USA

Henrique GomesMendes
Federal University of Minas Gerais (UFMG), Belo Horizonte, MG, Brazil

Gustavo Cancela e Penna
Federal University of Minas Gerais (UFMG), Belo Horizonte, MG, Brazil
Federal University of Rio de Janeiro, Rio de Janeiro, RJ, Brazil

Division of Endocrinology, Hospital Mater Dei, Belo Horizonte, MG, Brazil

Cynthia Koeppel Berenstein
Federal University of Minas Gerais (UFMG), Belo Horizonte, MG, Brazil
Division of Pathology, Instituto Roberto Alvarenga, Belo Horizonte, MG, Brazil

Adele O. Kraft
Department of Pathology, Virginia Commonwealth University, Richmond, VA, USA

Bernardo Fonseca
Division of Radiology, Spectra Institute, Belo Horizonte, MG, Brazil

Wagner José Martorina
Division of Endocrinology, Hospital Biocor, Belo Horizonte, MG, Brazil

Andreise Laurian N. R. de Souza
Division of Endocrinology, Hospital da Baleia, Belo Horizonte, MG, Brazil

Gustavo Meyer deMoraes
Division of Head and Neck Surgery, Hospital das Clinicas, UFMG, Belo Horizonte, MG, Brazil

Kamilla Maria Araújo Brandão Rajão
Division of Endocrinology, Hospital das Clinicas, UFMG, Belo Horizonte, MG, Brazil

Bárbara Érika Caldeira Araújo Sousa
Division of Endocrinology, Hospital Mario Pena, Belo Horizonte, MG, Brazil

Zeina C. Hannoush, Juan D. Palacios and Sabina Casula
Division of Endocrinology, Diabetes and Metabolism, Department of Medicine, University of Miami Miller School of Medicine, Miami, FL 33136, USA

Russ A. Kuker
Division of Nuclear Medicine, Department of Radiology, University of Miami Miller School of Medicine, Miami, FL 33136, USA

Roberto Cesareo and Alessandro Casini
Department of Internal Medicine, "S. M. Goretti" Hospital, Latina, Italy

Anda Mihaela Naciu, Silvia Manfrini, Gaia Tabacco, Angelo Lauria Pantano and Andrea Palermo
Department of Endocrinology, University Campus Bio-Medico, Rome, Italy

Valerio Pasqualini, Giuseppe Pelle and Roberto Cianni
Department of Radiology, "S. M. Goretti" Hospital, Latina, Italy
Yuka Muraoka and Hiroshi Arima Department of Endocrinology and Diabetes, Nagoya University Graduate School of Medicine, Nagoya 466-8550, Japan

Shintaro Iwama
Department of Endocrinology and Diabetes, Nagoya University Graduate School of Medicine, Nagoya 466-8550, Japan
Research Center of Health, Physical Fitness and Sports, Nagoya University, Nagoya 464-8601, Japan

Hye In Kang and Chan Yong Seong
Department of Surgery, Seoul National University Hospital and College of Medicine, 101 Daehak-ro, Jongno-gu, Seoul 110-744, Republic of Korea

Jin Wook Yi, Su-jin Kim and Kyu Eun Lee
Department of Surgery, Seoul National University Hospital and College of Medicine, 101 Daehak-ro, Jongno-gu, Seoul 110-744, Republic of Korea
Cancer Research Institute, Seoul National University College ofMedicine, 101 Daehak-ro, Jongno-gu, Seoul 110-744, Republic of Korea

Young Jun Chai
Department of Surgery, Seoul National University Boramae Medical Center, 20 Boramae-ro 5-gil, Dongjak-gu, Seoul 156-70, Republic of Korea

June Young Choi
Department of Surgery, Seoul National University Bundang Hospital, Seoul National University College of Medicine, Seongnam, Republic of Korea

Moon-Woo Seong and Sung Sup Park
Department of Laboratory Medicine, Seoul National University Hospital and College of Medicine, 101 Daehak-ro, Jongno-gu, Seoul 110-744, Republic of Korea

Andrew J. Spiro
Department of Internal Medicine, Walter Reed National Military Medical Center, Bethesda, MD, USA

Katherine N. Vu and Alicia Lynn Warnock
Department of Endocrinology, Metabolism and Diabetes, Walter Reed National Military Medical Center, Bethesda, MD, USA
Uniformed Services University of Health Sciences, Bethesda, MD, USA

KaeMorishita, Chika Kyo, Takako Yonemoto, Rieko Kosugi, Tatsuo Ogawa and Tatsuhide Inoue
Center for Diabetes, Endocrinology and Metabolism, Shizuoka General Hospital, No. 4-27-1, Kita-Ando, Aoi-ku, Shizuoka, Shizuoka 420-8527, Japan

MandanaMoosavi
Vancouver Coastal Health, Canada

Stuart Kreisman
Division of Endocrinology, St. Paul's Hospital, 1081 Burrard Street, Vancouver, BC, Canada V6Z 1Y6

Óscar Alfredo Juárez-León, Miguel Ángel Gómez-Sámano, Daniel Cuevas-Ramos, Paloma Almeda-Valdés, Alfredo Adolfo Reza-Albarrán and Francisco Javier Gómez-Pérez
Endocrinology and Metabolism Department, Instituto Nacional de Ciencias M´edicas y Nutrici´on Salvador Zubir´an, 14080 Mexico City, Mexico

Manuel Alejandro López-Flores A La Torre
School of Medicine, Universidad Panamericana, 03920 Mexico City, Mexico

Lauren LaBryer
Division of Endocrinology, Department of Internal Medicine, University of Oklahoma Health Sciences Center, Oklahoma City, OK 73104, USA
Oklahoma City VA Health Care Systems, Oklahoma City, OK 73104, USA

R. Hal Scofield
Division of Endocrinology, Department of Internal Medicine, University of Oklahoma Health Sciences Center, Oklahoma City, OK 73104, USA
Oklahoma City VA Health Care Systems, Oklahoma City, OK 73104, USA
Oklahoma Medical Research Foundation, Oklahoma City, OK 73104, USA

Ravindranauth Sawh
Oklahoma City VA Health Care Systems, Oklahoma City, OK 73104, USA
Department of Pathology, University of Oklahoma Health Sciences Center, Oklahoma City, OK 73104, USA

Colby McLaurin
Oklahoma City VA Health Care Systems, Oklahoma City, OK 73104, USA
Department of Otolaryngology, University of Oklahoma Health Sciences Center, Oklahoma City, OK 73104, USA

Marianne S. Elston
Department of Endocrinology, Waikato Hospital, Private Bag 3200, Hamilton 3240, New Zealand
Faculty of Medicine and Health Sciences, University of Auckland, Waikato Clinical Campus, Private Bag 3200, Hamilton 3240, New Zealand

John V. Conaglen
Faculty of Medicine and Health Sciences, University of Auckland, Waikato Clinical Campus, Private Bag 3200, Hamilton 3240, New Zealand

Goswin Y. Meyer-Rochow
Faculty of Medicine and Health Sciences, University of Auckland, Waikato Clinical Campus, Private Bag 3200, Hamilton 3240, New Zealand
Department of Surgery, Waikato Hospital, Private Bag 3200, Hamilton 3240, New Zealand

Michael Dray
Department of Pathology, Waikato Hospital, Private Bag 3200, Hamilton 3240, New Zealand

Michael Swarbrick
Department of Radiology, Waikato Hospital, Private Bag 3200, Hamilton 3240, New Zealand

Rifki Ucler, Murat Atmaca and Murat Alay
Department of Endocrinology and Metabolism, Medical Faculty, Yuzuncu Yil University, 65080 Van, Turkey

Erdal Kara
Department of Hematology, Medical Faculty, Yuzuncu Yil University, 65080 Van, Turkey

Sehmus Olmez
Department of Gastroenterology, Medical Faculty, Yuzuncu Yil University, 65080 Van, Turkey

Yaren Dirik
Department of Internal Medicine, Medical Faculty, Yuzuncu Yil University, 65080 Van, Turkey

Aydin Bora
Department of Radiology, Medical Faculty, Yuzuncu Yil University, 65080 Van, Turkey

Index

A

Acromegalic, 23, 26-27

Adrenocorticotropic Hormone, 32, 44-45, 50, 85, 88, 97, 170, 173, 201

Agranulocytosis, 104-105, 108

Aldosteronism, 9-12, 93-96

Anaplastic Thyroid Carcinoma, 113-114, 147, 149-150, 166, 169

Androgen Insensitivity Syndrome, 193-194, 197

C

Camp, 59, 61, 63-64, 79, 140, 189

Carotid-cavernous Fistulas, 160, 162, 164

Central Diabetes Insipidus, 13, 15, 73, 76

Cerebral Malaria, 13-16

Cholestatic Hepatitis, 23, 25-27

Chronic Hyperthyroidism, 147, 149-150

Computed Tomography, 8, 18, 37, 41, 65, 70, 74, 82, 84, 94, 121, 124, 131, 159, 166-168, 170, 184-185, 207, 216-217, 221-222, 242

Cryptococcosis, 41, 216-219

Cushing's Syndrome, 33-39, 60, 85, 88, 97-100, 170, 174, 198, 201

D

Ddavp, 14, 73-76

Diabetes Mellitus, 11-12, 38, 98, 143, 145-146, 151-152, 154, 171, 258, 260

Dka, 151-154

E

Ectopic Acth Secreting, 85-87, 99

Esthesioneuroblastoma, 170, 173-174

G

Ganglioneuroblastoma, 124-127, 130

Gastric Cancer, 183-184, 186-187

Gigantomastia, 77-80

Glucocorticoid Remediable Aldosteronism, 9-10

Glucocorticoid Replacement, 36, 38, 174

Glucokinase-activating Mutation, 230

Glycemic Control, 143-144, 228

Gonadotropinoma, 89-92

Graves Thyrotoxicosis, 179

Graves' Disease, 28, 30-31, 104-105, 118, 135-139, 141, 179, 181-182, 212, 214, 246

H

Hashimoto's Thyroiditis, 70, 115-116, 119, 121-123, 135, 139, 141-142, 159

Hctc, 65-67

Hip Replacement, 40-43

Hnf4a Mutation, 226, 228-229

Humoral Hypercalcemia, 55, 58, 183, 188

Hypercalcemia, 54-58, 82, 84, 181, 183-185, 187-188, 218, 240-241

Hyperprolactinemia, 14, 77, 79-80, 101-103

Hyperthyroidism, 3, 28, 30-31, 60, 71, 104-105, 108-109, 115-116, 135-138, 142, 147-150, 179, 181, 212, 214, 247

Hypertriglyceridemia, 151-154, 226, 228

Hypocalciuric Hypercalcemia, 82, 84

Hypopituitarism, 16, 47, 90, 160, 163-164

Hypovolemic Shock, 73-76, 91

I

Idiopathic Basal Ganglia Calcification, 1-3

Igg4 Immunostaining, 69-71

Impulse Control Disorder, 1-3

Intermittent Porphyria, 40

Intrahepatic Cholangiocarcinoma, 183, 185

L

Lenvatinib, 166-169

Liver Metastasis, 65-68

Lymph Node Biopsy, 133, 236

Lymphoma, 56-58, 119, 121-123, 133, 138, 160, 163, 165, 185

M

Macroprolactinemia, 77-81

Malignancy Diseases, 82

Metastatic Melanoma, 28, 30-31

Metastatic Papillary Thyroid, 131-134

Mifepristone, 174, 198-201

Mucosa-associated Lymphoid Tissue, 119, 123

Myelomonocytic Leukemia, 32-33

O

Osteolysis, 56, 59-60, 63

P

Papillary Carcinoma, 110-114, 157-158, 202-206, 237

Paraganglioma, 5-8, 220, 224-225, 248

Parotid Tumour, 85-87

Pheochromocytoma, 5-8, 97-100, 126, 129, 217, 220, 224-225

Pituitary Adenoma, 24, 49-52, 78-79, 85, 89, 91-92, 101, 103, 163-164, 243

Plummer Adenoma, 212, 214

Pneumothorax, 166-169

Posaconazole, 32-35
Postpartum Fever, 5, 7
Prop1 Gene, 44-48
Protracted Hungry Bone Syndrome, 240, 245
Pseudohypoparathyroidism Type 1a, 64, 189, 192

R
Radioactive Iodine Uptake, 175
Radiotherapy, 49-53, 71, 92, 113-114, 126, 150
Riedel's Thyroiditis, 69-72

S
Spindle Cell Squamous Carcinoma, 110

T
Temozolomide, 49, 51-53
Thoracoabdominal Aneurysms, 9, 11
Thymic Carcinoma, 54-55, 57
Thymic Cyst, 175-178
Thyroid Dysfunction, 15, 115, 135, 137-139
Thyrotoxicosis, 31, 68, 104-105, 108, 115-117, 136-137, 139-141, 147, 149-150, 179-182, 212-213

www.ingramcontent.com/pod-product-compliance
Lightning Source LLC
Chambersburg PA
CBHW080455200326
41458CB00012B/3974